PRINCIPLES OF RADIOGRAPHIC IMAGING

AN ART AND A SCIENCE

NOTICE TO THE READER

Cover illustration by Roy E. Schneider

Delmar Staff
Executive Editor: Barbara E. Norwitz
Associate Editor: Marion Waldman
Project Editor: Judith Boyd Nelson
Production Coordinators: Bruce Sherwin/Teresa Luterbach
Design Supervisor: Susan Mathews
Art Supervisor: John Lent

For information, address Delmar Publishers Inc.
Two Computer Drive West, Box 15–015
Albany, New York 12212

COPYRIGHT © 1992
BY DELMAR PUBLISHERS INC.

Printed in the United States of America
Published simultaneously in Canada
by Nelson Canada,
A Division of the Thomson Corporation

10 9 8 7 6 5 4 3 2 1

Library of Congress Cataloging-in-Publication Data

Carlton, Richard R.
    Principles of radiographic imaging: an art and a science /
Richard R. Carlton, Arlene McKenna Adler; contributors, Mary Ann
Hovis . . . [et al.]
        p.   cm.
    Includes bibliographical references.
    Includes index.
    ISBN 0–8273–3605–5
    1. Radiography, Medical.   I. Adler, Arlene McKenna.   II. Title.
    [DNLM: 1. Radiography.   2. Technology, Radiologic. WN 200 C285p]
RC78.C34 1992
616.07′572—dc20
DNLM/DLC
for Library of Congress   90–3449
                                                                CIP

PRINCIPLES OF RADIOGRAPHIC IMAGING

AN ART AND A SCIENCE

Richard R. Carlton, M.S., R.T. (R)
Director of Radiography
Lima Technical College
Lima, Ohio

Arlene McKenna Adler, M.Ed., R.T. (R)
Director, Radiologic Technology Program
Indiana University Northwest
Gary, Indiana

Contributors
Mary Ann Hovis, Raymond P. Rossi,
Roger Smith, Norlin T. Winkler

 DELMAR PUBLISHERS, INC.

THE FOUNDERS OF RADIOGRAPHY

WILHELM CONRAD RÖNTGEN (1845–1923)
Wilhelm Conrad Röntgen became the first radiographer when he discovered x-rays on November 8, 1895, in his laboratory at the University of Würzburg in Germany. For his discovery he received the first Nobel prize in physics in 1901 and was decorated by Prussia, Bavaria, Great Britain, Austria, Mexico, Germany, France, the Netherlands, Sweden, Italy, Turkey, and the United States.

(Portrait courtesy of the Historical Collections of the Library, College of Physicians of Philadelphia.)

EDDY CLIFFORD JERMAN (1865–1936)
In the United States Ed. C. Jerman is known as "The Father of Radiography" because he was its first teacher. He began teaching x-ray techniques in 1897. He founded the American Association of Radiological Technicians (now known as the American Society of Radiologic Technologists) and personally examined the first 1,000 members of the American Registry of X-Ray Technicians. He brought order to the principles of radiographic exposure technique by naming the qualities of the radiographic image: density, contrast, detail and distortion. In 1928 he published "Modern X-Ray Technic," the first book on radiographic principles.

(Portrait courtesy of the American Society of Radiologic Technologists.)

ARTHUR WOLFRAM FUCHS (1895–1962)
Arthur W. Fuchs is known as the inventor of the fixed kilovoltage technique of radiography. His father established the first x-ray laboratory in Chicago in 1896. He performed radiography for the United States Army in both World Wars I and II. During World War II he wrote the U.S. Army training manual, "Principles of Radiographic Exposure," in which he outlined his success with the optimal fixed kVp technique system. In 1955 he first published his book, "Principles of Radiographic Exposure and Processing."

(Portrait courtesy of the family of Arthur Fuchs.)

CONTRIBUTORS

Mary Ann Hovis
Associate Professor
Engineering Technologies
Lima Technical College
Lima, Ohio

Raymond P. Rossi
Assistant Professor of Radiology
University of Colorado Health Sciences Center
Denver, Colorado

Roger Smith
Medical Imaging—Radiography
British Columbia Institute of Technology
Burnaby, British Columbia

Norlin T. Winkler
Assistant Professor
Radiology
Mayo Medical School
Mayo Clinic Foundation
Rochester, Minnesota

To Sidney Finkleman and Quentin Garlets
for teaching us to be radiographers,

to LaVerne Ramaeker, Kay Shriver, and our students
for teaching us to be teachers,

and most importantly,
to our families and friends
for sustaining us throughout.

CONTENTS

UNIT III: ANALYZING THE IMAGE

UNIT IV: COMPARING EXPOSURE SYSTEMS

UNIT V: SPECIAL IMAGING SYSTEMS

FOREWORD

"State-of-the-art" is the best term I can think of to describe this textbook. It is an excellent book written **by** radiographers **for** radiographers. This book truly reflects what radiographers should be learning in their educational process. Ms. Adler and Mr. Carlton have done a superb job of explaining not only what occurs in radiography but also how it occurs and why it occurs. The art of radiography has come a long way in 95 years and with this in mind this book was written to prepare radiographers for the 21st century.

When I reviewed the table of contents for this book, I became intrigued immediately by the titles of the units. Upon reviewing these units I found that they live up to the promise of the table of contents. The authors have used a new approach in teaching the very information that is needed by radiographers.

Throughout the book students are encouraged to use critical thinking skills in solving problems presented by their professional practice. Students are encouraged to make independent decisions and the authors provide ways to support the decision-making process. Not only is the radiographer given "the rules" in this book, but in many cases the authors also discuss the exceptions to the rules. The authors emphasize that the responsibility of a radiographer is to create an image and analyze its quality, while the responsibility of the radiologist is to make a diagnosis from the image. Each of these professionals working together comprises the profession of radiology.

The method that has been used to write the book is educationally sound. Each of the 42 chapters has an outline, objectives, a summary, a set of review questions, and a very detailed bibliography for further reference material. Additionally, a large number of illustrations have been used in the book to further explain the content.

Ms. Adler and Mr. Carlton are to be commended for the depth of the subject matter they have incorporated into this textbook and for the clear, concise manner in which it is presented. *Principles of Radiographic Imaging* is an insightful contribution to the profession of radiologic technology and fortunate is the student who has the opportunity to learn from this book.

Marilyn Holland, B.S., R.T. (R)
Director of Radiologic Technology Education
The University of Iowa Hospitals and Clinics
Iowa City, Iowa

PREFACE

As radiography educators, we designed this textbook with educators and students in mind. As a result, each chapter contains an outline, objectives, a summary, review questions, and a detailed bibliography. Literary epigraphs begin each chapter and as an enjoyable finale, many chapters include interesting cases. Although the order of the chapters was based on our experiences in teaching our students, most chapters stand alone and can be used in the order which is most appropriate within a given program. In addition, supporting materials, including an instructor's guide and laboratory workbook have been developed.

We have made a special effort to represent our belief that professional development should be a prime objective of any radiography curriculum. This is best achieved through the demonstration of technical competence. This book is designed to assist students in developing this cornerstone of professionalism. Through technical competence and a professional demeanor students will be ready to assume their role as experts in the radiographic imaging process. In addition, we believe that true professionals take immense pride in their work, to the extent that it becomes an art as well as a science.

Both the *Curriculum Guide for Radiography* by the American Society of Radiologic Technologists and the *Curriculum Guide for Radiography* prepared by the Council on Education, Radiography, of the Canadian Association of Medical Radiation Technologists have been used extensively to assure both educators and students that all the material necessary for successful professional practice would be addressed.

A special attempt was made to provide an introduction to physics and the imaging modalities while exploring the details of the principles of radiographic exposure techniques

The overall design of the book separates the 42 chapters into five units: Creating the Beam, Creating the Image, Analyzing the Image, Comparing Exposure Systems, and Special Imaging Systems. This design was selected to help organize the contents for students.

Although we assume full responsibility for any errors, including those which may be construed as having arisen from quoting other works out of context, we have made every effort to ensure the accuracy of the information. However, appropriate information sources should be consulted, especially when new or unfamiliar procedures are involved. It is the responsibility of every practitioner to evaluate the appropriateness of a particular procedure in the context of actual clinical situations. Consequently, neither the authors nor the publisher take responsibility or accept any liability for the actions of persons applying the information contained herein in an unprofessional manner. This information is designed to supplement and enhance the instructional methodologies of educators in CAHEA (USA) and CAMRT (Canada) approved radiography programs and should not be applied, especially to human subjects, without this background. In committing this book to print we fully realize that it is never finished, merely abandoned for the time being.

Finally, your perceptions as a reader are important to us. We encourage you to communicate with us regarding facets of the book you appreciate or would like to see changed. We especially appreciate constructive comments and notice of errors. Our intention is to present the principles of radiography in an interesting format that provides a base from which true professionalism will develop. Any commentary readers care to make toward this end will be valued and welcomed.

—Rick Carlton
—Arlene McKenna Adler

February 1991

ACKNOWLEDGMENTS

The production of this book would not have been possible without the support of our spouses, Don and Lynn, Delmar Publishers in the persons of Dave Prout, Leslie Boyer, Marion Waldman, Judith Boyd Nelson, John Lent and Terrel Broiles, Indiana University Northwest, Lima Technical College, and St. Rita's Medical Center of Lima, Ohio, and we gratefully acknowledge their roles in this work. Special thanks are due Dr. LaVerne Ramaeker, Sam Bassitt, Marlene Ledbetter, and Dennis Spragg for their continued support. A major contribution to the accuracy of the information and illustrations was made by the consistent presence of Eugene Frank, of the Mayo Clinic Foundation, throughout.

We are in debt to many who inspired us, taught us, and collaborated with us throughout the years. Much of what is contained in this work is a direct result of their efforts. Those to whom we are especially indebted are Tracy Ahdel, Janice Akin, Judy Baron, Karen Brinkman, John Cortez, Marion Frank, Mick Jagger, Karen Jefferies, Robin Jones, Dr. George Koptik, Judy Koptik, Jon Lilly, Dr. Marzuto, Kathy Miller, Joe Mosqueda, Traci O'Donnell, Karen Schmidl, Tracy Thegze, Jean Widger, Rob Wilcoxen, and Sue Wilson. And, of course, our students at Indiana University Northwest, Lima Technical College, Wilbur Wright College, and Michael Reese Hospital and Medical Center.

Like our colleagues and students—past, present, and future—we owe much to the institutions that contributed to our professional expertise. We wish to thank Michael Reese Hospital and Medical Center, Lutheran General Hospital, Mercy Hospital and Medical Center (Chicago), and Wilbur Wright College, Illinois Central College, Carl Sandburg College, Evanston Hospital, Methodist Medical Center (Peoria), and Community Memorial Hospital (Monmouth).

We owe special thanks to many people for sharing their personal expertise and material collections. One of the highest forms of professionalism, the willingness to give freely of time and knowledge, was demonstrated again and again by all of the radiologic technologists from whom we requested assistance in our compilation of the multitude of photographs, drawings, radiographs, and other illustrative materials in the text, and who assisted in the numerous reviews of our writing. Among those deserving special thanks are Norlin Winkler of the Mayo Clinic and Raymond Rossi of the University of Colorado Health Sciences Center for their commentary and technical assistance above and beyond the normal bonds of friendship; Philip W. Ballinger of The Ohio State University; Terry West, Secretary-General of the International Society of Radiographers and Radiological Technicians; Stewart Bushong of Baylor College of Medicine; Terry Eastman of Dallas; Joe Fodor of the University of Cincinnati Medical Center; Nina Kowalczyk of Riverside Methodist Hospital, Columbus, OH; and Denise Moore of Sinclair Community College, Dayton, OH; Tim Penning of Athens Regional Medical Center, GA; Bob Kobistek in Cleveland and Martin Ratner and Steve Szeglin in Carle Place, NY, of Victoreen, Inc./Nuclear Associates; Robert Trinkle, formerly of Du Pont; Robert Lockery and Walter Weigl of Siemens; William Conklin of Orangeburg, SC; Jerry Conlogue of Gulf Coast Community College, FL; Bruce Long of Indiana University Medical Center; Charles R. Griffith of FGHB Certified Radiation Physicists; Pat Sharp of Gannon University, Erie, PA; Seymour Sterling of Eastman Kodak; Jerome Taubel of the Mayo Clinic Foundation; Terry Hanby of Du Pont; Mike Wilsey of AGFA Matrix; Robert Busic of GE

Medical Systems; Toshinori Komba of Komazawa University, Tokyo; Barb Imber of St. Rita's Medical Center; Rick Halker of Lima Memorial Hospital; Radiology Department at Van Wert County Hospital; John Stone of Emory University Medical School, Atlanta; Gene Craft, Tom Beery, Will Wells, Doug Raver, Chris Inskeep, Beverly Thomas, Jan Krietemeyer, Julia Moore, Amy Schmershal and especially Judy Shaw of Lima Technical College; David Jenkins of Leicestershire, England; Lois Dowdell of X-ray Imaging Consultants, Ltd., Orangeville, Ontario, and Linda Benson.

EPIGRAPH SOURCES AND CREDITS

Chapter 1 "Helping with the Math Homework," reprinted with permission of Louisiana State University Press, from *In All This Rain*, by John Stone. Copyright 1980 by John Stone.

Chapters 2, 3, 4, 8, 32 and **34** From Otto Glasser, *Dr. W. C. Röntgen*, 2nd edition (Springfield, Illinois, 1972), by permission of Charles C. Thomas, Publisher.

Chapters 5, 26, and **39** From Thomas Mann, *The Magic Mountain (Der Zauberberg)*, originally published by S. Fischer Verlag, Berlin, 1924; translated from the German by H. T. Lowe-Porter (New York: Alfred A. Knopf, 1965).

Chapter 6 From Patricia Goedicke, "One More Time," by permission of the author. Copyright by Patricia Goedicke.

Chapters 7, 24, and **35** From W. D. Coolidge, "Experiences with the Roentgen-Ray tube," *American Journal of Roentgenology* 54, 6, 1945.

Chapter 9 "X-Ray," reprinted with permission of Celia Gilbert from *Queen of Darkness*, by Celia Gilbert. Copyright 1977 by Celia Gilbert.

Chapters 10, 23, 27, and **31** From E. C. Jerman, "An analysis of the end-result: The radiograph," *Radiology* 6, 59–62, 1926.

Chapter 11 From A. H. Compton, preface to the first edition of *X-Rays and Electrons*, reprinted in *X-Rays in Theory and Experiment*, by A. H. Compton and H. K. Allison, 2nd edition (New York: Van Nostrand and Company, 1935).

Chapter 12 From Lawrence K. Russell, " " *Life*, March 12, 1896.

Chapter 13 From Moon Martin, Pete Sinfield, and Terry Taylor, "X-Ray Vision," from the Capitol-EMI album, *Mystery Ticket*. Copyright 1982 by Paper Music, Ltd.

Chapter 14 Reprinted with permission of New Directions Publishing Corporation, from *The Autobiography of William Carlos Williams*, by William Carlos Williams. Copyright 1951 by William Carlos Williams.

Chapter 15 From John Lennon and Paul McCartney, "I'm Looking Through You," from the Capitol-EMI album, *Rubber Soul*. Copyright 1965 by EMI Records, Inc.

Chapter 16 From Hollis E. Potter, "The Bucky diaphragm principle applied to roentgenography," *The American Journal of Roentgenology* 7, 292–95, 1920.

Chapter 17 From Arthur W. Fuchs, *Jerman Memorial Lecture*, given during the 1950 Annual Meeting of the American Society of X-Ray Technicians in Cincinnati, Ohio.

Chapter 18 From "This Is A Photograph of Me" by Margaret Atwood, *Selected Poems I* (Boston, MA: Houghton Mifflin, 1987) and *Selected Poems 1966–1984* (Toronto: McClelland and Stewart, 1987), by permission of the author.

Chapter 19 "In The X-Ray Room," reprinted with permission of the estate of Howard Moss, from *New Selected Poems*, by Howard Moss. Copyright 1985 by MacMillan Publishing Company.

Chapter 20 From E. R. N. Grigg, "From Immigrant to Inventor," the autobiography of Michael I. Pupin, in *Trail of the Invisible Light* (Springfield, Illinois: Charles C. Thomas, Publisher, 1965).

Chapter 21 From Arthur W. Fuchs, *Pall Mall Gazette* (March 1896), reprinted in "Radiography of 1896," *Image* 9:4–17, 1960.

Chapter 22 From Gerhart S. Schwarz, *Unit-Step Radiography* (Springfield, Illinois: Charles C. Thomas, Publisher, 1961), by permission of the publisher.

Chapter 25 From radiologist Merrill C. Sosman, in *Familiar Medical Quotations*, edited by Maurice B. Strauss (Boston: Little, Brown & Co., 1968).

Chapter 28 From William B. Hendee and Raymond P. Rossi, *Quality Assurance for Radiographic X-Ray Units and Associated Equipment* (Rockville, MD: U.S. Department of Health, Education, and Welfare, Public Health Service, Food and Drug Administration, Bureau of Radiological Health, HEW Publication FDA 79–8094, 1979).

Chapter 29 From Arthur W. Fuchs, preface to *Principles of Radiographic Exposure and Processing*, 1st edition (Springfield, Illinois: Charles C. Thomas, Publisher, 1955).

Chapter 30 From John B. Cahoon, Jr., *Jerman Memorial Lecture*, given during the 1961 Annual Meeting of the American Society of X-Ray Technicians in Montreal, Quebec.

Chapter 33 From the text of the chapter.

Chapter 36 From William Shakespeare, *Hamlet*, III, iv, 18.

Chapter 37 From Arthur W. Fuchs, "Edison and Roentgenology," *The American Journal of Roentgenology and Radium Therapy*, 57:2, 145–56, 1947.

Chapter 38 From Andre-Edmund-Marie-Bocage, *Method of, and Apparatus for, Radiography on a Moving Plate*, French patent 536464, June 3, 1921, reprinted in *Tomography: Physical Principles and Clinical Applications*, by J. T. Littleton, *Section 17: Golden's Diagnostic Radiology Series* (Baltimore, Maryland: Williams & Wilkins, 1976).

Chapter 40 From Christopher C. Kuni, *Introduction to Computers and Digital Processing in Medical Imaging* (Chicago: Mosby-Year Book, Inc., 1988); by permission of the author.

Chapter 41 From Allan Cormack, upon being informed that he and Godfrey Hounsfield were to share the 1979 Nobel Prize for Medicine for the invention of computed tomography.

Chapter 42 From Edward M. Purcell, "Research in nuclear magnetism," *Nobel Lectures: Physics 1942–1962* (Amsterdam: Elsevier Publishing Company, 1964), 210–31.

UNIT I: CREATING THE BEAM

An inherent quality of a professional is the possession of expertise, far above that of a nonprofessional, in the technical aspects of a field. Knowledge of the principles of radiographic image production is part of the technical expertise of the professional radiographer. Radiography programs provide students with classroom instruction, laboratory experience, and clinical practice in this subject. No other medical professional experiences are as intensive or comprehensive as the study of radiographic imaging. This unit is designed to provide the foundation for this discipline by building a framework of information regarding the creation of the diagnostic x-ray beam.

The framework begins with a review of **basic mathematics** and **radiation concepts**, including atomic theory, x-ray properties and necessary units of measurement. Although this may be a review of previous science course work for many readers, it is important to make sure everyone is on the same wavelength before using this information for the remainder of the book.

An understanding of **basic radiation protection** is required before beginning to use this information in a clinical setting. **Electricity** and **electromagnetism** are covered in two long chapters that lay the foundation for controlling the x-ray beam. Chapters 6–8, on **x-ray equipment**, the **x-ray tube** and **x-ray production**, provide an understanding of exactly how physics is used to create x-rays. The chapters on **filtration** and **the prime factors** explain how to shape and mold the beam to obtain the best results. Finally, Chapter 11, on **x-ray interactions**, opens the door to exactly what occurs to the biological systems that are being imaged, and lays the groundwork for future understanding of problems in image production.

1 BASIC MATHEMATICS

Mary Ann Hovis

In the beginning
there were polynomials

differences of squares
trial and error

and the sum of two cubes.
X² minus Y²

has always had
the same meaning

John Stone, "Helping with the Math Homework."

OUTLINE

ARITHMETIC
ALGEBRA
SEMILOGARITHMIC GRAPHING
UNITS OF MEASUREMENT

OBJECTIVES

Upon completion of this chapter, the student should be able to:

1. Perform functions with fractions and decimals.
2. Determine significant digits in a number.
3. Perform calculations in scientific notation with signed numbers and exponents.
4. Simplify algebraic expressions.
5. Differentiate between semilogarithmic and arithmetic graph axes.
6. Convert units within the SI system.

Mathematics is the language of science. Radiographers need to be able to speak this language. This math review is intended to refresh essential skills in this area.

ARITHMETIC

Fractions

Addition and Subtraction To add or subtract two fractions with **like** denominators, add or subtract the numerators and keep the like denominator.

Examples:

$$\frac{3}{8} + \frac{2}{8} = \frac{5}{8}$$

$$\frac{7}{8} - \frac{4}{8} = \frac{3}{8}$$

$$\frac{a}{b} + \frac{c}{b} = \frac{a+c}{b}$$

$$\frac{a}{b} - \frac{c}{b} = \frac{a-c}{b}$$

To add or subtract two fractions with **unlike** denominators, rewrite each fraction with a like or common denominator. Then add or subtract the numerators and keep the like or common denominator.

Examples:

$$\frac{1}{4} + \frac{5}{6} = \frac{3}{12} + \frac{10}{12} = \frac{13}{12}$$

$$\frac{7}{5} - \frac{1}{3} = \frac{21}{15} - \frac{5}{15} = \frac{16}{15}$$

$$\frac{a}{b} + \frac{c}{d} = \frac{ad}{bd} + \frac{bc}{bd} = \frac{ad+bc}{bd}$$

$$\frac{a}{b} - \frac{c}{d} = \frac{ad}{bd} - \frac{bc}{bd} = \frac{ad-bc}{bd}$$

Multiplication Multiplication can be written in several ways (see Table 1–1). To multiply

---

TABLE 1–1

MULTIPLICATION NOTATION

Throughout this review the algebraic notation for multiplication will be used.

Example: 3×4 will be written as $3 \cdot 4$.
A $\cdot$ (dot) is used as a symbol for multiplication.

Example: $a \times b$ will be written as $a \cdot b$ or as ab.
When two letters are used the dot is usually omitted.

Example: $3 \times a$ will be written as $3a$ or as $3 \cdot a$.
Parentheses can also be used to represent multiplication.

Example: 3×4 can be written as $(3)(4)$.

---

two fractions, multiply the numerators and multiply the denominators.

Examples:

$$\frac{2}{5} \times \frac{3}{7} = \frac{2 \times 3}{5 \times 7} = \frac{6}{35}$$

$$\frac{a}{b} \times \frac{c}{d} = \frac{a \times c}{b \times d}$$

Division To divide two fractions, rewrite the division problem as a multiplication problem by multiplying the first fraction by the second fraction inverted.

Examples:

$$\frac{2}{5} \div \frac{3}{7} = \frac{2}{5} \times \frac{7}{3} = \frac{2 \times 7}{5 \times 3} = \frac{14}{15}$$

$$\frac{a}{b} \div \frac{c}{d} = \frac{a}{b} \times \frac{d}{c} = \frac{a \times d}{b \times c}$$

Decimals

Decimal number place value (columns) is determined as shown in Figure 1–1.

Decimal number place value (columns)

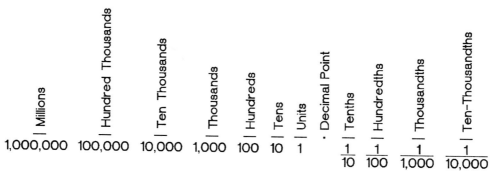

Figure 1–1. Decimal number place values.

Addition and Subtraction To add or subtract two decimal numbers, line up the decimal points in each number, adding or subtracting as with whole numbers. Remember to add in zeros to fill out the decimal positions if necessary. The decimal point must remain in the same position.

Examples:

Add:

$$\begin{array}{r} 76.81 \\ +384.1 \\ \hline 460.91 \end{array}$$

Subtract:

$$\begin{array}{r} 76.1 \\ -2.96 \\ \hline \end{array}$$

rewrite as:

$$\begin{array}{r} 76.10 \\ -2.96 \\ \hline 73.14 \end{array}$$

Multiplication To multiply two decimal numbers, multiply the numbers as if they were whole numbers. Place the decimal point in the product so the number of places in the product equals the sum of the number of decimal places in each number.

Example:

Multiply:

$$\begin{array}{r} 2.31 \\ \times 6.8 \\ \hline 1848 \\ 1386 \\ \hline 15.708 \end{array}$$

2 decimal positions
1 decimal position

3 decimal positions

Division To divide two decimal numbers, set up as if doing whole number division. Move the decimal point in the divisor to the right to make the divisor a whole number. Move the decimal point in the dividend the same number of places to the right (as was done for the divisor). Add zeros if necessary to maintain the position of the decimal. Divide the numbers as if they were whole numbers. Place the decimal point in the quotient directly above the decimal point in the dividend. Add zeros if necessary to maintain the position of the decimal.

Examples:

$$.25\,\overline{)1250}$$

$$.25\,\overline{)1250.00}^{5000.}$$

$$1.3\,\overline{)733.2}$$

$$\begin{array}{r} 564. \\ 1.3\,\overline{)733.2} \\ \underline{65} \\ 83 \\ \underline{78} \\ 52 \\ \underline{52} \\ 0 \end{array}$$

Convert a Fraction into a Decimal Number To convert a fraction into a decimal, divide the denominator into the numerator.

Example:
Convert 7/8 into a decimal:

```
       .875
  8 )7.000
      64
      ──
       60
       56
       ──
        40
        40
        ══
```

Calculator and Decimals To use a calculator, follow the following key strokes.

Example:

$\boxed{7}$ $\boxed{\div}$ $\boxed{8}$ $\boxed{=}$ .875

Example:
Convert 1/5 into a decimal using the calculator. There are two methods to do this:

1. $\boxed{1}$ $\boxed{\div}$ $\boxed{5}$ $\boxed{=}$ .2
2. Use the reciprocal key. $\boxed{5}$ $\boxed{1/x}$ = $\boxed{.2}$
   (The $\boxed{1/x}$ key is the reciprocal key.)

Convert a Percent to a Decimal To convert a percent to a decimal move the decimal point two places to the left.

Example:
Convert 78.5% to a decimal:
78.5% = .758

Convert a Decimal to a Percent To convert a decimal to a percent move the decimal point two places to the right.

Example:
Change .452 to a %
.452 = 45.2%

Computation with Values (Numbers)

Exact Some numbers are exact values, like the counting numbers (1,2,3, . . .). For example, there are exactly four legs on a chair. Exact numbers in computations are as accurate or as precise as is needed.

Significant Digits Some values are obtained by measurement and are only as accurate as the measuring device. The last digit in the reading is usually estimated. **When dealing with these values in computations, the results will only be as accurate as the least accurate value.** This is the concept of significant digits.

To determine the number of significant digits in a value (number):

1. Count all nonzero digits.
2. Count all zeros between nonzero digits.
3. Count all zeros at the end of a decimal value.

The number of significant digits in a value is the sum of the numbers obtained in steps one, two and three.

Examples:
The following are measured values from a radiation dose meter (dosimeter).
7.14 mR has three significant digits.
90.104 mR has five significant digits.
0.048 mR has two significant digits.
7300 mR has two significant digits.
6.900 mR has four significant digits.

Precision The precision of a value refers to the decimal position of the last significant digit.

Example:
.0218 is precise to the ten-thousandths.

Rounding Off To round a number the last digit to be retained is:

1. Left unchanged if the digit to the right of the last digit to be retained is less than 5.
2. Is increased by one if the digit to the right of the last digit to be retained is 5 or greater.

Examples:
75.2581 rounded to 4 significant digits is 78.26.
6836.66 rounded to 2 significant digits is 6800.
0.0381 rounded to 2 significant digits is 0.038.
0.0299 rounded to 2 significant digits is 0.030.

Multiplication and Division of Approximate Values
When multiplying or dividing two or more approximate values, the number of significant digits in the final answer is no greater than the number of significant digits in the values with the least number of significant digits.

Example:
Using the calculator, $(103.81) \cdot (1.34) = 139.1054$. However, since 1.34 has only three significant digits, the answer has only 3 significant digits. Therefore 139.1054 needs to be rounded to 3 significant digits, making it 139.

Addition and Subtraction of Approximate Values
When adding or subtracting two or more approximate values, the final answer should be no more precise than the **least** precise of the values.

Example:
Add the following:

123.1
 89.123
103.3456
―――――
315.5686

Since the least precise number is 123.1, the answer should be rounded to 315.6.

Powers of Ten
The decimal system is based on powers of ten, as is the metric system. These are very important systems to the radiographer. When a^n is written, a is called the base and n is the exponent.

Positive Exponents
Definition: $a^n = \underbrace{a \cdot a \cdot a \cdots a}_{n \text{ times}}$ (multiply n times)

Examples:
$10^1 = 10$
$10^2 = 10 \cdot 10 = 100$
$10^3 = 10 \cdot 10 \cdot 10 = 1000$
$10^n = 10 \cdot 10 \cdot 10 \cdots 10 = 100 \ldots 0$ (n zeros)

Negative Exponents
Definition: $a^{-n} = \dfrac{1}{a^n}$ (for $a \neq 0$)

$10^{-1} = \dfrac{1}{10} = .1$

$10^{-2} = \dfrac{1}{10^2} = .01$

$10^{-3} = \dfrac{1}{10^3} = .001$

$10^{-n} = \dfrac{1}{10^n} = .00 \ldots .001$ (n − 1, zeros)

Zero Exponents
Definition: $a^0 = 1$ (for $a \neq 0$)

Example:
$10^0 = 1$

Scientific Notation
A number written in scientific notation is written as the product of a number between 1 (including 1) and 10 times, a power of 10. In other words, $N \times 10^p$, where $1 \leq N < 10$ and p is an integer. Integers are defined as the numbers . . . −3, −2, −1, 0, 1, 2, 3, ...

Examples:
7.15×10^4 is a number in scientific notation.
1.598×10^{-5} is a number in scientific notation.
7.58×10^0 is a number in scientific notation.

Converting Numbers from Ordinary to Scientific Notation
To write a number in scientific notation, the decimal point must be moved to the position following the first nonzero digit.

Examples:

$$70.57 = 7.057 \times 10^1 \ (p = 1)$$
$$.00815 = 8.15 \times 10^{-3} \ (p = -3)$$
$$7.58 = 7.58 \times 10^0 \ (p = 0)$$

In the first example, the decimal point is moved one digit to the left, making the power of ten, one. In the second example, the decimal point is moved three digits to the right, making the power of ten, negative three. In the third example, the decimal point is not moved and the power of ten is zero.

In general, when moving the decimal point to the left the power of ten will be the number of positions moved. When moving the decimal point to the right the power of ten will be negative the number of positions moved. When the decimal point is not moved, the power of ten will be zero.

Converting Numbers from Scientific to Ordinary Notation

To convert a number in scientific notation to ordinary notation, the decimal position is moved according to the following:

1. If the power of ten is positive move the decimal point to the right the number of positions in the exponent.
2. If the power of ten is negative move the decimal point to the left the number of positions in the exponent.
3. If the power of ten is zero the decimal remains in the same position.

In all of the above, once the decimal point has been moved, the ten and its power are dropped. Zeros are added if necessary.

Examples:

$$3.7 \times 10^4 \ = 37,000$$
$$5.56 \times 10^{-5} = .0000556$$
$$1.34 \times 10^0 \ = 1.34$$

Calculator and Scientific Notation

Numbers can be entered in a calculator in sci-entific notation by using the EXP or EE key. These keys represent the exponent key on the calculator. (To learn the correct key, read the manual that came with the calculator.)

Examples:

Enter 7.81×10^4 $\boxed{7.81}$ $\boxed{\text{EXP}}$ $\boxed{4}$ $\boxed{=}$ 78,100

Enter 7.81×10^{10} $\boxed{7.81}$ $\boxed{\text{EXP}}$ $\boxed{10}$ $\boxed{=}$ 7.81 10

Enter 7.81×10^{-4}

     $\boxed{7.81}$ $\boxed{\text{EXP}}$ $\boxed{4}$ $\boxed{+/-}$ $\boxed{=}$ .000781

To change by calculator an ordinary decimal number to a number in scientific notation, the FSE key is used (or consult the manual). The FSE key converts a number from fixed (ordinary notation) to scientific notation to engineering notation (powers are multiples of 3).

Example:

Convert 70.57, .00815, and 7.58 to scientific notation.

$\boxed{70.57}$ $\boxed{=}$ $\boxed{\text{FSE}}$ $\boxed{\text{FSE}}$ 7.057000000 01

$\boxed{.00815}$ $\boxed{=}$ $\boxed{\text{FSE}}$ $\boxed{\text{FSE}}$ 8.150000000 −03

$\boxed{7.58}$ $\boxed{=}$ $\boxed{\text{FSE}}$ $\boxed{\text{FSE}}$ 7.580000000 00

To change the calculator to ordinary notation again, the FSE key must be used twice.

It should be noted that when two very large or very small numbers are multiplied on the calculator, the result will automatically appear in scientific notation. (Multiplying or dividing numbers in scientific notation is discussed under exponents.)

Dimensional Analysis

The concept of dimensional analysis is very useful when converting from one set of units to another. The principle is based on fractions whose quotients are 1.

Example:

$$\frac{12 \text{ in}}{1 \text{ ft}} = 1 \quad \text{or} \quad \frac{1 \text{ ft}}{12 \text{ in}} = 1$$

Recall that multiplying a quantity by 1 does not change the value of the quantity. In order to convert from one set of units to another, algebraic operations are performed with units in the same way they are with algebraic symbols.

Example:

Convert 7.0 ft to inches.

$$7.0 \text{ ft} = 7.0 \text{ ft} \cdot \frac{12 \text{ in}}{1 \text{ ft}} = 7 \cdot 12 \text{ in} = 84 \text{ in}$$

Note that it is possible to "cancel" the feet unit, leaving the inches unit.

Convert 70.0 km/hr to m/s.

$$70.0 \frac{\text{km}}{\text{hr}} =$$

$$70.0 \frac{\text{km}}{\text{hr}} \cdot \frac{1000 \text{ m}}{1 \text{ km}} \cdot \frac{1 \text{ hr}}{60 \text{ min}} \cdot \frac{1 \text{ min}}{60 \text{ s}} =$$

$$70.0 \cdot 1000 \cdot \frac{1}{60} \cdot \frac{1 \text{ m}}{60 \text{ s}} = 19.4 \frac{\text{m}}{\text{s}}$$

Recall that 1 km = 1000 m, 1 hr = 60 min, and 1 min = 60 s. Note that it is possible to "cancel" the km unit, the hr unit, and the min unit.

When converting cubic units or square units, extra attention needs to be given to the conversion factors. Study the following example carefully.

Example:

Convert 3.8000 ft³ (cubic feet) to cubic inches (in³).

$$3.8000 \text{ ft}^3 = 3.8000 \text{ ft}^3 \cdot \frac{12 \text{ in}}{1 \text{ ft}} \cdot \frac{12 \text{ in}}{1 \text{ ft}} \cdot \frac{12 \text{ in}}{1 \text{ ft}}$$
$$= 6566.4 \text{ in}^3$$

or

$$3.8000 \text{ ft}^3 = 3.8000 \text{ ft}^3 \cdot \left(\frac{12 \text{ in}}{1 \text{ ft}}\right)^3 = 6566.4 \text{ in}^3$$

Example:

Convert 10 roentgens per hour to roentgens per minute.

$$10.0 \frac{\text{roentgens}}{\text{hour}} = 10.0 \frac{\text{roentgens}}{\text{hour}} \cdot \frac{1 \text{ hour}}{60 \text{ minute}}$$

$$= .167 \frac{\text{roentgens}}{\text{minute}}$$

ALGEBRA

Signed Numbers

Numbers are not always positive. For example, the thermometer indicates that it is very cold at −20°F. Negative numbers can be illustrated by using a number line (see Figure 1–2). Positive numbers are assigned to the right of the zero point and negative numbers to the left of the zero point. A statement that seven is less than ten (written as 7 < 10) indicates that 7 is to the left of 10 on the number line. A statement that minus five is greater than minus nine (written as −5 > −9) indicates that −5 is to the right of −9 on the number line.

Absolute Value The absolute value of a number is the distance from 0 to that number on the number line. Since distance is a nonnegative quantity, that means that the absolute value of a number is always positive or zero. The notation used for absolute value is two vertical bars.(| |)

Examples:

$$|-2| = 2 \quad |4| = 4 \quad |0| = 0$$

Since −2 is two units from zero on the number line, the absolute value is 2. Since 4 is four units from zero on the number line, the absolute value is 4. Since 0 is zero units from zero on the number line, the absolute value is 0.

Addition To add two positive numbers, add their absolute values and attach a positive sign to the result. The positive sign is usually omitted.

Example:

$$(+7) + (+8) = +15 \qquad 7 + 8 = 15$$

Figure 1–2. Number line.

To add two negative numbers, add their absolute values and attach a negative sign to the result.

Example:

$(-7) + (-8) = -15 \qquad -7 + (-8) = -15$

To add two numbers with unlike signs, subtract the smaller in absolute value from the larger in absolute value and attach the sign of the larger in absolute value to the result.

Examples:

$(-10) + (3) = -7 \qquad 4 + (-9) = -5$
$(8) + (-5) = 3 \qquad -3 + (7) = 4$

Negative of a Number The negative of a number is the opposite of the number in sign.

Examples:

The negative of 7 is -7; the negative of -7 is 7.
If $b = 7$, then $-b = -7$.
If $b = -7$, then $-b = -(-7) = 7$.

Subtraction Subtraction is rewritten as addition, as in $a - b = a + (-b)$.

Example:

$8 - 10 = 8 + (-10) = -2$
$8 - (-10) = 8 + 10 = 18$
$-8 - 10 = -8 + (-10) = -18$
$-8 - (-10) = -8 + 10 = 2$

All of the above subtraction problems are rewritten as addition and then the rules for addition of signed numbers are used.

Multiplication To multiply two numbers, multiply their absolute values. If both numbers are positive or both numbers are negative, attach a positive sign to the result. If the numbers are opposite in sign, attach a negative sign to the result.

Examples:

$(2)(3) = 6$
$(-2)(-3) = 6$
$(2)(-3) = -6$
$(-2)(3) = -6$

Division To divide two numbers, divide their absolute values. If both numbers are positive or both numbers are negative, attach a positive sign to the result. If the numbers are opposite in sign, attach a negative sign to the result.

Examples:

$8 \div 2 = 4$
$-8 \div -2 = 4$
$8 \div (-2) = -4$
$-8 \div 2 = -4$

To use the calculator with signed numbers, the change of sign key needs to be used (or consult the calculator manual).

Example:

Enter -2

$\boxed{2}\ \boxed{+/-}$

Then use the signed number as needed.

Order of Operation

Order-of-operation problems may occur when parentheses are not indicated. For example, evaluate $2 + 3 \cdot 4$. Depending on whether addition or multiplication is performed first the answer might be 20 or 14. The answer depends on the order of operation. Rules have been established that make the correct result 14.

The difference between the unary minus sign $(-)$ and the subtraction sign $(-)$ and the difference between the unary plus sign $(+)$ and the addition sign $(+)$ must be understood before order-of-operation rules can be learned.

A subtraction sign $(-)$ is used between two numbers:

Example:

$7 - 8$ (subtraction sign)

A unary minus sign $(-)$ is used before one number.

Example:

-7 (unary minus sign)

An expression can have both a subtraction sign and a unary minus sign.

Example:
$-7 - 8$ (the first is a unary minus, the second a subtraction sign)

An addition sign (+) is used between two numbers:

Example:
$8 + 10$ (addition sign)

A unary plus sign (+) is used before one number.

Example:
$+8$

Rules for order of operation

1. Perform all operations inside grouping symbols (parentheses, radical symbols, fraction bar, brackets, etc.)
2. Exponentiation (raising to a power or roots)
3. Unary minus ($-$) or unary plus (+)
4. Multiplication and division
5. Addition and subtraction

Operations are performed from smallest to largest levels in the order from the lowest level (#1) to the largest level (#5).

Operations on the same level are evaluated left to right.

Examples:

$2 + \underline{3 \cdot 4}$ (multiplication first)

$= 2 + 12$ (addition)

$= 14$

$\underline{8 \cdot 6} - \underline{12 \div 2}$ (multiplication & division first)

$= \underline{48 - 6}$ (subtraction)

$= 42$

$\dfrac{8 + 7}{2 + 3}$ (bar acts as grouping symbol)

$= \dfrac{15}{5}$ (add numerator and add denominator first)

$= 3$ (divide)

$(-2)^3$ (exponentiation first)
$= -8$

$-(2)^4$ (exponentiation first)
$= -(16)$ (unary minus sign)
$= -16$

$3(\underline{7 + 4})$ (add inside parenthesis first)

$= \underline{3 \cdot 11}$ (multiply)

$= 33$

$2(\underline{6 + 1})^2$ (add inside parenthesis first)

$= 2\underline{(7)^2}$ (exponentiation next)

$= 2 \cdot 49$ (multiply)
$= 98$

Algebraic Expressions

Algebraic expressions are letters and/or numbers that are multiplied, divided, added, subtracted or raised to a power.

Examples:
$3x^3 + 5x^2 - 7x + 8$

$\dfrac{x + 5}{y - 7}$

There are several rules for combining algebraic expressions.

Distributive Law The statement of the distributive law is: $a(b + c) = a \cdot b + a \cdot c$

Examples:

$7(x + y) = 7x + 7y$

$7(3 + 5) = 7 \cdot 3 + 7 \cdot 5 = 21 + 35 = 56$

$p(x + 4) = px + 4p$ (The numeral is normally written in front of the letter.)

If the addition sign were a subtraction sign, then: $a(b - c) = a \cdot b - a \cdot c$

Examples:

$7(x - y) = 7x - 7y$

$7(3 - 5) = 7 \cdot 3 - 7 \cdot 5$
$\qquad\quad = 21 - 35 = 21 + (-35) = -14$

$p(x - 4) = px - 4p$

Care needs to be taken when one or two negative signs are involved.

Examples:

$\begin{aligned}
-7(x + y) &= -7x + (-7y) \quad \text{(distributive law)}\\
&= -7x - 7y \quad \text{(the reverse definition of subtraction)}\\
-7(x - y) &= -7x - (-7y) \quad \text{(distributive law)}\\
&= -7x + 7y \quad \text{(definition of subtraction)}\\
-7(-3 - 8) &= (-7)(-3) - (-7)(8) \quad \text{(distributive law)}\\
&= 21 - (-56) \quad \text{(multiply)}\\
&= 21 + 56 \quad \text{(definition of subtraction)}\\
&= 77
\end{aligned}$

Addition and Subtraction of Like Terms

Like terms are terms with identical literal factors. A literal factor is a factor denoted by a letter. Like terms may be added or subtracted.

Example:

$7x + 3x = 10x$ $\qquad\qquad$ (like terms)

Example:

$7x + 3y = 7x + 3y$ $\qquad$ (unlike terms may not be added)

Example:

$7x - 3x = 4x$

Example:

$\begin{aligned}
-7x - 3x &= -7x + (-3x) \quad \text{(definition of subtraction)}\\
&= -10x \quad \text{(combine like terms)}
\end{aligned}$

Example:

$\begin{aligned}
-7x - (-3x) &= -7x + 3x \quad \text{(definition of subtraction)}\\
&= -4x \quad \text{(combine like terms)}
\end{aligned}$

Parentheses When an algebraic expression involves parentheses, the parentheses need to be removed in order to simplify the expression.

Example:

$\begin{aligned}
&7(x + y) + 4(x + y)\\
&= 7x + 7y + 4x + 4y \quad \text{(distributive law)}\\
&= 11x + 11y \quad \text{(combine like terms)}
\end{aligned}$

Example:

$\begin{aligned}
&7(x + y) - 4(x + y)\\
&= 7(x + y) + (-4)(x + y) \quad \text{(definition of subtraction)}\\
&= 7x + 7y + (-4x) + (-4y) \quad \text{(distributive law)}\\
&= 3x + 3y \quad \text{(combine like terms)}
\end{aligned}$

Example:

$\begin{aligned}
&7(x - y) - 4(x - y)\\
&= 7(x - y) + (-4)(x - y) \quad \text{(definition of subtraction)}\\
&= 7x - 7y + (-4x) - (-4y) \quad \text{(distributive law)}\\
&= 7x + (-7y) + (-4x) + (4y) \quad \text{(definition of subtraction)}\\
&= 3x + (-3y) \quad \text{(combine like terms)}\\
&= 3x - 3y \quad \text{(reverse of definition of subtraction)}
\end{aligned}$

Example:

$\begin{aligned}
x - (y - x) &= x + (-1)(y - x)\\
&= x + (-y) - (-x)\\
&= x + (-y) + x\\
&= 2x - y
\end{aligned}$

If an expression involves parentheses within parentheses, then it is simplified from the innermost parentheses out.

Example:

$7 - [6x - (x - 4)]$
$= 7 - [6x - x + 4]$ (remove innermost parentheses)
$= 7 - [5x + 4]$ (simplify within parentheses)
$= 7 - 5x - 4$ (remove parentheses [square bracket])
$= 3 - 5x$ (combine like terms)

Exponents

Definition: $a^n = \underbrace{a \cdot a \cdot a \cdots a}_{n\ times}$ where a is the base and n is the exponent

Example:

$3^4 = 3 \cdot 3 \cdot 3 \cdot 3 = 81$

Laws of Exponents

Law 1: $a^m \cdot a^n = a^{m+n}$

Examples:

$a^4 \cdot a^3 = a^{4+3} = a^7$
$a \cdot a^5 = a^{1+5} = a^6$

Law 2:
$$a^{\frac{m}{n}} = \begin{cases} a^{m-n} & \text{if } m \geq n \\ \dfrac{1}{a^{n-m}} & \text{if } n > m \end{cases}$$

Examples:

$\dfrac{x^5}{x^2} = x^{5-2} = x^3$

$\dfrac{x^7}{x^{10}} = \dfrac{1}{x^{10-7}} = \dfrac{1}{x^3}$

Law 3: $(ab)^m = a^m b^m$

Example:

$(ab)^4 = a^4 b^4$

Law 4: $\left(\dfrac{a}{b}\right)^m = \dfrac{a^m}{b^m}$

Example:

$\left(\dfrac{a}{b}\right)^5 = \dfrac{a^5}{b^5}$

Law 5: $(a^m)^n = a^{m \cdot n}$

Example:

$(a^4)^5 = a^{4 \cdot 5} = a^{20}$

Definition: $a^0 = 1$ for $a \neq 0$

Examples:

$5^0 = 1$
$x^0 = 1$
$(5x)^0 = 1$
$5x^0 = 5 \cdot 1 = 5$

Definition: $a^{-n} = \dfrac{1}{a^n}$ for $a \neq 0$

Examples:

$x^{-7} = \dfrac{1}{x^7}$

$2^{-3} = \dfrac{1}{2^3} = \dfrac{1}{8}$

It can also be shown that: $\dfrac{1}{a^{-n}} = a^n$ for $a \neq 0$.

Examples:

$\dfrac{1}{x^{-5}} = x^5$

$\dfrac{1}{5^{-2}} = 5^2 = 25$

Calculator and Exponents To evaluate exponents using a calculator, the y^x key is used (y is the base and x is the exponent).

Example:

$5^3 = 5 \cdot 5 \cdot 5 = 125$

To use the calculator, press the following keys (or consult the manual).

$\boxed{5}\ \boxed{y^x}\ \boxed{3}\ \boxed{=}\ 125$

Example:
$5^{-3} = 1/5^3 = 1/125 = .008$
Calculator method:
$\boxed{5}\ \boxed{y^x}\ \boxed{3}\ \boxed{+/-}\ \boxed{=}$ .008

Example:
$(-5)^3 = (-5)(-5)(-5) = -125$
Calculator method:
$\boxed{5}\ \boxed{+/-}\ \boxed{y^x}\ \boxed{3}\ \boxed{=}$ -125

Example:
$1/5^{-3} = 5^3 = 125$
Calculator method:
$\boxed{5}\ \boxed{y^x}\ \boxed{3}\ \boxed{+/-}\ \boxed{=}\ \boxed{1/x}$ 125

Multiplying Numbers in Scientific Notation
When multiplying two numbers in scientific notation, the Ns are multiplied and the powers of ten are added. This is simply using the rule of exponents when the bases are the same.

Example:
$(2.4 \times 10^3)(3.8 \times 10^{11})$
$= (2.4 \cdot 3.8) \times 10^{3+11}$
$= 9.1 \times 10^{14}$

Dividing Numbers in Scientific Notation
When dividing two numbers in scientific notation, the Ns are divided and the exponents are subtracted. This is another of the rules of exponents.

Example:
$(8.3 \times 10^4) \div (2.7 \times 10^{11})$
$= 8.3 \div 2.7 \times 10^{4-11}$
$= 3.1 \times 10^{-7}$

Evaluating Algebraic Expressions
To evaluate an algebraic expression, replace each unknown with the given value and then perform the indicated operations.

Example:
Evaluate $2a^2 + 4b$ for $a = 3$ and $b = 4$.
$2a^2 + 5b = 2(3)^2 + 5(4)$
$\qquad\qquad = 2 \cdot 9 + 20$
$\qquad\qquad = 18 + 20$
$\qquad\qquad = 38$

Formulae are examples of equations where algebraic expressions are evaluated.

Example:
Convert 60.0° F to C.
The formula involved is $C = 5/9(F - 32°)$.
Determine C when $F = 60.0°$.
$C = 5/9(F - 32°)$
$C = 5/9(60.0° - 32°)$ (substitute 60.0° for F)
$C = 5/9(28°)$
$C = 15.6°$ C

Equations
An equation is a statement that contains an equal sign. For example, $A = B$ is an equation. An equation can be either a true or a false statement.

Examples:
$5 + 3 = 7$ (false statement)
$5 + 3 = 8$ (true statement)

Both of these statements are equations but only one is true.

An equation that contains at least one unknown (variable) is an open equation.

Examples:
$x + 5 = 7$
$3x + 5 = 7 - 2x$

An open statement becomes either true or false when the unknown (variable) is replaced (substituted) with a numeric value.

Examples:
In $x + 5 = 7$, replace x with 3.
$\quad 3 + 5 = 7$ is a false statement.
In $x + 5 = 7$, replace x with 2.
$\quad 2 + 5 = 7$ is a true statement.

The solution of an equation is that numeric value which, when substituted in the equation, gives a true statement. In the example above, 2 is the solution to the equation.

There may be many solutions to an equation. For example, in the equation $x + 5 = x + 5$, all numeric values for x will give a true statement. **This type of equation is called an identity.**

There may be no solutions to an equation. For example, in the equation $x + 5 = x + 6$, there are no numbers that, when substituted in the equation, give a true statement. Therefore there are no solutions to the equation.

Equivalence Principles The principles of equivalence are needed to solve equations. **Equivalent equations are equations that have the same solutions.**

Addition and Subtraction Principle If the same number is added to each side or subtracted from each side of an equation, the equation remains equivalent.

Example:

$$x - 5 = 7 \qquad \text{(add 5 to both sides)}$$
$$x - 5 + 5 = 7 + 5 \qquad \text{(equivalent equation to}$$
$$x = 12 \qquad x - 5 = 7)$$

Example:

$$x + 3 = 12 \qquad \text{(subtract 3 from both sides)}$$
$$x + 3 - 3 = 12 - 3 \qquad \text{(equivalent equation to}$$
$$x = 9 \qquad x + 3 = 12)$$

Multiplication and Division Principle
If the same nonzero number is multiplied or divided by each side of the equation, the equation remains equivalent.

Example:

$$\frac{x}{5} = 6 \qquad \text{(multiply each side by 5)}$$
$$\frac{5 \cdot x}{5} = 5 \cdot 6 \qquad \text{(equivalent equation)}$$
$$x = 30$$

Example:

$$3x = 12 \qquad \text{(divide each side by 3)}$$
$$\frac{3x}{3} = \frac{12}{3} \qquad \text{(equivalent equation)}$$
$$x = 4$$

To find a solution to an equation, the unknown (variable) must be isolated on one side of the equation.

Example:

Solve: $x + 7 = 12$ for x.

$$x + 7 = 12$$
$$x + 7 - 7 = 12 - 7 \quad \text{(subtract 7 from each side)}$$
$$x = 5$$

Check:

$$x + 7 = 12$$
$$5 + 7 = 12 \qquad \text{(substitute value for x)}$$
$$12 = 12 \qquad \text{(statement is true; therefore}$$
$$5 \text{ is solution to equation)}$$

Example:

Solve: $\dfrac{x}{6} = 18$ for x.

$$\frac{x}{6} = 18$$
$$6 \cdot \frac{x}{6} = 6 \cdot 18 \qquad \text{(multiply both sides by 6)}$$
$$x = 108$$

Check:

$$\frac{x}{6} = 18$$
$$\frac{108}{6} = 18 \qquad \text{(substitute 108 for x)}$$
$$18 = 18 \qquad \text{(statement is true)}$$

Example:

Solve: $5a = 30$ for a.

$$5a = 30$$
$$\frac{5a}{5} = \frac{30}{5} \qquad \text{(divide both sides by 5)}$$
$$a = 6$$

Check:

    5a = 30
    5(6) = 30   (substitute 6 for a)
    30 = 30   (statement is true)

Example:
Solve: $7x - 5 = 3x + 7$ for x.

    7x - 5 = 3x + 7
    7x - 5 + 5 = 3x + 7 + 5   (add 5 to both sides)
    7x = 3x + 12
    7x - 3x = 3x + 12 - 3x   (subtract 3x from
                                both sides
    4x = 12
    $\frac{4x}{4} = \frac{12}{4}$ (divide both sides by 4)
    x = 3

Check:

    7x - 5 = 3x + 7
    7(3) - 5 = 3(3) + 7   (substitute 3 for x)
    21 - 5 = 9 + 7
    16 = 16   (statement is true)

To solve an equation with parentheses, the parentheses need to be eliminated using some correct procedure, usually the distributive law.

Example:
Solve: $7(x + 6) = 21$ for x.

    7(x + 6) = 21   (distributive law)
    7x + 42 = 21   (subtract 42 from each side)
    7x = -21   (divide each side by 7)
    x = -3

Check:

    7(x + 6) = 21   (substitute -3 for x)
    7(-3 + 6) = 21
    7(3) = 21
    21 = 21   (statement is true)

Sometimes a formula needs to be rearranged. This is just like solving an equation for an unknown (variable).

Example:
Solve for t when $a = bt + c$

    a = bt + c
    a - c = bt + c - c   (subtract c from
                                  each side)
    a - c = bt   (divide by b)
    $\frac{a-c}{b} = \frac{bt}{b}$
    $\frac{a-c}{b} = t$

Check:

    a = bt + c
    $a = b \cdot \frac{a-c}{b} + c$ (substitute
                                     $\frac{a-c}{b}$ for t)
    a = a - c + c
    a = a   (statement is true)

Variation

There are two types of variation that will be discussed here—direct and inverse.

Direct Variation Direct variation means that one quantity is a multiple of a second quantity. An example of direct variation is $y = kx$ where k is the constant of proportionality. Here y is a multiple of x, making y directly proportional to x.

Another example is $y = kx^2$ where k is the constant of proportionality, making y directly proportional to the square of x. Another way to think of direct variation is that the quotient of the two quantities is always a constant. It is possible, knowing the values for the quantities, to find the constant.

Inverse Variation Inverse variation means that when two quantities are multiplied their product is a constant.

An example of inverse variation is $y = k/x$ where k is the constant of proportionality. Here the product of x and y is a constant, namely k. This is usually read as y is inversely proportional to x.

Another example is $y = k/x^2$ where k is the constant of proportionality. Here the product of x^2 and y is a constant. This is usually read as y is inversely proportional to the square of x (or x^2).

It is also possible to combine the above. As an example, consider $y = kx/z^2$. Here y is directly proportional to x and inversely proportional to the square of z.

SEMILOGARITHMIC GRAPHING

Semilogarithmic graphing is useful in recording data when one variable is much greater than the other. Radiography often uses semilogarithmic graphs with ordinary increments on the y axis (vertical axis) and logarithmic increments on the x axis (horizontal axis). Analysis of the curve is easier because data which would exhibit a nearly straight line on ordinary graph paper will demonstrate characteristics that otherwise would not be seen. The data from Table 1–2 produces the graph in Figure 1–3A on ordinary graph paper while the graph in Figure 1–3B is produced on semilogarithmic paper.

UNITS OF MEASUREMENT

In order to quantify scientific phenomena, standard units of measurement have been established. These units allow scientists to describe quantities. In physics, the primary or fundamental units of measurement are **mass, length and time.** These units, although they have the same meaning and have been standardized by international organizations, are measured by the use of two widely different systems. These are the British (foot-pound-second) system, also called the United States customary system, and the metric [MKS (meter-kilogram-second) or CGS (centimeter-

TABLE 1–2	
DATA FOR GRAPHING A RADIOGRAPHIC FILM SENSITIVITY CURVE	
Step Number	Density Value
1	0.16
2	0.16
3	0.17
4	0.17
5	0.18
6	0.20
7	0.24
8	0.37
9	0.59
10	0.93
11	1.46
12	2.13
13	2.61
14	2.90
15	3.11
16	3.26
17	3.39
18	3.47
19	3.50
20	3.52
21	3.54

gram-second)] system. Although most countries utilize the metric system of measurement, attempts to switch to this system in the United States have not been very successful. In the United States, length is measured in inches and feet rather than meters and kilometers. Nearly all other countries utilize the metric system. By combining one or more of the fundamental units, scientists arrive at secondary or derived units. For example, the area of an object is derived from the fundamental unit of length. The area of a rectangle is determined by multiplying the lengths of the two sides of the object.

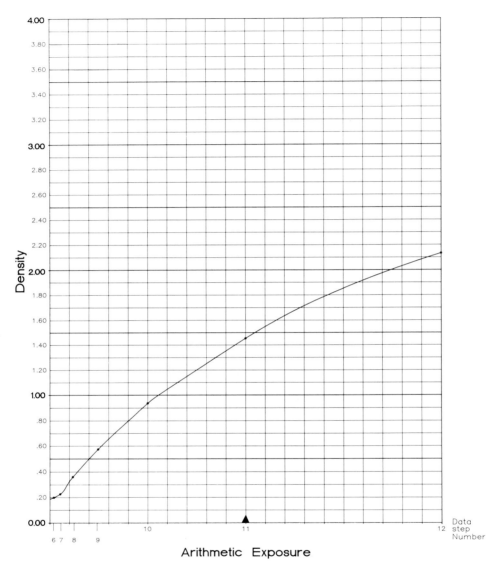

Figure 1–3A.   x and y axis arithmetic.

SI Units

In 1960, at the Eleventh General Conference of Weights and Measures, the Système Internationale d'Unites (SI) was defined and officially adopted. This system of units, used to measure various quantities, is now accepted as the metric system. In the SI system, there are seven base units (Table 1–3). All other units are derived from these units, although some derived units are given special names. It is important to become familiar with SI units since they have been internationally adopted.

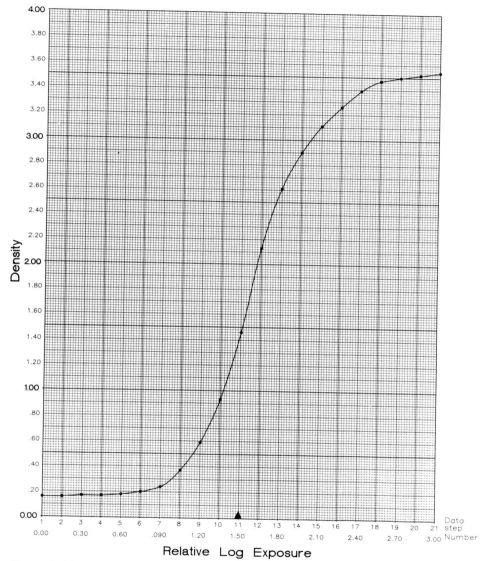

Figure 1–3B.   x axis arithmetic; y axis logarithmic.

In addition, although the United States does not use SI/metric units for the public, all scientific inquiries utilize the SI system. The seven base SI units are mass, length, time, electric current, temperature, amount of substance and luminous intensity. Radiologically important derived units are the **coulomb per kilogram** (C/kg), formerly the roentgen (R); the **gray** (Gy), formerly the rad (radiation absorbed dose); and the **seivert** (Sv), formerly the rem

TABLE 1–3	SI UNITS OF MEASUREMENT			
BASE UNITS				
Quantity	**Unit Name**	**Symbol**		
Mass	kilogram	kg		
Length	meter	m		
Time	second	s		
Electric current	ampere	A		
Temperature	kelvin	K		
Amount of substance	mole	mol		
Luminous intensity	candela	cd		
DERIVED UNITS				
Quantity	**Unit Name**	**Symbol**	**British Units**	
Absorbed dose	gray	Gy	rad	
Charge	coulomb	C	esu	
Electric potential	volt	v		
Dose equivalent	seivert	Sv	rem	
Energy	joule	J	erg	
Exposure	coulomb/kilogram	C/kg	roentgen	
Frequency	hertz	Hz	cycles per second	
Force	newton	N		
Magnetic flux	weber	Wb		
Magnetic flux density	tesla	T	gauss	
Power	watt	W		
Radioactivity	becquerel	Bq	curie	

(radiation equivalent man). These radiologic units will be described in greater detail in the next chapter.

Fundamental Units

Mass Mass is the amount or quantity of matter. The standard unit of mass is the **kilogram** (kg). It is represented by a cylinder of platinum-iridium which is kept in a vault at the International Bureau of Weights and Measures in Paris, France.

Length The unit of length is the **meter** (m). The meter was defined in 1983 as the distance that light travels in a vacuum in $\frac{1}{299,792,485}$ second

Time The unit of time is the **second** (s). The second was originally defined in terms of the rotation of the earth on its axis (the mean solar day) but, like the meter, the need for greater accuracy resulted in redefining the unit. Time is now measured by the vibrations of cesium–133 atoms. This method is sometimes called the atomic clock.

Prefixes

The metric system uses prefixes to units to denote different orders of magnitude, as shown in Table 1–4.

To convert from grams to kilograms or micrograms, or to grams with any other prefix, the decimal point is moved. If the prefix moves up the table, the decimal point is moved to the left the number of exponent positions moved. If the prefix moves down the table, the decimal point is moved to the right the number of ex-

TABLE 1–4

SI UNIT VALUES

Factors	Prefixes	Symbols
10^{12}	tera	T
10^9	giga	G
10^6	mega	M
10^3	kilo	k
10^2	hecto	h
10^1	deka	da
10^{-1}	deci	d
10^{-2}	centi	c
10^{-3}	milli	m
10^{-6}	micro	μ
10^{-9}	nano	n
10^{-12}	pico	p
10^{-15}	femto	f
10^{-18}	atto	a

TABLE 1–5

COMMONLY USED SI PREFIXES

Unit	Symbol	Meaning
kilovolt	kV	10^3 volts
centimeter	cm	10^{-2} meter
milliampere	mA	10^{-3} amp
millirem	mrem	10^{-3} rem
nanosecond	ns	10^{-9} second

view for the procedure to convert from one set of units to another.

SUMMARY

A basic review of arithmetic, algebra, semilogarithmic graphing and units of measurement has been presented. The arithmetic review includes fractions, decimals, computation with values, powers of ten, scientific notation and dimensional analysis. The algebra review includes signed numbers, order of operation, algebraic expressions, exponents, evaluating algebraic expressions, equations, and variation. Semilogarithmic graphing is explained and both SI and British (U.S. customary) units of measurement are introduced.

In order to quantify science, standard units of measurement were established. The fundamental units of measurement are mass, length and time. Units of measurement were officially defined on an international level through the adoption of the SI units. The seven base SI units are mass, length, time, electric current, temperature, amount of substance and luminous intensity. Radiologically important derived units are the coulomb per kilogram (C/kg), formerly the roentgen (R); the gray (Gy), formerly the rad (radiation absorbed dose); and the seivert (Sv), formerly the rem (radiation equivalent man).

ponent positions moved. Dimensional analysis can also be used.

Examples:

23.4 g = 0.0234 kg	Move the decimal point 3 positions left.
23.4 g = 23,400 mg	Move the decimal point 3 positions right.
23.4 mg = 0.0000234 kg	Move the decimal point 6 positions left.
23.4 kg = 2,340,000 cg	Move the decimal point 5 positions right.

Using dimensional analysis:

$$23.4 \text{ g} = 23.4 \text{ g} \ \frac{1 \text{ kg}}{1000 \text{ g}} = 0.0234 \text{ kg}$$

Some commonly used prefixes are shown in Table 1–5. Conversion from one system to another is needed from time to time. For example, 1 inch = 2.54 cm is the conversion fact for changing inches to centimeters. See the section on dimensional analysis under the math re-

REVIEW QUESTIONS

1. $\dfrac{4}{7} + \dfrac{1}{2} =$

2. $\dfrac{2}{9} \cdot \dfrac{3}{8} =$

3. $571.1 - 182.572 =$

4. $725 \div 0.25 =$

5. Change .325 to a percent.

6. What are the significant digits of each of the following:
   a. 20.10
   b. 192
   c. 38.04
   d. 2,700
   e. 1,800.004

7. Add the following numbers, leaving the results with the correct number of significant digits if each number is assumed to be approximate.
   a. $2.1 + 2.824$
   b. $3.2 + 4.19$

8. Change the following numbers to scientific notation:
   a. .0081
   b. 7,811.2
   c. .00024
   d. 78,432

9. Change the following numbers to ordinary notation:
   a. 3.614×10^2
   b. 1.876×10^{-4}
   c. 1.823×10^3
   d. 5.67×10^6

10. Convert 1,500 seconds to hours.

11. Convert 10 meters^2 to centimeters^2.

12. Simplify the following algebraic expressions:

   a. $-3(x + y) + 7(2x + 1)$
   b. $-4(x + 2y) - 8(2x - y)$

13. Simplify the following expressions, leaving the answer with only positive exponents:
   a. $a^2 \cdot b^3 \cdot a^4 \cdot b^2$
   b. $(a^4)^3 \cdot (a^2)^{-3}$

14. Evaluate the expression for $a = 5$ and $b = 3$
$$\frac{3}{8}(a^2 - b^2)$$

15. Evaluate the expression for $a = 2$, $b = -4$, and $c = 6$.
$$3(a + b) - c$$

16. Solve for x: $2x - 8 = 4$

17. Solve for x: $2(3x - 8) = 3(4 - x) + 6x$

18. Solve for a: $\dfrac{2}{3} = \dfrac{a}{15}$

REFERENCES AND RECOMMENDED READING

Aufmann, Richard N., and Vernon C. Barker. *Basic College Mathematics*. 3rd ed. Boston, MA: Houghton Mifflin Company, 1987.

Austin, Gill, and Isern. *Technical Mathematics*. 4th ed. Saunders College Publishing Company, 1988.

Burns, J. E. The new SI units—problems with conversion. *The Canadian Journal of Radiography, Radiotherapy, and Nuclear Medicine* 10:2, 60–70, 1979.

The SI for the health professions. *The Canadian Journal of Medical Radiation Technology* 10:4, 138, 1979.

Washington, Allyn J. *Basic Technical Mathematics*. 5th ed. Redwood City, CA: The Benjamin/Cummings Publishing Company, Inc., 1990.

Wyckoff, Harold O. The international system of units (SI). *Radiology* 128, 833–835, 1978.

2 RADIATION CONCEPTS

I have discovered something interesting, but I do not know whether or not my observations are correct.

W. C. Röntgen to his friend Theodor Boveri in early December 1895.

OUTLINE

MATTER AND ENERGY
ATOMIC THEORY
TYPES OF ENERGY
ELECTROMAGNETIC SPECTRUM
THE DISCOVERY OF X-RAYS
X-RAY PROPERTIES

OBJECTIVES

Upon completion of this chapter, the student should be able to:

1. Describe the branches of science.
2. Differentiate between matter and energy.
3. Describe the basic structure of matter.
4. Identify the various types of energy.
5. Explain the basic concepts of atomic theory.
6. Differentiate between the radiations along the electromagnetic spectrum.
7. Describe the wave and particle theories for electromagnetic radiation.
8. Identify the properties of x-rays.
9. Explain the standard units of measurement.

MATTER AND ENERGY

Radiography is the recording of images created by the use of x-ray energy. It is both an art and a science. In order to perform the du-ties of a radiographer it is necessary to understand the art of the profession as well as the science.

Science is the use of knowledge in an organized and classified manner. The scientific method has been used by man to understand the world in which we live. This method systematically involves collecting facts, studying their relationships and arriving at conclusions based on analysis. Natural science is the study of the universe and its contents. It can be divided into two categories: 1) the study of nonliving matter, known as physical science, and 2) the study of living matter, known as biological science. Radiographers learn about biological science through a study of human anatomy and physiology and about physical science through a study of x-ray production and imaging processes.

Physics is a branch of physical science which studies matter and energy and their interrelationships. Matter is defined as anything that has mass and occupies space. Energy is the ability to do work.

Matter

Matter is a very general term used to describe the substance which comprises all physical objects. It has shape, form and occupies space. A principle characteristic of matter is **mass**. Mass is the quantity of matter contained in an object. It is best described by its energy equivalence although the term weight is generally used to mean the same thing. **Weight** is the force that an object exerts under the influence of gravity. An object may be weightless in a zero gravity environment, such as in space, but the mass of that object would remain unchanged.

The unit of mass is the kilogram, which equals 1,000 grams. The kilogram represents the weight of a standard piece of platinum-iridium kept at the International Bureau of Weights and Measures in Paris, France. It is equal to the mass of 1,000 cm^3 of water at 0° Celsius (C) or Centigrade.

The structure of matter has been studied throughout history. In nature, matter is most commonly found as a mixture of substances (Table 2–1). A **substance** is defined as a material which has a definite and constant composition. When two or more substances are combined they form a **mixture**. For example, air is a mixture of oxygen, hydrogen, nitrogen and a variety of other substances.

Substances may be either simple or complex. Simple substances are known as **elements** and complex substances are known as **compounds**. An element is a substance that cannot be broken down into any simpler substances by ordinary means. There are 92 naturally occurring elements which are identified on the periodic table of elements (Table 2–2). Elements include such substances as hydrogen, oxygen, carbon, calcium, copper, silver, gold, lead and barium. When two or more elements are chemically united in definite proportion, compounds are formed. Water and salt are both examples of compounds. Water is formed by the chemical union of two hydrogen atoms and one oxygen atom and is referred to as H_2O (Figure 2–1). Each element has an abbreviated letter or letters to identify it. These abbreviations for the elements are outlined on the periodic table. For example, in the compound salt, the element sodium (Na) is chemically combined with the element chlorine (Cl), in equal proportions, to form sodium chloride (NaCl).

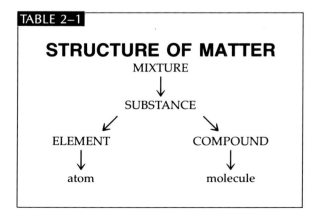

TABLE 2–1

STRUCTURE OF MATTER

MIXTURE
↓
SUBSTANCE
↙   ↘
ELEMENT   COMPOUND
↓   ↓
atom   molecule

TABLE 2-2

PERIODIC TABLE OF THE ELEMENTS

Period	Outer Electrons located in	Group I	Group II	Group III	Group IV	Group V	Group VI	Group VII	Group VIII
1	K shell	1 · 1.09 · **H** · Hydrogen							2 · 4.00 · **He** · Helium
2	L shell	3 · 6.94 · **Li** · Lithium	4 · 9.02 · **Be** · Beryllium	5 · 10.82 · **B** · Boron	6 · 12.01 · **C** · Carbon	7 · 14.09 · **N** · Nitrogen	8 · 16.00 · **O** · Oxygen	9 · 19.00 · **F** · Fluorine	10 · 20.18 · **Ne** · Neon
3	M shell	11 · 23.0 · **Na** · Sodium	12 · 24.32 · **Mg** · Magnesium	13 · 26.97 · **Al** · Aluminum	14 · 28.06 · **Si** · Silicon	15 · 30.98 · **P** · Phosphorus	16 · 32.06 · **S** · Sulfur	17 · 35.46 · **Cl** · Chlorine	18 · 39.99 · **A** · Argon
4	N shell	19 · 39.096 · **K** · Potassium	20 · 40.08 · **Ca** · Calcium	21 · 45.10 · **Sc** · Scandium	22 · 47.90 · **Ti** · Titanium	23 · 50.95 · **V** · Vanadium	24 · 52.01 · **Cr** · Chromium	25 · 54.93 · **Mn** · Manganese	26 · 55.85 · **Fe** · Iron; 27 · 58.94 · **Co** · Cobalt; 28 · 58.69 · **Ni** · Nickel
4	N shell	29 · 63.57 · **Cu** · Copper	30 · 65.38 · **Zn** · Zinc	31 · 69.72 · **Ga** · Gallium	32 · 72.60 · **Ge** · Germanium	33 · 74.91 · **As** · Arsenic	34 · 79.00 · **Se** · Selenium	35 · 79.92 · **Br** · Bromine	36 · 83.7 · **Kr** · Krypton
5	O shell	37 · 85.48 · **Rb** · Rubidium	38 · 87.63 · **Sr** · Strontium	39 · 88.92 · **Y** · Yttrium	40 · 91.22 · **Zr** · Zirconium	41 · 92.91 · **Cb** · Columbium	42 · 96.0 · **Mo** · Molybdenum	43 · 99 · **Tc** · Technetium	44 · 101.7 · **Ru** · Ruthenium; 45 · 102.9 · **Rh** · Rhodium; 46 · 106.7 · **Pd** · Palladium
5	O shell	47 · 107.88 · **Ag** · Silver	48 · 112.41 · **Cd** · Cadmium	49 · 118.70 · **In** · Indium	50 · 118.70 · **Sn** · Tin	51 · 121.77 · **Sb** · Antimony	52 · 127.6 · **Te** · Tellurium	53 - 126.92 · **I** · Iodine	54 · 131.3 · **Xe** · Xenon
6	P shell	55 · 132.9 · **Cs** · Cesium	56 · 137.4 · **Ba** · Barium	Rare Earths 57–71	72 · 178.6 · **Hf** · Hafnium	73 · 180.9 · **Ta** · Tantalum	74 · 183.9 · **W** · Tungsten	75 · 186.3 · **Re** · Rhenium	76 · 190.2 · **Os** · Osmium; 77 · 193.1 · **Ir** · Iridium; 78 · 195.2 · **Pt** · Platinum
6	P shell	79 · 197.2 · **Au** · Gold	80 · 200.6 · **Hg** · Mercury	81 · 204.4 · **Tl** · Thallium	82 · 207.2 · **Pb** · Lead	83 · 209.0 · **Bi** · Bismuth	84 · 210 · **Po** · Polonium	85 · 211 · **At** · Astatine	86 · 222 · **Rn** · Radon
7	Q shell	87 · 224 · **Vi** · Virginium	88 · 226.05 · **Ra** · Radium	Actinide Series 89–103					

Rare Earth Series

57 · 138.91 · **La** · Lanthanum	58 · 140.12 · **Ce** · Cerium	59 · 140.91 · **Pr** · Praseodymium	60 · 144.24 · **Nd** · Neodymium	61 · 147 · **Pm** · Promethium	62 · 150.35 · **Sm** · Samarium	63 · 151.96 · **Eu** · Europium	64 · 157.25 · **Gd** · Gadolinium	65 · 158.92 · **Tb** · Terbium	66 · 162.50 · **Dy** · Dysprosium	67 · 164.93 · **Ho** · Holmium	68 · 167.26 · **Er** · Erbium	69 · 168.93 · **Tm** · Thulium	70 · 173.04 · **Yb** · Ytterbium	71 · 174.97 · **Lu** · Lutetium

Actinide Series

89 · 227 · **Ac** · Actinium	90 · 232.04 · **Th** · Thorium	91 · 231 · **Pa** · Protactinium	92 · 238.03 · **U** · Uranium	93 · 237 · **Np** · Neptunium	94 · 242 · **Pu** · Plutonium	95 · 243 · **Am** · Americium	96 · 245 · **Cm** · Curium	97 · 249 · **Bk** · Berkelium	98 · 251 · **Cf** · Californium	99 · 254 · **Es** · Einsteinium	100 · 254 · **Fm** · Fermium	101 · 255 · **Md** · Mendelevium	102 · 256 · **No** · Nobelium	103 · 257 · **Lr** · Lawrencium

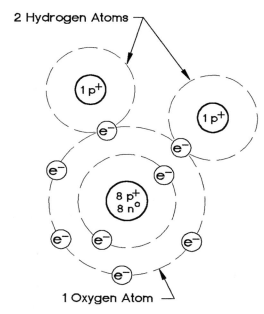

2 Hydrogen Atoms

1 Oxygen Atom

Figure 2–1.   A water molecule is formed when 2 atoms of hydrogen combine with one atom of oxygen.

When broken down and examined in its purest form, matter is actually comprised of very small invisible particles known as atoms. An **atom** is the smallest particle of an element that still possesses the characteristics of that element. When two or more atoms are chemically united they form a **molecule**, which is the smallest particle of a compound that still possesses the characteristics of the compound. For example, in the compound water, two hydrogen (H) atoms combine with one oxygen (O) atom to form one water (H_2O) molecule. With salt, one sodium (Na) atom combines with one chlorine (Cl) atom to form one sodium chloride (NaCl) molecule.

Atoms are tightly bonded to one another when a molecule is formed. These bonds cannot be broken by ordinary physical means, such as crushing. Atoms and molecules are, however, bound to one another by varying degrees of attraction. The degree of attraction be-

tween atoms or molecules will determine if the substance is a solid, a liquid or a gas. The attraction is weakest with a gas and strongest with a solid. For example, depending on the degree of molecular attraction, water can exist in its usual state as a liquid, or it can exist as a gas (steam) or a solid (ice). The state is determined by the heat or thermal energy that the substance possesses.

Energy

Energy is defined as the ability to do work. When energy is emitted and transferred through matter it is called **radiation**. Radiation is a term applied to many forms of energy, such as heat and light. When the burner on a stove is lit, it can be described as radiating heat. A light bulb is capable of radiating light. When any form of matter is struck by a form of radiant energy, it is described as being exposed or radiated.

There is a unique relationship between matter and energy. They are interchangeable. This relationship was described in 1905 by the American physicist, Albert Einstein (1879–1955), in his well-known theory of relativity. Einstein mathematically described the relationship between matter and energy in the equation:

$$E = mc^2$$

where: E = energy
  m = mass
  c = constant (the speed of light in a vacuum)

At the basis of Einstein's work is the Law of Conservation. This law states that the sum total of all matter and energy in the universe is a constant: matter and energy cannot be created or destroyed but can be converted from one form to another. Although recent research has demonstrated certain circumstances when Einstein's theory has been disproved, for practical purposes it is essentially true.

ATOMIC THEORY

Matter is comprised of very small particles known as atoms. Atoms can be further subdivided into three basic subatomic particles: **protons (p$^+$)**, **neutrons (n^0)** and **electrons (e$^-$)**.

Historical Overview

The composition of the atom has been a topic of scientific investigation for thousands of years. The Greeks theorized that matter has four basic components: air, water, earth and fire. They named the smallest division of these components the atom. This theory was accepted until the early 1800s, when an English schoolteacher named John Dalton (1766–1844) published his work on atomic theory. Dalton concluded that all elements could be differentiated from one another based on the characteristic of mass. He further concluded that each of the elements was composed of atoms which behaved in an identical fashion during a chemical reaction. During the mid-1800s a Russian scientist, Dmitri Mendeleev (1834–1907), developed the first periodic table of the elements. This table arranges the elements in order of ascending atomic mass and on the basis of the repetition of similar chemical properties (see Table 2–2).

Investigation of the structure of matter continued and, in 1911, English physicist Ernest Rutherford (1871–1937) developed a model for the atom which contained a central, small, dense nucleus, which possessed a positive charge and was surrounded by a negative cloud of randomly placed electrons, which had a negative charge. In 1913 Niels Bohr (1885–1962), a Danish physicist, expanded on Rutherford's work and proposed a model for the atom which is considered the most representative of

the structure of matter. Bohr's atom is likened to a miniature solar system where electrons orbit around a central nucleus just as the planets revolve around the sun.

Although the atom is far more complex than Bohr's simple model suggests, this model is still the most widely used in explaining the composition of matter. One key distinction between Bohr's model and an actual atom is that electrons orbit the nucleus in many planes, while the planets orbit the sun in essentially the same plane.

Basic Atomic Particles

The atom is best described as having a small, dense center, known as the **nucleus**, which is surrounded by electrons that orbit it at various levels (Figure 2–2). The nucleus contains two of the three basic particles of the atom, protons and neutrons, which are responsible for almost all of the mass of an atom. **Protons** and **neutrons** together are referred to as **nucleons**. The third basic particle, the **electron**, is located outside the nucleus and has a relatively insignificant mass, 1/1,828 that of a proton.

These subatomic particles possess electrical charges. There are two types of electrical charges: positive and negative. The proton is a positively charged particle and the electron is a negatively charged particle. The neutron contains no charge and is said to be electrically neutral. When the number of positively charged protons equals the number of negatively charged electrons, the atom is neutral or stable. Because of its electrical nature, the atom is dynamic and ever moving. It is in a constant, vibrating motion because of the strong positive nuclear force field which is surrounded by the negatively charged spinning and orbiting electrons.

Each of the elements has its own specific number of nuclear protons. This is the key characteristic which distinguishes one element from another. The number of nuclear protons

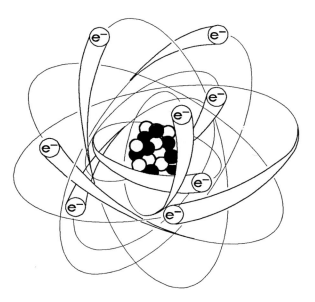

Figure 2–2. A three-dimensional diagram of an atom of oxygen, which contains 8 protons, 8 neutrons located within the center nucleus, and 8 electrons within orbital shells moving around the nucleus.

in an atom is known as the **atomic number** or **Z** number. The simplest element, hydrogen, possesses only one proton and therefore has an atomic number of 1. Helium comes next on the periodic table and has two protons, giving it an atomic number of 2. Lead has an atomic number of 82, indicating that within the nucleus of an atom of lead there are 82 protons. The periodic table lists the elements in ascending order according to the element's atomic number (see Table 2–2). In a neutral atom the number of protons is equal to the number of electrons. For example, in a stable, neutral atom of hydrogen there is one proton and one electron. In a stable atom of lead there are 82 protons and 82 electrons.

Although not a common occurrence in nature, when an atom of a given element loses or gains a proton that atom becomes a different element. For example, if an atom of carbon with atomic number 6 gains a proton, the atom then becomes an atom of nitrogen with atomic number 7. Atoms of one element do change to atoms of another element during the natural process of radioactive decay. Radium, with an atomic number of 88, decays over a very long period of time to form the element radon, which has atomic number 86. Radon is a naturally occurring gas which is also radioactive. Recent studies have found increased radon levels in homes around the country. Radon testing kits are now commercially available to measure radon levels in the home.

Changes in the number of protons change the identity of the element completely, but this is not the case with changes in the number of neutrons or electrons. If an atom gains or loses neutrons, the result is an atom called an **isotope**. Isotopes are atoms which have the same number of protons in the nucleus but differ in the number of neutrons. Deuterium is an isotope of hydrogen. It contains the same number of protons as hydrogen but also contains one neutron. If an atom gains or loses an electron, it is called an **ion** and the atom is said to be ionized.

Ionization is the process of adding or removing an electron from an atom. When an electron is removed from an atom, the atom becomes a positive ion; that is, the atom possesses an extra positive charge. When an electron is added to an atom, the atom becomes a negative ion; that is, it possesses an extra negative charge (Figure 2–3).

Atomic Mass

The mass of an atom is extremely small; however, it is important to understand the differences in the mass of each of the basic parti-

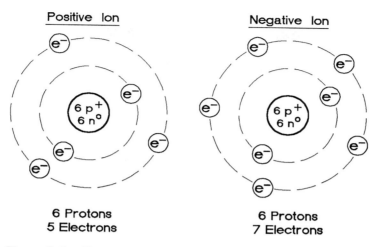

Positive Ion

6 p⁺
6 n°

6 Protons
5 Electrons

Negative Ion

6 p⁺
6 n°

6 Protons
7 Electrons

Figure 2–3. The ionization process: When an electron is either added or removed from an atom, the atom is ionized. A neutral carbon atom contains 6 protons and 6 electrons; a positive ion of carbon would contain more protons than electrons and a negative ion of carbon would contain more electrons than protons.

cles of an atom. Each individual particle has its own unique mass. As stated earlier, the mass of an atom is almost entirely concentrated in the nucleus. The mass of a proton is approximately 1.673×10^{-27} kilograms and the mass of a neutron is almost identical, at 1.675×10^{-27} kilograms. While these numbers seem remarkably small, they are still significantly greater than the mass of an electron, at 9.109×10^{-31} kilograms. Protons have approximately 1,836 times the mass of electrons and neutrons have approximately 1,838 times more. The mass of the particles of an atom is sometimes described in **atomic mass units (amu)**.

In order for science to be as exact as possible, scientists defined an atomic mass unit as equal to one twelfth of a carbon 12 atom. The amu of a proton is approximately 1.00728, a neutron has an amu of approximately 1.00867, and an electron has an amu of approximately 0.000549. When precision is not necessary, the mass of an atom is described by an **atomic mass**

number symbolized by the letter **A**. The atomic mass number is equal to the number of protons and neutrons in the nucleus. For our purposes, each proton and neutron can be considered to have a mass number of one and an electron has a mass number of zero (Table 2–3).

Orbital Electrons

Each of the electrons around the nucleus is in continuous motion in an orbit or path. The orbits are each at a particular distance from the nucleus. This distance determines the energy level or **shell** that the electron occupies. This energy level is also referred to as the **electron binding energy (E_b)**. The closer an electron is to the nucleus, the more tightly it is bound to its path. Certain forces are responsible for maintaining the electron's position and motion in its orbit. The electron is in motion around the nucleus and maintains a specific distance from the nucleus through **centripetal force**. In the atom centripetal (center-seeking)

TABLE 2–3		ATOMIC PARTICLES		
Particle	**Mass Number**	**Mass (Kilograms)**	**amu**	**Charge**
Proton	1	1.673×10^{-27}	1.00728	Positive
Neutron	1	1.675×10^{-27}	1.00867	Neutral
Electron	0	9.109×10^{-31}	0.000549	Negative

force is the result of one of the basic laws of electrical charges: like charges repel and unlike charges attract.

Recall that the nucleus carries a positive charge and the electron a negative one. The electron is not pulled into the nucleus because a balance exists between the centripetal force and the electron's velocity in its given path. The end result is an electron that is in motion in a specific circular path or orbit around the nucleus. The closer an electron is to the nucleus, the higher the electron binding energy is and the more difficult it is to remove the electron from its path (Figure 2–4). Conversely, the further an electron is from the nucleus, the greater the electron's velocity will be in order for it to maintain its position in orbit. An analogy to this concept would be cars circling a race track. The car that is closest to the center is "bound" more tightly to the center and, compared to the outer circle cars, is less likely to lose its position. For the outer circle cars to keep pace with the inner circle cars, they must travel at a greater speed.

The orbital shell which sits closest to the nucleus is called the **K-shell**, the next shell is called the L-shell, then M-, N-, O-, P-, and finally the Q-shell. In a neutral atom, the number of protons and electrons is equal. This means that each element has a different number of orbital electrons. The element hydrogen has only one proton and one electron. The electron of a hydrogen atom orbits in the K-shell. There is a maximum number of electrons which can occupy a given shell. The maximum number is determined by the formula $2n^2$,

where n equals the shell number, starting with K as the first shell. According to this formula, the maximum number of electrons in each of the shells would be:

$$K = 2(1)^2 = 2$$
$$L = 2(2)^2 = 8$$
$$M = 2(3)^2 = 18$$
$$N = 2(4)^2 = 32$$
$$O = 2(5)^2 = 50$$
$$P = 2(6)^2 = 72$$
$$Q = 2(7)^2 = 98$$

Electrons may begin to appear in the next shell before a shell contains its maximum number of electrons. For example, electrons may appear in the N-shell before the M-shell has 18 electrons in it. This is because the number of electrons in the outermost shell never exceeds eight electrons. This is commonly referred to as the **octet rule**. Atoms that contain exactly eight electrons in their outermost shell are considered inert and chemically stable. The specific electron configuration will determine an element's position within the groups of the periodic table.

As the number of electrons increases, so does the binding energy of a given electron. This means that the electrons in atoms of high atomic number elements are bound more tightly than the electrons in atoms of lower atomic number elements. The binding energy of electrons in the K-shell of lead is much higher than the binding energy of the K-shell electrons in hydrogen or oxygen. In addition, the binding energy of an electron decreases as

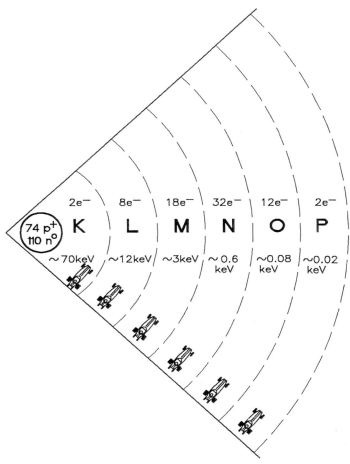

Figure 2–4. The closer an electron is to the nucleus, the greater will be the binding energy of the electron. However, outer shell electrons must travel at greater velocities in order to maintain their position in orbit around the nucleus. The negative electrons are maintained at specific distances from the positive nucleus by centripetal force.

the distance from the nucleus is increased. It takes more energy to remove a K-shell electron from its path than it would to remove an electron from a shell at a greater distance from the nucleus, such as the L-, M-, or N-shell. This will become important to remember when studying the effect of x-rays on atoms.

The binding energy of an electron is measured in a unit called the **electron volt (eV)**. This is the same unit used to describe x-ray energies. The electron volt is the energy one electron will have when it is accelerated by an electrical potential of one volt. Because x-ray and binding energies are great, the usual unit used to express these energies is the kilo-electron volt (keV). One keV equals 1,000 electron volts.

The atomic configuration and the approximate binding energies of certain elements are important because of their significance in radiology. These elements include hydrogen (H), carbon (C) and oxygen (O) because they are the principle elements which comprise the human body; iodine (I) and barium (Ba) because these elements are used as contrast media for a variety of radiologic examinations; tungsten (W) because it is the x-ray tube target material; and lead (Pb) because it is the element used for radiation protection devices. A diagram of these elements shows that as the atomic number of an element increases, the K-shell binding energy of the element increases (Figure 2–5). This means that a K-shell electron of lead (Pb) is more tightly bound and more difficult to remove from the atom than a K-shell electron of smaller atomic number elements, such as hydrogen (H) or oxygen (O).

To remove the K-shell electron from an atom of tungsten or lead requires much more energy than would be necessary to remove a K-shell electron from an atom of hydrogen, carbon or oxygen. When an electron is removed from an atom, the atom is said to be ionized. X-rays are capable of ionizing atoms. The x-ray energy must be greater than the binding energy of the electron in order for ionization to occur (Figure 2–6).

The Periodic Table

The present-day periodic table lists the 92 naturally occurring elements and an additional 11 elements that have been created in the laboratory through scientific investigation (see Table 2–2). The elements are listed in ascending order based on the atomic number located in the upper left corner. The atomic mass of the element is identified in the upper right corner.

Each of the elements is also arranged into one of seven horizontal periods and one of eight vertical groups. The periods represent elements with the same number of electron shells and the groups represent elements with the same number of electrons in the outermost shell. For example, each element in the eighth group has eight electrons in its outermost shell. These elements are chemically very stable atoms.

The number of electrons in the outermost shell of an atom determines the chemical combining characteristic or **valence** of the element. An element that has only one electron in the outermost shell is described as having a valence of $+1$ and would be located in Group I on the periodic table. This element will freely give up this electron to bind with another element to form a compound. An element that has seven electrons in its outermost shell has a valence of -1 and would be located in Group VII. This element will freely accept an electron to form a chemical bond because atoms prefer the stable octet configuration. An example of this bond, known as an ionic bond, is the salt molecule. Sodium (Na), having a valence of $+1$, can easily combine with Chlorine (Cl), with a valence of -1, to form sodium chloride (NaCl), salt (Figure 2–7). The valence of an element determines the way the atoms will combine in definite proportions. Because of the element's valence number, **two** hydrogen atoms combine with **one** oxygen atom to form water. Hydrogen has a valence of $+1$ while oxygen has a valence of -2. Oxygen has room for two hydrogen atoms and will share electrons, a type of bond known as a covalent bond (Figure 2–8).

TYPES OF ENERGY

Energy is the ability to do work. It exists in many different forms. Regardless of form, all types of energy possess an actual or poten-

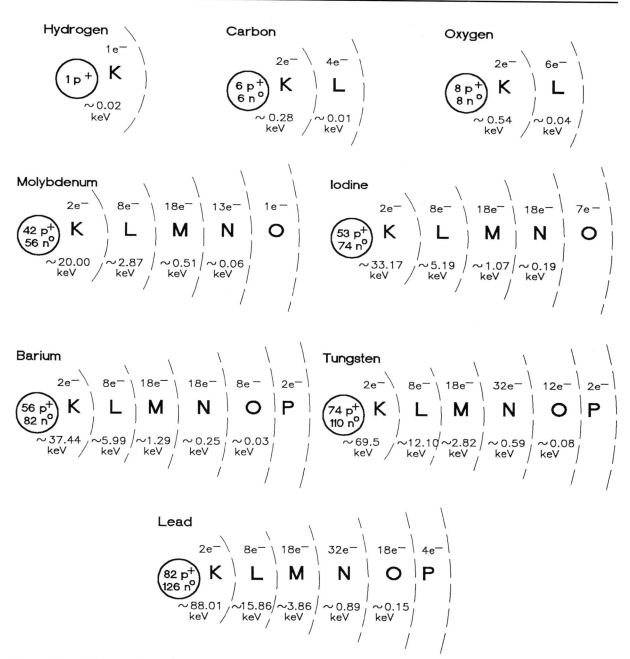

Figure 2–5. The atomic configurations and binding energies of elements which have significance in radiology.

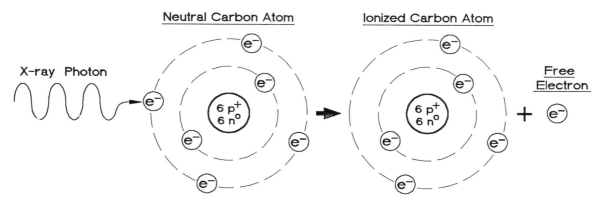

Figure 2–6.   An x-ray photon can interact with an electron and eject it from an atom. This removal of an electron results in the ionization of the atom.

tial ability to do work. Work is the result of a force acting upon an object over a distance. It is expressed in the equation **work = force × distance**. When a force acts upon an object over a distance, energy is expended. For example, when a book is lifted one foot above a table, work is done and energy is expended. If the same book is lifted two feet above the table, twice as much work and energy are expended.

Mechanical Mechanical energy is the result of the action of machines or physical movement. There are two types of mechanical energy: potential and kinetic. **Potential energy** is the energy which an object has because of its position. It is stored, by virtue of its position, in the object until it is converted to another form of energy. A car located at the top of a hill possesses more potential energy than the same car located at the bottom of a hill. If the

Figure 2–7.   An ionic bond is formed between sodium (Na) and chlorine (Cl) to form table salt, sodium chloride (NaCl).

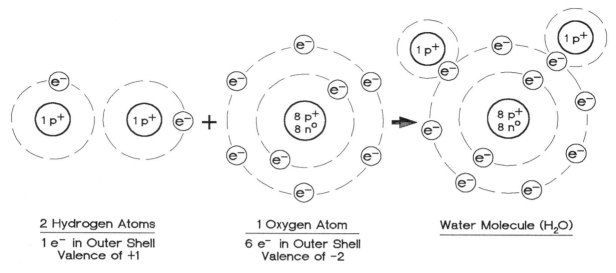

2 Hydrogen Atoms
1 e⁻ in Outer Shell
Valence of +1

1 Oxygen Atom
6 e⁻ in Outer Shell
Valence of −2

Water Molecule (H_2O)

Figure 2–8.   A covalent bond is formed between two hydrogen atoms and one oxygen atom to form water, H_2O.

car's brakes are released, the potential energy is then converted to kinetic energy as the car moves to the bottom of the hill (and a lower energy state). **Kinetic energy** is the energy of motion. An object in motion is able to perform work because it is moving. For example, the energy of water as it moves in a river can be used to perform work. When a dam is built across a river, the kinetic energy of the moving water can be used to produce electric energy. No electricity will be produced if the water is not moving.

Chemical Chemical energy is the form of energy released during a chemical reaction. A battery operates using chemical energy. The purpose of a battery is to convert chemical energy into electrical energy.

Heat Heat, also called **thermal energy**, is the result of the motion of atoms and molecules. The faster the atoms and molecules within a substance are moving or vibrating, the greater the thermal energy of the substance. **Tempera-** ture is a measure of thermal energy. As the temperature of a substance increases, the motion of the atoms in the substance increases. When a pan of water is placed on an electric burner, the electrical energy is converted to heat energy, which raises the temperature of the water and increases the motion of its atoms and molecules.

Electrical Electrical energy, or **electricity**, is the result of the movement of electrons (electrical charges). Electricity is the study of resting or moving electrical charges. There are numerous appliances which operate by the use of electrical energy. When a lamp is turned on, a flow of electrons passes along a wire in a light bulb. The light bulb is a device which converts electrical energy to light, which is a form of electromagnetic energy. In a toaster, electrical energy is converted to heat, or thermal energy.

Nuclear Nuclear energy is stored in the nucleus of each atom and holds the nuclear particles in a tight bond. A tremendous amount of energy is stored in the nucleus of an atom. In the 1940s scientists working at the University of Chicago learned how to control the release of this energy and, as a result of this knowledge, developed the atomic bomb. Today, nuclear power plants convert nuclear energy, within a very controlled environment, to electricity.

Electromagnetic Electromagnetic energy is a form of energy that is the result of electric and magnetic disturbances in space (Figure 2–9). This type of energy travels through space as a combination of electric and magnetic fields and is produced by the acceleration of a charge. There are many very familiar forms of electromagnetic energy, including radio waves, microwaves, infrared light, visible light, and cosmic rays. X-rays are a form of man-made electromagnetic energy that is created in an x-ray tube when high-speed electrons are suddenly stopped. Physically they are identical to gamma rays, differing only in origin. Gamma rays originate from the nucleus of radioactive materials, while x-rays originate in an x-ray tube.

ELECTROMAGNETIC SPECTRUM

Electromagnetic radiation is a natural part of the environment in which we live. Although the term may not be a common one, we are all familiar with many forms of this energy. The nature of electromagnetic radiation was discovered in scientific experiments using visible light. Visible light was shown to have both electric and magnetic properties and was therefore described as being electromagnetic. Shortly after these investigations, other forms of electromagnetic radiation, invisible to man, were studied and a theory to explain this form of energy was proposed.

Electromagnetic radiation (EM) spans a continuum of wide ranges of magnitudes of energy. This continuum is termed the **electromagnetic spectrum** (Figure 2–10). (See the end pages in the back of the book.) The electromagnetic spectrum details all of the various forms of EM radiation. One of the common properties of all forms of EM radiation is velocity. The velocity of EM energy is equal to the speed of light

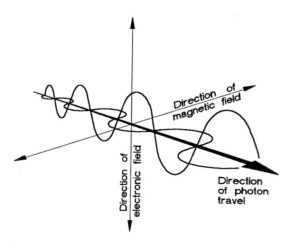

Figure 2–9.   Two overlapping sine waves, one representing an electric field and the other a magnetic field, illustrate electromagnetic radiation.

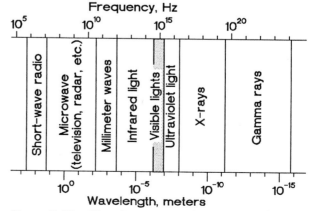

Figure 2–10.   The electromagnetic spectrum. See the end pages at the back of the book for the complete electromagnetic spectrum.

(c), which is 3×10^8 meters/second (186,400 miles per second). In studying EM radiation scientists found that under certain circumstances it behaved as a wave and at other times it behaved as a particle. **This dual nature is known as the wave-particle duality of radiation. To best understand x-rays, it is necessary to consider them as both waves and particles of energy.**

Wave Theory Electromagnetic energy travels through space in the form of waves. Waves are disturbances in a medium. Ocean waves and sound waves are examples of disturbances of the mediums of water and air. When a rock is dropped into water, waves result. During speech, sound waves are created as disturbances in the air. **Electromagnetic waves are unique in that no medium is required.** They can travel in a vacuum.

All types of waves have an associated wavelength and frequency. To illustrate the wave concept, a sine wave is used because electromagnetic waves travel in the form of a sine wave (Figure 2–11). Sine waves can be mathematically described but these definitions are beyond the scope of this book. Instead, we will use the primary descriptions of electromagnetic waves: wavelength and frequency. The **wavelength** is the distance between any two successive points on a wave. Wavelength is usually measured from crest to crest or trough to trough. It is represented by the Greek letter **lambda** (λ), the character for length. Wavelengths vary from kilometers to Angstroms. The Angstrom (represented by the symbol Å) is equal to 10^{-10} meters, which is one ten-billionth of a meter. The Angstrom is of special interest because the wavelength of diagnostic x-rays is 0.1–0.5 Å. The **frequency** is the number of waves that pass a particular point in a given time frame, or the number of cycles per second. It is represented by the Greek letter **nu** (ν), the initial for number. The unit of frequency is the hertz (Hz) or cycles per second (cps).

A relationship exists between the frequency, wavelength and velocity of a wave. This relationship is expressed by the formula:

$$\text{velocity} = \text{frequency} \times \text{wavelength},$$
$$\text{or } c = \lambda \nu$$
$$\text{where: } c = \text{constant (the speed of light)}$$
$$\lambda = \text{the frequency}$$
$$\nu = \text{the wavelength}$$

This is known as the wave equation. Recall that with electromagnetic waves, velocity was a constant equal to the speed of light. Because velocity is a constant, an increase in frequency would result in an associated decrease in wavelength and vice versa. Therefore, **frequency and wavelength are inversely proportional.**

Radiation along the electromagnetic spectrum will vary according to the associated frequency and wavelength. Low frequencies and long wavelengths are at the bottom end of the spectrum with radio waves and microwaves, visible light is in the center of the spectrum, and at the top of the spectrum are gamma and x-rays, with associated high frequencies and short wavelengths.

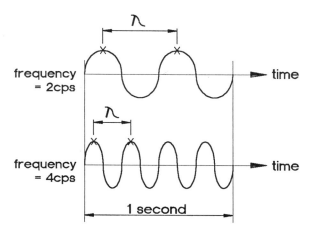

Figure 2–11. Two sine waves. With electromagnetic waves, if wavelength decreases, frequency will increase.

Particle Theory When high-frequency electromagnetic radiation interacts with matter, it behaves more like a particle than a wave. With this model, electromagnetic radiation acts like a small bundle of energy, known as a **photon** or **quantum**. The photon carries a specific amount of energy which is dependent upon frequency. **Photon energy and frequency are directly proportional.** If the frequency of an x-ray is doubled, the energy is doubled. This relationship was first described by the German physicist Max Planck (1858–1947). The relationship between photon energy and frequency is mathematically described in the formula:

$$E = h\lambda$$

where:　E = photon energy (eV)
　　　　h = Planck's constant
　　　　　　$(4.15 \times 10^{-15}$ eV-sec)
　　　λ = photon frequency (Hz)

From this formula, it is possible to calculate the frequency of an x-ray when given the x-ray photon's energy.

Example: What is the frequency of a 72 keV x-ray photon?

Answer: $E = h\lambda$

$$\lambda = \frac{E}{h}$$

$$\lambda = \frac{72\text{keV}}{4.15 \times 10^{-15} \text{ eV-sec}}$$

$$\lambda = \frac{7.2 \times 10^4 \text{ eV}}{4.15 \times 10^{-15} \text{ eV-sec}}$$

$$\lambda = 1.73 \times 10^{19} \text{ Hz}$$

THE DISCOVERY OF X-RAYS

On November 8, 1895, the German physicist Wilhelm Conrad Röntgen discovered an unusual phenomenon while working at his laboratory at the University of Würzburg.

Röntgen had been repeating various experiments with cathode rays, notably those of his colleagues Hertz, Hittorf, Crookes and Lenard. These investigators had developed equipment for exploring the effects of high tension discharges in evacuated glass tubes. By late 1895 this small group of physicists was beginning to explore the properties of cathode rays outside the tubes. Early in November of 1895 Röntgen was repeating an experiment with one of Lenard's tubes in which a thin aluminum window had been added to permit the cathode rays to exit the tube. Lenard had supplied the tube with a tightly fitting cardboard covering to protect the aluminum window from damage by the strong electrostatic field necessary to produce the cathode rays. This covering also prevented any visible light from escaping. Röntgen had successfully repeated the experiment and had observed that the invisible cathode rays caused a fluorescent effect on a small cardboard screen painted with barium platinocyanide when it was placed very close to the aluminum window.

It occurred to Röntgen that the Hittorf-Crookes tube, which had a much thicker glass wall than the Lenard tube, might also cause this fluorescent effect. In the late afternoon of November 8 he determined to test his idea. He carefully constructed a black cardboard covering similar to the one he had used on the Lenard tube. He covered the Hittorf-Crookes tube with the covering and attached electrodes to the Ruhmkorff coil to generate an electrostatic charge. Before setting up the barium platinocyanide screen to test his idea, Röntgen darkened the room to test the opacity of his cardboard cover. As he passed the Ruhmkorff coil charge through the tube, he determined that the cover was light-tight and turned to prepare the next step of the experiment. It was at this point that he noticed a faint shimmering from a bench a meter away from the tube. To be sure he tried several more discharges and saw the same shimmering effect each time. Striking a match, Röntgen discovered the shimmering had come from the location of the barium platinocyanide screen he had been intending to use next.

Röntgen spent the next few hours repeating the experiment again and again. He quickly determined that the screen would fluoresce at a distance from the tube much greater than in his previous tests. He speculated that a new kind of ray might be responsible. November 8 was a Friday, and Röntgen took advantage of the weekend to repeat his experiments and make his first notes. In the following weeks he investigated nearly all the known properties of the rays, even eating and sleeping in his laboratory.

Röntgen's discovery of x-rays was no accident and he was not working alone. With the investigations he and his colleagues in various countries were pursuing, the discovery was imminent. The idea that he just happened to notice the barium platinocyanide screen totally misrepresents his investigative powers. He had planned to use the screen in the next step of the experiment.

At one point while he was investigating the ability of various materials to stop the rays, he brought a small piece of lead into position while a discharge was occurring. Imagine Röntgen's astonishment as he saw the first radiographic image, his own flickering ghostly skeleton. He later reported it was at this point that he determined to continue his experiments in secrecy, because he feared for his professional reputation if his observations were in error.

Röntgen became the first radiographer when he produced a series of four photographs to accompany the first draft of his paper: the hand of his wife (Figure 2–12), a set of weights, a compass, and a piece of metal. Röntgen's original paper, "On a New Kind of Rays," was published 50 days later on December 28. It is translated in Appendix A. Röntgen assigned the mathematical term for an unknown, X, to the rays he discovered. In later years they were officially given his name to honor his work. Today either term, x-rays or Röntgen rays, is acceptable. Röntgen published a total of three papers on x-rays between 1895 and 1897. His investigative powers were so phenomenal that none of his conclusions have yet been proven false. Röntgen received many honors for his discovery, including, in 1901, the first Nobel prize for physics. He died of carcinoma of the bowel in 1923.

X-RAY PROPERTIES

When Röntgen began his study of the invisible x-rays, it was unlikely that he would be able to identify all of the properties of this new discovery. Röntgen's investigation was so thorough, however, that no scientist since has been able to add to the list of properties Röntgen identified.

Through his use of the scientific method, Röntgen found that x-rays:

1. Are highly penetrating, invisible rays which are a form of electromagnetic radiation.
2. Are electrically neutral and therefore not affected by either electric or magnetic fields.
3. Can be produced over a wide variety of energies and wavelengths (polyenergetic and heterogeneous).
4. Release very small amounts of heat upon passing through matter.
5. Travel in straight lines.
6. Travel at the speed of light, 3×10^8 meters per second in a vacuum.
7. Can ionize matter.
8. Cause fluorescence (the emission of light) of certain crystals.

Figure 2–12. The first x-ray image of the human body. This radiograph was taken by Dr. Röntgen of his wife's hand.

9. Cannot be focused by a lens.
10. Affect photographic film.
11. Produce chemical and biological changes in matter through ionization and excitation.
12. Produce secondary and scatter radiation.

SUMMARY

The physical universe can best be understood through physics—the study of matter and energy and their interrelationships. Matter is the substance which comprises all physical objects. The smallest subdivision of matter is the atom, which is comprised of three basic subatomic particles: the proton, the neutron and the electron. Energy is the ability to do work. There are many forms of energy, including x-rays, which are a form of electromagnetic radiation. Matter and energy cannot be created or destroyed but are interchangeable, as described in Einstein's theory of relativity ($E = mc^2$).

The atom is best described as having a small, dense center, known as the nucleus, that is surrounded by electrons located within orbital shells. Protons and neutrons are located within the nucleus and are responsible for almost all of the mass of an atom. The electron is located outside the nucleus and has a relatively insignificant mass. Protons possess a positive charge, electrons possess a negative charge and neutrons are electrically neutral.

Each of the elements has its own specific number of nuclear protons. This is the key characteristic which distinguishes one element from another. The number of nuclear protons in an atom is known as the atomic number or Z number. The periodic table lists the elements in ascending order according to the element's atomic number.

Electromagnetic radiation behaves as both a wave and a particle. As a wave, EM radiation has an associated frequency and wavelength. As a particle, it behaves as a bundle of energy, called a photon. X-rays are a man-made form of electromagnetic radiation which is created when high-speed electrons are suddenly stopped. X-rays were discovered by Wilhelm Conrad Röntgen on November 8, 1895, in Germany. From his thorough investigation, 12 properties of x-rays were identified.

REVIEW QUESTIONS

1. What are the two major branches of natural science?

2. How do matter and energy differ?

3. Define an atom and a molecule.

4. What are the three basic subatomic particles?

5. What is ionization?

6. What is the formula used to determine the maximum number of electrons that can be contained in a given shell? How many electrons can be contained in the N-shell?

7. The periodic table of elements arranges the elements into periods and groups. How are the elements similar within each period? within each group?

8. How do radiations differ along the electromagnetic spectrum?

9. List five types of energy.

10. For electromagnetic radiation, what is the relationship between frequency and wavelength? between frequency and photon energy?

11. List five properties of x-rays.

REFERENCES AND RECOMMENDED READING

Ball, J. L., and A. D. Moore. *Essential Physics for Radiographers.* 2nd ed. Oxford: Blackwell Scientific Publications, 1986.

Bushong, Stewart C. *Radiologic Science for Technologists: Physics, Biology, and Protection.* 4th ed. St. Louis, MO: C. V. Mosby Company, 1988.

Curry, Thomas S. III, James E. Dowdey, and Robert C. Murry. *Christensen's Introduction to the Physics of Diagnostic Radiology.* 3rd ed. Philadelphia, PA: Lea and Febiger, 1984.

Fuchs, Arthur W. Radiography of 1896. *Image* 9:4–17, 1960.

Funke, Thomas. William Conrad Roentgen, the German museum, and you. *The X-ray Technician* 32:Nov., 193–194, 1961.

Glasser, Otto. *Dr. W.C. Roentgen.* 2nd ed. Springfield, IL: Charles C. Thomas, 1958.

Handbook of Chemistry and Physics. 69th ed. Boca Raton, FL: C.R.C. Press, 1989.

Johns, Harold E., and John R. Cunningham. *The Physics of Radiology.* 4th ed. Springfield, IL: Charles C. Thomas, 1983.

Meredith, W. J., and J. B. Massey. *Fundamental Physics of Radiology.* 3rd ed. Chicago, IL: Yearbook Medical Publishers, 1977.

Ridgway, Arthur, and Walter Thumm. *The Physics of Medical Radiography.* Reading, MA: Addison-Welsey Publishing Company, 1973.

Röntgen, W.C. On a new kind of rays. *Nature* 53:1369, 274–276, 1896.

Röntgen, W.C. On a new kind of rays. *Science* 3:59, 227–231, 1896.

Selman, Joseph. *The Fundamentals of X-ray and Radium Physics.* 7th ed. Springfield, IL: Charles C. Thomas, 1985.

Sprawls, Perry. *Physical Principles of Medical Imaging.* Rockville, MD: Aspen Publishers, 1987.

Ter-Pogossian, Michel M. *The Physical Aspects of Diagnostic Radiology.* New York: Hoeber Medical Division, Harper & Row, 1967.

Thumm, Walter. Röntgen's discovery revisited. *Canadian Journal of Radiography, Radiotherapy, and Nuclear Medicine* 5:1, 22–28, 1974.

Wilks, Robin J. *Principles of Radiological Physics.* Edinburgh: Churchill Livingstone, 1981.

THE CASE OF THE UNIDENTIFIED FLYING OBJECT IN THE SKULL

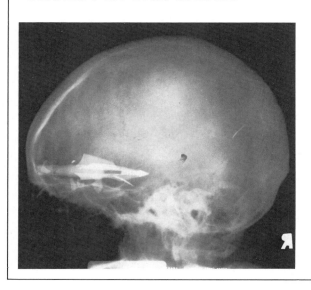

This lateral skull radiograph was obtained on a patient in the emergency room. What could this rocket-shaped object be?

Answers to the case studies can be found in Appendix E.

3 BASIC RADIATION PROTECTION

Raymond P. Rossi

One aspect of the wide use of the x-rays perturbed Röntgen greatly. From laboratories in the United States, England, Germany, and France came more and more reports of a peculiar skin reaction similar to a sunburn in persons working with the rays, some of these reactions being particularly serious. . . . It distressed Röntgen to believe that these effects were due to x-rays. . . . Röntgen almost from the beginning had conducted all his experiments in his big zinc box. . . . Then he had added a lead plate to the zinc between the tube and himself, and in doing so he had unknowingly protected himself completely. With an accurate appreciation of the import of these unexplained effects, Röntgen foresaw the suffering consequent to the careless handling of the rays.

Otto Glasser from the biography, *Dr. W. C. Röntgen.*

OUTLINE

THE BASICS OF RADIATION PROTECTION PRINCIPLES AND PRACTICE

QUANTITIES AND UNITS RELEVANT TO RADIATION PROTECTION

DETECTION AND MEASUREMENT OF RADIATION EXPOSURE

DOSE-EQUIVALENT LIMITS AND REGULATIONS

PROTECTION OF PERSONNEL

PROTECTION OF THE PATIENT

OBJECTIVES

Upon completion of this chapter, the student should be able to:

1. Describe the nature of ionizing radiation.
2. Identify the types of biological effects of ionizing radiation.
3. Identify the principle sources of ionizing radiation.
4. Define the quantities and units used for measurement of radiation.

5. Describe devices used to detect and measure radiation, including personnel-monitoring devices and ionization-chamber instruments.
6. Explain the concept of dose-equivalent limits related to the use of radiation.
7. Discuss the precautions that should be taken to minimize potential fetal exposures.
8. Describe the ALARA concept.
9. Explain the basic principles for reducing exposure to radiation.
10. Describe techniques used to minimize radiation exposure to patients and personnel.

THE BASICS OF RADIATION PROTECTION PRINCIPLES AND PRACTICE

In medical applications, exposure to ionizing radiation carries with it both a benefit and a risk. The benefit of information from an x-ray examination regarding the clinical management of the patient is weighed against the risk when a physician requests the examination. The diagnostic benefit of a radiological procedure far outweighs the risk resulting from the associated x-ray exposure. The information about the clinical condition of a patient received by the physician from a radiologic examination is an essential part of the practice of modern medicine.

It is the responsibility of the radiographer to ensure that each patient receives the minimum dose of radiation that will produce a diagnostic image consistent with the requirements of the examination. Radiographers must also ensure that all individuals are properly protected from unnecessary radiation exposure.

The Nature of Ionizing Radiation

Ionizing radiation arises from both natural and man-made sources and has the ability, as a consequence of its interactions with matter, to affect the various organs and tissues within the body. The energy possessed by ionizing radiation is capable of displacing atomic electron bonds and breaking the electron bonds that hold the molecules of matter together, resulting in chemical changes which can lead to harmful effects.

Ionizing radiations are grouped as **particulate radiations** or **electromagnetic** radiations. Particulate radiations include high-energy electrons, neutrons and protons which produce ionization in matter by direct atomic collisions. Photon radiations include x-rays and gamma rays, which produce ionization in matter by other types of interactions.

For electromagnetic radiation in the medically useful x-ray energy range (<200 keV), the transfer of energy from the photon to matter, resulting in ionization, may occur by processes known as **photoelectric absorption** and **Compton scattering.**

During such photon interactions with matter, photon energy is transferred by a two-step process. First, the incident photon interacts with an atom, causing an electron to be set in motion, which results in kinetic energy being released in the material. Second, the absorption of the released kinetic energy from the electron occurs via excitation and ionization. The excitations and ionizations which occur along the tracks of the charged particles set in motion give rise to biological damage in tissue. The biological damage may be a result of a direct interaction between the charged particle set in motion by the photons, in which cellular macromolecules are directly excited or ionized, or may be a result of an indirect interaction in which the absorption of radiation occurs in a water molecule, producing high reactive species such as free radicals, which diffuse from the site of origin and subsequently cause biological damage. For x-rays and gamma rays, approximately two-thirds of the biological effects on tissue are the result of indirect actions.

Biological Effects of Ionizing Radiation

Exposure to ionizing radiation affects various organs and tissues in the body and may result in a finite probability of radiation-induced disease in persons exposed to the radiation, and in their descendants. Health effects are known to be influenced by radiation characteristics and biological factors and include cancer induction, genetically determined ill health, developmental abnormalities and degenerative diseases. The effects from the exposure to ionizing radiation may be classified as either **somatic** or **genetic.**

Somatic effects are those which may become evident in the irradiated individual. Such effects are not usually to be expected in individuals exposed in the course of their work in the medical environment.

Genetic effects are those which do not produce any significantly observable effect in the exposed individual, but may appear in descendants of the exposed individual. They may not be manifest in the children of the exposed individual, but may lie dormant for several generations and, eventually, may be eliminated completely from the genetic pool. Such effects result from alterations in the reproductive cells which can lead to defects in the offspring. Detectable radiation-induced mutations can result if the individual's reproductive cells have been exposed to an appreciable amount of radiation. It is unlikely that any worker in the medical environment would be exposed to ionizing radiation at a level high enough to cause the transmission of appreciable genetic effects.

Among the many factors which will influence the effect of exposure to ionizing radiation are the total dose received, the rate at which the dose was received, the age at exposure, the type of radiation, the sensitivity of the irradiated cells and the portion of the body which was irradiated.

When x-rays were initially investigated, scientists were unaware of any harmful effects of their use and a number of the early radiation workers suffered injuries that are easily prevented today. Injuries from exposure were reported in Europe within the first year of investigation of x-radiation. In 1904 the first radiation fatality, a radiation-induced cancer, was reported in the United States. Over the next decade blood disorders such as leukemia and anemia, cancerous skin lesions and cancer deaths were reported among radiation workers and linked to x-ray exposure. As a result of the high rate of documented radiation-related injuries, the British X-Ray and Radium Protection Committee was formed in 1921 to study ways to reduce radiation exposure to patients and medical personnel.

The goal of radiation protection is to limit human exposure to ionizing radiation to a degree that is reasonable and acceptable in relation to the benefit gained from the activities that involve the exposure, thereby reducing the likelihood of the occurrence of somatic and genetic effects.

Sources and Magnitude of Ionizing-Radiation Exposure

Everyone is exposed to sources of ionizing radiation. Some individuals will be exposed to a wide variety of such sources, while others will be exposed to only a few. The sources include those of **natural origin**, either undisturbed by human activities or which have somehow been affected by human activities, and **man-made** sources.

Natural sources include cosmic radiation, terrestrial radiation from naturally occurring radioactive sources in the ground, radionuclides naturally present in the body and inhaled and ingested radionuclides of natural origin, such as radon. Human exposure to these natural sources varies depending on locality and other circumstances. When human exposure to natural sources increases as a result of man's actions, deliberate or otherwise, the natural sources are known as enhanced.

Man-made sources of radiation result from various man-made materials and devices and include such sources as x-rays and radiopharmaceuticals in medicine, consumer products containing radioactive materials, such as some smoke detectors and static eliminators,

nuclear fuel production for power, air travel and such catastrophic events as atmospheric fallout from nuclear weapons testing and accidents in nuclear power plants.

The magnitude of exposure from these sources for the average member of the United States population has been studied and the results are summarized in Table 3–1.

QUANTITIES AND UNITS RELEVANT TO RADIATION PROTECTION

Various quantities, units and radiation dosimetry concepts have been developed and defined in order to quantify the amount of radiation received by individuals. Historically

TABLE 3–1

ANNUAL EFFECTIVE DOSE EQUIVALENT AND GENETICALLY SIGNIFICANT DOSE IN THE U.S. POPULATION

Source	Average Annual Effective Dose Equivalent		Average Annual Contribution to the GSD	
	mSv	mrem	mSv	mrem
Natural Sources				
Radon	2.0	200	0.1	10
Other	1.0	100	0.9	90
Occupational	0.009	0.9	≈0.006	≈0.6
Nuclear Fuel Cycle	0.0005	0.05	<0.005	<0.5
Consumer Products				
Tobacco	———		———	
Other	0.05–0.13	5–13	≈0.05	<5
Miscellaneous				
Environmental Sources	0.0006	0.06	<0.001	<0.1
Medical				
Diagnostic x-ray	0.39	39	0.2–0.3	20–30
Nuclear Medicine	0.14	14	0.02	2
Rounded Total	3.6	360	1.3	130

Adapted from NCRP Report No. 93: Ionizing Radiation Exposure of the Population of the United States (Tables 8.1 and 8.2)

the quantities and units associated with radiation dosimetry have included: the **roentgen (R)**, used for specifying exposure; the **rad** (radiation-absorbed dose), used for specifying energy absorbed; and the **rem** (radiation equivalency in man), used for specifying the biologically equivalent dose.

In 1948 the International Committee for Weights and Measures was charged with developing an international system of units based on the metric system. The committee developed the **Système Internationale d'Unites** or **SI** units. In recent years the international system of units has been adopted for radiation protection, and within this system of units the older units are no longer applicable. Although the National Council on Radiation Protection and Measurement (NCRP) adopted the SI units for use with ionizing radiation in 1985, traditional units are still very much in use. The following discussion will serve to review the conventional and more familiar units and to introduce the new SI units. Table 3–2 provides conversions from conventional units to SI units.

Exposure

The roentgen (R) represents a unit of exposure in air and was defined as that quantity of x-rays or gamma rays required to produce a given amount of ionization (charge) in a unit mass of air. One roentgen creates 2.08×10^9 ion pairs per cubic centimeter of air to produce a total ion charge of 2.58×10^{-4} coulomb (C) per kilogram (kg). The roentgen is limited to the measurement of exposure in air only and is not applicable to photons of energy above 3 Mev or to particulate radiations. The roentgen has no direct equivalent or special unit in the SI system of units and is no longer used. Exposure may be expressed directly in C/kg^{-1}.

Absorbed Dose

The rad was developed as a unit of absorbed energy or dose and is applicable to any material. The rad was defined as 100 ergs of energy absorbed in one gram of absorbing material. In the SI system of units the rad has been replaced by the **gray (Gy)**, which is defined as 1 joule (J) of energy absorbed in each kilogram (kg) of absorbing material. One gray is equivalent to 100 rads; therefore 1 rad equals 10 mGy. This unit is not restricted to air and can be measured in other absorbing materials.

Dose Equivalent

Different types of radiation, such as alpha and beta particles and neutrons, produce different degrees of biological damage as compared to gamma or X-radiation. In order to account for the fact that the same absorbed dose of radiation may result in different biological responses for different types of radiation, a unit known as the rem was developed. This unit of **dose equivalence** (H) was determined as the product of the absorbed dose, in rads,

TABLE 3–2		
CONVERSIONS BETWEEN CONVENTIONAL AND SI UNITS		
Conventional Unit (Column A)	Conversion Factor (Column B)	SI Unit (Column C)
roentgen	2.58×10^{-4}	coulomb/ kilogram
rad	0.01	gray
rem	0.01	sievert
curie	3.7×10^{10}	becquerel

Column A amount multiplied by Column B equals Column C amount.
Column C amount divided by Column B equals Column A amount.

and a **quality factor** (Q) which is specific to certain types of radiation and accounts for the biological effectiveness of the specific radiation. The quality factor for gamma or X-radiation equals one. This means that 1 rad equals 1 rem for gamma or X-radiation. For alpha particles, however, the quality factor is 20. This means that 1 rad equals 20 rem for alpha particle absorption. In the SI system of units the rem has been replaced by the **sievert (Sv)**, which is defined as the product of the absorbed dose in gray and the quality factor. One sievert is equal to 100 rem, and 1 rem is equal to 10 mSv.

Other dosimetry concepts have been derived specifically for use in radiation protection and include the **effective dose equivalent** (H_E) and the **collective dose equivalent** (S).

Since exposure received from ionizing radiation is rarely uniform over the entire body, the concept of effective dose equivalent has been developed. The effective dose equivalent is used to compare the detriment from irradiation of a limited portion of the body with the detriment from irradiation of the entire body and employs weighting factors for the relative risks associated with irradiation of various body tissues. The effective dose equivalent is

determined as the sum of the products of the dose equivalent for each organ or tissue of interest and the weighting factor for the respective organ or tissue.

The collective dose equivalent is used to express low doses of radiation delivered to a population. It is determined as the product of the dose equivalent for a member of the exposed group of individuals and the number of individuals in the exposed subgroup.

Further information regarding the international system of units and its application in radiation protection and measurements may be found in *NCRP Report No. 82: SI Units in Radiation Protection and Measurements*. A comparison between SI units and conventional ones is set out in Table 3–3.

DETECTION AND MEASUREMENT OF RADIATION EXPOSURE

A number of different dose-measuring devices, known as dosimeters, are employed for detection and measurement of radiation exposure from x-rays. These **dosimeters** may be classified as either **personnel monitoring devices** or **ionization chamber instruments**.

TABLE 3–3

COMPARISON BETWEEN SI AND CONVENTIONAL UNITS

Quantity	Symbol for Quantity	Expression in SI Units	Expression in Symbols for SI Units	Special Name for SI Unit	Symbol Using Special Name	Conventional Unit	Symbol for Conventional Unit	Value of Conventional Unit in SI Units
Activity	A	1 per second	s^{-1}	becquerel	Bq	curie	Ci	3.7×10^{10} Bq
Absorbed Dose	D	joule per kilogram	J/kg^{-1}	gray	Gy	rad	rad	0.01 Gy
Dose Equivalent	H	joule per kilogram	J/kg^{-1}	sievert	Sv	rem	rem	0.01 Sv
Exposure	X	coulomb per kilogram	C/kg^{-1}			roentgen	R	2.58×10^{-4} C/kg^{-1}

Adapted from NCRP Report No. 82: SI Units in Radiation Protection and Measurements.

Personnel Monitoring Devices

Individuals who are regularly exposed to ionizing radiation should be provided with personnel-monitoring devices in order to provide an estimate of the exposure received. Personnel monitoring is recommended whenever a possibility exists that an individual will receive more than 1/10 of the recommended dose-equivalent limit as a result of his occupational activities. A personnel-monitoring device measures the quantity of exposure it has received. It is not a radiation protection device. The two most common types of personnel-monitoring devices are the **film badge** and the **thermoluminescent dosimeter** (TLD).

Film Badges Film badges are the most commonly used form of personnel-monitoring devices and are usually issued on a monthly basis (Figure 3–1). Two pieces of film having different sensitivities to x-rays are contained within a light-tight envelope. This film packet is placed within a holder which contains a number of different filter elements held in a fixed position with respect to the film. Printed on the front of the film packet is the name of the in-

Figure 3–1. (Left to right) A typical film badge, thermoluminescent dosimeter ring, and collar badge. (Courtesy of Tech/Ops Landauer, Inc.)

dividual, the beginning date for which the film badge is issued and other coded information.

When the badge is exposed to ionizing radiation, deposits of silver atoms are distributed in the film emulsion which, upon development, becomes dark in proportion to the degree of radiation exposure received. The resultant optical density can be measured with a densitometer and calibrated to the degree of radiation exposure received.

The filters in the film badge holder provide a means of determining the energy of the incident radiation. Because the absorption of radiation by a specific thickness of given material will depend on the energy of the radiation, the measurement of the relative film densities under the different filters provides a means of estimating the energy of the exposing x-ray beam.

Film badges are capable of measuring exposures over the range of approximately 10 mrem (0.1 mSv) to 2,000 rem (20 Sv) and are most commonly used to measure the total body exposure of the individual. Readings of less than 10 mrem (0.1 mSv) are generally not detectable and may be reported as minimal (M).

When only one film badge or other personnel-monitoring device is issued it should be worn on the anterior surface of the body between the chest and waist level. When a lead apron is worn and only one film badge or other personnel-monitoring device is issued, it is recommended that it be worn under the lead apron. Because of the considerable controversy regarding the proper location of the film badge when a lead apron is worn, the local radiation safety officer should be contacted for specific guidance.

An additional film badge, usually designated as a collar badge, may be worn in addition to the whole-body badge when the potential for significant exposure to the thyroid or eyes exists. This badge is usually positioned near the collar outside of the lead apron (but not on top of it) and may be used in conjunction with the whole-body badge to determine the effective dose equivalent. The whole-body badge and collar badge must never be interchanged.

Thermoluminescent Dosimeter (TLD) Badges
Personnel-monitoring devices using thermoluminescent dosimeters are similar in appearance to film badges (see Figure 3–1). Instead of using film to measure the radiation exposure, TLD badges contain small chips of a thermoluminescent material, usually lithium fluoride (LiF). When exposed to radiation, a portion of the absorbed energy is stored in the crystal structure of the LiF chips in what are known as metastable states. This absorbed energy will remain in these states for long periods of time. If the LiF chips are heated, the absorbed energy is released as visible light. The heating and measurement of the LiF chips are carried out in a device called a reader, and the amount of measured light is proportional to the absorbed radiation dose. TLDs provide approximately the same measurement range as film badges and can be used as whole-body badges or collar badges. Because of their small size, TLDs are commonly used for monitoring exposure to the extremities in the form of ring badges.

Ionization Chamber Instruments
Ionization chamber instruments are commonly employed for the measurement of the primary and secondary radiation beam for purposes of evaluation of equipment performance, environmental exposure assessment of scatter and leakage radiation and for measurement of patient exposure. An ionization chamber works on the principle that when radiation interacts with air electrons, positive ions are produced giving rise to an electrical charge which can be measured.

A typical ionization chamber dosimeter consists of a chamber with a known volume of

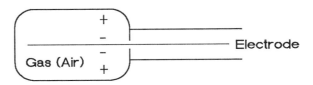

Figure 3–2. An ionization chamber dosimeter. The chamber encloses a known volume of air, inside which a chargeable electrode is positioned to attract electrons freed by the ionization of the gas by the radiation. The difference in the electrode's charge before and after exposure is measured by an electrometer and displayed in radiation units.

air and an electrode (Figure 3–2). A small voltage is applied between the electrode and the wall of the chamber so that the electrode is positive and the chamber wall is negative. As x-ray photons pass through the chamber they ionize the air. The free electrons from these ionizations are attracted to the positive electrode, where they can be measured with a device called an electrometer. The intensity of the signal that is produced on the electrode is proportional to the radiation exposure that occurred in the air volume of the chamber. This relationship can be displayed on a digital readout in R or C/kg units.

Ionization dosimeters can be designed to measure specific ranges of radiation intensity. Some of these devices are Geiger-Müller (GM) counters, "cutie pie" survey meters, automatic exposure control (AEC) ion chambers and computed tomography detectors.

A special type of ionization chamber used for personnel dosimetry is known as a **pocket dosimeter** (Figure 3–3). When irradiated, the radiation ionizes the air in the chamber, which discharges the previously charged electrode, causing a pointer to move on a scale. The amount of ionization and movement of the pointer is proportional to the radiation exposure to the chamber. Such devices are usually charged and read out on a special charger-reader device. Pocket dosimeters are occasionally used for personnel monitoring in

Figure 3–3. A pocket ionization chamber. (Courtesy of Nuclear Associates division of Victoreen, Inc., Carle Place, NY)

situations where the convenience of an immediate readout is desired (for example, after each procedure in a cardiac catheterization laboratory). However, they provide no permanent record of personnel exposure and are not routinely used.

Care of Personnel Monitoring Devices

Proper care and handling of personnel monitoring devices are essential in order to obtain accurate results. The personnel monitoring device must be worn only by the individual to whom it is assigned, must be worn in the proper location for the prescribed time period and must be turned in for processing when due.

Both film badge dosimeters and TLD dosimeters may be adversely affected by heat, humidity, mechanical pressure, inadvertent exposure to light and prolonged delay between exposure and processing. Exposure from the rear or from oblique angles may also result in inaccurate results.

Generally, groups of personnel dosimeters are provided with a control that must be stored in an unexposed area at the facility and returned with the group for processing. This control provides an unexposed level against which the personnel dosimeters are evaluated.

Personnel monitoring devices should not be worn during medical or dental exams and should never be intentionally exposed to the primary radiation beam. Individuals should be aware of the exposure they receive by reviewing their exposure readings on the reports posted in the facility on a routine basis. Should any aspect of the reported exposure be unclear or cause concern, the individual should seek the counsel of the facility radiation safety officer.

DOSE EQUIVALENT LIMITS AND REGULATIONS

It is important to set limits for the protection of the radiation worker and the general public because of the known biological effects of exposure to ionizing radiation. For radiation protection purposes, individuals may be divided into two groups. First are those classified as radiation workers, who incur, as an occupational risk, a certain likelihood of exposure to ionizing radiation in the course of their normal duties.

Radiation workers may be further classified as **occupationally exposed workers** and **occasionally exposed workers.** Occupationally exposed workers are individuals who have a significant potential for exposure to radiation in the course of their employment. Occasionally exposed workers are individuals whose duties may occasionally bring them into areas where radiation exposure may occur. Both occupationally exposed workers and occasionally exposed workers should receive instruction and training regarding hazards of radiation exposure and radiation protection practices.

Dose Equivalent Limits

Radiation exposure limits pertinent to the protection of radiation workers are known as **dose equivalent limits** and are specified for both **total body** exposure and for exposure to **certain critical organs.** The term maximum permissible dose (MPD) is no longer acceptable terminology because no dose is considered permissible. Dose equivalent limits replace MPD and reflect this philosophy.

A number of advisory groups have shared in the establishment of these limits, including: the International Commission on Radiological Protection (ICRP), the National Council on Radiation Protection and Measurement (NCRP), the National Academy of Sciences Advisory Committee on the Biological Effects of Ionizing Radiation (NAS-BEIR) and the United Nations Scientific Committee on the Effects of Atomic Radiation (UNSCEAR). Currently recommended values for dose equivalent limits are given in Table 3–4 and reflect the recommendations of the National Council on Radiation Protection and Measurments as put forth in *NCRP Report No. 91: Recommendations on Limits for Exposure to Ionizing Radiation.*

The dose equivalent limit for whole-body exposure of a radiation worker is 5 rem (50 mSv) per year. Prior to the release of *NCRP Report No. 91* in 1987, the maximum cumulative whole-body dose for radiation workers was determined by the formula:

$$H = 5(N-18) \text{ rem}$$
where: H = dose equivalent limit
N = age in years

Under the new recommendations, the maximum cumulative dose equivalent is age in rem, which is determined in SI units by the formula:

$$H = 10 \text{ N mSv}$$
where: H = dose equivalent limit
N = age in years

Example: What is the dose equivalent limit (H) for a 19-year-old radiation worker using both the old and new formulas?

Answer:
$$H = 5(N-18) \text{ rem}$$
$$H = 5(19-18) \text{ rem}$$

TABLE 3–4

EFFECTIVE DOSE EQUIVALENT LIMIT RECOMMENDATIONS

Occupational Exposures (annual)

— Effective dose equivalent limit	50 mSv	(5 rem)
— Dose equivalent limits for tissues and organs		
— lens of eye	150 mSv	(15 rem)
— all others (e.g., red bone marrow, breast, lung, skin and extremities)	500 mSv	(50 rem)
— Guidance: Cumulative exposure	10 mSv × age	(1 rem × age in years)
Public Exposures (annual)		
— Effective dose equivalent limit, continuous or frequent exposure	1 mSv	(0.1 rem)
— Effective dose equivalent limit, infrequent exposure	5 mSv	(0.5 rem)
— Dose equivalent for lens of eye, skin and extremities	50 mSv	(5 rem)
Embryo-Fetus Exposures		
— Total dose equivalent limit	5 mSv	(0.5 rem)
— Dose equivalent limit in one month	0.5 mSv	(0.05 rem)
Education and Training Exposures (annual)		
— Effective dose equivalent limit	1 mSv	(0.1 rem)
— Dose equivalent for lens of eye, skin and extremities	50 mSv	(5 rem)

Adapted from NCRP Report No. 91: Recommendations on Limits for Exposure to Ionizing Radiation (Table 22.1).

Old   H = 5(1) rem
H = 5 rem (50 mSv)

New   H = 10 N mSv
H = 10 × 19 mSv
H = 190 mSv (19 rem)

Example: What is the dose equivalent limit (H) for a 35-year-old radiation worker using both the old and new formulas?

Answer:

Old   H = 5(N–18) rem
H = 5(35–18) rem
H = 5(17) rem
H = 85 rem (850 mSv)

New   H = 10 N mSv
H = 10 × 35 mSv
H = 350 mSv (35 rem)

Irradiation at the upper level of the dose equivalent limits is not to be considered as desirable and in every case efforts to reduce exposures to the lowest possible level should be taken.

Individuals not classified as radiation workers are considered as members of the **general public.** For purposes of protection of these individuals, the level of recommended dose equivalent limits, exclusive of any exposure received as the result of a medical procedure, has been established as one-tenth of the dose equivalent limit for radiation workers—0.5 rem (5 mSv) per year.

Radiation Exposure and Pregnancy

A situation which deserves special consideration is that of the possibility of radiation exposure during the early weeks of pregnancy, generally before the woman is aware of her condition. Here, the dose to the fetus is of concern, particularly in the early stages of development, when certain tissues and organs are especially sensitive to radiation. Recent studies, as summarized in the report, *BEIR V*, suggest that the fetus may be particularly radiosensitive during the period of 8 to 15 weeks post-conception. As a result, care must be taken to reduce radiation exposure to any pregnant individual, including pregnant (or potentially pregnant) patients and personnel. It is currently recommended by the NCRP that the total dose equivalent limit (excluding medical exposure) for the embryo not exceed 0.5 rem (5 mSv) during the entire gestation period and not exceed 0.05 rem (0.5 mSv) in any month once the pregnancy becomes known.

For the female radiation worker wearing a personnel monitoring device, it is possible to determine the exposure and so regulate the pregnant radiographer's duties in order to limit radiation to the fetus. For women who are not radiation workers, the dose equivalent limit of 0.5 rem (5 mSv) per year will suffice to maintain acceptable levels during pregnancy.

To minimize the possible exposure to an embryo in the earliest days of a pregnancy, a guideline known as the ten day rule was recommended by a number of advisory agencies. This guideline states that elective abdominal x-ray examinations of fertile women should be postponed until the ten day period following the onset of menstruation, as it would be improbable that a women would be pregnant during these ten days.

The application of this guideline within the radiology department has always proven difficult. In the event a postponed examination is needed, and pregnancy has been determined, the exposure of the fetus might occur during a period of increased radiosensitivity. It is now the general belief that postponement of abdominal x-ray examinations is not necessary when the physician requesting the examination has considered the entire clinical state of the patient, including the possibility of pregnancy. The potential pregnancy status of all female patients of childbearing age should always be determined, and, in the event of known pregnancy, steps should be taken to minimize exposure to the fetus. A diagnostic radiological physicist should perform calculations to estimate the actual fetal dose in those cases where such a procedure is necessary.

NCRP Report No. 54: Medical Exposure of Pregnant and Potentially Pregnant Women discusses the risks associated with fetal exposure:

> This risk is considered to be negligible at 5 rad or less when compared to other risks of pregnancy, and the risk of malformations is significantly increased above control levels only at doses above 15 rad. Therefore, the exposure of the fetus to radiation arising from diagnostic procedures would very rarely be cause, by itself, for terminating a pregnancy. If there are reasons, other than the possible radiation effects, to consider a therapeutic abortion, such reasons should be discussed with the patient by the attending physician, so that it is clear that the radiation exposure is not being used as an excuse for terminating the pregnancy.

When a radiation worker becomes pregnant, special care must be taken to minimize the radiation exposure to the embryo/fetus. The annual occupational dose equivalent limits for the worker no longer apply and are reduced to reflect the dose equivalent limits for the embryo/fetus, as discussed above. The pregnant radiation worker should take all of the expected radiation safety precautions and carefully monitor the radiation exposure to ensure that it is kept to a minimum.

Maintaining Exposure As Low As Reasonably Achievable (ALARA)

A basic philosophical principle of radiation protection concerning the use of ionizing radiation emphasizes the need to maintain exposure to ionizing radiation at a level **As** **L**ow **A**s **R**easonably **A**chievable (ALARA), with economic and societal factors being taken into consideration. This premise has been accepted by advisory and regulatory agencies, and requires that radiological personnel take on the responsibility of minimizing the exposure to their patients and any other individuals involved in a radiological procedure. Implementation of the ALARA principle is achieved by application of the basic principles of radiation protection and a thoughtful approach to all work involving exposure to ionizing radiation.

PROTECTION OF PERSONNEL

When radiological procedures are performed, there is a possibility that individuals other than the patient will receive some radiation exposure. While the patient should be the only person exposed to the primary beam, others involved in the procedure may be exposed to radiation scattered from the primary beam or to leakage radiation from the x-ray tube. This occurs particularly during fluoroscopy, mobile examinations, interventional special procedures and cardiac catheterization. For most radiographic exposures, personnel should be behind protective barriers. Radiologic personnel should not be involved in holding patients who are unable to cooperate during an x-ray exposure. Immobilization devices should be used or, if absolutely necessary, assistance should be requested from the patient's family or friends.

Principles of Personnel Exposure Reduction

Reduction of an individual's exposure to ionizing radiation may be accomplished by the application of three basic principles: (1) reduce the amount of **time** spent in the vicinity of the radiation source while it is operating, (2) increase the **distance** between the radiation source and the individual to be protected and (3) interpose a **shielding** material which will attenuate the radiation from the source.

Time X-ray imaging equipment produces radiation only during the actual exposure which is used to form the image during a procedure. The time of exposure on a per image basis is very short (typically much less than one second) during radiographic procedures. During fluoroscopic procedures, which are used when dynamic information is required, the x-ray source may be on (usually intermittently) for several minutes to as long as an hour. To minimize exposure to radiation, individuals should reduce the amount of time they spend in the vicinity of an operable radiation source. The simplest way to do this is to ascertain whether their presence is needed during the procedure.

Distance Increasing the distance between the individual and the source of radiation is an effective method to reduce exposure to radiation. As distance from the source of radiation is increased, the radiation level will decrease significantly. Maximizing the distance from an operable source of radiation is a particularly effective method of exposure reduction during mobile radiographic and fluoroscopic procedures.

Shielding Shielding is used when neither time nor distance is effective in achieving the desired degree of reduction in exposure. By interposing any material between the source of radiation and the point at which it is desired to reduce the exposure, a certain reduction in exposure will be achieved. The degree of exposure reduction will depend on the physical characteristics of the material (atomic number, density and thickness). For fixed x-ray imaging facilities the most common materials are lead and concrete. Such facilities are designed in accordance with specific recommendations

(*NCRP Report No. 49*) depending on the configuration of the equipment, its intended use and the surrounding area. Additional devices, such as mobile shields, lead equivalent aprons, and lead equivalent gloves should be used when it is not possible to take advantage of fixed structural barriers.

Protective Barriers

During the design of fixed x-ray imaging facilities it is necessary to ensure that the layout of the equipment and shielding of the room are such that the exposure to personnel and members of the public within adjacent areas is within the recommended dose equivalent limits. This is accomplished through the use of **structural protective barriers** made of materials having effective x-ray attenuating properties and of thicknesses sufficient to reduce exposure to the desired levels. Commonly used barrier materials include lead sheet, concrete, lead glass, steel and leaded acrylic.

Protective barriers are classified as either **primary barriers** or **secondary barriers**. Primary barriers are defined as those which can be struck by the primary or useful beam exiting the x-ray tube. Secondary barriers are defined as those which can only be struck by scattered and leakage radiation.

The design of structural shielding for x-ray imaging facilities is treated in detail in *NCRP Report No. 49: Structural Shielding Design and Evaluation for Medical Use of X Rays and Gamma Rays of Energies Up to 10 MeV*. Barrier requirements are dependent upon the type of equipment, its layout within the room, the occupancy of adjacent areas and other factors. Such shielding is usually designed by a qualified diagnostic radiological physicist.

Protective Devices

When it is not possible for personnel to remain behind a protective barrier, it is the radiographer's responsibility to ensure that **protective devices** are worn by all personnel, including physicians, nurses, aides, etc. These situations arise frequently during fluoroscopy and some mobile procedures. The most common protective devices are lead aprons and lead gloves. Special devices include leaded glasses and thyroid shields.

During fluoroscopy and mobile radiography, personnel should always wear a protective apron. Lead gloves should also be worn if the hands will be in close proximity to the primary beam. Protective aprons and gloves are usually made of lead-impregnated vinyl within the range of 0.25–1.0 mm of lead equivalency. The greater the lead equivalence, the greater will be the protective ability and the weight of the item. Aprons vary in weight from a few pounds to over 20 pounds, depending on design and lead content. For example, a lead apron that wraps completely around the body, extending from shoulders to knees and having a 1 mm lead equivalent, will possess a significant weight. This weight can be a serious consideration if personnel are expected to wear the apron for long periods of time. The protective aprons must possess a minimum of a 0.25 mm lead equivalent if the peak energy of the x-ray beam is 100 kVp. Most departments use aprons with a 0.5 mm lead equivalent to provide personnel with a balance between protection and weight. Lead gloves usually possess 0.25 mm of lead equivalency.

PROTECTION OF THE PATIENT

Proper radiation protection of the patient is achieved through both medical and technical decisions. Medical decisions lie with the patient and are based on the professional judgment of physicians and other practitioners of the healing arts in consultation with the patient.

A number of factors affect the amount of radiation a patient receives during a diagnostic x-ray examination. Many of these factors are under the direct control of the radiographer. It is a radiographer's responsibility to understand these factors and to minimize patient exposure while producing a satisfactory diagnostic image.

While it is desirable to minimize the exposure to a patient undergoing a radiological procedure, it must be kept in mind that the goal of any radiological imaging procedure is to provide information about the medical condition of the patient to aid in clinical management. Overzealous attempts to reduce patient exposure may significantly compromise the information to be obtained from the examination. Keeping these concepts in mind, the following principles should be applied to minimize exposure to the patient.

Beam Limitation

The size of the x-ray beam should always be restricted to the area of clinical interest and should never exceed the size of the image receptor. Proper collimation not only reduces patient exposure but also improves the overall quality of the radiographic image. Ideally, evidence of proper collimation, as demonstrated by an unexposed border on all sides of the radiographic image, should be present.

Technique Selection

Technique factors for a given examination should be selected to minimize exposure to the patient. Higher kVp techniques are preferred. However, the selected kVp should be chosen so the required contrast in the radiographic image is not compromised as a result of a more penetrating x-ray beam or because of an increase in the amount of scatter radiation reaching the film, which can impair image quality. Tube current and exposure time should be chosen to minimize the degrading effects of anatomical motion. Proper technical factor selection is the responsibility of the radiographer. This decision must take into account the information needed to make a proper diagnosis.

Filtration

Filters are placed at the x-ray port to selectively absorb low-energy photons which would be absorbed by the patient and not contribute to the image. These low-energy photons absorbed by the patient would result in an increase in the patient dosage. Specialized filtration is also available which allows for additional exposure reduction by the selective removal of photons from the beam.

Grids

Radiographic grids are placed between the patient and the image receptor to preferentially absorb scatter radiation. Because grids absorb primary as well as scatter radiation, technical factors must be increased to produce an image of acceptable optical density. This increase in technical factors results in an increase in patient exposure but image quality is significantly improved. The lowest possible grid ratio consistent with effective scatter removal should be utilized.

Gonadal Shielding

Shielding the gonads (ovaries or testes) is especially important in order to minimize the possibility of any genetic effect on the future children of an exposed individual. Special attention should be paid to shielding the gonads of children and of adults of childbearing age.

Proper collimation is important when decreasing gonadal dose, but special gonadal shields should be used any time the gonads are within 4 to 5 cm of the primary beam. The three basic types of gonadal shields are **flat contact shields, shaped contact shields** and **shadow shields** (Figure 3–4).

Flat contact shields are usually made of various sizes of lead-impregnated vinyl and are placed directly over the patient's gonads. It may be necessary to secure them in place to ensure correct placement in a variety of patient positions.

Shaped contact shields are cup-shaped and designed to enclose the male gonads. These shields provide maximum protection in a number of patient positions.

Shadow shields are mounted to the tube and are placed in the x-ray beam near the collimator. The collimator's light field must be accurate for accurate shield placement. The device casts a shadow on the patient which is adjusted over the patient's gonads.

Image Receptors

The speed of the image receptor should be chosen to be the highest possible, consistent with the required information of the radiologic procedure. The use of intensifying screens in conjunction with film greatly reduces patient exposure by reducing the quantity of x-ray photons needed to create an image. Intensifying screens convert x-ray photons to light photons which expose the film within the cassette. The speed of the image receptor is influenced by the type of intensifying screen and type of film. Intensifying screens, which provide efficient absorption of the incident radiation, allow the production of a satisfactory image with less radiation exposure to the patient.

Projection

The projection used for a particular examination will have an impact on patient dosage to specific body tissues. For example, the lens of the eye receives a greater dose during antero-posterior (AP) projections of the cranium than it does if the postero-anterior (PA) projection is used. Or, a contrast-filled bladder will serve as a gonadal shield for females if the exposure is made with the patient in the AP

Figure 3–4.   Gonadal shields: (left to right) flat shield, shadow shield, contact shield.

projection but will not shield the ovaries in the PA projection.

Repeat Radiographs

Any time a radiograph must be repeated, patient exposure increases as a direct result of the exposure from the poor radiograph. Radiographers must possess a complete understanding of the entire radiographic process in order to minimize repeat exposures. Radiographs generally need to be repeated for such reasons as improper exposure factor selection, poor positioning (tube/part/film alignment), poor patient instruction or improper film processing. Radiographs should only be repeated when the quality of the radiograph compromises the diagnostic information of the procedure.

Patient Exposure Estimates

Estimates of the exposure received by patients undergoing radiographic procedures should be available. These estimates should be developed for the average patient based on standard technique charts and measured exposure characteristics of the radiological imaging equipment.

Equipment

All radiological imaging equipment should be surveyed periodically by a diagnostic radiological physicist to assess its radiation safety characteristics. Such surveys should normally be conducted in conjunction with scheduled preventive maintenance and performance surveys and should be performed at least annually. The results of such surveys should be documented. Any deficiencies found during such surveys should be corrected prior to returning the equipment to clinical service.

SUMMARY

Exposure to ionizing radiation carries with it both a benefit and a risk. With few exceptions, the diagnostic benefit of a radiologic procedure far outweighs the minimal risk resulting from the x-ray exposure. The information received by the physician from a radiologic examination about the clinical condition of the patient is an essential part of the practice of modern medicine.

Ionizing radiation is any form of radiation which possesses energy capable of displacing atomic electron bonds and breaking the electron bonds which hold the molecules of matter together. The potential biological damage from the ionization process is the reason for the need to understand proper radiation protection practices. Ionizing radiation comes from two major sources: natural background radiation and man-made radiation.

The biological effects of radiation exposure are either somatic, occurring in the individual exposed, or genetic, occurring in the descendants of the individual exposed. It is the responsibility of the radiographer to ensure that each patient receives the minimum dose of radiation necessary to produce a diagnostic image. Radiographers must also be properly shielded from unnecessary radiation exposure.

Radiation quantities and units that are important in radiation protection are exposure, absorbed dose and dose equivalent. The SI units that correspond to these quantities are the coulomb per kilogram (C/kg), the gray (Gy) and the sievert (Sv). The corresponding traditional units are the roentgen (R), the rad and the rem.

Various devices are available to detect and measure exposure to ionizing radiation. Personnel monitoring devices include the film badge and thermoluminescent dosimeter. Ionization chamber instruments are commonly used to measure the primary and scatter x-ray beam and may also be used for personnel monitoring in the form of pocket dosimeters.

The basic principles of time, distance and shielding should be applied in order to minimize exposure to personnel. For fixed x-ray installations, protective barriers, either primary or secondary, are used. Primary protective barriers are designed to protect against the direct exposure of the primary x-ray beam. Secondary protective barriers are designed to protect against exposure from scatter and leakage radiation. When it is not possible for personnel to remain behind a protective barrier, protective devices, such as lead aprons and gloves, should be worn.

To minimize patient exposure while creating a diagnostic image, the radiographer must understand the factors which have a significant relationship to patient dosage, such as beam limitation, exposure factors, filtration, gonadal shielding, grids, intensifying screens and repeat radiographs.

REVIEW QUESTIONS

1. What are the primary sources of ionizing radiation? Give examples of each.
2. What are the basic quantities of radiation measurement and their associated units?
3. Explain the ALARA concept.

4. List the three types of personnel monitoring devices.

5. Describe the function of an ionization chamber survey instrument.

6. What are the basic principles used for minimizing exposure to ionizing radiation?

7. How can a radiographer minimize radiation exposure to the patient?

8. What is the difference between primary and secondary protective barriers?

REFERENCES AND RECOMMENDED READING

Burhart, R. L., R. E. Gross, R. G. Jans, J. L. McCrohen, Jr., M. Rosenstein, and F. A. Reuter (eds.). *Recommendations for Evaluation of Radiation Exposure from Diagnostic Radiology Examinations.* HHS Publication 85–8247, 1985.

Bushong, Stewart C. *Radiologic Science for Technologists: Physics, Biology, and Protection.* 4th ed. St. Louis, MO: C. V. Mosby Company, 1988.

Bushong, Stewart C. Radiation exposure in our daily lives. *The Physics Teacher* March, 135–144, 1977.

Caprio, Michael L. The pregnant x-ray tech—providing adequate radiation safety for the fetus. *Radiologic Technology* 52:2, 161, 1980.

Curry, Thomas S., James E. Dowdey, and Robert C. Murry. *Christensen's Introduction to the Physics of Diagnostic Radiology.* 4th ed. Philadelphia, PA: Lea & Febiger, 1990.

Detain, J. Is it time to question the 10-day rule? *Radiography* 50:592, 149–150, 1984.

Doust, C. Personal monitoring period for radiographers. *Radiography* 52:603, 109–112, 1986.

Frank, Eugene, John Stears, Joel Gray, Norlin T. Winkler, and Alan D. Hoffman. Use of the

P.A. projection: A method of reducing x-ray exposure to specific radiosensitive organs. *The Canadian Journal of Medical Radiation Technology* 15:2, 63, 1984.

Fry, Orvis E., and Cesare Gianturco. Bedside radiography—reduction of patient exposure and orientation of grid cassettes. *Radiologic Technology* 31:4, 387, 1960.

Gibbs, S. Julian. Approaches to radiation risk estimation. *The Physical Basis of Medical Imaging.* 329–342. Editors: Coulam, Craig M., John J. Erickson, David F. Rollo, and A. Everette James, Jr. New York: Appleton-Century-Crofts, 1981.

Glaze, Sharon, Adrian D. LeBlanc, and Stewart C. Bushong. Defects in new protective aprons. *Radiology,* 217, 1984.

Gray, Joel E., John G. Stears, and Eugene D. Frank. Shaped, lead-loaded acrylic filters for patient exposure reduction and image-quality improvement. *Radiology,* 825, 1983.

Hall, Eric J. *Radiobiology for the Radiologist.* 3rd ed. Philadelphia, PA: J. B. Lippincott Company, 1988.

Health Effects of Exposure to Low Levels of Ionizing Radiation BEIR V. Washington, D.C.: National Academy Press, 1990.

Hendee, William R. (ed.). *Health Effects of Low-Level Radiation.* Norwalk, CT: Appleton-Century-Crofts, 1984.

Hilger, Martin T. J. Radiation exposure to nursing personnel from portable radiographic procedures. *Radiology Management* 6:2, 16, 1983.

Huda, Walter, and Karen Gordon. Radiation risks to medical radiation technologists during pregnancy. *The Canadian Journal of Medical Radiation Technology* 17:3, 121, 1986.

International Commission on Radiation Protection. Publication Number 16. *Protection of the*

Patient in X-ray Diagnosis. Oxford, England: Pergamon Press, 1970.

Jankowski, Carol B. Radiation exposure of nurses in a coronary care unit. *The Journal of Critical Care* 13:1, 55–58, 1984.

Light, Mary C., Sabee Y. Molloi, Donald R. Yandouo, and Frank N. Ranallo. Scatter radiation exposure during knee arthrography. *Radiology*, 867, 1987.

Miller. Biological effects of diagnostic irradiation. *Radiologic Technology* 48:1, 11–16, 1976.

Mole, R. H. The 10-day rule: A misnomer. *Radiography* 50:593, 229–230, 1984.

Mole, R. H. Consequences of pre-natal radiation exposure for post-natal development. A review. *International Journal of Radiation Biology* 42:1, 1–12, 1982.

Mole, R. H. Radiation effects on pre-natal development and their radiological significance. *The British Journal of Radiology* 52:614, 89–101, 1979.

NCRP Report No. 49: Structural Shielding Design and Evaluation for Medical Use of X-Rays and Gamma Rays of Energies Up to 10 Mev. Bethesda, MD: National Council on Radiation Protection and Measurements, 1976.

NCRP Report No. 54: Medical Exposure of Pregnant and Potentially Pregnant Women. Bethesda, MD: National Council on Radiation Protection and Measurements, 1977.

NCRP Report No. 82: SI Units in Radiation Protection and Measurements. Bethesda, MD: National Council on Radiation Protection and Measurements, 1985.

NCRP Report No. 91: Recommendations on Limits for Exposure to Ionizing Radiation. Bethesda, MD: National Council on Radiation Protection and Measurements, 1987.

NCRP Report No. 93: Ionizing Radiation Exposure of the Population of the United States. Bethesda, MD: National Council on Radiation Protection and Measurements, 1987.

NCRP Report No. 102: Medical X-Ray, Electron Beam and Gamma-Ray Protection for Energies Up to 50 Mev (Equipment Design, Performance and Use). Bethesda, MD: National Council on Radiation Protection and Measurements, 1989.

Novitch, Mark. Evaluation of radiation exposure in diagnostic radiology examinations. *Radiology Management* 5:4, 33, 1983.

Omran, Hanan. Thermoluminescent dosimeters for in vivo measurement of radiation exposure and related dose in mammography. *Radiologic Technology* 53:5, 383, 1982.

Osborn, S. B. Radiation doses received by diagnostic x-ray workers. *British Journal of Radiology* 28, 650–654, 1955.

Radiation exposure from diagnostic radiology exams: General recommendations. *Radiology Management* 8:2, 49, 1986.

Raeside, David E., and D. W. Anderson. Thermoluminescent dosimetry in the radiological sciences. *Radiologic Technology* 46:1, 20, 1974.

Ragozzino, Mark W. Average fetal depth in utero: Data for estimation of fetal absorbed radiation dose. *Radiology*, 513, 1986.

Selman, Joseph. *The Fundamentals of X-ray and Radium Physics.* 7th ed. Springfield, IL: Charles C. Thomas, 1985.

Statement from the 1985 Paris meeting of the International Commission on Radiological Protection. *Radiology* September, 1985.

Statkiewicz, Mary Alice, and E. Russell Ritenour. *Radiation Protection for Student Radiographers.* Denver, CO: Multi-Media Publishing, Inc., 1983.

Stewart, A., and G. W. Kneale. Radiation dose effects in relation to obstetric x-rays and childhood leukemias. *Lancet* 1, 1185–1188, 1970.

Travis, Elizabeth LaTorre. *Primer of Medical Radiobiology.* 2nd ed. Chicago, IL: Yearbook Medical Publishers, 1989.

Winkler, Norlin T. Minimizing radiation exposure of patients and personnel (screen-film, TFD, filters, shields, grid ratios). *Radiologic Technology* 41:3, 142, 1969.

Wochos, John F., and John R. Cameron. Effect of operator training on patient exposure: An analysis of the NEXT data. *Radiologic Technology* 48:1, 19–22, 1976.

THE CASE OF THE WEIRD X-RAY MACHINE

(Photograph courtesy of Philip W. Ballinger)

The ancient x-ray unit was discovered in the corner of a museum. What purpose did it serve during the production of x-rays?

Answers to the case studies can be found in Appendix E.

4 ELECTRICITY

The experience of life itself is the real test . . . for any . . . profession.

W. C. Röntgen.

OUTLINE

ELECTROSTATICS
ELECTRODYNAMICS
SERIES AND PARALLEL CIRCUITS

OBJECTIVES

Upon completion of this chapter, the student should be able to:

1. Explain the atomic nature of electricity.
2. State the elementary laws of electrostatics.
3. Describe the methods of electrification.
4. Interpret the results of various electrostatic interactions.
5. Differentiate conductors from insulators.
6. Describe the basic factors of electrodynamics.
7. Calculate the effect of changes in voltage, amperage and resistance according to Ohm's law.
8. Calculate voltage, amperage and resistance in a simple series and parallel circuit.

To control x-rays it is necessary to understand how they are produced. X-rays exist when extremely high-energy electricity forces electrons to interact with matter. Electricity must be understood at the subatomic level for this process to become clear. The distribution and movement of electrons, along with their associated charges, make up electricity. Under-

standing atomic structure, including how electrons interact both in and outside of atoms, becomes the key to understanding electricity. It is the distribution and movement of atomic charges that can cause forces to interact.

Atoms contain both kinds of electrical charges, the **positive charge** of the proton, which is locked within the nucleus by very strong forces, and the **negative charge** of the electron, which is located outside the nucleus, bound by relatively weak forces. Electrons may not be associated with a nucleus at all, in which case they are called "free" electrons. In either case, **the positive charge of the proton and the negative charge of the electron are equal in strength**. Because electrons, with their negative charges, are free to move between atomic orbital shells and even between atoms, electricity concerns the distribution and movement of electrons and has little to do with the protons locked within the atomic nucleus.

ELECTROSTATICS

Electrostatics is the study of the distribution of fixed charges, or electrons that are at rest. Just as all atoms are charged (neutral, positive, negative), objects become charged by their composite individual atomic charges. Some atoms include electrons in their outer shells, or beyond the outer shell but within the atom's sphere of influence, that are very easily removed. There are instances, as when walking across a heavy rug in winter, when electrons are easily transferred (literally scooped up) onto another object. It is this type of distribution and redistribution of charged electrons that makes up electrostatics.

The term **electrification** is used to describe the process of electron charges being added to or subtracted from an object. When one object has more electrons than another it also has more negative charges. Therefore it can be considered to be negatively electrified, or to have a **negative charge**. The concept of positive electrification, a positive charge, is more complicated because protons, which carry true positive charges, are not easily distributed. Therefore a **positive charge** usually refers to something with a weaker negative charge, or fewer electrons. The so-called positively electrified, charged, object has a nega-

tive charge; it is just a weaker negative charge than the object with which it is being compared. It is less negative, and therefore termed positive, by comparison. It is important to remember that electrification is a relative term and that nearly all objects have negative charges. **When discussing electricity, the terms negative and positive refer to the relationship between two objects, not to their true atomic charges**.

In conjunction with the idea that negative and positive charges are relative to each other, another concept is required in order to establish a neutral reference point. This is done by defining the earth as **zero or ground potential**. Because the earth contains what is essentially an infinite number of charges, both positive and negative, in equal distribution, it is considered to be neutral and is the reference point for discussing charges. It has zero potential because the equally balanced charges have no potential to perform work and release energy. The symbol for ground is $\perp\!\!\!\!\perp$.

Laws of Electrostatics

Before attempting to understand how objects are electrified, it is helpful to learn five fundamental **laws of electrostatics**. These important laws have many corollaries in physics and will be used again and again throughout this book. The five laws are:

1. **Repulsion-attraction** (Figure 4–1). Like charges repel; unlike charges attract.
2. **The inverse square law** (Figure 4–2). The force between two charges is directly proportional to the product of their magnitudes and inversely proportional to the square of the distance between them. As a charged object gets further away, the influencing charge decreases because of the increased area it affects. The law is expressed as:

$$\frac{I_1}{I_2} = \frac{D_2^2}{D_1^2}$$

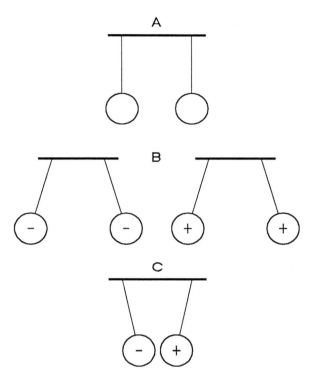

Figure 4–1. Repulsion-attraction law: (A) neutral charges, (B) repulsion of like charges and (C) attraction of unlike charges.

where: I_1 = old intensity
I_2 = new intensity
D_1^2 = old distance squared
D_2^2 = new distance squared

Example: If an object has a charge of 4 coulombs at 4 mm, what will the charge be at 8 mm?

Answer:

$$\frac{I_1}{I_2} = \frac{D_2^2}{D_1^2}$$

$$\frac{4 \text{ coulombs}}{x} = \frac{8mm^2}{4mm^2}$$

$$\frac{4}{x} = \frac{64}{16}$$

$$64x = 64$$
$$x = 1 \text{ coulomb}$$

In this example, as the distance doubled, the charge was reduced to 25 percent of its original value. Although this inverse square formula is usually sufficient for radiographic needs, it is important to understand that the true relationship of the force between two charges is accurately expressed in Coulomb's law:

$$F = \frac{kq_1 \times q_2}{R^2}$$

where: F = electrostatic force in newtons
k = constant of proportionality (9×10^9 for coulombs and meters)

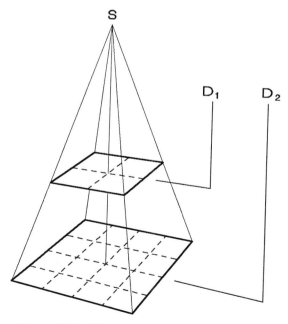

Figure 4–2. The inverse square law: if S is the source and D_2 is twice the distance of D_1, the area covered by the diverging field at D_2 is four times the area covered at D_1.

q_1 and q_2 = charges in coulombs

R = distance in square meters

This formula takes into account the true definition: the force between two charges (q_1 and q_2) is directly proportional to the product of their magnitudes ($q_1 \times q_2$), and inversely proportional to the square of the distance between them (($q_1 \times q_2$)/R^2). Ironically, although the French physicist Coulomb (1736–1806) received the credit for development of this law, the original inquiry was initiated by the American scientist Benjamin Franklin (1706–1790).

3. **Distribution** (Figure 4–3). Charges reside on the external surfaces of conductors and equally throughout nonconductors. This law is a result of the effect of the repulsion-attraction law as electrons, all with negative charges, attempt to repel each other as much as possible. In a solid conductor this results in equal distribution on the surface, which is the point where electrons can ob-

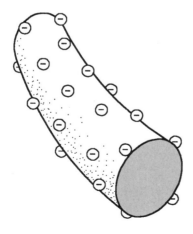

Figure 4–3. The law of distribution of charge: as individual electrons are repelled from one another, they distribute at the outer limits of a conductor.

tain maximum distance from each other. In a nonconductor, such as a cloud, charge movement is not facilitated and equal distribution throughout the object results.

4. **Concentration** (Figure 4–4). The greatest concentration of charge will be on the surface where the curvature is greatest. If enough electrons congregate they can induce ionization of the surrounding air and even discharge to the nearest point of lower concentration. Therefore x-ray tubes, which are subjected to extremely high charges, must not have sharp or rough edges where concentrations of electrons could occur and discharge at the wrong moment or in an undesirable direction. Consequently, the interior components of x-ray tubes are rounded and highly polished to eliminate sharply curved surfaces.

5. **Movement**. Only negative charges move along solid conductors. Because the positive charges, the protons, are tightly bound inside the atomic nuclear field, only the electrons, which exist outside the nucleus, are easily moved along conductors.

Electrification

Objects can be electrified by three methods: **friction**, **contact** and **induction**.

Friction Electrification by **friction** occurs when one object is rubbed against another and, due to differences in the number of electrons available on each, electrons travel from one to the other. Ideal conditions for electron transfer occur during the winter when low humidity removes stabilizing atoms from the air, decreasing the resistance to electron movement between objects. An example is a common trick that delights children—rubbing a balloon against a wool sweater will permit the balloon to stick to a wall. In low humidity, electrons will transfer from the wool to the balloon, giving it a negative charge which can cause it to

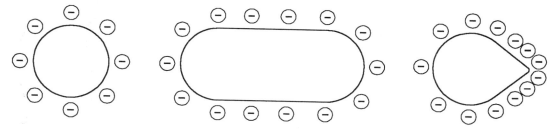

Figure 4–4.   The law of concentration of charge: because each negative charge is repelled by all other negative charges, they tend to concentrate at points of greatest curvature.

stick to a smooth wall with a relatively positive charge. This is an example of opposites attracting one another. A common example of like charges repelling one another occurs when hair is electrified by friction during combing in low humidity conditions. The comb removes electrons from the strands of hair, often accompanied by crackling sounds, leaving each more positively charged. The strands are then repelled by those adjoining, which now also have stronger positive charges. The result is wild strands of hair standing straight out from your head. The solution to the problem is to increase the humidity, or the amount of water in the air, causing a slight condensation on all surfaces. This thin film of moisture becomes a pathway for the distribution of electrons. The use of a humidifier in a radiographic darkroom during cold weather thus helps eliminate electrostatic discharges that can cause artifacts on film.

Contact Electrification by **contact** occurs when two objects touch, permitting electrons to move from one to the other. This process is a simple equalization of charges, with both objects having similar charges after the contact. Walking across a woolen carpet in the winter may cause shoes to scoop from the carpet fibers electrons that would be distributed over the entire body. This is an example of electrification by friction. However, when a positively charged object with fewer electrons

is touched, the contact will cause electrons to move to the less negatively charged object in an attempt to equally distribute the charges. A metal doorknob or another person are examples of positively charged objects that would attract electrons from a person who had just walked across a rug. After the contact both objects would have a more equal distribution of electrons. This is caused by the individual force fields of the electrons satisfying the repulsion-attraction law over the entire surface of the conductors. In many instances actual physical contact does not occur before the electrons equalize. As soon as the oppositely charged objects are in close proximity, the electrons often jump the gap in the form of a **static discharge**. This occurs as soon as the difference in charges becomes sufficiently great and the intervening distance sufficiently small. In most cases the static discharge releases excess energy in the form of light photons. When this occurs between a piece of radiographic film and a cassette, darkroom bench or the body of the person handling the film, the light forms an image on the film. Figure 4–5 illustrates one of the common types of static discharge that appears as a radiographic film artifact.

An electroscope is a simple device that illustrates the laws of electrostatics. It consists of a rod connected to a pair of thin, easily charged metallic leaves which are protected from air currents by a glass flask (Figure 4–6A). When a charged object (such as the

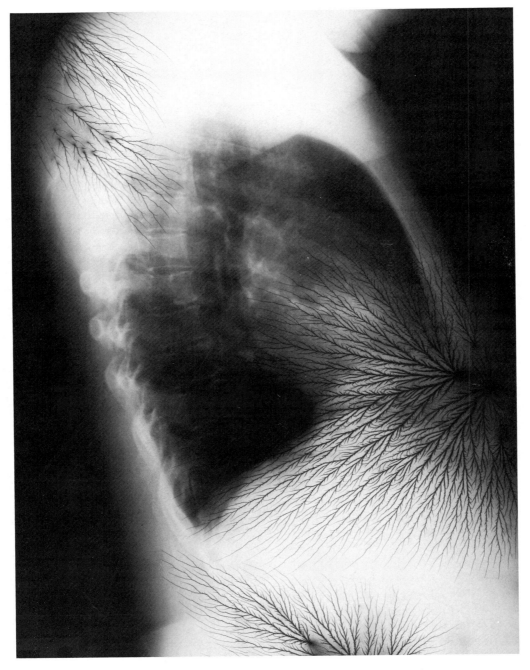

Figure 4–5.   A typical tree-branch static discharge artifact on a radiograph.

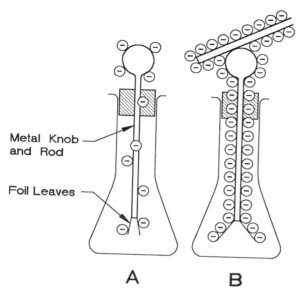

Metal Knob and Rod

Foil Leaves

A   B

Figure 4–6. (A & B) Charging an electroscope by contact: electrons distribute equally when they are permitted to move from one object (the rod) to another (the electroscope) by contact.

metallic rod shown in Figure 4–6B) is brought into contact with the rod, the excess electrons obey the third law of electrostatics and distribute equally throughout the rod and leaves. The resultant increase in the number of electrons present on both leaves causes the two leaves to obey the first law of electrostatics and, since they possess like charges, repel each other. Consequently, it is possible to see the two leaves move further apart.

If an electroscope is subjected to an intense beam of ionizing x-ray photons, the air becomes ionized. The ionized atoms draw excess electrons from the leaves, thus causing the charge on the leaves to be reduced. Consequently, the electroscope leaves relax and move closer together.

Induction Electrification by **induction** is the most important method because it is the one used in the operation of electronic devices. **Induction is the process of electrical fields acting on one another without contact**. Every charged body is surrounded by a force field, much like the fields that surround individual atoms. Like atoms, force fields are a result of the composite forces of the charges residing within the object. These force fields are called **electric fields** and they can cause induction. When a strongly and a weakly charged object come close to one another, the electrical fields will begin to act on one another before contact occurs (Figure 4–7A). As can be seen in Figure 4–7B, charges will migrate to one end of an object in anticipation of contact. However, as seen in Figure 4–7C, when the stronger object is removed before contact, the charges in the weaker object will redistribute themselves as they were before the induction occurred. This temporarily induced movement of charges is useful in many electronic devices, such as motors, transformers and solenoids.

With an understanding of friction and induction electrification it becomes possible to understand one of the greatest of natural phenomena—lightning. Lightning discharges occur as the masses of atoms making up the water vapor in clouds move rapidly through the atmosphere. Under conditions where many electrons are available, such as when there are numerous storm clouds, the movement of the water vapor atoms tends to cause electrons to be picked up or lost. As an individual cloud becomes predominantly positively or negatively charged, it becomes a candidate for a huge electrostatic discharge. Clouds often pick up electrons on their upper edges and lose them on their lower edges and vice versa. In these instances the difference in charges makes the cloud a candidate for a cloud-to-cloud discharge as soon as the insulating effect of the vapor between the two surfaces has been overcome. But the most interesting part of lightning is cloud-to-ground discharges. The ground often develops a temporary opposite charge from the underside of the cloud because of the induction effect of the cloud on

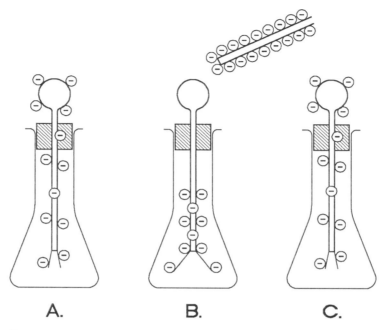

A.   B.   C.

Figure 4–7.   Charging an electroscope by induction: electrons are induced to move away from the heavily charged rod (B) but return to their normal distribution when the rod is removed (A & C).

the ground. This causes the electrons to spread out, which in turn tends to rapidly increase the difference in charges between cloud and ground and can quickly overcome the insulating effect of the air between the cloud and the ground. The result is lightning discharges occurring much more rapidly than if induction had not taken place. Lightning discharges do not occur as a single transfer of electrons from one area to another. Instead, vast numbers of electrons may be transferred from cloud to ground, overloading the ground, which in turn transfers electrons back to the cloud, which again transfers them to the ground, over and over until the charges are somewhat equally distributed. A short lightning discharge often transfers electrons back and forth between cloud and ground many times within a microsecond.

ELECTRODYNAMICS

Electrons that are moving in predominantly the same direction are often referred to as an **electric current**. A number of conditions encourage electron movement, thus permitting the flow of electric current. A **vacuum** is a space from which air has been removed. Since it has few atoms to oppose electron flow, it is especially useful in permitting electrons to reach the speed necessary to produce x-rays. Some **gasses** (such as neon) will promote the drift of electrons from a negative electrode (cathode) to a positive electrode (anode). These gasses also promote the drift of positive ions toward the negative cathode while negative ions move toward the positive anode. **Ionic solutions** can cause electrons to migrate to positive or negative poles during electrolysis, when they are subjected to an electric current.

Electrolysis becomes possible when two neutral atoms with complementary valences (i.e., −1 and +1) are brought together in a solution. They become ions in the solution when the positive valence atom gives up an outer-shell electron to the negative valence atom. The atom missing an electron becomes a positive ion (because a negative charge has been removed) while the one receiving the electron becomes a negative ion (because a negative charge has been added). When metallic rods are connected to a battery and immersed in the solution, the negative pole will attract the positive ions while the positive pole will attract the negative ions. This migration of electrons during the electrolytic process comprises an electrical current. **Metallic conductors**, such as copper wire, are the most common pathways provided for the movement of electrical current. The atoms of metallic conductors permit valence electrons to drift. In common household wiring the actual physical movement is about 2 mm per second (Figure 4–8). The electrical current, as a whole, is similar to a tube filled with balls, as in Figure 4–9. If the tube is full and a new ball is pushed into one end, a ball will drop instantly from the far end, although each ball moved or drifted only a short distance. Electrons move along a conductor with a similar domino effect, resulting in movement of electrons at the far end. This movement occurs extremely rapidly, nearly at the speed of light (3×10^8 meters/second).

Figure 4–9. As when balls are pushed into a tube, each electron needs to move only a short distance for the effect of current movement to be achieved at the other end.

The movement of electrons is facilitated by materials that easily permit electrons to flow. These materials are called **conductors** and **superconductors**. Examples of conductors are metals such as copper and aluminum. Conversely, electron movement is inhibited by materials that resist the flow of electrons. These nonconducting materials are called **insulators**. Examples of insulators are plastic, rubber and glass. The third classification of materials is **semiconductors**. They have the ability to conduct under certain conditions and insulate under others. The actual conditions causing these changes in conductivity are complex and are addressed later in this chapter. They result primarily from changes in the energy states of atoms, causing outer-shell electrons to move in a particular direction (Table 4–1).

An **electrical circuit** is a pathway (commonly copper wire) that permits electrons to move in a complete circle from their source, through resisting electrical devices and back to the source. As in electrostatics, an electrical

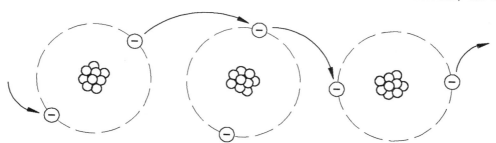

Figure 4–8. Electron drift along a conductor.

TABLE 4–1	PROPERTIES OF CONDUCTING MATERIALS	
State	**Material**	**Characteristics**
Insulator	Plastic Rubber Glass	Large energy difference between conduction and valence bands Resists electron flow
Semiconductor	Silicon Germanium	Small energy difference between conduction and valence bands Conducts OR resists, depending on temperature and other conditions
Conductor	Copper Aluminum	Overlapping conduction and valence bands Conducts with minor resistance, varying depending on temperature and other conditions
Superconductor	Titanium	Greatly overlapping conduction and valence bands Conducts with little or no electrical potential Most current systems require extreme cold to function although research indicates room temperature superconductors may be developed soon.

circuit must have an excess charge at one end and a comparative deficiency at the other to allow electrons to flow. There are several sources of the excess electrons necessary to cause current flow. Examples include **batteries**, which convert chemical energy to electrical; **generators**, which convert mechanical energy to electrical; **solar converters**, which convert solar photons to electrical energy; and **atomic reactors**, which convert nuclear energy to electrical. Only batteries and generators are efficient devices at present. Solar converters and atomic reactors have yet to be developed to directly convert energy for widespread commercial use. Solar converters remain expensive while nuclear reactors, although efficient on a large scale, continue to meet significant public opposition. They operate simply by using the massive energy of the atom to produce steam, which is used to run turbine generators.

Describing Current Flow

Electrons move from the highest concentration to the lowest. There is much confusion regarding how to describe their movement because early pioneers in electrical phenomena assumed that the moving charges were positive when actually they were negatively charged electrons. The negative pole is the source of electrons which move toward the positive receiving pole. Consequently, **conventional electric current is described as going from positive to negative poles while electron flow is actually from negative to positive poles**.

It is important to specify whether descriptions are of electrical current or electron flow, as they are exact opposites. It may be useful to think of negative charges moving in one direction as being equivalent to a positive charge effect in the opposite direction. The importance of these definitions will become apparent later in this text, especially when discussing the interactions of both electrical and magnetic forces.

The nature of the flow of electrons that make up an electric current can be described in many different ways. The most common factors used as descriptors are the **quantity** of electrons flowing, the **force** with which they travel, the amount of **opposition** to the current flow in the circuit and the **direction** of travel.

The **direction** of travel of the electrons is defined as either **direct current (DC)**, when all electrons move in the same direction, or **alternating current (AC)**, when electrons move first in one direction and then reverse and move in the opposite direction. Through the use of various electrical devices, which we will investigate later, it is possible to change the current from DC to AC and back, as necessary.

Current

The **quantity**, or number, of electrons flowing is sometimes referred to as the **current**. It is useful to think of the measurement of current as the number of electrons flowing past a given point per unit of time (usually per second). The French scientist André Ampère (1775–1836) did much original work in defining electricity and magnetism. Consequently, the unit of current bears his name. The **ampere** is sometimes called the **amp** for short and is represented by the symbol **A**. It consists of the movement of 6.24×10^{18} **electrons per second** past a given point; therefore the technical definition is **one coulomb of electrical charge flowing per second (1 ampere = 1 coulomb/1 second)**. Earlier the drift of electrons was given as less than 1 mm per second. The fact that one ampere flowing in a household wire causes 6,240,000,000,000,000,000 electrons to move less than 1 mm per second should help in understanding the small size of electrons. Diagnostic radiographic equipment utilizes milliamperage units to regulate the number of electrons available to produce x-ray photons. The milliamperage (**mA**) is found on nearly all x-ray machines and adjustment by the radiographer operating the equipment will cause the number of electrons and the number of x-ray photons produced to vary. The adjustment of an x-ray machine to add an additional 100 mA

(a common increment) causes 6.24×10^{17} more electrons per second to pass through the x-ray tube.

Example: If an x-ray machine is operating at 0.01 seconds and the amperage is increased by 100 mA, how many more electrons would move through the tube?

Answer:
$(6.24 \times 10^{17}$ electrons/second$) \times 0.01$ seconds$=$ 6.24×10^{15} (6.24 million billion or 6,240,000,000,000,000)

The word current is used to describe the presence of electron flow as well as to describe exactly how much current is flowing. It is important to distinguish which use of the word is intended.

Potential Difference

The **force** with which the electrons travel is a function of the difference between the number of electrons in excess at one end of the circuit and the deficiency at the other end. The attempt of the unequal forces to balance is the cause of the force of electron movement. Because the difference is present while the source is connected into the circuit, **there does not have to be an actual flow of current for the difference to exist**. Therefore the simple potential for a difference is used to describe the force, or strength of movement, behind electrons.

Potential difference is the best term to describe the **force** or **strength** of electron flow. It should be remembered that potential difference continues to exist even when a switch is opened in a circuit, breaking the actual flow of electrons (current). Because potential difference is the prime force causing electrical devices to convert electrical energy to mechanical, the term **electromotive force (emf)** has also been used. Electromotive force is actually the total maximum difference of potential between the positive and negative ends of the electron source, but it is not incorrect to use the term in place of potential difference.

The unit of potential difference is the **volt**, represented by the symbol **V** (named for the Italian physicist Alessandro Volta [1745–1827]). The term voltage is also used to describe potential difference. The technical definition of a volt is **1 joule (J) of work done on one coulomb of charge (1 volt = 1 joule/1 coulomb)**. A joule is the SI unit for both mechanical energy and work.

Thus, for the reasons stated above, the force with which electrons travel can be described by the terms **potential difference, electromotive force (emf)** and **voltage (V)**.

As the current flows along the circuit, the potential difference is reduced because the closer the electrons come to the deficient end of the circuit, the further they are from the excess end (the driving source) and the closer they are to becoming part of the deficiency themselves. With this understanding of potential difference, the concept of grounding electrical circuits for safety should become clear. When equipment is properly grounded and the radiographer, who is also grounded, comes in contact, there is no potential difference. However, when equipment is not properly grounded, the radiographer may become a better path to ground. The passage of electrons (voltage) through the radiographer may be shocking, to say the least.

Resistance

The amount of opposition to the current in the circuit is called the **resistance**. Research into the interrelationships of current, potential difference, and resistance was done by the German physicist Georg Ohm (1787–1854). As a result, the unit of resistance is called the **ohm**. It is represented by the symbol Ω (omega). The technical definition of an ohm is the resistance to a flow of current provided by a column of mercury 106.3 cm long with a diameter of 1 mm^2 at 0° C. A practical definition of an ohm will be provided later, based on the interaction of several characteristics of a conductor. Resistance and impedance are the terms used to describe current opposition. There are numerous factors that impede the flow of electrons, thus increasing resistance. The primary factors for electrical circuits are the **ability to conduct** electrons, the **length** of the conductor, the cross-sectional **diameter** and **temperature**.

When the expression $\frac{1}{R}$ is used, the resistance of a DC circuit is measured as **conductance** while that of an AC circuit is measured as **admittance**. The SI unit for conductance and admittance is the siemens, which is represented by the symbol S and is named after the English electrical engineer Sir William Siemens (1823–1883), brother of Werner von Siemens, founder of the German electrical and x-ray equipment corporation.

The **ability to conduct** electrons has already been discussed enough to define a **conductor** as a material that permits electrons to flow easily, and an **insulator** as one that inhibits their movement. The tendency of an atom to permit electrons nearby or within one of the orbital shells is the prime factor in determining conductivity, semiconductivity and insulation properties. The **valence energy band** (the outermost and sometimes next-to-outermost orbital shell) not only determines the chemical properties of the atom, as discussed previously, but has much to do with conductivity as well. Orbital shells lower or closer to the nucleus (and of less energy) than the valence band are normally completely full (see Figure 4–10). Valence has much to do with the ability of a material to conduct electrons. Any element with one valence electron is a good conductor (i.e., copper, silver and gold). In addition, the further the valence electron is

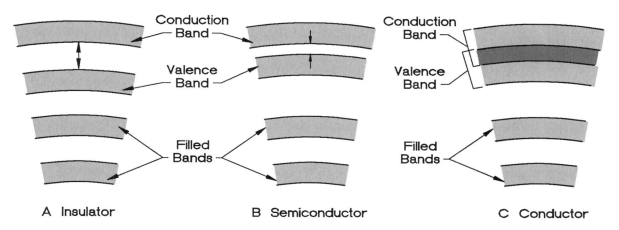

Figure 4–10. The arrows demonstrate the difference between the energy levels of conduction and valence bands in an insulator (A), semiconductor (B) and conductor (C). Note that the conduction and valence bands overlap in a good conductor.

from the nucleus, the better a conductor it is. For example, gold is a better conductor than silver because its valence electron is in the sixth shell while silver's is in the fifth. Silver is a better conductor than copper because copper's valence electron is in the fourth shell. Since copper has a higher melting point and is much cheaper, it is more commonly used than silver or gold.

There is also an area beyond the valence band that is referred to as the **conduction band**. The conduction band is not an orbital shell but is within the force field (area of influence) of the atom (Figure 4–10). Conductors have conduction bands that are populated by free electrons and, in solid materials, they are able to move freely from one atom's conduction band to another's, as in Figure 4–10C. This is why many of the best conductors are solids. Conversely, insulators have very poor or nonexistent conduction bands. The number of electrons in the conduction band is determined by the energy difference between the valence band and the conduction band. Although the conduction band is always at a higher energy level than the valence band, the

energy required of an individual electron to place it in the conduction band will determine how many electrons can possibly exist there. In fact, the difference between the energy levels required of conduction band electrons as compared to valence band electrons is the factor that differentiates conductors from semiconductors from insulators. In Figure 4–10, the differences are shown as (C) a good conductor with overlapping valence and conduction bands, (B) a semiconductor with closely related bands, and (A) a good insulator with a wide gap between the bands. Metals often have overlapping bands with conduction bands including portions of the valence bands, thus placing large numbers of electrons into the conduction bands. Therefore metals, especially silver and copper, make the best conductors. The best insulators are materials with complex molecular structures, such as wood, plastic, glass, and rubber.

The **length** of the conductor has a directly proportional relationship to resistance. In other words, as the length of the conductor doubles, the resistance will also double. Just as a short garden hose will spray water with greater force than a long hose, so a short conductor will permit a greater force to electrons while a longer conductor offers greater resistance.

The cross-sectional **diameter** of the conductor has an inversely proportional relationship to resistance. In other words, as the cross-sectional diameter doubles, the resistance will be halved. A garden hose with a small diameter will impede water flow more than a large-diameter hose, just as a small-diameter conductor will resist electron flow more than a conductor with a large diameter.

Finally, the **temperature** of the conductor can also influence the resistance. Heat is simply a measurement of the amount of atomic and molecular energy, often seen as vibration. As temperature increases, atomic collisions provide enough energy to some electrons to permit them to jump into the atom's conduction band. In conductors, increased temperature increases free electron collisions and this in turn lessens electrical current flow. In insulators the increased number of collisions because of increased temperature causes some electrons to lose energy and fall back into the

valence band, thus decreasing the energy difference between the bands and consequently decreasing the insulating ability of the material. Semiconductors become more conductive as temperature increases, for the same reason, with a resultant narrowing of the gap between their already close bands.

An approximation of these relationships is shown in Figure 4–11. A close examination of this figure illustrates that increased resistance from heat is significant. In fact, it becomes a major problem with the large heat-producing transformers used in x-ray equipment, and unique methods have been adopted to overcome its effect. In addition, extrapolation of the conductor curve to the left illustrates that if conductors can be supercooled, as they are in modern magnetic resonance imaging equipment, a significant increase in conductivity can be achieved.

In recent years, superconductivity has been achieved to reduce resistance to the point where current is apparently flowing without potential difference or current. Table 4–1 provides information on the conductive properties of materials important in electronics.

The total resistance is calculated as:

$$R = \frac{\rho L}{A}$$

where: R = resistance in ohms
ρ = resistivity (a function of atomic structure and temperature) (ρ is the Greek letter rho)
L = length in meters
A = area in square meters

This total resistance formula is the true technical definition of an ohm as a unit.

Ohm's Law

Georg Ohm discovered a mathematical relationship between the factors of current, potential difference, and resistance that applies to

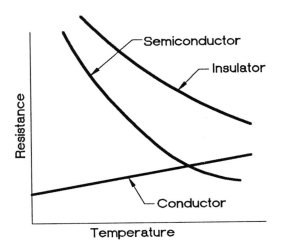

Figure 4–11.   The effect of temperature on conductors, semiconductors and insulators.

all resistance circuits and is known as Ohm's law. The law describes the relationship between current and potential difference as **the current along a conductor is proportional to the potential difference**. It is easier to remember this relationship as a formula:

$$\frac{V}{I}$$

V = potential difference in volts
I = current in amperes

This expression does not include the resistance factor, which is a critical element. Therefore, Ohm's law is usually expressed as the algebraic derivation with resistance times current equal to potential difference, or:

$$V = IR$$

where: V = potential difference in volts
I = current in amperage
R = resistance in ohms

This version solves for voltage when the current and resistance are known. Of course, Ohm's law can also be stated in its other forms to solve for unknown currents and resistances:

$$I = \frac{V}{R}$$

and

$$R = \frac{V}{I}$$

Example: What is the amperage in a circuit of 20 volts and 10 ohms?

Answer:
$$I = V/R$$
$$I = 20 \text{ volts}/10 \text{ ohms}$$
$$I = 2 \text{ amperes}$$

Example: What is the voltage in a circuit of 100 amperes and 5 ohms?

Answer:
$$V = IR$$
$$V = 100 \text{ amperes} \times 5 \text{ ohms}$$
$$V = 500 \text{ volts}$$

Example: What is the resistance in a circuit of 80 kilovolts and 200 milliamperes?

Answer:
$$R = V/I$$
$$R = 80 \text{ kV}/200 \text{ mA}$$
$$R = 80,000 \text{ volts}/0.2 \text{ ampere}$$
$$R = 400,000 \text{ ohms}$$

It is useful to be able to calculate the total amount of power used in an electric circuit. **The unit of power is the watt**. Because the total amount of energy available in a circuit is determined by the current (amperage) and potential difference (voltage), **the watt is defined as one ampere flowing through one volt per second**. Power is calcuated with the following formula:

$$P = IV$$

where: P = power in watts
I = current in amperes
V = potential difference in volts

Common household appliances tend to operate between 500 and 2,000 watts (most have labels indicating their wattage ratings) and all circuits in buildings have wattage safety limitations. The use of equipment whose total wattage ratings exceed the safety limit of the circuit will cause the circuit to overload and shut down because of excessive heat generation. Radiographic equipment capabilities can be measured by the power rating, usually by calculating the greatest possible energy output.

Example: What is the power rating, in kilowatts, of an x-ray generator capable of 800 milliamperes at 100 kilovolts?

Answer: $P = IV$
$$P = 800 \text{ mA} \times 100 \text{ kV}$$

$$P = 0.8 \text{ A} \times 100,000 \text{ V}$$
$$P = 80,000 \text{ watts}$$
$$P = 80 \text{ kilowatts}$$

An interesting historical note for anyone who has seen car engines rated by horsepower is that one horsepower = 746 watts. We could say that an 80 kW generator is a 107 horse-power x-ray machine.

Example: If a mobile x-ray machine operates from a 110 V wall receptacle and is rated at a total resistance of 12 Ω, how much current does it draw during a one-second exposure?

Answer:
$$I = \frac{V}{R}$$

$$I = \frac{110 \text{ V}}{12 \ \Omega}$$

$$I = 9.2 \text{ A}$$

Example: How much power does it use per second?

Answer: $P = IV$
$$P = 9.2 \text{ A} \times 110 \text{ V}$$
$$P = 1,012 \text{ W}$$

With this information it is also possible to calculate the expense of the power for a radiographic examination.

Example: If the power company charges 5¢ per kW/hour, what is the cost of the power for 10 minutes of fluoroscopy at 5 mA and 100 kV?

Answer:
The power per second is calculated as:
$$P = IV$$
$$P = 5 \text{ mA} \times 100 \text{ kV}$$
$$P = 0.005 \text{ a} \times 100,000 \text{ V}$$
$$P = 500 \text{ W}$$

The total power is calculated as:
total power = power × seconds
total power = 500 W × 10 minutes
total power = 500 W × 600 seconds
total power = 300,000 W/sec
total power = 300 kW/sec

The total cost is calculated as:
total cost = total power used × $0.05/kW/hr
total cost = 300 kW/second × $0.05/kW/hr
total cost = 5 kW/minute × $0.05/kW/hr
total cost = 0.08 kW/hr × $0.05/kW/hr
total cost = $0.004, or
total cost = 0.4¢

The heat that is produced during the operation of electrical equipment becomes of great concern as power use increases. The importance of changes in resistance to heat output can best be understood if the power formula, $P = IV$, is converted to what is sometimes called the **power loss formula, $P = I^2R$**. This is calculated from:

the power formula, $P = IV$
substituting IR for V
(because Ohm's law states that $V = IR$)
resulting in $P = I \times IR$
or $P = I^2R$ (watts per second).

This equation clarifies that power loss from current heat is proportional to the resistance, and heat power loss increases very rapidly with current increase. As illustrated in the formula, heat power loss is proportional to the square of the amperage. In other words, doubling the amperage increases power loss by a factor of 4, etc.

SERIES AND PARALLEL CIRCUITS

An electric circuit can be designed to send electrons through various resistance devices by linking them one after the other in a **series circuit** (Figure 4–12A) or by giving each component an individual branch in a **parallel circuit** (Figure 4–12B). The effect of each type of circuit on current, potential difference, and resistance is summarized in Table 4–2. The best way to understand the effects of both series and parallel circuitry is to work through a series of problems that demonstrate these differences.

A.   Series Circuit

B.   Parallel Circuit

Figure 4–12.   Series (A) and parallel (B) circuits.

Example: What is the total current in a series circuit supplied with 10 amperes?

Answer: $I_t = I_1 = I_2 = I_3$
$I_t = 10\ A = 10\ A = 10\ A$
$I_t = 10$ amperes

Example: What is the total current in a parallel circuit with 3 resistances, each supplied with 10 amperes?

Answer: $I_t = I_1 + I_2 + I_3$
$I_t = 10\ A + 10\ A + 10\ A$
$I_t = 30$ amperes

Note that the series circuit supplies a current of 10 amperes while the parallel circuit supplies 30 amperes. Parallel circuits supply a greater total current than series circuits when all other factors are the same. An interesting phenomenon occurs when the effect on voltage is compared, instead of current, using resistances.

Example: What is the total voltage in a series circuit supplied with 10 volts?

Answer:
$$V_t = V_1 + V_2 + V_3$$
$$V_t = 10\ V + 10\ V + 10\ V$$
$$V_t = 30\ volts$$

Example: What is the total voltage in a parallel circuit with 3 resistances, each supplied with 10 volts?

Answer:
$$V_t = V_1 = V_2 = V_3$$
$$V_t = 10\ V = 10\ V = 10\ V$$
$$V_t = 10\ volts$$

TABLE 4–2

EFFECT OF CIRCUIT TYPE ON CURRENT, POTENTIAL DIFFERENCE AND RESISTANCE (with an example circuit of 3 resistances)

	Series	Parallel
Current	Same in each element, each element same as total circuit, $I_t = I_1 = I_2 = I_3$	Sum of all elements equals total circuit, $I_t = I_1 + I_2 + I_3$
Voltage	Sum of all elements equals total circuit, $V_t = V_1 + V_2 + V_3$	Same in each element, each element same as total circuit, $V_t = V_1 = V_2 = V_3$
Resistance	Sum of all elements equals total circuit, $R_t = R_1 + R_2 + R_3$	Sum of reciprocal of each element is inversely proportional to the total, $$\frac{1}{R_t} = \frac{1}{R_1} + \frac{1}{R_2} + \frac{1}{R_3}$$

NOTE: A reciprocal ohm, as in $\frac{1}{R}$, is known as a siemens.

Note that the series circuit supplies 30 volts while the parallel circuit supplies 10 volts. Series circuits supply greater total potential difference than parallel circuits when all other factors are the same. The difference between series and parallel circuits when the same resistances are used is also notable.

Example: What is the total resistance of a series circuit with resistances of 2.5 Ω, 4.2 Ω and 6.8 Ω?

Answer:
$$R_t = R_1 + R_2 + R_3$$
$$R_t = 2.5 \ \Omega + 4.2 \ \Omega + 6.8 \ \Omega$$
$$R_t = 13.5 \ \Omega$$

Example: What is the total resistance of a parallel circuit with resistances of 2.5 Ω, 4.2 Ω and 6.8 Ω?

Answer:
$$\frac{1}{R_t} = \frac{1}{R_1} + \frac{1}{R_2} + \frac{1}{R_3}$$
$$\frac{1}{R_t} = \frac{1}{2.5 \ \Omega} + \frac{1}{4.2 \ \Omega} + \frac{1}{6.8 \ \Omega}$$
$$\frac{1}{R_t} = 0.4 \ S + 0.24 \ S + 0.15 \ S$$
$$\frac{1}{R_t} = 0.785 \ S$$
$$R_t = \frac{1}{0.7 \ S}$$
$$R_t = 1.274 \ \Omega$$

Note that the series circuit provides 13.5 Ω of resistance while the parallel circuit has only 1.274 Ω. Parallel circuits offer less total resistance to electrical current when all other factors are the same. In addition, parallel circuits are not broken when a single resistance is interrupted (as when a light bulb burns out). Series circuits require all resistances to be operable, otherwise there is no pathway for the current to take. The classic example of the dif-

ference is illustrated by comparing strings of Christmas lights in series versus parallel circuits. When a single series-wired light burns out, it breaks the circuit and all the lights go out. When a single parallel-wired light burns out, it breaks the circuit in its parallel branch only and the other lights continue to operate. Electrical devices use a wide variety of both types of circuits, including complicated combinations of both. It is also interesting to calculate the effect of both circuit types on amperage by figuring resistance and then applying Ohm's law.

Example: What is the total amperage in a series circuit with resistances of 2.5 Ω, 4.2 Ω and 6.8 Ω with a potential difference of 10 volts?

Answer:
The total resistance is calculated as:
$$R_t = R_1 + R_2 + R_3$$
$$R_t = 2.5 \ \Omega + 4.2 \ \Omega + 6.8 \ \Omega$$
$$R_t = 13.5 \ \Omega$$
The total amperage is calculated with Ohm's law:
$$I = \frac{V}{R}$$
$$I = \frac{10 \ V}{13.5 \ \Omega}$$
$$I = 0.74 \ \text{amperes}$$

Example: What is the total amperage in a parallel circuit with resistances of 2.5 Ω, 4.2 Ω and 6.8 Ω and a potential difference of 10 volts?

Answer:
The total resistance is calculated as:
$$\frac{1}{R_t} = \frac{1}{R_1} + \frac{1}{R_2} + \frac{1}{R_3}$$
$$\frac{1}{R_t} = \frac{1}{2.5 \ \Omega} + \frac{1}{4.2 \ \Omega} + \frac{1}{6.8 \ \Omega}$$

$$\frac{1}{R_t} = 0.4\ S + 0.24\ S + 0.15\ S$$

$$\frac{1}{R_t} = 0.785\ S$$

$$R_t = \frac{1}{0.7\ S}$$

$$R_t = 1.274\ \Omega$$

The total amperage is calculated with Ohm's law:

$$I = \frac{V}{R}$$

$$I = \frac{10\ V}{1.274\Omega}$$

$$I = 7.85\ amperes$$

Note that the series circuit operates with a current of 0.74 amperes while the parallel circuit operates with a current of 7.1 amperes. Parallel circuits operate with greater current when all other factors are the same. It is also interesting to study the effect of both circuit types on voltage by calculating resistance and then applying Ohm's law.

Example: What is the total voltage of a series circuit with resistances of 2.5 Ω, 4.2 Ω and 6.8 Ω with a current of 50 amperes?

Answer:
The total resistance is calculated as:
$$R_t = R_1 + R_2 + R_3$$
$$R_t = 2.5\ \Omega + 4.2\ \Omega + 6.8\ \Omega$$
$$R_t = 13.5\ \Omega$$
The total voltage is calculated with Ohm's law:
$$V = IR$$
$$V = 50\ A \times 13.5\ \Omega$$
$$V = 675\ volts$$

Example: What is the total voltage of a parallel circuit with resistances of 2.5 Ω, 4.2 Ω and 6.8 Ω and a current of 50 amperes?

Answer:
The total resistance is calculated as:

$$\frac{1}{R_t} = \frac{1}{R_1} + \frac{1}{R_2} + \frac{1}{R_3}$$

$$\frac{1}{R_t} = \frac{1}{2.5\ \Omega} + \frac{1}{4.2\ \Omega} + \frac{1}{6.8\ \Omega}$$

$$\frac{1}{R_t} = 0.4\ S + 0.24\ S + 0.15\ S$$

$$\frac{1}{R_t} = 0.785\ S$$

$$R_t = \frac{1}{0.7\ S}$$

$$R_t = 1.274\ \Omega$$

The total voltage is calculated with Ohm's law:
$$V = IR$$
$$V = 50\ A \times 1.274\ \Omega$$
$$V = 63.68\ V$$

Note that the series circuit operates at 675 volts while the parallel circuit operates at 64 volts. Parallel circuits operate at lower voltage than series circuits when all other factors are the same.

Parallel circuits are used for the electrical wiring of buildings because the failure of a single device does not break the electrical supply to other devices. As can be seen from these problems, the addition of current-using devices to a series circuit causes the voltage to drop, thus reducing the potential difference to the other devices in the circuit. In a series circuit of lights, for example, the addition of more bulbs will cause all the bulbs to burn dimmer. **As more resistances are added to a parallel circuit, total resistance drops, total amperage increases and total voltage remains unchanged**.

A disadvantage to parallel circuits is that with the addition of resistances, the increasing amperage can short circuit the entire system. This creates the possibility of wires becoming hot enough to start a fire. To prevent this from occurring, either a **circuit breaker** or a **fuse** is placed in the line. These devices are constructed to permit the breaking of the circuit before a dangerous temperature is reached. Circuit breakers simply pop open and can be reset once the cause of the problem has been located and removed from the circuit. Fuses are constructed with a metal tab that, when dangerously heated, will melt, thus breaking the circuit. Fuses are not reusable and must be replaced.

A variable resistor called a **potentiometer** or **rheostat** permits a variable contact to slide along a series circuit of resistance coils. When resistors are connected in a series circuit Ohm's law dictates that an increase in resistance will result in a decrease in voltage and vice versa if the amperage remains unchanged. When a knob is connected to the variable slide contact (as in a radio volume control), a simple twist permits voltage and amperage regulation (with a corresponding increase or decrease in speaker volume). Unfortunately, rheostats cause significant energy waste in heat, and the direct application of Ohm's law results in voltage changing when only an amperage change is desired and vice versa. For these reasons, rheostats are not practical in high-voltage situations. Their prime use is to control current but they have never been adaptable to high-voltage transformers.

SUMMARY

The distribution and movement of electrons, along with their associated charges, make up electricity. Electrostatics is the study of the distribution of fixed charges that are at rest. When one object has more electrons than another, it also has more negative charges and is considered to have a negative charge. A positive charge refers to something with a weaker negative charge, or fewer electrons. The terms negative and positive refer to the relationship between two objects, not to their true atomic charges. Because the earth contains what is essentially an infinite number of charges, it is considered to be neutral, or at zero ground potential. The five laws of electrostatics are: 1) repulsion-attraction, 2) the inverse square law, 3) distribution, 4) concentration and 5) movement. Objects can be electrified by friction, contact and induction.

The movement of electrons is facilitated by materials that permit electrons to flow easily. These materials are called conductors or superconductors. Nonconducting materials are called insulators, while materials that conduct under certain conditions and insulate under others are known as semiconductors.

An electrical circuit is a pathway that permits electrons to move in a complete circle from their source, through resisting electrical devices, and back to the source. Electrons move from the highest concentration to the lowest. Conventional electric current is described as going from positive to negative poles, while electron flow is actually from negative to positive poles. It is important to specify whether descriptions are of electrical current or electron flow, as they are exact opposites.

The quantity of electrons flowing is referred to as the current and is measured in amperes. The force with which the electrons travel is referred to as the potential difference, electromotive force or voltage and is measured in volts. There does not have to be current flow for voltage to exist. The opposition to the current flow is referred to as resistance and is measured in ohms. The relationship between these factors is expressed in Ohm's law: $V = IR$. The resistance of metallic conductors is affected by length, diameter and temperature. When $1/R$ is used to express resistance in an AC circuit, it is measured in siemens.

The valence energy band of an atom has much to do with the ability of a material to conduct electrons. There is also an area beyond the valence band that is referred to as the conduction band. Conductors have conduction bands that are populated by electrons that are able to move freely from one atom's conduction band to another's. Insulators have widely separated valence and conduction bands, while semiconductors have intermediate properties.

Circuits are known by several parameters. These include the direction the electrons travel, which is defined as either direct current (DC) or alternating current (AC). It is possible to change the current from DC to AC and back, as necessary. The total amount of energy in a circuit is described as the power of the circuit and is measured in watts so that $P = IV$. Circuits can be described as series or parallel, depending on how the components are connected. The total resistance of a series circuit is measured in ohms, as $R_t = R_1 + R_2 + R_3$. The total resistance of a parallel circuit is measured in siemens, as

$$\frac{1}{R_t} = \frac{1}{R_1} + \frac{1}{R_2} + \frac{1}{R_3}$$

Parallel circuits operate with greater current through resistances and they supply a greater total current from the power supply than series circuits when all other factors are the same. Parallel circuits are often used because the failure of a single device does not break the electrical supply to other devices. Circuit breakers and fuses prevent damage to electrical components by permitting the breaking of an overloaded circuit before a dangerous temperature is reached. A potentiometer or rheostat is a variable resistor.

REVIEW QUESTIONS

1. State the five elementary laws of electrostatics.

2. Describe the three methods of electrification.

3. How are conductors different from insulators?

4. Explain the difference between conventional electrical current and actual electron flow.

5. State the four basic factors that are used to describe the nature of the flow of electrons in electrodynamics.

6. What are the units used to describe potential difference, current flow and opposition to current flow?

7. State Ohm's law.

8. What is the potential difference in a circuit of 20 amperes and 10 ohms? 30 amperes and 6 ohms? 100 mA and 5 ohms?

9. What is the power rating of an x-ray generator capable of 1,000 mA at 110 kV?

10. What is the voltage in a parallel circuit of 20 amperes with resistances of 6, 10 and 15 ohms?

11. What is the amperage in a series circuit of 110 volts with resistances of 5, 10 and 20 ohms?

REFERENCES AND RECOMMENDED READING

Ball, J. L., and A. D. Moore. *Essential Physics for Radiographers*. 2nd ed. Oxford: Blackwell Scientific Publications, 1986.

Bushong, Stewart. *Radiologic Science for Technologists*. 4th ed. St. Louis, MO: C. V. Mosby Co. 1988.

Chesney, D. Noreen, and Muriel O. Chesney. *X-Ray Equipment for Student Radiographers*. 3rd ed. Oxford: Blackwell Scientific Publications, 1984.

Dendy, P. P., and B. Heaton. *Physics for Radiologists*. Oxford: Blackwell Scientific Publications, 1987.

Gates, Earl D. *Introduction to Electronics: A Practical Approach*. Albany, NY: Delmar Publishers, 1987.

Gifford, Derek. *A Handbook of Physics for Radiologists and Radiographers*. New York: John Wiley & Sons, 1984.

Glasser, Otto, Edith H. Quimby, Lauriston S. Taylor, J. L. Weatherwax, and Russell H. Morgan. *Physical Foundations of Radiology*. 3rd ed. New York: Paul B. Hoeber Division of Harper & Brothers, 1961.

Hay, George A., and Donald Hughes. *First-Year Physics for Radiographers*. London: Bailliere Tindall, 1972.

Johns, Harold E., and John R. Cunningham. *The Physics of Radiology*. 4th ed. Springfield, IL: Thomas, 1983.

Meredith, W. J., and J. B. Massey. *Fundamental Physics of Radiology*. 3rd ed. Chicago, IL: Yearbook Medical Publishers, 1977.

Nadon, John M., Bert J. Gelmine, and Edward D. McLaughlin. *Industrial Electricity*. 4th ed. Albany, NY: Delmar Publishers, 1989.

Ridgway, Arthur, and Walter Thumm. *The Physics of Medical Radiography*. Reading, MA: Addison-Wesley, 1973.

Selman, Joseph. *The Fundamentals of X-Ray and Radium Physics*. 7th ed. Springfield, IL: Thomas, 1985.

Sprawls, Perry. *Principles of Radiography for Technologists*. Rockville, MD: Aspen Publishers, 1990.

Sprawls, Perry. *Physical Principles of Medical Imaging*. Rockville, MD: Aspen Publishers, 1987.

Stockley, Sybil M. *A Manual of Radiographic Equipment*. Edinburgh: Churchill Livingstone, 1986.

Ter-Pogossian, Michel M. *The Physical Aspects of Diagnostic Radiology*. New York: Hoeber Medical Division, Harper & Row, 1967.

Thompson, Thomas T. *A Practical Approach to Modern Imaging Equipment*. 2nd ed. Boston, MA: Little, Brown, and Co., 1985.

van der Plaats, G. J. *Medical X-Ray Techniques in Diagnostic Radiology*. 4th ed. The Hague: Martinus Nijhoff Publishers, 1980.

Wilks, Robin J. *Principles of Radiological Physics*. Edinburgh: Churchill Livingstone, 1981.

5 ELECTROMAGNETISM

He expressed his satisfaction and, going back to Joachim, warned him to draw in his breath and hold it until all was over. Joachim's rounded back expanded and so remained; the assistant, at the switch-board, pulled the handle. Now, for the space of two seconds, fearful powers were in play—streams of thousands, of a hundred thousand of volts.

Thomas Mann, *Der Zauberberg* (The Magic Mountain).

OUTLINE

**MAGNETISM
ELECTROMAGNETISM
CONTROLLING ELECTRICAL CURRENT
RECTIFICATION**

OBJECTIVES

Upon completion of this chapter, the student should be able to:

1. Explain the atomic nature of magnetism.
2. Classify materials according to their magnetic properties.
3. State Fleming's hand rules of electromagnetics.
4. Explain how a solenoid and an electromagnet function.
5. Describe magnetic and electromagnetic induction.
6. List the types of movement that will produce electromagnetism.
7. State the factors that regulate the strength of electromagnetic induction.
8. Explain self-induction.
9. Illustrate the generator and motor principles.
10. Explain the waveform produced by direct- and alternating-current generators and motors.
11. Describe the function of a transformer.
12. Calculate voltage and amperage according to the transformer law.
13. Discuss various factors affecting transformer efficiency and construction.
14. Explain the function of an autotransformer and a capacitor.

15. Describe the function of a silicon-controlled rectifier at the atomic level.
16. Describe the process of thermionic emission.
17. Explain the waveforms that are produced by half-wave and full-wave rectification.

MAGNETISM

Magnetism is one of the fundamental forces. Materials that have the ability to attract iron are classified as having a strong magnetic force. To understand magnetism it is important to return to atomic structure for a detailed examination of the effects of particle movement around the nucleus. **When a charged particle is in motion, a magnetic force field perpendicular to the motion will be created** (Figure 5–1). In the case of the negatively charged electrons orbiting the nucleus of an atom, the closed loop of the orbit cancels all but the field that is perpendicular to the plane of the motion (Figure 5–2). This perpendicular magnetic force is called **orbital magnetic moment**.

A magnetic effect is also established by electrons spinning on their axes. The effect created by the movement of these electrons is called **spin magnetic moment**. The disruption of this axial spinning and the energy released as it reorients itself are the physical basis that permits magnetic resonance imaging (see Chapter 42).

Atoms having a significant number of electrons with their magnetic moments in the same direction, especially when the outer shells are involved, will exhibit a net magnetic field in a distinct direction (Figure 5–2A). Groups of atoms with this net magnetic field are known as **magnetic dipoles** or **magnetic domains**. This is the basis of the domain theory of magnetism. It has been theorized that 10^{15} (10,000,000,000,000,000 or 10 thousand billion) atoms make up a single dipole. This is not a standard number, as it has been shown that dipoles vary in size and actually grow or shrink, depending on local conditions. In nonmagnetic objects the magnetic dipoles are randomly arranged, essentially cancelling out each other. If an external force field has the time or strength to orient enough of the dipoles in the same direction and/or cause those dipoles to grow in size, the object exhibits a uniformly strong magnetic field and is referred to as a **magnet** (Figure 5–2B).

The force fields that are created when magnetic dipoles orient to create a magnet are called **lines of force**, **lines of flux** or the **magnetic field**. These lines of force flow not only through the magnet itself but outside the magnetic material, forming a three-dimensional field surrounding the magnet (Figure 5–2B). The stronger the magnetic field, the more lines of flux. Placing small iron filings on a surface under which a strong magnet is placed will

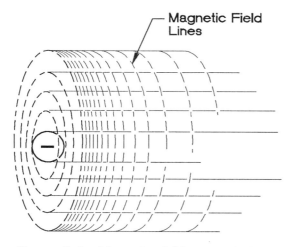

Figure 5–1. Magnetic field created by a charged particle in motion. The movement of a charged particle creates a magnetic field perpendicular to the motion of the particle.

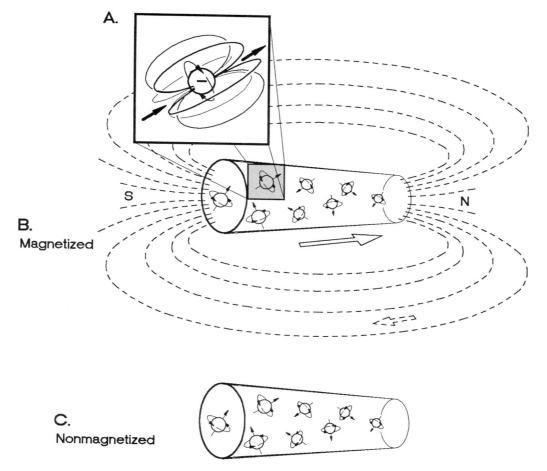

Figure 5–2. The concept of magnetism: (A) The spinning of an individual electron is the spin magnetic moment, and the magnetic field created by the spin is the orbital magnetic moment (heavy arrows). Groups of atoms with most of the magnetic moment force in a single direction form a magnetic dipole or domain. (B) When the magnetic dipoles or domains are in a predominant direction a magnet is formed with an external magnetic field. (C) When the magnetic dipoles or domains are not in a predominant direction the object is not magnetized.

map out the magnetic lines of flux. Figure 5–3 illustrates the lines of flux emanating from the poles of a bar and a horseshoe magnet. The ends of a magnet are defined as the north and south poles; **lines of force always flow from north to south outside a magnet and from** **south to north within a magnet** (Figure 5–2B). It is important to remember that **lines of force never intersect**. In some cases they are described as being parallel. However, many circumstances may cause the magnetic field to contract or expand. Under these conditions the

Figure 5–3.   Strong permanent magnets placed under a surface containing loose iron filings will demonstrate magnetic lines of flux as the filings orient to the magnetic field (forming the initials of an Indiana university).

lines of force bend closer or further from one another, no longer making them truly parallel.

The stronger the magnetic field, the greater the number of lines of flux or the greater the **flux density**. Flux density is determined both by field strength and by the area in which the lines of flux are located.

$$\text{magnetic flux} = \frac{\text{field strength}}{\text{area}}$$

There are two primary units used to measure the strength of magnetic fields. **The SI unit for magnetic flux is the Weber**, represented by the symbol Wb, (for the German physicist Wilhelm Weber [1804–1891], who proposed the basic theory of magnetism discussed above). 1 Wb = 10^8 lines of flux. **The units for magnetic flux density are the tesla**, represented by the symbol T (for the American physicist Nikola Tesla [1857–1943]), and the gauss, represented by the symbol G (for the German mathematician Johann Gauss [1777–1855]). **1 tesla = 10,000 gauss**. 1 T = 1 Wb/m^2, or 1 Wb per square

meter. The earth's magnetic field averages about 0.0001 T (1 G or 100,000 lines of flux per square meter), while an ordinary household magnet (used, for example, to keep papers on a refrigerator) might have a strength of 0.1 T (1,000 G or 100,000,000 lines of flux per square meter). Modern magnetic resonance imaging (MRI) equipment often operates in the range of 0.3–2.0 T (3,000 to 20,000 G or 300,000,000 to 2,000,000,000 lines of flux per square meter).

Because the earth itself is a magnet, with a north and a south pole, lines of force, although relatively weak, are present everywhere. This fact is used in the design of a magnetic compass. The pointer is simply a small piece of permanent magnet which will align itself with the earth's magnetic lines of force and indicate direction. Because of this, a compass is a useful tool in detecting magnetic lines of force, including those induced by electrons moving in electrical circuits and devices. Worth noting is the fact that the earth's true magnetic poles are not located in Antarctica and the Arctic Ocean. Instead, the true magnetic north pole is located in Canada's far north while the true magnetic south pole is near Australia. Both poles tend to drift to new locations as geological conditions beneath the earth's crust change.

Magnets can be classified by type of production as **natural**, **artificial permanent** and **electromagnets**. **Natural magnets** are created when iron oxide (magnetite) remains in the earth's magnetic field for ages, slowly orienting the magnetic dipoles in the same direction. These natural magnets are called lodestones. They were recognized by primitive man and investigated by Greek academics. In some regions entire mountains of iron ore that have remained undisturbed for eons have magnetic properties. Natives of Thunder Bay, Ontario, delight in watching tourists follow signpost instructions to place their cars in neutral gear at the bottom of a magnetic mountain's gentle grade in hopes that the magnetic field will pull their cars up the hill.

Artificial permanent magnets are manufactured from a steel alloy called alinco, composed of aluminum, nickel and cobalt. While it is hot, alinco is subjected to the field of a strong commercial magnet to permit easier orientation of the magnetic dipoles. Upon cooling, the magnetic field becomes relatively permanent.

Electromagnets are temporary magnets produced by moving electric current. Because the electrons comprising the flow of current create magnetic fields in exactly the same manner as do the orbiting and spinning atomic electrons, any flow of current produces a magnetic field. When the current ceases flowing, the magnetic field collapses, making these electrical magnets temporary.

It is possible to create a fourth type of magnet by vibration. Prior to the 20th century, experienced blacksmiths were easy to spot because the tongs they used to handle heated metals had become magnetized. After many years of standing in the same position (in orientation to the earth's magnetic lines of force), heating the tongs in the forge, and then pounding the hot metal into shape on the anvil, the tongs had become well magnetized. A request to see a horseshoe hanging from a rafter would prove a smith's experience when he used the magnetized tongs to easily lift it down.

The laws governing magnetism are similar to the laws of electrostatics. However, only three are of importance for this text:

1. **Repulsion-attraction**. Like poles repel; unlike poles attract. In addition, like lines of force repel and unlike lines of force attract, when placed within each other's force fields (Figure 5–4).
2. **The inverse square law**. The force between two magnetic fields is directly proportional to the product of their magnitudes and in-

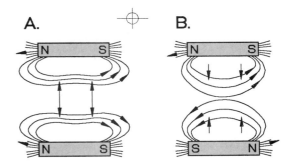

Figure 5–4. Repulsion-attraction of magnetic lines of force: (A) Lines of force in the same direction will repel each other. (B) Lines of force in opposite directions will attract each other.

versely proportional to the square of the distance between them. Exactly as with electrostatics, as an object gets further away, the influencing field decreases because of the increased area it affects.

3. **Magnetic poles**. Every magnet has two poles, a north and a south, as discussed earlier. No matter how much a magnet is divided, even into individual moving electrons, both poles continue to exist.

Because the laws of electrostatics, magnetism, and gravity have so many similarities, physicists have long searched for a mathematical theory to relate the three forces into a unified field theory. Albert Einstein worked unsuccessfully toward this goal until he died and the search continues to the present time, led by Stephen Hawking.

Magnetic Induction

When a nonmagnetized iron bar is brought within the lines of force of a strong magnet, the dipoles will temporarily align themselves with the lines of force passing through the iron bar. If the bar is removed from the field after a short time, the dipoles will return to their random orientation, thus leaving the bar unmagnetized. This process is termed magnetic induction and operates like electromagnetic induction. Instead of temporary repulsion of electrons, magnetic poles are induced through the temporary orientation of the dipoles.

The ease with which sensitive devices can be magnetized or demagnetized by stray electrical fields makes magnetic shielding desirable in many situations. Because there is no magnetic insulator, shielding is accomplished by providing a highly permeable ferromagnetic material, such as iron, through which stray magnetic fields can be directed, thus protecting sensitive devices from exposure to the stray field. This technique is used to shield some magnetic resonance imaging (MRI) units although they require radio frequency (RF) shielding as well.

Magnetic Classification of Materials

Permeability is the ease with which a material can be magnetized, while **retentivity** is the ability of a material to stay magnetized. These two factors are inversely proportional because if it is difficult to orient the dipoles (low permeability) it is also difficult to disorient them (high retentivity). The major classifications of the magnetic properties of materials according to their relative permeabilities are:

1. **Ferromagnetic** (or simply magnetic) materials such as iron, cobalt and nickel are highly permeable and greatly susceptible to induction. These materials have a majority of their dipoles lying in the same direction, thus setting up a natural magnetic field. In addition, the material must permit the atoms to be oriented, thus permitting the growth of magnetic dipoles in predominantly the same direction. Specialized alloys such as alinco, permalloy or mumetal (some alloys, strangely enough, contain no ferromagnetic elements) are designed to en-

hance permeability and exhibit dramatically increased magnetic field strength.

2. **Paramagnetic** materials, such as platinum and aluminum, have low permeability and weak attraction to magnetic fields. These materials have only a slight majority of dipoles in the same direction and there is little tendency for the size of the dipoles to grow.

3. **Diamagnetic** materials, such as beryllium, bismuth and lead, are actually weakly repelled by all magnetic fields, including both north and south poles. Strangely, water is slightly diamagnetic. This property is so weak that it is easily obscured by other types of magnetic induction.

4. **Nonmagnetic** materials, such as wood, glass, rubber and plastic, are not affected by magnetic fields and cannot be magnetized. Nonmagnetic materials are most often composed of atoms locked into crystalline or molecular patterns, thus forming ionic and covalent bonds and eliminating the ability of electrons to freely orient themselves to external magnetic lines of force. This classification includes most materials.

ELECTROMAGNETISM

Electricity and magnetism are actually different aspects of the same force, electromagnetism. Although the study of magnetism dates to ancient times, and the study of electricity to Queen Elizabeth I's physician, William Gilbert (1540–1603), it was not until 1820, when the Danish physicist Hans Oersted (1777–1851) observed the deflection of a compass during a classroom demonstration of electrical phenomena, that the relationships between the two began to be established. Oersted's discovery, and subsequent investigations by many others, permitted the generation, control and practical use of electricity and initiated the electronic revolution that continues today.

Oersted's experiment proves that when there is no current flowing in the wire, the compass needle aligns itself with the earth's magnetic field (Figure 5–5). However, when

A. Without Current Flow

B. With Current Flow

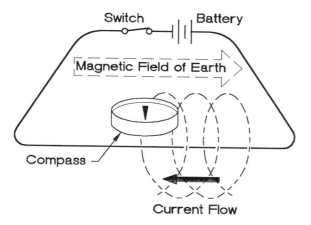

Figure 5–5. Oersted's experiment: A compass placed near a wire conductor will indicate the direction of the earth's magnetic field (A) when no current is flowing in the wire. Because flowing current creates a magnetic field around the wire conductor that is stronger than the earth's field, the compass will indicate the direction of the current-induced field while the switch is closed (B).

current is flowing, the needle is deflected toward the wire and when the current stops, the needle returns to alignment with the earth's field. This led to the conclusion that **any moving charge produces a magnetic field**. As was stated earlier in the section on magnetism, this applies to even a single electron's negative charge in orbit around an atom. A slightly different arrangement of Oersted's experiment (Figure 5–6) permits the mapping of the magnetic field surrounding the flow of current.

The English scientist John Fleming (1849–1945) developed a series of easily remembered aids to help with the relationship between electricity and magnetism. They are known as **Fleming's hand rules**. There are several "hand" rules that are quite useful for remembering various electromagnetic relationships. The rules are divided into four groups: (1) **hand thumb rules along a conductor**, (2) **hand thumb rules for solenoid and electromagnet poles**, (3) **hand generator effect rules** and (4) **hand motor principle rules**. These are summa-

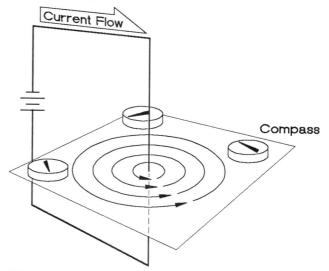

Figure 5–6. Relationship of induced magnetic field to direction of current flow: a variation of Oersted's experiment maps out the magnetic field induced by flowing current.

TABLE 5–1	FLEMING'S HAND RULES FOR ELECTROMAGNETIC RELATIONSHIPS		
		Conventional Current Flow	Electron Flow
Along a Conductor			
thumb = conventional current or electron flow		right-hand thumb rule (see Figure 5–7)	left-hand thumb rule (left-hand version)
fingers = magnetic field			
Solenoid and Electromagnet Poles			
thumb = direction of north pole		right-hand thumb rule (see Figure 5–9)	left-hand thumb rule (left-hand version)
fingers = conventional current or electron flow			
Generator Effect			
thumb = movement of conductor on armature		right-hand generator rule (see Figure 5–12)	left-hand generator rule (left-hand version)
index finger = magnetic lines of force field			
middle finger = current or electron flow			
Motor Principle			
thumb = movement of conductor on rotor		left-hand motor rule (see Figure 5–18)	right-hand motor rule (right-hand version)
index finger = magnetic lines of force field			
middle finger = current or electron flow			

rized in Table 5–1. Before learning any of the rules, it is critical to remember that **hand rules which are based on current flow (conventional current direction) and hand rules which are based on electron flow (actual direction of electron movement) will be exact opposites**. For example, the right-hand thumb rule applies to conventional current flow. This is identical to the left-hand thumb rule applied to actual electron flow.

The hand thumb rule, the first of the hand rules, applies to remembering the relationship between the direction of current along a conductor and the direction of the resulting magnetic lines of force field. **Fleming's right-hand thumb rule states that if the right hand is used to grasp a conducting wire with the thumb in the direction of the current flow, the fingers will indicate the direction of the magnetic field lines of force surrounding the conductor** (Figure 5–7). (If the thumb points in the direction of actual electron flow, then a left-hand thumb rule must be used to show the direction of the magnetic field lines of force surrounding the conductor.) Table 5–1 compares this rule with the other "hand" rules.

Solenoids and Electromagnets

An interesting phenomenon occurs when conducting wire is looped (Figure 5–8A). Using the right-hand thumb rule to determine the direction of the magnetic lines of flux, it is apparent that inside the loop the magnetic fields from both sides join to double the magnetic flux density. If a series of loops are made, creating a coil (Figure 5–8B), the flux density is

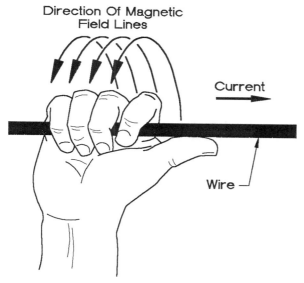

Direction Of Magnetic
Field Lines

Current

Wire

Figure 5–7. Fleming's right-hand thumb rule: When the right hand is positioned so the thumb points in the direction of conventional current flow, the fingers indicate the direction of the induced magnetic field. Fleming's left-hand thumb rule does the same for actual electron flow. (Adapted from Gates, Earl D. *Introduction to Electronics: A Practical Approach*. Albany: Delmar Publishers, 1987.)

greatly increased. When current is flowing through this type of coil it is called a **solenoid**. The flux density can be increased further still by adding a ferromagnetic core. This configuration is called an **electromagnet**. **The strength of solenoids and electromagnets is determined by the number of loops (or turns) of wire, the current strength and the permeability of the core**. The right-hand thumb rule can also be applied to a solenoid or an electromagnet to determine the location of the magnetic poles. **If the fingers point in the direction of the current, the thumb will point toward the north pole** (Figure 5–9). (If the fingers point in the direction of actual electron flow, then a left-hand thumb rule must be used for the thumb to point toward the north pole.) Table 5–1

above compares this rule with the other "hand" rules.

Both the solenoid and the electromagnet demonstrate magnetic properties only while electric current is flowing. If the current stops flowing, the magnetic properties vanish, and if the current is adjusted up or down, the magnetic strength changes accordingly. The factors that govern the effectiveness of solenoids and electromagnets are the **diameter** of the coil, its **length** and the **current** passing along the coil. Electromagnets are used as remote control devices in circuit breakers and in the temporary locks, sometimes called detents, on radiographic equipment. In a typical circuit breaker configuration a wire from the circuit to be protected is incorporated into an electromagnet which, when the current becomes dangerously high, has been calculated to attract a movable contact which breaks the circuit.

Solenoids are often used as detent locks on the overhead crane of x-ray tubes. The detent can be activated by a switch at the x-ray tube controls. The switch activates the magnetic properties of the solenoid, which in turn attracts a metal latch or bolt. This temporarily locks the tube to the center of the x-ray table or at the proper distance from a film holder. **Electromagnetic relays** are similar to circuit breakers. They are used to protect radiographers from electrical shock by isolating control buttons on the x-ray console from the actual circuit in which high voltage is flowing.

Electromagnetic Induction

Once it became known that electrical current could generate a magnetic field, the obvious question was whether the reverse was true. The fact that it is was demonstrated by the English physicist Michael Faraday (1791–1867) the year after Oersted's discovery. The simple presence of a magnetic field is not sufficient to cause electrons to move along a wire. Faraday discovered that the magnetic lines of

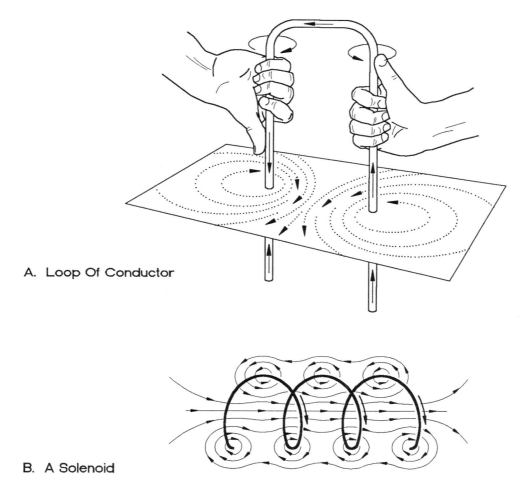

A. Loop Of Conductor

B. A Solenoid

Figure 5–8.   A solenoid: (A) When a conductor is looped to form a coil, the magnetic fields from both sides join to double the magnetic field strength inside the loop. (B) A solenoid is a helix coil through which current is flowing; it uses the coil loops to produce a greatly strengthened magnetic field.

force and the wire must have a motion relative to each other to induce an electrical current (Figure 5–10). There are three ways to create the motion between lines of force and a conductor:

1. **Move the conductor** through a stationary, unchanging strength magnetic field.

2. **Move magnetic lines of force** through a stationary conductor with an unchanging strength magnetic field.

3. **Vary the magnetic flux strength** from a stationary magnet through a stationary conductor. As the flux strength varies, the lines of force will expand and contract, in effect

Figure 5–9. Fleming's right-hand thumb rule applied to determining the pole of a solenoid or electromagnet. When the fingers point in the direction of the current, the thumb will point toward the north pole.

A. Without Relative Motion

B. With Relative Motion

Figure 5–10. Faraday's experiment: a meter will not indicate current flow (A) until the magnetic lines of force from the magnet and wire have a motion relative to one another (B).

causing the relative motion necessary to induce current.

The exact definitions of "magnetic flux strength" and "lines of force" are critical to understanding these differences.

There are two primary laws that govern the induction of current by magnetic fields. Faraday's law (sometimes called The First Law of Electromagnetics) states that four factors regulate the strength of induced current when magnetic lines of force and a conductor are in motion relative to one another:

1. the **strength** of the magnetic field,

2. the **speed** of the motion between lines of force and the conductor,

3. the **angle** between the magnetic lines of force and the conductor and

4. the **number of turns** in the conducting coil.

This law makes it possible to determine the direction in which the induced current will flow.

This application of the law was established by the Russian scientist Heinrich Lenz (1804–1865). Lenz's law (sometimes called The Second Law of Electromagnetics) states that induced current flow sets up a magnetic field opposing the action that produced the original current, or, simply, that induced current opposes any flux change.

These two laws apply to both forms of induction: mutual induction and self-induction. **Mutual induction** occurs when two coils are placed in proximity and a varying current supplied to the first coil (as an electromagnet) induces a similar flow in the second coil (Figure 5–11). The coil supplied with current is called the **primary** coil while the coil in which the

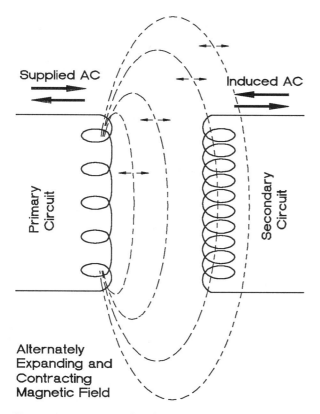

Figure 5–11. Mutual induction: A varying current supplied to the primary coil induces a similar flow in the second coil. The constantly expanding and contracting magnetic lines of force induced in the primary coil provide the relative motion with the secondary coil necessary to induce current flow in the secondary circuit.

current is inducted is called the **secondary** coil. The flow occurs in the secondary coil because the primary current alternates. This follows the rule that moving lines of force from a varying intensity current will induce electron flow in the wire through which it passes. In this case the secondary coil is cut by the varying (and therefore moving) lines of force from the current in the primary coil.

Self-induction is much more complicated but is more understandable when comparing a coil supplied with direct current, where there is no self-induction, with a coil supplied with alternating current, where self-induction occurs. Alternating current is present when the electrons constantly change direction. A coil supplied with alternating current permits a steady flow of electrons and establishes an electromagnetic effect for half the cycle. However, at the instant the current supply reverses, the previously established electromagnetic north and south poles will induce an opposing potential difference, thus attempting to induce against the incoming supply of electrons. This tendency of an alternating current is called **inductive reactance** and is measured in ohms of resistance. Self-induction is useful when it is desirable to permit direct current to flow while at the same time hindering alternating current.

An important relationship is that between the direction of movement of a wire coil (the armature), the direction of the magnetic lines of force field and the direction in which the induced current will flow. This relationship is best remembered by the use of another "hand" rule (Figure 5–12). **Fleming's right-hand generator rule states that if the thumb points in the direction the conductor (or armature) is moving and the index finger points in the direction of the magnetic lines of force field, then the middle finger will indicate the direction of the conventional current.** (If the direction of actual electron flow is desired,

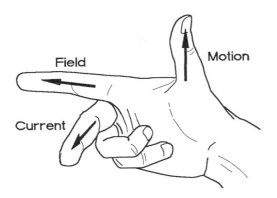

Figure 5–12. Fleming's right-hand generator rule: When the thumb points in the direction the conductor (or armature) is moving and the index finger points in the direction of the magnetic lines of force field, the middle finger indicates the direction of conventional current flow. Fleming's left-hand generator rule does the same for actual electron flow.

then a left-hand generator rule must be used.) Table 5–1 compares this rule with the other "hand" rules.

Generators

A **generator**, or dynamo, is a device that converts mechanical energy to electrical energy using Faraday's discovery of moving lines of flux in relationship to a conductor to induce current. This process converts the mechanical energy of the motion (any of the three ways) to electrical energy. A simple generator is composed of a conductor and magnets arranged as shown in Figure 5–13. The conductor is a coil of wire, called an **armature**, set between opposing magnetic poles so that it encounters the strongest lines of force. If the armature is rotated by a strong source of mechanical energy (such as a steam or water turbine), the generator can produce massive amounts of electrical energy. It is important to note the method that is used to convey the electrical current from the armature to the circuit. A set of **slip rings**

and brushes permits the circuit to remain stationary while the armature rotates without breaking the electrical contact between them. This allows the electrons to flow without interruption. **Each slip ring connects to one end of the armature wire** (See Figure 5–13.)

To understand exactly how the current is produced it is necessary to follow the production step by step (Figure 5–14). Notice that the armature coil wire is shown in cross-section at the top, three-dimensionally in the middle, and that the graph at the bottom represents the voltage produced. It is important to understand the relationship of the angle between this wire's motion and the lines of force between the stationary magnets. In Figure 5–14A the wire's motion is parallel to the lines of force. This produces no emf, as shown on the graph. In Figure 5–14B the rotation of the armature has changed the wire's motion until it is at a 45° angle to the lines of force. Fleming's right-hand generator rule demonstrates that the conventional electrical current is moving into the page (electron flow would be out of the page). Because of the 45° angle, the magnitude of the emf, although rising, has not yet reached its peak. In Figure 5–14C, the motion of the wire is 90° to the lines of force (the maximum angle), resulting in the peak emf. As the wire begins to turn back to parallel in Figure 5–14D, the emf begins to drop back toward zero. When the wire reaches a parallel position, as in Figure 5–14E, the emf has returned to zero. As the wire begins to move into a 270° position (which is a 90° position in the opposite direction), notice that the relationship between the wire's motion and the lines of force has changed. Using Fleming's right-hand generator rule again, it is simple to see that the conventional electrical current has now reversed and is moving out of the page (while the electron flow has reversed to move into the page). **It is at this point that alternating current is produced**. This has occurred be-

Rotating Shaft (Attached to turbine or other
source of mechanical energy)

Figure 5–13.   An AC generator: Mechanical energy rotates the shaft
to which the armature is attached. As the wires of the armature rotate, they cut through the magnetic lines of flux from the magnets
and produce electrical current. The slip rings and brushes permit the
armature to rotate while maintaining contact with the wires of the
circuit.

cause **alternating current is produced when the wire's motion relative to the lines of force is reversed**. In Figures 5–14F, G, H, and I, the rise to peak and drop back to zero emf is repeated but in the opposite direction. This explains not only why generator-produced current must be alternating but also accounts for its pulsating nature.

The type of curve produced by an AC generator will always appear as in Figure 5–14. It is called a **sine wave** because it depends on the mathematical sine between the plane of the armature and a plane perpendicular to the lines of force. **One complete turn of the generator armature represents one cycle**. The sine wave illustrates one complete turn of the armature as the distance between two corresponding points. Note that this would be represented by the distance between a and i in

Figure 5–14. **The frequency of the sine wave is determined by the number of cycles per second (cps). The unit of frequency is the Hertz, represented by the symbol Hz. 1 cps = 1 Hz**. American and Canadian generators operate at 60 Hz. Most of the rest of the world operates at 50 Hz.

Example: How many times per second do the electrons in a 60 Hz alternating current change their direction of movement?

Answer:
60 Hz × 2 directions = 120 changes per second

From Figure 5–14, it also becomes apparent that the **peak voltage is not the same as the average voltage** throughout the entire sine wave. The same is true of amperage and resistance (Ohm's law). This makes the mea-

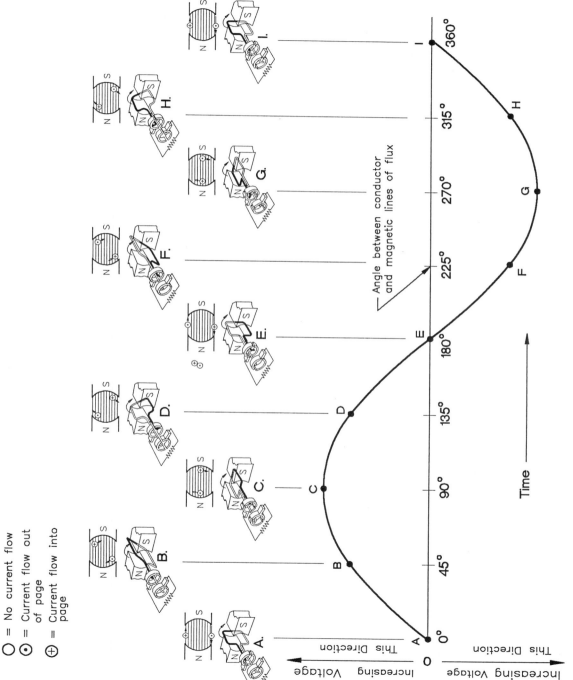

O = No current flow

⊙ = Current flow out of page

⊕ = Current flow into page

Figure 5–14. The production of alternating current: Armature coil wire is shown in cross-section (*top*). Three-dimensional view of generator (*middle*). Graph of the voltage produced (*bottom*). See text for step-by-step description.

surement of all factors very difficult in pulsating alternating current because of the constant fluctuation of the sine wave. This is solved by using the root mean square (rms) values of the amperage and voltage. **Root mean square (rms) values of the total voltage and amperage in an alternating current are equivalent to the effect that would be produced in a direct current resistance by the same factors**. Resistance in alternating currents is calculated from a complicated series of factors, resulting in measurement of the apparent total resistance. **Apparent total resistance of an alternating current is called impedance, which is represented by the symbol Z**. This permits a revised version of Ohm's law to be applied for alternating current as:

$$I = \frac{V}{Z}$$

where: I = rms amperage
V = rms voltage
Z = impedance

When using an x-ray machine, it is worth remembering that the **kilovoltage settings represent peak kilovoltage, not average or rms values**.

A **direct-current generator** is made by exchanging the slip rings for a commutator ring,

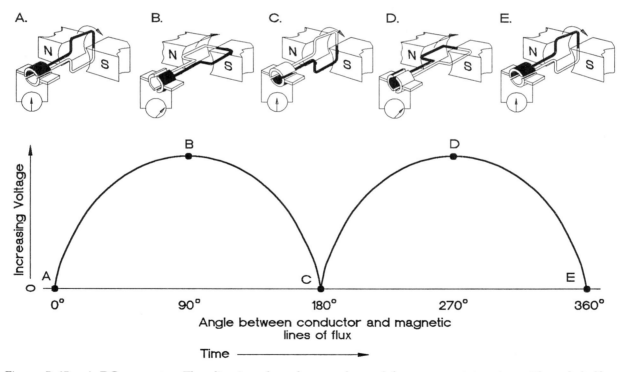

Figure 5–15. A DC generator: The slip rings have been exchanged for a commutator ring with each half connecting to one end of the armature wire. Although the armature turns exactly as in an AC generator, the commutator routes the current as shown on the graph. See text for step-by-step description. (Adapted from Loper, Orla E., Arthur F. Ahr, and Lee R. Clendenning. *Introduction to Electricity and Electronics*. Albany: Delmar Publishers, 1973.)

as shown in Figure 5–15. **A commutator is a single ring that is divided in half, with each half connected to one end of the armature wire**. The single commutator's two halves replace the pair of slip rings. Instead of each end of the armature wire being connected to its own slip ring, each end of the armature wire is connected to half of the commutator ring.

Figure 5–16. Multiple coil, split commutator, DC generator: more than one coil, or armature, with a split commutator (A) will produce DC current as shown in the graph (B). (Adapted from Loper, Orla E., Arthur F. Ahr, and Lee R. Clendenning. *Introduction to Electricity and Electronics*. Albany: Delmar Publishers, 1973.)

When a generator has its armature connected to a commutator, the sine wave of the output is dramatically different from that produced by a pair of slip rings. Although the armature turns exactly as in an alternating current generator, the commutator routes the current very differently. This current produces a sine wave exactly as in an alternating current generator (Figures 5–15A–C). The use of Fleming's right-hand generator rule demonstrates that the conventional electrical current is moving into the page (electron flow would be out of the page). In Figure 5–15D the wire has begun to move toward the second phase of the cycle. As in the alternating-current generator, the relationship between the wire's motion and the lines of force has changed. Using Fleming's right-hand generator rule again, it is simple to see that the conventional electrical current has now reversed and is moving out of the page (while

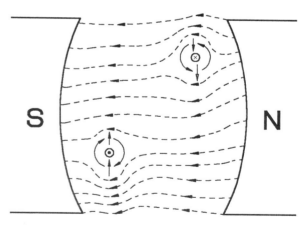

Figure 5–17. The motor principle: Because the conducting wires of the armature lie within the lines of force from the stationary magnets, when current begins to flow through the armature, the induced lines of force will be attracted downward for the left wire and upward for the right wire while at the same time being repelled in the other direction (upward for the left wire and downward for the right wire). The net result is that the conductor begins to move in the direction of the arrows.

the electron flow has reversed to move into the page). However, it is extremely important to note that in Figure 5–15D, the commutator ring has also changed the brush with which it was in contact. This has the same effect as switching the exiting connections on the armature wires. **Although Fleming's right-hand generator rule demonstrates the change in direction of current within the armature wire, the commutator ring has also reversed the exiting connections, thus keeping the current in the circuit flowing in the same direction. It is at this point that direct current is produced.** Note that the direct current is not as steady as would be expected with a battery source. Instead a pulsating direct current has been produced.

Multiple-coil direct-current generators are used in place of the simple single-coil generators diagrammed in Figures 5–14 and 5–15. These DC generators utilize numerous coils and a commutator divided into a corresponding number of segments, as shown in Figure 5–16A. This type of generator produces a sine wave, as shown in Figure 5–16B. The combined current generated never drops to zero and has the advantage of a much steadier flow, although the pulsations have not been completely eliminated.

Motors

A device that is supplied with electrical current to produce mechanical motion is called a motor. Motors have essentially the same parts as generators and operate on the same principles, but in reverse. In addition, some of the parts have been slightly redesigned and carry names different from those in a generator.

The motor principle is a result of the interaction of magnetic fields when an electric current is sent along a conductor that is residing in a magnetic field. As current flows through the conducting coil, a magnetic field is established, according to Fleming's right-hand thumb rule (Figure 5–17). Because the conducting coil lies within the lines of force from the stationary magnets, the induced lines of force will be attracted in one direction (downward for the left wire and upward for the right wire) while at the same time being repelled in the other direction (upward for the left wire and downward for the right wire). The net result is that the conductor begins to move in the direction of the arrows.

Fleming's left-hand motor rule states that if the index finger points in the direction of the magnetic lines of force field and the middle finger points in the direction of the conventional current, the thumb will indicate the direction the conductor will move (Figure 5–18). (This would be a right-hand motor rule if the direction of electron flow is being considered.) Table 5–1 compares this rule with the other "hand" rules.

Different motor configurations are required depending on whether alternating or direct current is supplied. **Direct-current motors use commutator rings**. As with a DC generator, the commutator is required in order to switch the flow of current when the conducting coil begins to reach a 180° position, where the induced and stationary lines of force no longer attract or repel one another. When the current flow is switched by the commutator ring, the magnetic lines of force also reverse. Continuing this switching of current flow results in the conductor continually being simultaneously repelled and attracted in a circle, thus turning a shaft and supplying the mechanical motion as a conversion of the applied electrical energy.

These direct-current motors use many turns of wire in the conductor coil to increase the strength of the field. This requires numerous pairs of stationary magnets to force the conductor coil to cut the stationary lines of force as near to 90° (the maximum inducing angle) as often as possible (Figure 5–19).

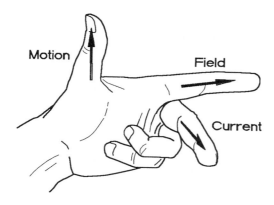

Figure 5–18. Fleming's left-hand motor rule: If the index finger points in the direction of the magnetic lines of force and the middle finger points in the direction of the conventional current flow, the thumb will indicate the direction the conductor will move. (This would be a right-hand motor rule if the direction of actual electron flow is being considered.)

Alternating-current motors use slip rings. Unlike direct-current motors, the incoming current switches direction, making the commutator unnecessary. There are two major types of alternating current motors.

Synchronous alternating-current motors have conducting coils that turn at the same speed as the generator armature supplying the current (or a multiple of the armature's speed). Synchronous motors are useful when a steady speed is necessary, as in a timing device. They tend to be relatively weak because insufficient motor principle force is established at the conducting coil.

Alternating-current induction motors utilize a rotor coil with the exterior magnetic field supplied by several pairs of electromagnets, thus producing a strong magnetic field, increasing the power of the motor and permitting it to run at any desired speed. Instead of supplying current to the coil in the magnetic field, an induction motor uses a device called a rotor. **A rotor consists of bars of copper around**

an iron core (see Figure 5–19). No commutator or slip rings are required. Instead, a device called a stator is used. **A stator consists of pairs of stationary magnets (or, more commonly, electromagnets) arranged around the rotor. The stator must be supplied with multiphase current.** The stator electromagnets are energized in sequence. As the copper bars of the rotor reach a point where the motor principle forces are equalized, the multiphase current activates the next pair of electromagnets and the motor principle forces pull the rotor around to the next position. This continuing sequential energization causes the motor principle forces to continually turn the rotor. Extremely powerful induction motors are made by increasing the strength and number of pairs

Figure 5–19. Alternating-current induction motor: The rotor windings obey the motor principle as they move perpendicular to the magnetic lines of flux, in the direction of the arrows. The stator electromagnets are supplied with multiphase current to activate them in sequential pairs to maintain maximum perpendicular motor principle force.

of electromagnets; these motors are popular for industrial and consumer uses.

Induction motors are used in rotating anode x-ray tubes where the target anode is attached to the induction motor rotor inside the glass vacuum tube. Because magnetic lines of force will pass through glass and a vacuum, the electromagnets can be positioned outside the vacuum tube, thus avoiding interference with the high voltages required to produce x-rays.

The motor principle is also used in meters: **galvanometers for direct current**, when permanent magnets are used, to indicate current and **dynamometers for alternating current**, when electromagnets are used (Figure 5–20A). To a great extent they are being replaced by digital meters that provide numerical indications of current. **When a meter is connected in parallel**, it measures current in amperes and is called an **ammeter (Figure 5–20B). When connected in series, it measures potential difference in volts and is called a voltmeter** (Figure 5–20C).

CONTROLLING ELECTRICAL CURRENT

Transformers

Alternating current, because of its changing direction, constantly establishes, collapses, re-establishes and re-collapses its surrounding magnetic field. This aspect can be used to change electricity by combining electromagnetic mutual induction with an application of Ohm's law to form a device called a **transformer**. Transformers are composed of two coils placed near one another (but without electrical connection). If current is supplied to one coil, the lines of force that are induced will pass through the other coil and induce a flow of electrons (see Figure 5–11). The coil that is supplied with current is the **primary**, while the coil in which current is induced is the **secondary**.

The number of turns of wire in the primary coil is designed to be different from the number of turns of wire in the secondary. This causes the induced current to be different in

    A. A Galvanometer   B. Ammeter in Circuit   C. Voltmeter in Circuit

Figure 5–20.   (A) A simple galvanometer uses an electromagnet to attract a coil of wire to which a needle is attached. When a scale is calibrated, amperage or voltage can be measured. (B) Ammeter connection. (C) Voltmeter connection.

the secondary coil. For example, the lines of force induced by a single primary coil loop may cut two loops of the secondary. In this case the voltage in the primary would be induced in **both** secondary loops, thus doubling the secondary voltage. When the voltage is increased from primary to secondary it is called a **step-up transformer**. When the voltage is decreased from primary to secondary it is called a **step-down transformer**. The **transformer law** expresses this phenomenon:

$$\frac{V_s}{V_p} = \frac{N_s}{N_p}$$

where: V = potential difference in volts
N = number of turns of wire in the coil
p = primary coil
s = secondary coil

Example: If a transformer is supplied with 400 volts to the primary coil, has 100 turns of wire on the primary coil and 20,000 turns of wire on the secondary coil, what will the voltage be in the secondary coil?

Answer:

$$\frac{V_s}{V_p} = \frac{N_s}{N_p}$$

$$\frac{V_s}{400 \text{ V}} = \frac{20,000 \text{ turns}}{100 \text{ turns}}$$

$$100 \, V_s = 400 \text{ V} \times 20,000 \text{ turns}$$

$$V_s = \frac{8,000,000}{100}$$

$$V_s = 80,000 \text{ volts or 80 kilovolts}$$

Example: If a transformer has 120 turns of wire on the primary coil, 80 volts in the primary coil and 20 volts in the secondary coil, how many turns of wire must there be in the secondary coil?

Answer:

$$\frac{V_s}{V_p} = \frac{N_s}{N_p}$$

$$\frac{20 \text{ V}}{80 \text{ V}} = \frac{N_s}{120 \text{ turns}}$$

$$\frac{2,400 \text{ turns}}{80} = N_s$$

$$N_s = 30 \text{ turns}$$

Transformers are used to change voltage. However, Ohm's law is in effect and the effect of the transformer on amperage, voltage and number of turns in the coils can be calculated by combining the transformer law with Ohm's law:

$$\frac{I_s}{I_p} = \frac{V_p}{V_s}$$

and:

$$\frac{I_s}{I_p} = \frac{N_p}{N_s}$$

It is helpful to remember that voltage and number of turns are directly proportional, while voltage and amperage are inversely proportional. Therefore, the number of turns and amperage must also be inversely proportional. It is also important to note that a step-up transformer increases voltage from primary to secondary while decreasing amperage. Conversely, a step-down transformer decreases voltage from primary to secondary while increasing amperage. Because transformers are designed to change voltages, the descriptive terms step-up and step-down refer to the voltage change, not the amperage change. You should remember that Ohm's law requires the consideration of resistance and this is indeed an important factor. However, this book will not address that aspect. **All transformers must** operate on alternating current to provide the establishing and collapsing magnetic fields that induce the voltage changes in the secondary coil.

Although transformer efficiency, the ability of a transformer to avoid power loss, is usually above 95 percent, a number of factors influence how much energy is lost. Because the high voltage transformer used in x-ray equipment must step up voltage into the kilovolt range, it uses large amounts of secondary coil windings. This massive amount of wire and the high induced voltage cause several problems that greatly affect the efficiency of the transformer.

1. **I^2R loss**, sometimes called copper loss, is caused by the inherent resistance to current flow that is found in all conductors. The power lost due to this resistance is proportional to the square of the current. It is minimized by using low-resistance wire, such as large-diameter copper, and by using high voltage and low amperage. Lost power is given off as heat. This is the reason why power transmitted long distances between cities is carried on high-voltage power lines. The high voltage permits low amperage and greatly reduced I^2R loss. Because high voltages are extremely dangerous, they are carried on high towers. Step-down transformers are used at receiving stations to lower the voltage (and increase the amperage) to make the power safe for use in buildings.

2. **Hysteresis loss** (lagging loss) in the core occurs because energy is expended as the continually changing AC current magnetizes, demagnetizes and remagnetizes the core material. Demagnetization leaves some dipoles in the original orientation, and this residual magnetism causes the remagnetic effort to lag. The characteristic that requires energy to carry out this constant reorientation of the magnetic dipoles is called **coer-**

civity. Coercivity can be minimized by using a core material such as silicon iron.

3. **Eddy current loss** in the core is a result of currents opposing the cause which produced them, according to Lenz's law, as discussed earlier. They are produced in any conducting material subjected to changing magnetic fields. Laminating the transformer core reduces the eddy current loss by dividing the core into thin layers. This reduces the strength of the eddy currents (Figure 5–21).

These factors result in a great amount of heat build-up which can be felt by placing your hand on the exterior of the transformer cabinet in a diagnostic x-ray room. Although the transformer is highly insulated and immersed in insulating dielectric oil, there is a definite warmth to the cabinet after the machine has been in use for a few hours. The size of the x-ray transformer makes its efficiency an important factor.

There are numerous types of transformer configurations. The simple arrangement of two coils of wire in proximity to facilitate induction, that has been used so far to explain transformer function, is called an **air core** transformer. If the primary and secondary coils are filled with an iron core, the strength of the magnetic field is greatly increased, forming an **open-core** transformer. Various types of cores have been designed to enhance the lines of force and thereby increase the magnetic field strength (Figure 5–22). The field from an open core tends to diverge as it forms the external lines of force. Closing the core to form a **closed-core** transformer (by placing a top and bottom to the cores) will direct the lines of force from primary and secondary cores toward each other and result in a significant system net increase in field strength. The **shell type** transformer goes one step further by converging both the inside and outside lines of force through an iron core. In addition, a great efficiency is obtained by insulating the wiring and wrapping the primary and secondary coils atop one another, thus minimizing the distance between coils and maximizing the coupling effectiveness of the induction. X-ray generators use laminated core, shell type transformers.

Autotransformers

It is possible to construct a variable transformer, called an **autotransformer**, by connecting both primary and secondary coils in series instead of insulating them. This also permits a single coil on a central core. Connections are made along a single coil at different points for primary and secondary. The secondary side has a selection of taps available to permit a variable number of turns in the secondary coil (Figure 5–23). When the connections to the taps are attached to control buttons, an effective means of changing voltage is available.

Autotransformers are not suitable for use in the high-voltage transformers in x-ray machines. However, they are suitable for controlling voltage on the low-voltage side of the x-ray circuit before it has been increased by the main step-up transformer, thereby varying the voltage on the high-voltage side as well.

There are three important transformers in the x-ray circuit (Figure 5–24). The autotransformer is used to vary the incoming-line voltage to an appropriate level for the high-voltage step-up transformer. The high-voltage step-up transformer is used to raise the incoming-line voltage to the kilovoltage range necessary for x-ray production. The filament step-down transformer is used to decrease the incoming-line voltage to the 5–15 volt and 3–5 ampere range used to heat the x-ray tube filament.

Capacitors

A **capacitor** is a device capable of accumulating and storing an electrical charge. A simple capacitor consists of two insulated metal plates with opposite charges (Figure 5–25). The repulsion between the charges on the

A. Closed Core Transformer

B. Non Laminated Core

C. Eddy Currents

D. Laminated Core

E. Eddy Currents

Figure 5–21. (A) A Closed-core transformer, (B) nonlaminated core, (C) nonlaminated core eddy currents, (D) laminated core, and (E) laminated core eddy currents.

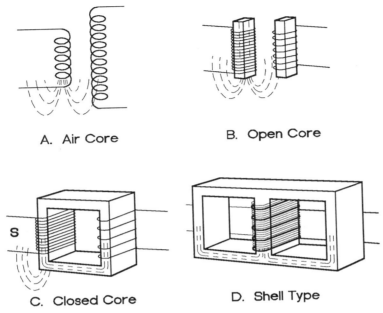

A. Air Core   B. Open Core

C. Closed Core   D. Shell Type

Figure 5–22. Various types of transformer core configurations: (A) air core, (B) open core, (C) closed core, and (D) shell type.

two plates permits a greater number of electrons to be stored on each. The insulation between the plates is called the **dielectric** and its value is determined by the insulating ability as well as the plate size, distance between the plates, and charge. The unit of capacitance is named for Faraday but has been shortened to **farad**. It is represented by the symbol **f** and is expressed as:

$$C = \frac{q}{V}$$

where: c = capacitance in farads
q = charge on either plate in coulombs
V = potential difference between plates in volts

Because of the immense size of the coulomb, the farad is very large, making the microfarad (μf) the more common unit.

Capacitors must be charged to be operable; this is done by applying a direct-current voltage. The capacitor will accept a charge until it equals the DC voltage. When discharged, the capacitor has the ability to deliver the stored charge in short and easily controlled intervals. This uniform direct current is especially useful in mobile x-ray units where it is convenient to have a battery charge a capacitor and then initiate a burst of high voltage for the x-ray exposure. Capacitors are also used to supply a more constant voltage to the x-ray tube in some stationary units.

RECTIFICATION

X-ray tubes operate best when receiving direct current. In fact, there is a danger in supplying alternating current because if a flow of electrons occurs in the wrong direction the tube may be damaged beyond repair. **Rectification is the process by which alternating cur-**

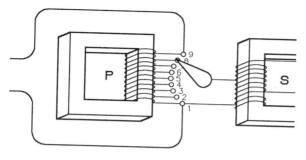

Figure 5–23. An autotransformer.

rent is changed to pulsating direct current, and requires the use of one-way electrical devices called rectifiers. Although solid-state semiconductor diodes are most commonly used, it is easier to understand the operation of a vacuum-tube rectifier. Both of these devices create electrical "one-way streets" by permitting electrons to flow easily in one direction while offering a high resistance to movement in the other direction.

The operation of semiconductors was mentioned earlier, in Chapter 4, during the discussion of conductor valence bands. There are numerous types of semiconductors but they all operate in the same manner. The sim-

Figure 5–24. Three critical transformer locations in the diagnostic x-ray circuit. The autotransformer permits selection of the voltage (by controls labeled kV on the console). The high-voltage transformer steps the incoming-line voltage up to the kV range before sending it to the x-ray tube. The filament transformer steps the incoming-line voltage down to heat the x-ray tube filament.

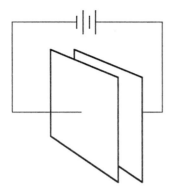

Figure 5–25. A simple parallel plate capacitor.

plest to explain is the p-n junction semiconductor, which is composed of solid materials of two predominant categories, n-type and p-type. N-type materials have loosely bound electrons that move freely between an atom's conduction bands. P-type materials have electron traps made up of positively charged holes that tend to attract and hold electrons instead of permitting them to move freely to another atom. Both types of materials are affected by slight amounts of impurities which are intentionally added to change the conduction properties. For example, arsenic has a valence that permits it to form covalent bonds with silicon crystals, but it makes an extra electron available for conduction, thus forming an n-type material. Conversely, gallium also has a valence permitting covalent bonding with silicon, but it leaves a need for an additional electron, thus forming an electron "hole" and a p-type material.

A rectifying semiconductor called a **diode** is made by sandwiching a p-type crystal with an n-type to form a p-n junction (Figure 5–26). When a potential difference is established with the positive charge at the p side of the junction and the negative charge at the n side, the positive holes from the p side are attracted to the junction, as are the available electrons from the n side. This permits easy movement of elec-

trons into the p holes. **In a diode, electrons flow from the n to the p side of the p-n junction and conventional electrical current moves from the p to the n side**. When alternating current reverses and the positive charge is at the n side of the junction and the negative charge is at the p side, the positive holes from the p side are repelled from the junction, as are the available electrons from the n side. This makes movement of electrons from the n side of the junction to the p side very unlikely, as both the repulsion-attraction of the charges and the distance between p holes and electrons are working against the electron movement. The result is that no electrons move across the junction, thus creating a one-way street for electrons. The electronic symbol for a diode reflects this movement for conventional electrical current (Figure 5–26D). Remember that electron flow will be opposite the direction of the arrow.

A thyristor, or silicon-controlled rectifier (SCR), is a more complex semiconductor that has proven useful for high-speed switching of the primary high-voltage x-ray circuit. SCRs are composed of two p-type and two n-type layers, making three p-n junctions (Figure 5–27). Both n-p-n-p and p-n-p-n sequences are possible. In either case, the third section serves as a gate. This gate can change the polarity of the entire SCR by receiving a given charge. Rapid pulses of current to the gate permit it to hold or release large amounts of current. The SCR functions extremely rapidly and has replaced mechanical switchers and thyratrons (gas-filled predecessors to thyristors) in high kilowattage x-ray generators.

A valve tube was a vacuum tube that operated in the same manner as a diode but was constructed like an x-ray tube. Although they are no longer used in x-ray circuitry, they are a useful example in learning how a modern diode circuit functions. The difference between a valve tube and an x-ray tube is that a valve tube operated at energies below the range nec-

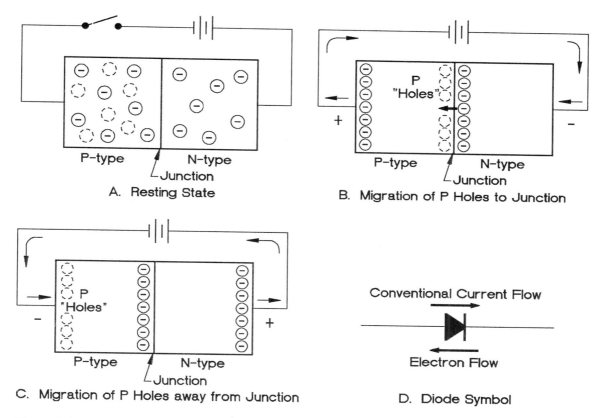

Figure 5–26.   The functioning of a p-n junction of a solid-state semiconductor diode.

essary to produce x-ray photons. The cathode and anode were arranged to permit electrons to jump without requiring the energy necessary to produce x-rays (Figure 5–28). Current could flow from cathode to anode because the jump to the massive anode was easy. However, as electrons repelled one another they spread out over the entire surface of the anode and could not develop sufficient repulsive force to jump to the cathode. This made the tube a one-way street for electrons to move from cathode to anode.

The **cathode included a coil of small-diameter tungsten wire, called the filament, through which current was passed**. Of course the small diameter of the wire caused a greatly increased resistance to the flow of electrons. This resulted in heat increase to the extent that electron movement actually ejected individual electrons from the surface of the wire. Sometimes this phenomenon is described as a boiling of electrons from the surface. The result was the formation of an electron cloud (Figure 5–28B). This process is called **thermionic emission** because the heat (therm) has caused ionization (ionic), resulting in electrons being expelled (emission) from the surface of the wire. This effect is sometimes called a **space charge cloud**. It is important to note that the small diameter of the cathode's thin filament wire makes it extremely fragile. At the high kilovoltages supplied to x-ray tubes, a single

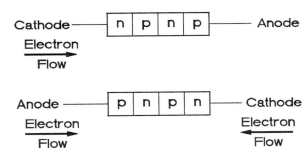

Figure 5–27. Silicon-controlled rectifier (SCR) n-p-n-p and p-n-p-n junctions.

A. Valve Tube Anode and Cathode

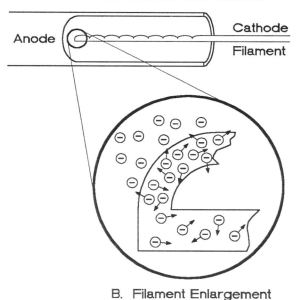

B. Filament Enlargement

Figure 5–28.   Anode and cathode of a valve tube.

electron striking the heated filament would cause it to break, thus rendering the tube useless. All modern x-ray machines use safety devices to prevent the anode side of the tube from receiving electrons, even during the opposing flow of alternating current.

The anode is a relatively large metallic surface, usually a cup, disk or flat plate, depending on the desired function of the tube. The shape of the anode varies between a valve tube and an x-ray tube and this accounts for the fact that x-ray tubes emit primarily x-ray range photons while valve tubes do not. Diagnostic x-ray tubes utilize angled disks, while dental x-ray tubes and other types of relatively low-voltage tubes use flat-plate anodes. A valve-tube anode consists of a cold metallic cup that surrounds the coiled filament (Figure 5–28).

Valve tubes permit electrons to flow from cathode to anode when a large enough potential difference exists to cause the electrons of the thermionically emitted cloud to be simultaneously repelled from the cathode and attracted to the anode. This is done by creating a **negative charge at the cathode and a positive charge at the anode (Figure 5–29). Remember that electron flow will always be from cathode to anode and this means conventional electrical current will always be from anode to cathode**. It is important to note that electrons cannot move from anode to cathode due to the charges and to the shapes of the anode and cathode. The anode is shaped much larger than the cathode filament and this causes the electrons to distribute themselves over the entire surface as they follow the law of repulsion in regard to one another (see Figure 5–29). With such a large distribution surface, the electrons should not build up enough repulsion or heat to make movement from anode to cathode possible. When direct current causes the anode to remain positive at all times, there is a force of attraction working to keep the electrons on the anode. On the other hand, the cathode is relatively small and carries a negative charge at all times. The small size not only causes heating, it also restricts the flow of electrons so much that thermionic emission is enhanced. The negative charge works to encourage thermionic emission by actively repelling the electrons from the filament surface.

Together these forces make the anode very attractive to electrons, while making the cathode undesirable. Consequently, as electron movement from cathode to anode is made easy, movement from anode to cathode is made extremely difficult. This creates a one-way street for electron flow, just as in a diode.

Half-Wave Rectification

In both solid-state diodes and valve tubes the forces create an electronic one-way street and effectively suppress the opposing half of the incoming current flow. A supply of alternating current to either type of rectifier will result in a pulsating direct current due to the supression of half of the incoming wave (Figure 5–30). This type of suppression rectification is called **half-wave rectification** because only half of the incoming alternating current is being converted to pulsating direct current.

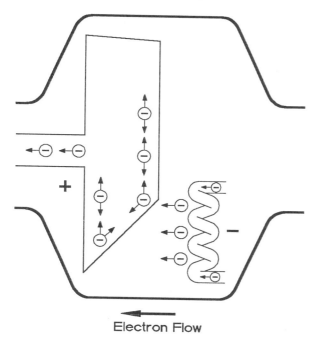

Electron Flow

Figure 5–29. Electron flow through an x-ray tube.

The opposing half of the flow is simply ignored and not utilized. In early radiography this type of circuit was called **self-rectification** (Figure 5–31). The danger was that overheating of the anode might cause thermionic emission. This condition could result in electrons moving to the cathode filament during the half of the alternating-current cycle when the anode was negatively charged. This of course would break the filament and destroy the x-ray tube. In even the simplest of modern x-ray equipment the x-ray tube is protected from this occurrence by the addition of a single rectifier on the anode side of the circuit (see Figure 5–30). This protects the x-ray tube anode from receiving a negative charge. In addition, if overheating should occur, the protecting rectifier would be destroyed and could be replaced, costing much less than it would to replace the x-ray tube.

Full-Wave Rectification

It is possible to convert the opposing half of the incoming current flow so that electrons are always moving in the same direction, instead of discarding half the cycle by suppression. This is done through an ingenious arrangement of four rectifiers in a bridge circuit called a **full-wave rectification circuit** (Figure 5–32). A full understanding of the circuit requires following the current completely from the secondary coil of the high-voltage step-up transformer to the x-ray tube during both halves of the AC cycle. Figure 5–32A illustrates the conventional current flow by the sequence of numbered arrows.

1. Conventional current flow is induced from the secondary coil of the high-voltage step-up transformer.

2. Current reaches the first circuit junction and flows both ways.

3. Current on this path reaches the anode of valve tube II and distributes over the large,

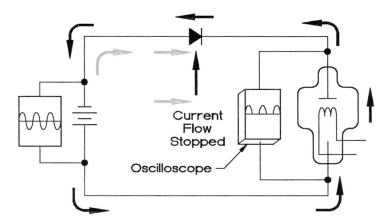

Figure 5–30. Half-wave rectification with one diode rectifier on the anode side of the x-ray tube circuit. Note the wave forms that would result if oscilloscopes were connected to the circuit.

unheated surface, attempting to build up enough charge to jump to the cathode.

4. Current on this path reaches the heated cathode of valve tube I and easily jumps to the anode (thus never permitting enough charge to accumulate for the current at arrow 3 to jump across valve tube II).

5. Current reaches the second junction and flows both ways.

6. Current on this path reaches the anode of valve tube III and distributes over the large, unheated surface, attempting to build up enough charge to jump to the cathode.

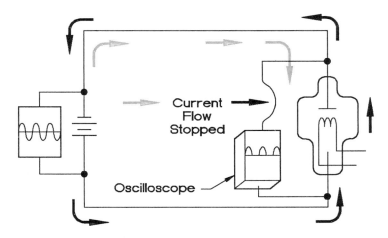

Figure 5–31. Half-wave rectification without a diode rectifier (self-rectification).

7. Current on this path moves without resistance toward the x-ray tube.

8. Current reaches the x-ray tube heated cathode and jumps to the anode.

9. X-rays are produced as a result of the current striking the anode.

10. Current from the anode moves without resistance back toward the rectification circuit.

11. Current reaches the third junction and flows both ways.

12. Current on this path reaches the heated cathode of valve tube II but cannot jump to

Figure 5–32. (A) A full-wave rectification circuit from within a basic diagnostic x-ray circuit. (See text for description of current flow.) (B) The full-wave rectified current sine wave.

the anode because the anode is still loaded with the charge moving at arrow 3. Because these are like charges, they repel one another.

13. Current on this path reaches the heated cathode of valve tube II and easily jumps to the anode.

14. Current reaches the fourth junction and flows both ways.

15. Current on this path reaches the heated cathode of valve tube III but cannot jump to the anode because the anode is still loaded with the charge moving at arrow 6. Because these are like charges, they repel one another.

16. From this point on, current on this path moves without resistance toward the secondary coil of the high-voltage step-up transformer. This completes the circuit.

Following the same logic, to trace the current path for the opposite half of the alternating current cycle in Figure 5–32 results in reorientation of the direction of current flow. This is full-wave rectification and it produces the sine wave shown in Figure 5–32B.

Note that **the x-ray tube will emit x-ray photons during both halves of the full-wave rectified AC cycle.** The double efficiency of full-wave rectification permits a significant increase in the power output capability of radiographic equipment. This results in an ability to use higher mA and kVp settings. Consequently, nearly all modern x-ray equipment is full-wave rectified.

SUMMARY

A magnetic force field surrounds all charged particles when they are in motion. These force fields are magnetic lines of force. Electromagnets are temporary magnets produced by moving electric current. The laws governing magnetism are similar to the laws of electrostatics. Electromagnetic induction is an important phenomenon basic to nearly all electrical devices. It is produced by movement between magnetic lines of force and a conductor.

A generator is a device that converts mechanical energy to electrical energy. Either AC or DC current can be produced through the use of either slip rings or a commutator ring. One complete turn of the generator armature represents one cycle (1 Hz). A device that is supplied with electrical current to produce mechanical motion is called a motor. Motors have essentially the same parts as generators and operate on the same principles, but in reverse. A meter may be connected in parallel to measure current or in series to measure voltage.

A transformer is used to change voltage through the use of Ohm's law. A capacitor is a device capable of accumulating and storing electrical charge. Rectification is the process by which alternating current is changed to pulsating direct current. Silicon-controlled rectifiers are solid-state semiconductors that are used for high-speed switching of the primary high-voltage x-ray circuit. Both self-wave and half-wave rectification are infrequently used in modern x-ray equipment. Diodes replaced valve tubes as one-way circuits that permit full-wave rectification.

REVIEW QUESTIONS

1. What is magnetism?

2. What is an electromagnet?

3. Explain the difference between electron flow and conventional current flow.

4. What is indicated by the direction of the thumb, forefinger, and fingers in one of Fleming's hand rules?

5. What are the three ways to induce electromagnetic current flow in a conductor?

6. Name the four factors controlling the strength of electromagnetically induced current.

7. What is the difference between a generator and a motor?

8. Describe the functions of slip rings and of a commutator ring.

9. How is an ammeter different from a voltmeter?

10. What is the function of a transformer?

11. State the transformer law.

12. What is the function of an autotransformer?

13. What is a diode?

14. What is rectification?

15. What components are necessary to produce a full-wave rectified circuit?

REFERENCES AND RECOMMENDED READING

Ball, J. L., and A. D. Moore. *Essential Physics for Radiographers*. 2nd ed. Oxford: Blackwell Scientific Publications, 1986.

Bushong, Stewart. *Radiologic Science for Technologists*. 4th ed. St. Louis, MO: C. V. Mosby Co., 1988.

Chesney, D. Noreen, and Muriel O. Chesney. *X-Ray Equipment for Student Radiographers*. 3rd ed. Oxford: Blackwell Scientific Publications, 1984.

Curry, Thomas S. III, James E. Dowdey, and Robert C. Murry. *Christensen's Introduction to the Physics of Diagnostic Radiology*. 3rd ed. Philadelphia, PA: Lea and Febiger, 1984.

DeFrance, J. J. *Electrical Fundamentals*. Englewood Cliffs, NJ: Prentice-Hall, 1969.

Del Toro, Vincent. *Principles of Electrical Engineering*. 2nd ed. Englewood Cliffs, NJ: Prentice-Hall, 1972.

Dendy, P. P., and B. Heaton. *Physics for Radiologists*. Oxford: Blackwell Scientific Publications, 1987.

Gates, Earl D. *Introduction to Electronics: A Practical Approach*. Albany, NY: Delmar Publishers, 1987.

Gifford, Derek. *A Handbook of Physics for Radiologists and Radiographers*. New York: John Wiley & Sons, 1984.

Glasser, Otto, Edith H. Quimby, Lauriston S. Taylor, J. L. Weatherwax, and Russell H. Morgan. *Physical Foundations of Radiology*. 3rd ed. New York: Paul B. Hoeber Division of Harper & Brothers, 1961.

Hay, George A., and Donald Hughes. *First-Year Physics for Radiographers*. London: Bailliere Tindall, 1972.

Johns, Harold E., and John R. Cunningham. *The Physics of Radiology*. 4th ed. Springfield, IL: Thomas, 1983.

Loper, Orla E., Arthur F. Ahr, and Lee R. Clendenning. *Introduction to Electricity and Electronics*. Albany, NY: Delmar Publishers, 1973.

Meredith, W. J., and J. B. Massey. *Fundamental Physics of Radiology*. 3rd ed. Chicago, IL: Yearbook Medical Publishers, 1977.

Nadon, John M., Bert J. Gelmine, and Edward D. McLaughlin. *Industrial Electricity*. 4th ed. Albany, NY: Delmar Publishers, 1989.

Ridgway, Arthur, and Walter Thumm. *The Physics of Medical Radiography*. Reading, MA: Addison-Wesley, 1973.

Selman, Joseph. *The Fundamentals of X-Ray and Radium Physics*. 7th ed. Springfield, IL: Thomas, 1985.

Sprawls, Perry. *Principles of Radiography for Technologists*. Rockville, MD: Aspen Publishers, 1990.

Sprawls, Perry. *Physical Principles of Medical Imaging*. Rockville, MD: Aspen Publishers, 1987.

Stockley, Sybil M. *A Manual of Radiographic Equipment*. Edinburgh: Churchill Livingstone, 1986.

Ter-Pogossian, Michel M. *The Physical Aspects of Diagnostic Radiology*. New York: Hoeber Medical Division, Harper & Row, 1967.

Thompson, Thomas T. *A Practical Approach to Modern Imaging Equipment*. 2nd ed. Boston, MA: Little, Brown, & Co., 1985.

van der Plaats, G. J. *Medical X-Ray Techniques in Diagnostic Radiology*. 4th ed. The Hague: Martinus Nijhoff Publishers, 1980.

Wilks, Robin J. *Principles of Radiological Physics*. Edinburgh: Churchill Livingstone, 1981.

THE CASE OF BLACK MEDIASTINUM

Upon processing a routine portable chest radiograph the patient's entire mediastinum appears black although all other densities are normal. What are some possible causes of this image?

Answers to the case studies can be found in Appendix E.

6 X-RAY EQUIPMENT

Suspended in icy silence
I look at myself from far off
Calmly, I feel free

Even though I'm not, now
Or ever:

The metal teeth of death bite
But spit me out

One more time:

When the technologist says breathe
I breathe.

Patricia Goedicke, "One More Time."

OUTLINE

TYPES OF X-RAY EQUIPMENT
POWER FOR X-RAY GENERATION
A BASIC X-RAY CIRCUIT
GENERATORS
AUTOMATIC EXPOSURE CONTROLS

OBJECTIVES

Upon completion of this chapter, the student should be able to:

1. Describe various diagnostic-equipment-table, tube-support, and ancillary-equipment configurations.
2. State incoming line current characteristics.
3. Describe the differences between single-phase and three-phase power.
4. Explain the functions of the basic components of the main and filament x-ray circuits.
5. Discuss the differences between single-phase, three-phase six- and twelve-pulse, and high-frequency waveforms on generator output.

6. Describe the function of capacitor discharge and battery-operated mobile units.
7. Explain the function of a falling load generator.
8. Differentiate phototimers from ionization chamber automatic exposure controls.
9. Describe the placement and function of a phototimer and an ionization chamber automatic exposure control.
10. Describe potential problems that could be caused by minimum reaction times.
11. Justify the use of backup time when using automatic exposure controls.

TYPES OF X-RAY EQUIPMENT

A vast number of uses for x-rays have been found in medicine and this has led to the development of a wide variety of categories and types of equipment (Figure 6–1). Medical x-ray units can be classified as **diagnostic** or **therapeutic**. Most diagnostic units are designed for specific procedures, such as general procedures, cardiac cathetererization, head procedures, fluoroscopy, etc. All of these units operate within the diagnostic x-ray range. This range is approximately 10–1,200 milliamperes (mA), 0.001–10 seconds, at a peak kilovoltage (kVp) of approximately 25 to 150. Therapeutic equipment operates at much higher energies, ranging from 4 to 40 million electron-volts (meV). Because of the extremely high voltages used, therapy equipment operates below 20 mA and with time settings in the range of 1 to 60 minutes.

Tables

The radiographic table is designed to support the patient in a position that will enhance radiographic examination. As any patient can attest, comfort is not the primary purpose of the table, although some institutions permit foam pads for lengthy examinations.

The tabletop must be uniformly radiolucent to easily permit x-rays to pass through. A Bakelite or similar surface is most common, although specialized applications, such as angiography, may use a carbon graphite fiber to reduce absorption of photons. Although flat tops are most common, curved tops are available. Curved (or dished) tops are usually used for fluoroscopic examinations. They are usually more comfortable for the patient and permit the body part to be placed slightly closer to the film for a more accurate image. Curved tops have two serious disadvantages. It is difficult for the radiographer to maintain a patient accurately in an oblique or lateral position on a curved top, and the top is entirely useless as a level support surface for a film cassette during tabletop radiography.

The tabletop must be **easily cleaned, hard to scratch, and without crevices where radiographic contrast media can accumulate**. It is sometimes necessary to remove body fluids after an examination and this must be possible to achieve in a quick and sanitary manner.

The table must **include space for a tray to hold film cassettes and a radiographic grid** (Figure 6–2). The tray is often called a "Bucky tray" in honor of Dr. Gustav Bucky (1880–1963), the inventor of the radiographic grid that is installed over the film cassette tray. The grid installation usually consists of a mechanism that will automatically move the grid during exposure. Many units include automatic exposure control sensors in the tray. Some tables use a stationary tray with a movable tabletop. Others use a tray that is movable along rails extending the length of the table with a stationary tabletop. Still others use a tray and top that are both partially movable. Some tabletops are motor driven and movable along their length. Others are floating tops which can be moved

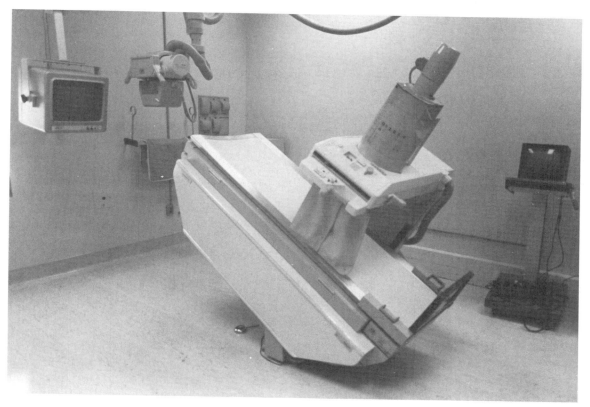

Figure 6–1.   A diagnostic radiographic unit.

along their length and width simultaneously when an electromagnetic brake is released. The brake may be controlled by hand, knee, or foot. Floating tops save radiographers significant amounts of time and effort, especially when positioning large patients.

Tables are available in **fixed** and **tilting** models. Fixed tables do not permit tilting the patient's head or feet down. They are designed for diagnostic radiographic work only. Tilting tables are sometimes described by their tilting capability (for example, 90–15 would indicate a table capable of tilting 90° in one direction and 15° in the other). Rooms designed to perform both diagnostic radiographic and fluoroscopic

(R&F) examinations are equipped with tilting tables, although some rooms designed only for radiographic examinations may also use them.

The table is usually at a height that reduces physical strain on the radiographer, who must stretch and bend over and around the table as the patient, ancillary equipment, film, and x-ray tube are positioned. This is usually 30–40 inches or 75–100 cm from the floor. This is not a safe or convenient height for patients and it causes problems for ambulatory patients who are not in good physical condition. A primary concern for all radiographers must be proper assistance to these patients when they are getting onto and down from the

Figure 6–2.   A diagnostic radiographic table. (Used by permission from Stockley, Sybil M. *A Manual of Radiographic Equipment.* Edinburgh: Churchill Livingstone, 1986.)

table. Fixed tables are available in adjustable models that can be lowered while a patient is assisted onto the table and then raised to a working height.

Ancillary equipment for tilting tables includes a **footboard** for patients to stand on when the table is upright. The footboard is often used for gastrointestinal studies when the patient begins the examination in a horizontal position and is then brought upright during the procedure, or vice versa. In these instances it is critical to ascertain that the footboard is securely in place and will support the full weight of the patient. This is best done when the table is horizontal by pulling hard on the footboard. Procedures requiring tilting the patient's head down, such as myelography, may require the use of **shoulder supports** to keep patients from sliding off the table. In these instances **handgrips** give the patient an added feeling of security.

Compression bands serve two functions: they restrain patients who are unable to cooperate, and they compress abdominal tissue for a more uniform subject density. Both functions improve radiographic image quality. A compression band should never be used as the sole restraint device.

Tube Supports

The tube support system is designed to permit the x-ray tube to be manipulated to the various locations necessary to obtain examination procedure projections and to hold the tube immobile during the exposure. Tube suspension systems are available in five versions: **overhead, floor-to-ceiling, floor, mobile and C-arm**. Both flexibility and cost are reflected in this order, with overhead supports being the most flexible and costly.

The **overhead suspension system**, sometimes called ceiling suspension, includes **two sets of rails** for controlling **longitudinal** and **transverse** positioning and a **telescoping column** for controlling vertical distance. The end of the telescoping column can be capable of **angling** up to a 300° arc toward the head or foot of the table, **rotating** up to 360° around the column, and **rolling or pitching** up to 60° transversely (side to side). A properly installed overhead suspension system will be perfectly counterbalanced and will not drift toward one side or corner of the room when the positioning locks are released. A well-designed system will permit the radiographer to remove the locks and "carry" the tube to any position within the room.

Each of these complex motions is locked into place by a solenoid with a control placed where it can be easily reached by the radiographer. Also included in the control mechanisms are "detents," or centering locks, to verify common tube positions (for example, centered to the film cassette in the Bucky tray or at a routine distance from the table or upright Bucky unit). Unfortunately, each manufacturer uses a different placement and labeling for these controls. For this reason, it is helpful to practice manipulating the controls prior to using the equipment to perform radiographic procedures.

The **floor-to-ceiling suspension system** uses a pair of rails, one on the ceiling and one on the floor, for longitudinal positioning. Rooms with extremely high ceilings may use an overhead rail suspended from a wall. This system uses a telescoping arm for transverse positioning and a main column collar that slides up and down for vertical distance and pivots for additional maneuverability. The tube may also be able to angle and roll or pitch but it is not capable of rotating. One of the disadvantages of a floor-to-ceiling tube is that rotation must be accomplished by pivoting the main column collar and then bringing the tube back into position by longitudinal and transverse adjustments.

A **floor suspension system** uses a tube-support column mounted on the floor. Stationary columns are fixed to the table while movable columns run on either one or two rails mounted on the floor. The operation of this system is similar to the operation of a floor-to-ceiling system. The system must be carefully counterbalanced to avoid tipping. This is usually accomplished by adding a counterweight to the back of the telescoping tube arm and requires that both tube system and table be installed further from the back wall than other systems. Some floor suspension systems are not designed to permit pivoting of the col-

lar, which limits their positioning capability severely.

There are many types of **mobile** systems. The tube suspension systems for mobile units vary tremendously but most are based on the floor suspension system. Another type of system is simply a tube mounted on a mobile stand for use during special procedures, such as angiography. The basic radiography system (BRS) developed by the International Society of Radiographers and Radiological Technicians (ISRRT) and the World Health Organization (WHO) for use in developing regions is a very simple system designed to facilitate the provision of services to these areas. This extremely portable system can be mounted on a tripod or patient lift support.

A **C-arm tube suspension system** utilizes a C-shaped arm to support the tube and image receptor. The tube and image receptor are fixed to opposite ends of the C-arm. When the clamp or lock holding the C-arm in position is released, it permits both tube and image receptor to be rotated to a new position. C-arms (or U-arms) are used in head units, mobile fluoroscopy units and ceiling-suspended angiography and surgical units.

Head Units

A **head unit** is a specialized adaptation of the floor-to-ceiling unit and is designed to enhance radiography of the cranium and facial bones. A head unit consists of an x-ray tube and a Bucky tray unit but does not include a table. The patient can be radiographed standing, sitting in a chair, or pulled over the Bucky tray from a locked cart. The advantage of a head unit is that it can be added to a radiographic room with an existing tube and table and can usually be operated from an existing generator and console. It improves head radiography by regulating tube angles, decreasing the distance from the patient to the film and minimizing the positioning of the patient (especially advantageous for trauma patients). The unit consists of a floor-to-ceiling tube mount with a C-arm or U-arm attachment on the pivoting collar.

Upright Units

An upright film cassette holder or Bucky unit is a common and useful ancillary piece of equipment in any radiographic room. Chest radiography should routinely be done in an upright position and there are numerous other procedures that are best done upright (for example, acromio-clavicular joints, abdominal obstructive procedures, cervical spine, etc.). Upright film cassette holders may or may not include a radiographic grid. Upright Bucky units may include the same equipment as the Bucky tray located in a table (movable radiographic grid, film cassette tray and automatic exposure control sensors).

Other Specialized Diagnostic Equipment

Other types of equipment have been developed to meet specialized needs. They include **chest units** designed to automate chest radiography by combining an upright Bucky unit with an automatic film handling mechanism, **mammography** units for breast studies, **tomography** units with tubes that move in an arc during exposure, **head units** for cranial studies (as previously discussed), **panoramic dental and facial units** for combined tomography of facial structures, **computed tomography** units for computerized sectional images, radiation therapy **simulator** units to verify radiation therapy treatment set-ups prior to actual treatment, **urologic** units to facilitate urological and genital studies and units custom built to nearly any specifications.

POWER FOR X-RAY GENERATION

A diagnostic x-ray generator is composed of numerous basic electrical devices. An x-ray circuit is established when these devices are connected in a sequence capable of accelerating electrons to the speed necessary to cause the production of x-ray photons within an x-ray tube. The incoming line power may be modified in several ways to establish these conditions.

Incoming Line Current

Electricity is usually supplied to buildings in the United States and Canada by 60 Hz alternating current with a nominal rms of 200–240 volts. These are termed nominal because, as users operate various resistances, the voltages constantly fluctuate, as illustrated by Ohm's law. This power is called the **incoming line current** (sometimes called the **mains**) and is supplied in the form of a three-phase power cycle (Figure 6–3). One of the "hot" wires is always half the incoming voltage above-ground potential while the other is always the same voltage below-ground potential. In the United States and Canada each carries 110–120 volts. With 60 Hz alternating current, the two hot wires reverse their polarity 120 times per second. Bringing incoming line current from the neutral (or ground) wire and one of the hot wires produces a potential difference of 110–120 volts. Because the two lines are not in phase with one another, using incoming cur-

Figure 6–3. Three-phase, 60 Hz, 240 V incoming line current.

rent from both hot wires produces a potential difference that is less than the sum of the two single phases. The usual result is about 210 V. Nearly all x-ray equipment operates from an incoming line of 210–220 volts.

Single-Phase Power

Single-phase power permits the potential difference to drop to zero with every change in the direction of current flow (Figure 6–4A) and is represented by the symbol 1φ. In a full-wave rectified circuit (direct pulsating current), this means the x-ray tube is experiencing no potential difference and is producing no x-ray photons 120 times each second on a 60 Hz line (Figure 6–4B). With the 60 Hz line, an exposure of 0.1 second with a single-phase full-wave rectified unit results in twelve intervals of no photon production (Figure 6–5). In addition, the photons produced during the low-voltage periods are of such low energy that they may not exit the tube, or they do not contribute to the radiographic image because they are absorbed before reaching the image receptor (film). The root mean square (rms) voltage

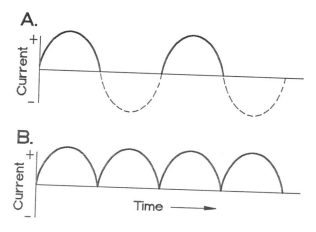

Figure 6–4. Single-phase power: (A) incoming line, (B) full-wave rectified.

of a single-phase sinusoidal wave is usually given as 70.7 percent of the peak voltage.

Example: What is the approximate rms voltage of a single-phase sine wave with a peak of 80 kVp?

Answer:

rms voltage = 70.7% peak kVp
rms voltage = 70.7% × 80 kVp
rms voltage = 56.6 kVp

Obviously this is not as efficient as desired. A solution is to combine several waveforms of current slightly out of step with one another to create **three-phase power**.

Three-Phase Power

Three-phase power is produced by the generator and is the common form in which power is supplied to users by power companies. Three-phase power is generated as is shown in Chapter 5 by Figure 5–16 and is represented by the symbol 3φ. As each wave peak begins to drop toward zero, the overall potential difference is boosted back to peak by the next phase wave. The result is that the sum of the phasing never drops to zero (Figure 6–6A). When full-wave rectification is applied, the net voltage produces a **voltage ripple**. Three-phase current produces a voltage ripple of 3 pulses per half cycle, which is 6 pulses per Hz and 360 pulses per second.

Whenever any of the phases is at zero, the other two phases are of equally opposite values so that the sum of the three currents is always zero. This fact is used in connecting the generator windings to combine the current. A **wye or star connection** (Figure 6–7A) combines phases 1, 2 and 3 to achieve the waveform seen in Figures 6–6A&B. Although the wye or star connection is more popular because it permits a single phase to be easily tapped from the same line, a **delta connection** is also possible (Figure 6–7B).

Figure 6–5. (A) X-ray photon production during an exposure of 0.1 second with a 1φ full-wave rectified unit. (B) Emission of photons from an x-ray tube during an exposure of 0.1 second with a 1φ full-wave rectified unit.

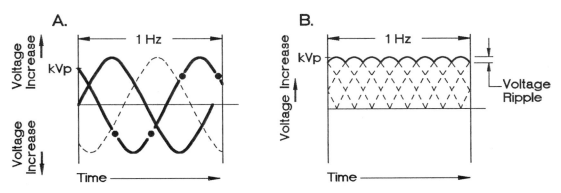

Figure 6–6. (A) Three-phase incoming line current. (B) Full-wave rectified three-phase current.

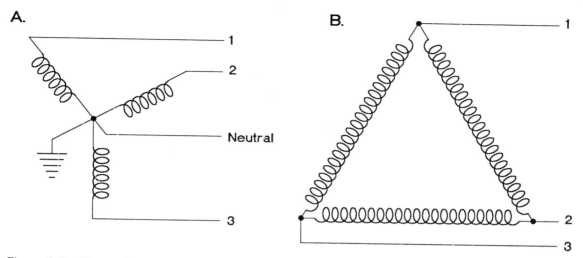

Figure 6–7. Three-phase connections: (A) wye or star, (B) delta. Phases 1, 2 and 3 are combined in a wye or delta configuration to achieve incoming three-phase power.

A BASIC X-RAY CIRCUIT

The basic x-ray circuit can be divided into the **main** and **filament** circuits. **The main circuit supplies the x-ray tube with properly modified power.** Its purpose is to produce x-rays. **The filament circuit supplies the filament of the x-ray tube with properly modified power.** Its purpose is to create the appropriate thermionically emitted electron cloud at the filament. These two circuits are distinct from each other although they are interconnected (Figure 6–8).

The Main X-ray Circuit

The main x-ray circuit modifies the incoming-line power to produce x-rays by a sequence of devices, as shown in Figure 6–9. The circuit must boost the voltage to the range necessary to produce x-rays and to permit the radiographer to adjust the amperage, voltage and length of exposure, as well as incorporate appropriate circuitry to increase the efficiency of x-ray production.

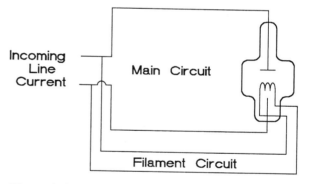

Figure 6–8. Main and filament circuits.

The **main switch** and **circuit breakers** are usually enclosed in an electrical power box. The **exposure switch** is simply a remote control switch that permits current to flow through the circuit. Diagnostic x-ray control exposure switches are designed to begin but not end exposures. The **timer** circuit is intended to end the exposure at an accurately measured, preset time. For this reason, whenever the exposure switch is depressed it must be held until both the audible and visible indicators (usually a buzzer and a light) have ceased. For example,

Figure 6–9.   The complete basic x-ray circuit: (1) main breaker, (2) exposure switch, (3) autotransformer, (4) timer circuit, (5) high-voltage step-up transformer, (6) four-diode rectification circuit, (7) filament circuit variable resistance, (8) filament step-down transformer, (9) x-ray tube and (10) rotor stator.

if a radiographer is accustomed to making short exposures of less than 0.5 second, failure to hold the exposure switch for a 2.5 second exposure of a large abdomen would prematurely terminate the exposure.

The Exposure Switch

The exposure switch can be connected to the switch that activates the rotating anode of the x-ray tube. The anode must be turning at a sufficiently high speed to avoid melting of the target area by the high kilovoltage exposure. To avoid the possibility of error, all x-ray units that utilize rotating anodes have circuitry that prevents an exposure until the anode is turning at the correct speed. It is usually convenient to combine the anode rotor and the exposure switch in a two-step button. Therefore, most exposure switches are depressed halfway to activate the anode rotation and then

depressed completely to initiate the x-ray exposure. Tube manufacturers recommend that these buttons be depressed completely in one motion. This helps to extend the life of the x-ray tube.

The exposure switch must be attached to the control console in such a manner that it is impossible for the operator to be exposed. In addition, the equipment must be designed to prohibit the x-ray tube from being manipulated into a position where it could expose the user. On mobile equipment the switch must be on a cord with a minimum length of six feet. This is to permit the radiographer to move as far as possible from the x-ray tube during an exposure. All exposure switches must be of the "dead-man" type, in which x-ray exposure may occur only while the switch is depressed. Release of the switch must terminate the exposure. This prevents the exposure from continuing when the operator enters the radiation area.

The Timer Circuit

The timer circuit can be of several types. All are designed to regulate the length of time the x-ray tube is part of the circuit and thereby control the number of x-ray photons produced.

Mechanical Timers Mechanical timers are simple spring-wound devices occasionally seen on older mobile or dental units. A dial, marked in time increments, is attached to a spring which will unwind at a known rate. Although inexpensive, they are not very accurate and are capable of exposures only to 0.25 second.

Synchronous Timers Synchronous timers operate from a simple motor that is turning at the same rate as the generator. The number or percentage of rotations can be converted into time increments. Units equipped with synchronous timers are easily recognized as the time increments tend to be multiples of 1/60th (1/30, 1/20, 1/15, etc.). They require a short recycling time and therefore cannot be used for serial exposures.

Impulse Timers Impulse timers count the number of sine wave pulses before opening the exposure switch. For example, a 1ϕ, full-wave rectified unit operates at 2 pulses per Hz. On 60 Hz current this is 1/120th second per pulse. Therefore 1 pulse would equal 1/120th second, 2 pulses would equal 1/60th second, etc.

Electronic Timers Electronic timers are the most common timers in use today. They are capable of accurate exposures as short as 0.001 second with only a 1 msec delay. Most electronic timers operate by charging a silicon-controlled rectifier (SCR) which then triggers the exposure. It is linked with a microprocessor that calculates the length of time the current will need to reach a trigger value. This level is set by the variation of the timer controls on the console unit by the radiographer.

Milliampere-Second Timers Milliampere-second timers are sometimes used in capacitor discharge units to monitor the product of mA and time on the secondary side of the high-voltage step-up transformer. When the desired mAs level is reached, these timers interrupt the circuit to stop the exposure. Because the high-voltage capacitor, timer and x-ray tube are operating on the same circuit, mAs value remains constant even when there is a slight fluctuation in the capacitor charging current.

Automatic exposure controls or automatic exposure devices are also used, as described later in this chapter. The **autotransformer**, with its taps controlled by the kVp selectors on the control console, modifies the incoming line voltage in anticipation of the kilovoltage that will be produced by the step-up transformer. Some units divide the kVp adjustments into major and minor regions. Usually a major adjustment will change in units of 10 kVp while minor adjustments will change in units of 1 or 2 kVp.

The Filament Circuit

The filament circuit modifies the incoming line power to produce the thermionic emission from the filament wire of the x-ray tube by a sequence of devices (Figure 6–9). The incoming line must be modified to about 3–5 amperes and 6–12 volts. The filament circuit's supply is drawn directly from the main circuit's supply. Current control devices regulate the amperage supplied to the filament in the x-ray tube. This control device can be adjusted by the radiographer at the control console. It is not labeled by the actual amperage it controls. Instead it is marked in increments representative of the mA that will be available at the filament when the high-voltage supply is released at exposure. Filament circuits are usually adjustable to the equivalent of mA ratings of 50, 100, 200, 300, 400, 500, 600, 800, 1,000 and 1,200. Not all equipment will have all mA settings and some may have other unusual settings, as discussed in the section on timers. Most 1 φ units do not go beyond 500 mA. Specialized tomographic equipment generators may also include 10, 15, 20, 25, 30 and 40 mA stations.

Many units include a meter at this point to provide an accurate reading of the amperage delivered. After regulation, the current is then sent to a step-down transformer that modifies it to the appropriate mA that will reach the filament itself. A very slight shift in the quantity of electrons in the thermionic cloud around the filament can have a dramatic effect on the quantity of x-ray photons produced when the kilovoltage exposure occurs. Therefore, filament circuits also incorporate several types of current stabilization devices, including frequency compensators, voltage stabilizers and space charge compensators.

The main and filament circuits are combined to form the complete basic x-ray circuit (Figure 6–9). The radiographer adjusts the various factors from a control console which must be located in a radiation-shielded location outside the radiographic exposure room. **All of the radiographer-operated controls are located on the low-voltage side of the circuit to protect operators from high-voltage shock hazards**. The controls that are likely to be located on this console are included in Table 6–1.

GENERATORS

Single-Phase Generators

Single-phase generators with full-wave rectification produce a voltage ripple of 2 pulses per Hz or 120 pulses per second (Figure 6–10A). This produces two usable pulses per cycle (1φ 2P waveform) with a ripple of 100 percent. This means the voltage in the tube drops to 0 twice per Hz.

Three-Phase Generators

When full-wave rectification is applied to 3φ current, it produces a voltage ripple of 6 pulses per Hz or 360 pulses per second (Figure 6–10B). This produces six usable pulses per cycle, which is known as a **three-phase, six-pulse** (3φ 6P) waveform. Three-phase, six-pulse power

---

TABLE 6–1

COMMON DIAGNOSTIC X-RAY CONSOLE CONTROLS

Control	Factor	Electrical Device and Location in Circuit
kVp selection	kVp level	Autotransformer (between incoming line and exposure switch)
mA selection	Filament current	Variable resistor (in filament circuit between incoming line and step-down transformer)
Time selection	Length of exposure	Timer circuit (between exposure switch and step-up transformer)
Rotor switch	Speed of rotating anode	Stator (separate circuit from stator of anode motor)
Exposure switch	Moment of exposure	Switch (between autotransformer and timer circuit)

Figure 6–10. Voltage waveforms: (A) 1φ 2P, (B) 3φ 6P, and (C) 3φ 12P.

Equipment is now available with a **three-phase, twelve-pulse** waveform. This is accomplished by a complicated combination of twelve diodes with one wye and two delta windings so as to create two transformer windings that are out of step with one another. The voltage peaks from one of the wye transformers are then inserted into the line to fill in the ripples between the voltage peaks from one of the delta transformers. When full-wave rectified, this configuration produces a voltage ripple of 4–10 percent, with tube voltage never dropping below 90–96 percent of the peak kilovoltage setting. **A full-wave rectified, three-phase, twelve-pulse waveform produces approximately 41 percent more average photon energy than full-wave rectified, single phase.** This is also an important point to remember when setting technical factors. Voltage ripple varies as higher voltage loads are applied; the percentage figures given are approximations under average loads.

Generator power ratings are determined by the greatest load the generator is capable of sending to the x-ray tube. Power is calculated as voltage times amperage. The unit of power is the watt, so V × A = W. This formula applies to a 3φ generator. Because 1φ generators have a lower average photon emission energy, the formula must be corrected by using a constant. For a 1φ generator the power rating formula is V × A × 0.7 = W. Since x-ray generators operate in the kilovoltage and milliamperage range, their power ratings are stated in kilowatts.

Example: What is the power rating for a 3φ generator capable of delivering 150 kVp at 1,000 mA to the tube?

Answer:

$$V \times A = W$$
$$150 \text{ kV} \times 1,000 \text{ mA} = W$$
$$150,000 \text{ V} \times 1.0 \text{ A} = 150,000 \text{ W}$$
$$= 150 \text{ kW}$$

produces a ripple of 13–25 percent. This means the voltage in the x-ray tube never falls below 75–87 percent of the peak kilovoltage setting on the console. **A full-wave rectified, three-phase, six-pulse waveform produces approximately 35 percent more average photon energy than full-wave rectified, single phase.** This will become an important point to remember when setting technical factors.

Example: What is the power rating for a 1ϕ generator capable of delivering 120 kVp at 300 mA to the tube?

Answer:

$$V \times A \times 0.7 = W$$
$$120 \text{ kV} \times 300 \text{ mA} \times 0.7 = W$$
$$120,000 \text{ V} \times 0.3 \text{ A} \times 0.7 = 25,200 \text{ W}$$
$$= 25.2 \text{ kW}$$

These ratings serve as a guideline for comparing the capability of various generators. Generator power often varies as kilovoltage changes so a high-power generator at 150 kVp may not be as powerful when the kVp is lowered into the middle diagnostic range.

High Frequency

High-frequency generators use AC and DC power converters to change the incoming-line voltage frequency from 60 Hz to the 6,000 Hz range (Figure 6–11A). When a high-frequency current is supplied with full-wave rectified power, a 12–13 MHz waveform can be produced. When this wave is applied to the x-ray tube, the peak kilovoltage is achieved in about 10 percent of the time necessary for 3ϕ generators (Figure 6–11B). Full-wave rectified high-frequency generator ripple ranges from 4–15 percent, depending on the total load, which is comparable to 3ϕ 12P generators. Because of the higher-frequency current, transformers for these units are significantly smaller.

Capacitor Discharge Mobile Units

It is also possible to operate an x-ray tube with the power generated from the discharge of a high-voltage capacitor. The capacitor operates exactly as explained in Chapter 3 but in the kilovoltage range necessary to produce x-rays. In these units, depression of a charge button causes the rectification circuit to charge a capacitor instead of the x-ray tube. A signal indicates readiness when the capacitor fills to the appropriate level, and depression of the exposure switch triggers a discharge to the x-ray tube.

The disadvantage of a capacitor discharge unit is that the capacitor may continue to discharge after the usable exposure. Figure 6–12A shows the charging curve, the exposure period, and the discharging curve. Exposure begins at the peak voltage and then decreases (Figure 6–12B). This is sometimes called wave-tail cutoff. **Capacitor discharge units provide an rms voltage significantly lower than the peak voltage**. The ending kVp is approximately 1 kV per mAs lower than the initial kVp. Therefore the rms voltage is about 0.5 kV/mAs lower than the initial kVp. Because capacitors discharge more slowly as potential difference decreases, considerable residual kVp may exist after the desired exposure time. This can create a leakage of radiation, although several devices help avoid the problem. Grid-biased x-ray tubes can be used to cut the photon emission at a set time by reversing the charge polarity of a wire grid in front of the filament. Additionally, the tube collimator can be designed to automatically close its lead shutters after the desired exposure, thus stopping radiation leakage.

Capacitor discharge units are most commonly used for mobile equipment. The capacitor circuit is supplied from batteries which are charged from line current. This permits the unit to be mobile without having to be plugged into a wall outlet. Instead, the batteries can be recharged periodically when the unit is parked.

Battery-Operated Mobile Units

Mobile units are also available that operate on nickel-cadmium (NiCd) battery-supplied AC current. The batteries supply nonpulsating direct current to a rotary converter which provides current similar to 3ϕ 12P or even greater

Figure 6–11. High-frequency waveforms: (A) Conversion of 1φ 2P to 3φ 6P to high frequency. (B) Comparison of time interval necessary to reach peak kV on 3φ 6P and high-frequency generators. (Courtesy of Siemens AG, Medical Engineering Group. Siemens high-frequency generators were in operation in the US as early as 1980, with all other (major) manufactures following since then.)

frequencies. Compared to capacitor discharge machines, these units have the obvious advantage of 3φ exposure consistency, higher rms voltage, and no leakage possibility. They also have all the advantages of mobility, with recharging capabilities, and for these reasons they have become extremely popular.

Falling Load Generators

The generators discussed so far have all been constant potential. In other words, the voltage and amperage have been constant throughout the exposure time. The concept of the falling load generator involves taking full advantage of the current loading capability of the x-ray tube by beginning the exposure with a high amperage and then allowing it to fall during the exposure.

Falling load generators are a solution to this problem as they permit greater use of the acceptable tube limits. They do so without requiring a higher-power (and more expensive) generator that would permit higher mA loading. A falling load generator permits the same

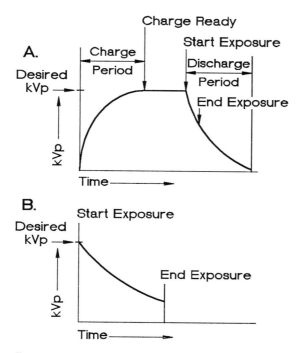

Figure 6–12. (A) Capacitor discharge unit waveform. (B) Wavetail cut-off.

tube to achieve 240 mAs in 0.5 second. This is accomplished by beginning the exposure at 600 mA for the first 0.1 second (Figure 6–13). At this time the 600 mA tube limit is reached and the generator is programmed to automatically reduce the mA to 500 until the tube limit is again reached (0.2 second later, or 0.3 second from exposure start). Once again the generator reduces the mA to 400 until the limit is reached (0.2 second later, or 0.5 second from exposure start). This produces 240 total mAs.

A falling load generator utilizes the tube's loading potential to a much greater extent than the constant-potential generator. This is made evident by comparing the falling load of the 240 mAs example with a constant-potential load for the same mAs. In actual practice a margin of error is allowed for the tube loading. Most falling load generators will step down the

mA at 70–80 percent of the tube loading capacity. This feature has a disadvantage in that constant-potential generators may actually make better use of tube loading capacity on very short exposures, where they may use 80–90 percent of the tube loading capacity.

Falling load generators begin exposures at the highest possible mA. This removes control of the mA from the radiographer, and there are instances when this is undesirable. For example, some examinations, such as those for the lateral thoracic vertebra (spine) and sternum, require a "breathing technique" in which low mA and long-time exposures are used to blur superimposing structures from the image. Unless falling load consoles are equipped with special controls to permit starting exposures at low mA, these examinations cannot be performed correctly.

There are several factors that should be understood before using falling-load generators. Because they function with an mA that is unknown to the operator, it is impossible for the operator to set the correct time to achieve the desired mAs. Therefore, falling load generators must be used with automatic exposure controls, as discussed in the next section. The kVp across the tube varies for a brief moment as the mA is adjusted. This is an Ohm's law effect during the mA step-downs and results in a slightly lower average kVp. Falling load generators can shorten x-ray tube life considerably as they use higher mA settings, thus causing the filament to wear out more quickly. The advantages of falling load generators are shorter times in heavy-load situations, and simpler operation.

AUTOMATIC EXPOSURE CONTROLS

All automatic exposure controls do exactly what their name indicates; they are programmed to terminate the radiographic exposure time. It is important to remember that automatic exposure controls do not control any factor except time. Milliampere-seconds and kVp remain under the control of the radiographer in all but falling load generators. Even falling-load units leave the kVp under the radiographer's control.

There are two types of automatic exposure controls: **phototimers and ionization chamber devices. The term phototimer is often used to refer to all automatic exposure controls.** They are also referred to as automatic exposure devices and the acronyms AEC and AED occasionally appear in professional literature. Actually, phototimers are seldom utilized in modern radiography. Most of the devices that are called phototimers today consist of ionization chambers.

All automatic exposure controls function by measuring a preset quantity of radiation and breaking the timer circuit when a dose sufficient to produce the desired film density has been reached. The exact method by which

Phototimers

Old-fashioned phototimer devices use a thyratron to regulate exposure automatically (Figure 6–14). The x-ray beam passes through the patient, tabletop, and cassette before it strikes a fluorescent screen that has the ability to absorb the x-rays and produce light photons. The light photons are then directed toward a photomultiplier tube. A photomulti-

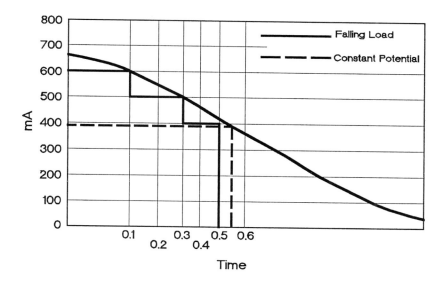

Figure 6–13. Falling load generator versus constant-potential tube limit curve. In the example shown the mAs is calculated as follows:

mA	Time in sec.	mAs achieved
600	0.1	60
500	0.2	100
400	0.2	80
TOTALS	0.5	240

Figure 6–14.   Phototimer AEC circuit.

Ionization Chambers

Ionization chamber automatic exposure control is quite different (Figure 6–15). The x-ray beam passes through the patient and table-top before striking the ionization chamber. Unlike with the old phototimers, the cassette and film are positioned under the ion chamber. Until the development of a thin, parallel-plate ionization chamber, it was impossible to locate the chamber in this position because it would cast an objectionable shadow artifact on the film. Because thin, parallel-plate chambers are only about 5 mm in thickness, this is not a problem (Figure 6–16). It is critical that the exact size, shape and position of the ionization chamber be known to the radiographer.

Minimum Reaction Time

All automatic exposure controls have a **minimum reaction (or response) time**, which is determined by the length of time necessary for the AEC to respond to the radiation and send the signal to terminate the exposure. Old

plier tube has the ability to produce multiple electrons from each light photon. The electrons then establish a charge on the capacitor. When the capacitor reaches its preset value, it discharges, triggering a thyraton and opening the relay to terminate the exposure. Phototimers are calibrated by setting the capacitor-discharge point (usually controlled by a set screw in the electronics cabinet) at a level that will produce a satisfactory density on the radiographic film in the cassette. This is done by a trial-and-error procedure with a radiographic phantom. Radiographs are exposed at various combinations of kVp, time, and mAs until a satisfactory diagnostic quality image is consistently obtained.

Figure 6–15.   Ionization chamber AEC circuit.

Figure 6–16. Parallel-plate ionization chamber AEC. (Courtesy of Siemens Medical Systems, Inc.)

phototimers had a minimum reaction time of 0.05 second or less. Modern ionization chambers with SCRs may have a minimum reaction time of less than 0.001 second. Automatic exposure controls are sometimes incapable of terminating exposures quickly enough, especially with extremely high-speed films and intensifying screens during high kVp chest radiography. In this instance, radiographic technology has outstripped itself and either a manual time or a slower film and screen combination must be used.

Backup Time

Nearly all automatic exposure equipped units permit (and may have electronic interlocks that require) a manual backup time to be set. There are numerous reasons why an automatic exposure control may be improperly set. For example, if one forgets to activate the AEC in a wall unit, this may leave an AEC in a table unit waiting for exposure by a tube that is directed toward the wall (and through a patient). Because the wall AEC is not receiving any radiation dose, the exposure would not cease until the tube overload protector activated. Not only is this an expensive waste of tube life, but the radiographer error causing

excessive radiation dose to the patient is completely unwarranted. The fact that the radiograph would be overexposed, requiring it to be repeated, adding to the patient's dose again, simply makes matters worse. Backup times cannot exceed the tube limit and should be set at 150 percent of the anticipated manual exposure mAs. According to U.S. Public Law 90–602, generators must terminate the exposure at 600 mAs for exposures above 50 kVp and 2,000 mAs for exposures below 50 kVp (primarily during mammography).

SUMMARY

Medical x-ray units can be classified as diagnostic or therapeutic. Diagnostic units operate within a range of 10–1,200 milliamperes (mA), 0.001–10 seconds and at a peak kilovoltage (kVp) of approximately 25 to 150.

Radiographic equipment includes a wide variety of units with different tube stand configurations, including ceiling suspension, floor-to-ceiling, floor mounted and C-arms. Nearly all x-ray equipment operates from an incoming line of 210–220 volts, which is then used for single-phase or three-phase power.

The basic x-ray circuit can be divided into the main and filament circuits. The main circuit supplies the x-ray tube with properly modified power, while the filament circuit supplies the filament of the x-ray tube with properly modified power. The basic circuit includes the exposure switch, timer, high-voltage step-up transformer and rectifier circuit.

Although waveforms differ depending on incoming line and rectification, differences occur in both voltage ripple and the interval between initiation of the exposure and the peak kilovoltage.

Generator power ratings are determined by the greatest load the generator is capable of sending to the x-ray tube. Power is expressed in watts and varies by incoming line current and rectification. Falling load generators permit more effective use of the tube loading capacity but eliminate mA and time settings from consideration.

Although often called phototimers, automatic exposure controls (AECs) today are almost always ionization chambers. When using an AEC, problems may be avoided by considering the minimum reaction time and the backup time.

REVIEW QUESTIONS

1. Name three types of diagnostic radiographic tube-support systems.

2. What are the two types of incoming line current?

3. How many pulses are there per Hz for 1ϕ and 3ϕ power?

4. What device in the x-ray circuit controls kVp? mA? time? rectification?

5. What is the approximate voltage ripple for 1ϕ 2P equipment? 3ϕ 6P? 3ϕ 12P?

6. What happens to the tube mA during an exposure using a falling load generator?

7. What is the difference between an ionization chamber and a phototimer?

8. What factor determines the minimum reaction time?

REFERENCES AND RECOMMENDED READING

Amman, Ernst. Update on technology of x-ray generators. Radiological Society of North America Refresher Course. Chicago, IL: December 1, 1986.

Baranoski, Dennis. High frequency and speed 500. *The Canadian Journal of Radiography, Radiotherapy, and Nuclear Medicine* 16:2, 55–59, 1985.

Barnes, Gary T., and Jack M. Tishler. Flouroscopic image quality and its implications regarding equipment selection and use. *The Physical Basis of Medical Imaging.* 93–106. Editors: Coulam, Craig M., John J. Erickson, F. David Rollo, and A. Everette James, Jr. New York: Appleton-Century-Crofts, 1981.

Chesney, D. Noreen, and Muriel O. Chesney. *X-ray Equipment for Student Radiographers.* 3rd ed. Oxford: Blackwell Scientific Publications, 1984.

Curry, Thomas S. III, James E. Dowdey, and Robert C. Murry. *Christensen's Introduction to the Physics of Diagnostic Radiology.* 3rd. ed. Philadelphia: Lea and Febiger, 1984.

Evans, S. A., Loyce Harris, C. P. Lawinski, and I. R. F. Hendra. Mobile x-ray generators: A review. *Radiography* 51:595, 89, 1985.

Gray, Joel E., Norlin T. Winkler, John Stears, and Eugene D. Frank. Radiologic exchange. *Radiologic Technology* August, 1988.

Gray, Joel E., Norlin T. Winkler, John Stears, and Eugene D. Frank. *Quality Control in Diagnostic Imaging.* Baltimore, MD: University Park Press, 1983.

Joseph, Edward S., and John E. Schneble. X-ray automatic exposure timing and control circuitry. *Application of Optical Instrumentation in Medicine, IV*, 70, 166–170, 1975.

Lin, Pei-Jan Paul. Phototimers, user's point of view. *Application of Optical Instrumentation in Medicine, IV*, 70, 196–200, 1975.

Morgan, James A. The development and application of multi-phase x-rays in medical radiography. *Radiologic Technology*, 40:2, 57, 1968.

Ridgway, Arthur, and Walter Thumm. *The Physics of Medical Radiography*. Reading, MA: Addison-Wesley, 1973.

Seeram, Euclid. *X-Ray Imaging Equipment*. Springfield, IL: Charles C. Thomas, 1985.

Selman, Joseph. *The Fundamentals of x-ray and Radium Physics*. 7th ed. Springfield, IL: Charles C. Thomas, 1985.

Sprawls, Perry. *Principles of Radiography for Technologists*. Rockville, MD: Aspen Publishers, 1990.

Sprawls, Perry. *Physical Principles of Medical Imaging*. Rockville, MD: Aspen Publishers, 1987.

Stears, John G., Joel E. Gray, William E. Webbles, and Eugene D. Frank. Radiologic exchange (automatic exposure control function). *Radiologic Technology* 59:6, 521–522, 1988.

Sterling. Automatic exposure control: A primer. *Radiologic Technology*, 59:5, 421–427, 1988.

Stockley, Sybil M. *A Manual of Radiographic Equipment*. Edinburgh: Churchill Livingstone, 1986.

Thompson, Thomas T. *A Practical Approach to Modern Imaging Equipment*. 2nd ed. Boston, MA: Little, Brown, & Co., 1985.

Weigl, Walter. A new high-frequency controlled x-ray generator system with multi-pulse wave shape. *Journal for Radiological Engineering* 1:1, 7–19, 1989.

Weigl, Walter. Design of falling load generators. Unpublished paper presented at American Association of Physicists in Medicine seminar, 1988.

Wilks, Robin J. *Principles of Radiological Physics*. Edinburgh: Churchill Livingstone, 1981.

7 THE X-RAY TUBE

. . . circumstances led me to the construction of experimental high vacuum tubes with a heated tungsten filament as cathode and a tungsten disc as anode . . . . The tube was then stable and controllable . . . .

W. D. Coolidge, "Experiences with the Roentgen-ray tube."

OUTLINE

THE CATHODE ASSEMBLY
THE ANODE ASSEMBLY
THE GLASS ENVELOPE
PROTECTIVE HOUSING
OFF-FOCUS RADIATION
RATING CHARTS AND COOLING CURVES
RECOMMENDATIONS FOR EXTENDING TUBE LIFE

OBJECTIVES

Upon completion of this chapter, the student should be able to:

1. Draw a complete dual-focus cathode assembly.
2. Discuss the necessary characteristics of filament metals and construction.
3. Describe the control of thermionic emission from the filament.
4. Select exposure factors and techniques that will extend tube life.
5. Explain the function and design of a grid-biased focusing cup.
6. Draw a complete rotating anode assembly.
7. Discuss the characteristics of anode targets.
8. Explain the line-focus principle and its effect on anode target design.
9. Explain the anode heel effect and its effect on primary beam intensity.
10. Explain the production of off-focus radiation.
11. Describe the function of a rotating anode induction motor stator and rotor.

12. Discuss the construction of the glass envelope and protective housing.
13. Calculate safe exposures when provided with a tube rating chart, anode cooling curve, and housing cooling curve.

The electrical production of x-rays is only possible under very special conditions including a source of electrons, an appropriate target material, a high voltage and a vacuum. The x-ray tube is the device that permits these conditions to exist, and it is within the tube that x-ray photons come into existence. The tube consists of a **cathode** and an **anode** enclosed within a **glass envelope** and then encased in a **protective housing** (Figure 7–1). X-ray tubes, whose useful life can be significantly extended by proper care and handling by professional radiographers, can cost over $10,000.

THE CATHODE ASSEMBLY

The cathode is the negative side of the x-ray tube. The function of the cathode is to produce a thermionic cloud, conduct the high voltage to the gap between cathode and anode

and focus the electron stream as it heads for the anode. The cathode is a complex device and can be referred to as the **cathode assembly**. This assembly consists of the **filament** or filaments, **focusing cup** and associated **wiring** (Figure 7–2).

The Filament

The filament is a small coil of thin thoriated tungsten wire. The wire is about 0.1–0.2 mm thick and the coil 1–2 mm wide by 7–15 mm long. It is set in the cathode assembly within the focusing cup (Figure 7–3). Tungsten is the material of choice because of its high melting point (3,370°C) and because it is difficult to vaporize (turn into a gas). Rhenium (melting point of 3,170°C) and molybdenum (melting point of 2,620°C) are also desirable materials. The high melting point permits the

Figure 7–1. A rotating anode x-ray tube.

Figure 7–2.   A cathode assembly.

Figure 7–3.   Dual filaments in a focusing cup.

filament to operate at the high temperatures required of an x-ray tube. In addition, tungsten is not easily vaporized. Vaporization produces particles that deposit on other surfaces and reduce the vacuum within the tube. The length and width of the filament have a great effect on the ability of the particular x-ray tube to image fine details.

Most diagnostic x-ray tubes have dual filaments called a **dual focus** arrangement (Figure 7–3). The wiring for dual filaments does not require separate ground conductors. Instead a common ground is used (Figure 7–4).

As we have discussed previously, the function of the filament is to provide sufficient resistance to the flow of electrons so that the heat produced will cause thermionic emission to occur. (A tungsten filament will not exhibit significant thermionic emission below 2,200°C.) This process causes electrons to leave the surface of the filament wire and form a thermionic cloud. When the high voltage is released at exposure the entire cloud is available to be driven toward the anode target where x-ray photons will be produced. This provides many more times the number of electrons than would be available from a cold cathode.

Not all of the electrons that are thermionically emitted from the filament are driven to the anode or return to the filament. A very small percentage of the electrons are permanently vaporized from the filament and they contribute to reducing the vacuum, thus making the tube gassy. Vaporized tungsten (from both filament and anode) is also gradually deposited on the inner surface of the glass enve-

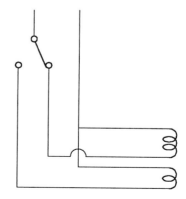

Figure   7–4.   Dual-filament wiring.

lope. This deposit causes old tubes to have a mirrored appearance and can eventually cause high-voltage arcing when sufficient current is attracted to a deposit during an exposure. Arcing of this type immediately destroys the tube. Evaporization deposits on the glass envelope also cause increased filtration of the primary beam and this decreases tube efficiency. Tubes with a metal or ceramic envelope can be grounded to significantly reduce this problem.

Another major cause of tube failure is the breaking of the filament itself. Filaments become increasingly thin as vaporization continues. When about 10 percent of the diameter has vaporized, a filament becomes subject to breaking, exactly the way a light bulb filament will burn out. However, older tubes are much more sensitive to rough handling and a thin filament that is jarred can break prematurely.

When the x-ray machine is first turned on, a mild current is sent to the filament. The filament remains in this preheated mode until immediately prior to an exposure. **When the switch labeled "rotor" is activated prior to an exposure**, not only does the rotor begin to turn but **a higher current is sent to the filament to bring the thermionic cloud to the proper size for the mA selected**. This increase in filament heating is what causes most of the vaporization of the filament. An average diagnostic x-ray tube filament life is only about 6–9 hours (10,000–20,000 exposures) at this heating level. One of the primary causes of premature tube failure is the radiographer's habit of holding the rotor switch prior to making exposures. Every second the rotor switch is depressed, life is removed from the filament. Routinely delayed exposures while the filament is enduring maximum current can shorten tube life by 50–60 percent (to 5,000–6,000 exposures).

Most tube manufacturers recommend that two-step exposure switches be **fully depressed in one motion**. For units with separate switches, the **exposure** switch should be depressed first,

then the rotor switch. All units have electronic interlocks that will not permit the exposure to occur until the rotor has brought the anode up to the proper speed. The only instance in which holding the rotor switch (and filament heat) can be justified is in cases where the patient is unable to cooperate. In these instances (such as with pediatric patients) the rotor and filament must be readied to permit an instant exposure to avoid patient breathing and motion. Single-phase generators are usually capable of initiating exposure within 10 milliseconds (0.01 second) and 3ϕ generators may be as quick 1 millisecond (0.001 second). Routine clinical examinations seldom need to be timed closer than these limitations.

Historical Notes In the earliest days of radiography a cold cathode with an unheated filament was used. It was not until the American physicist William D. Coolidge (1873–1975) developed the Coolidge tube for the General Electric Corporation in 1915 that the hot filament became available. Prior to the development of the Coolidge tube, the radiographer kept a selection of tubes of various mA values on a rack, usually in the darkroom (Figure 7–5). When a change of mA was required, the radiographer disconnected the tube and replaced it with a different one from the rack. Coolidge's contributions to radiography included not only the hot filament, but also the focusing cup, the imbedded anode target, and various anode cooling devices (including the unique water-cooled tube).

The Focusing Cup

The focusing cup is a shallow depression in the cathode assembly designed to house the filament (Figure 7–2). It is made of nickel and its purpose is to narrow the thermionic cloud as it is driven toward the anode. Because electrons all possess negative charges, their

Figure 7–5. A selection of cold filament tubes as displayed at the Deutsches Röntgen Museum, Remscheid-Lennep, Germany. (Photograph courtesy of Philip W. Ballinger.)

tendency is to diverge rather than to travel in straight lines. The focusing cup is provided with a low negative current which, because of its geometry, focuses the electrons toward one another in a convergence pattern (Figure 7–6). As more and more electrons build up in the area of the filament, their negative charges begin to oppose the emission of additional electrons. This phenomenon is called the **space charge effect** and it limits x-ray tubes to maximum mA ranges of 1,000–1,200.

Saturation current is another filament phenomenon that affects the efficiency of the x-ray tube. As kVp increases, a greater percentage of the thermionically emitted electrons are driven toward the anode. This relationship is shown by a filament emission chart (Figure 7–7). The filament amperage curve flattens out when the kVp is driving the entire thermionic cloud toward the anode. The filament saturation current has been achieved when there are

no further thermionic electrons to be driven toward the anode. At this point an increase in kVp will not increase the tube mA. Further mA increases must be achieved by increasing the filament amperage. Close examination of a

Figure 7–6. The geometry of the negative charge on the cathode focusing cup.

Figure 7-7. A filament emission chart showing saturation as a function of filament amperage, tube voltage and tube current. (Courtesy of Varian EIMAC.)

filament emission chart demonstrates that something must be done to compensate for the tube mA increase when kVp is changed. For example, an exposure at 100 kVp will produce a significantly greater tube mA than the same exposure at 60 kVp. The filament amperage must be adjusted to compensate for these changes and the x-ray circuitry does this automatically whenever factors are changed by the operator.

Grid-Biased Tubes In some applications, such as cine-film recording or capacitor discharge generators, it is desirable to quickly regulate the flow of electrons producing x-ray photons. The addition of a low positive current at the focusing cup causes the cup to attract the thermionic cloud. This attraction very cleanly removes electrons from use for x-ray production. When the focusing cup charge is pulsed from negative to positive in synchrony with another device (such as the shutter of a cine camera), it becomes possible to regulate,

pulse and synchronize x-ray production very precisely. A third wire to charge the focusing cup is the only physical difference between a normal and a grid-biased tube. In older tubes an actual grid of wires was placed between the filament and anode. These types of tubes are sometimes called **grid-pulsed, grid-biased or grid-controlled**.

THE ANODE ASSEMBLY

The anode is the positive side of the x-ray tube and has three functions: it serves as a target surface for the high-voltage electrons from the filament, thereby becoming the source of the x-ray photons; it conducts the high voltage from the cathode back into the x-ray generator circuitry and it serves as the primary thermal conductor. The anode target surface is where the high-speed electrons from the filament are suddenly stopped, resulting in the production of x-ray photons. The entire anode is a complex device referred to as the **anode assembly**. This assembly consists of the **anode, stator and rotor** (Figure 7-8) and serves as the path for the high-voltage flow during exposure.

Figure 7-8. The anode assembly with anode, target, rotor, bearings, and stator.

The Anode

Anodes are divided into two types: **stationary and rotating** (Figure 7–9). Rotating anodes, developed in 1936, turn during the exposure, thus presenting a much larger target area. Modern rotating anodes permit bombardment of a given area of the target for only 7–50 microseconds. The faster the anode rotates, the better the heat dissipation. The use of stationary anode x-ray tubes has become limited to low-power functions, such as those of dental units. Nearly all units designed for diagnostic radiography utilize rotating anodes because of their greater efficiency.

The anode is composed of several different metals, each designed to contribute the maximum to the overall function of the anode. Stationary anodes are composed of rhenium-alloyed tungsten imbedded in a 45° angled end of a copper rod. Rotating anode disks range from 5–13 cm in diameter and are composed of molybdenum. The anode's function as the source of x-ray photons and as the primary thermal conducting device is enhanced by the use of rhenium-alloyed tungsten as the target focal track material (Figure 7–10). Tungsten is the metal of choice for the source of x-ray photons for three primary reasons:

1. high atomic number,
2. high melting point and
3. heat-conducting ability.

Tungsten's atomic number (74) enhances the production of diagnostic-range photons. During normal use, the focal track reaches a temperature between 1,000–2,000°C but the temperature can go higher if the tube load increases. Because of tungsten's high melting point, it can withstand normal operating temperatures. Tungsten also conducts heat very well. The rhenium provides greater elasticity when the focal track expands rapidly due to the intense heat. To assist in the dissipation of heat in heavy load situations, specialized anodes may have the anode disk backed by a thicker layer of molybdenum or graphite. Graphite-backed anodes can double heat-loading capabilities without increasing bearing wear.

Specialized x-ray tubes for mammography utilize molybdenum (atomic number 42) as the primary target material due to its ability to emit a more uniform range of lower energy photons. The lower characteristic energy photons permit a better soft tissue image. Molybdenum also has a high melting point, as discussed above. These tubes also utilize a specialized glass envelope window made of beryl-

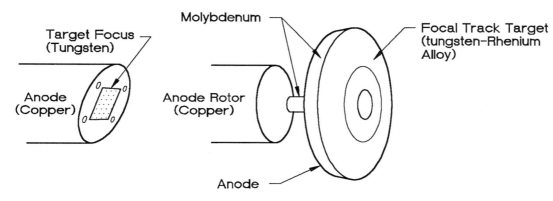

Figure 7–9.   A stationary and a rotating anode.

Figure 7–10. Rotating anode construction.

Figure 7–11. Pitting of a rotating anode focal track from extended use.

lium because the glass used in most x-ray tubes absorbs too much of the low-energy beam.

Normal use of a rotating anode will eventually vaporize sufficient target focal track material to roughen or pit the target area (Figure 7–11). Pitting reduces the efficiency of the tube; the term pitted or pitting is often used to describe an older tube's focal track.

When first activating an x-ray unit, it is important to use an **anode warm-up procedure**. These procedures are specified by the tube manufacturers and are designed to bring the anode heat from room temperature to near the range of operation. A normal procedure might require an average kVp and mA station for a one-second exposure to be followed by two more two-second exposures. Failure to follow the warm-up procedure can cause the entire anode to crack if the molybdenum absorbs the heat too rapidly and exceeds its expansion capability.

The Target Area The portion of the anode where the high-voltage electron steam will impact is called by various names: the **target**, the **focus**, the **focal point**, the **focal spot** or the **focal track** (although this last term has a more specific definition, it is the target area). This is

the precise point at which the x-ray photons are created. The target is considered to be a point source of x-ray photons and it is from this point that all tube-to-object and image-receptor (film) distances are measured. Some x-ray tube housings have a line drawn on them to indicate the exact level of the target within. All measuring devices have their zero point at this level. This is why a tape measure attached to the side or bottom of a tube collimator may begin at 12 cm. It is attached 12 cm from the target but is calculated to measure target-to-image-receptor distances.

Stationary anodes have a static target area. Rotating anodes have a dynamic target area and are designed to greatly increase the target area (see Figure 7–9). A rotating anode can increase the target area up to 300 times, depending on the diameter of the anode disk.

Rotating anodes have much greater heat loading capacities than stationary anodes. High-speed anodes have higher heating capacities than regular-speed anodes (often 50 percent greater).

When discussing a rotating anode target area, the term **focal track** is used to represent the circular path that will be impacted by the electron beam. The terms **target, focus, focal point** and **focal spot** refer to the area of the focal track that is impacted by the electron beam at one time. In addition, the term **actual focal spot** is used to describe the physical area of the focal track that is impacted. The term **effective focal spot** is used to describe the area of the focal spot that is projected out of the tube toward the object being radiographed (Figure 7–12).

Line-Focus Principle

The **line-focus principle** is used to reduce the effective area of the focal spot. This permits the best resolution of detail while permitting as large an actual area as possible (to increase thermal conductivity). **The effective focal-spot size is controlled by** the size of the actual focal spot (which is controlled by the length of the filament) and the anode target angle. As the actual focal-spot size increases, the effective focal-spot size also increases (Figure 7–12).

When the target angle is less than 45°, the effective focal spot is smaller than the actual focal spot (Figure 7–13). This is accomplished by the line-focus principle. This principle can best be understood by holding a pencil straight up and then sloping it towards oneself so that the pencil is seen end on. The perceived dimensions of the pencil change as the angle changes. In the x-ray tube, changing the angle of the target changes the effective focal spot.

The most common diagnostic radiography target angle is 12°. However, tubes are available with angles ranging from 7° to 17°. When the angle is decreased, smaller focal spots can be achieved. A disadvantage of extremely small target angles is that the geometry of the angle can limit the size of the primary beam field at short source-to-image

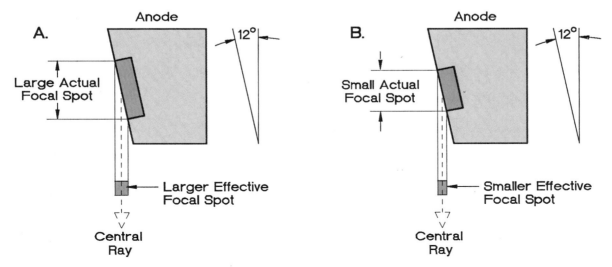

Figure 7–12.   Effect of actual focal-spot size on effective focal-spot size.

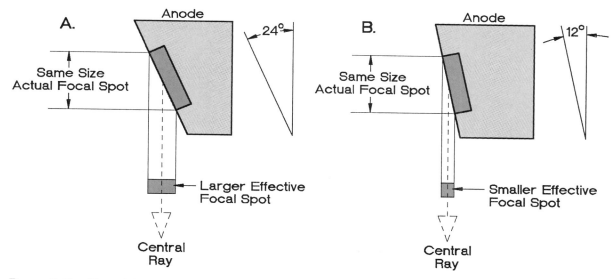

Figure 7–13. Use of the line-focus principle to obtain an effective focal spot smaller than the actual focal spot.

receptor distances (Figure 7–14). To cover a 14" × 17" field at 40", a 12° target angle is required. It has been shown that at large heat loads, target angles can decrease due to "warping" of the anode. In these instances, the anode end of the primary beam field can be reduced enough to cut off structures near the collimated edge. A slight angle of the tube will compensate for this effect. Some tubes have offset filaments with two different focal tracks, which can be set at different target angles.

X-ray tube focal spots are rectangular because the line-focus principle applies only in the direction of the angle. It does not apply horizontally across the anode focal track because there is no angle in this direction. X-ray tube targets must be narrow to maintain the small effective focal-spot size in the horizontal direction, usually not over 2 mm. The line-focus principle permits the actual focal spot's vertical dimension to be as much as 6 mm to gain the maximum thermal conductivity. **The effective focal spot's vertical dimension is the**

one that is stated as the focal-spot size. Diagnostic tubes are available with focal spots of 0.1 mm to 3.0 mm. Occasionally the term **fractional focal spot** is used to refer to a very small focal spot, one that is a fraction of a millimeter in size.

In normal usage, the term focal-spot size refers to the effective focal spot size. Most diagnostic x-ray tubes have dual focal spots to include one for fine detail studies and the other for heavy tube loads. The small focal spot will not permit the use of higher mA stations. If the x-ray unit allows the radiographer to choose the focal-spot size, an exposure cannot be made with a high mA station and the small focal spot. Automatic systems link the focal-spot size selection with the appropriate mA station. Therefore, the radiographer should realize that the focal-spot size may be mandated by the mA station. When a small focal spot is desired, it is important to use only low mA stations, even though this may require a longer exposure time.

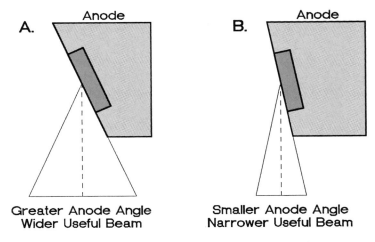

Figure 7–14. Anode target angle as a function of maximum primary beam field size.

Focal-spot size increases, or blooms, as milliamperage is increased. For example, the focal spot is slightly larger during an exposure of 80 kVp, 800 mA and 0.1 second than it is during an exposure of 80 kVp, 100 mA and 0.8 second. Although originally considered to be a significant factor, recent research has indicated that focal-spot blooming does not have a re-sounding effect on recorded detail.

Anode Heel Effect The use of the line-focus principle causes a problem that is known as the **anode heel effect** (Figure 7–15). Because of the geometry of an angled anode target, the **radiation intensity is greater on the cathode side**. As electrons bombard the target, x-rays are produced and most are emitted at angles between 45 and 90 degrees in the direction of the electron travel. These are absorbed by the anode itself or by the tube housing. Those photons that are emitted from the surface of the target are emitted in all directions. The intensity of the radiation which is emitted will vary between the cathode end of the tube and the anode end of the tube. This is because photons which are emitted toward the anode

end are more likely to be absorbed by the tar-get material itself than those which are emitted toward the cathode end (Figure 7–16). This can cause as many as 20 percent more photons at

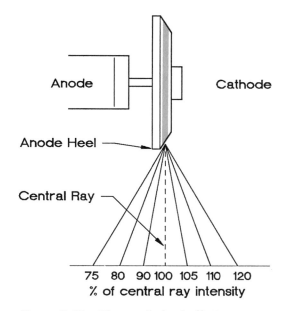

Figure 7–15. The anode heel effect.

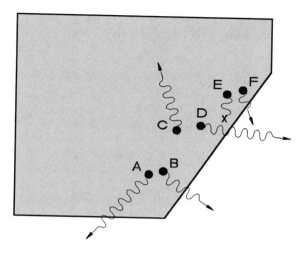

Figure 7–16. A-E represent photons created in the target. A exits at anode end of tube while B exits at cathode end of tube. Notice the greater distance photon A must travel through the target material itself as compared to photon B. Most photons are absorbed as in C, which is absorbed in anode, D, which exits anode but is absorbed in housing, and E, which is heading toward the anode end but does not exit anode. F exits at cathode end because it has a shorter distance to travel through the anode.

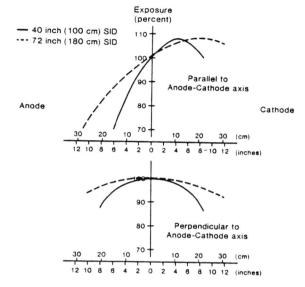

Figure 7–17. Variation in intensity of x-ray emissions parallel and perpendicular to anode-cathode axis. (By permission of Mayo Foundation, *Quality Control in Diagnostic Imaging*, Aspen Publishers, Inc., Rockville, 1983.)

the cathode end of the tube and 25 percent fewer photons at the anode end (Figure 7–17). A total variation of approximately 45 percent exists parallel to the anode-cathode axis. No significant variation occurs perpendicular to the anode-cathode axis.

The 45 percent variation is significant enough to cause a visible difference in film density during radiographic examinations when large film sizes are used at short distances. The anode heel effect is the reason why each radiographic table has a standard or natural "head" end. The tube anode is established at the head of the table to utilize the anode heel effect to best advantage. No significant variations will be seen in density from side to side.

Because the cathode end of the x-ray tube has a more intense beam, it should be positioned toward the denser (thicker) part of the body.

Example: In which direction should the cathode be placed for an anterior-posterior examination of the thoracic vertebral column?

Answer: Because the inferior thoracic region is more dense, the cathode's more intense beam should be positioned inferiorly to help increase the film density in that region.

The Stator

The induction-motor electromagnets comprise the stator that turns the anode. The stator is the only part of cathode or anode assemblies that is located **outside** the vacuum of the glass envelope (see Figure 7–8). The electromagnetic effect that causes the rotor to turn can function through the glass, permitting electrical isolation of the stator coils from the high voltage of the exposure. The kilovoltage range of the exposure would destroy the stator's electromagnets. The switch labeled "rotor" that must be activated prior to an exposure actually sends current to the stator, which then causes the rotor to turn the anode. If the stator fails, the rotor will cease to turn the anode, resulting in the immediate melting of a spot on the target because rotating anode targets are not designed to absorb the heat of a high-voltage exposure while stationary (Figure 7–18).

The Rotor

The rotor is located inside the stator and inside the glass envelope. It is composed of a hollow copper cylinder or cuff that is attached to the anode disk by a molybdenum shaft. The

Figure 7–18. Anode melt due to rotor-bearing failure.

cuff is the true rotor that is affected by the electromagnetic field of the stator, causing it to turn. Common rotating anodes revolve at 3,200–3,600 revolutions per minute (rpm). High-speed rotating anodes that operate at 10,000–12,000 rpm are also available to assist in dissipating heat.

The inside of the rotor contains silver-plated steel ball bearings around a shaft that is anchored to the glass envelope (see Figure 7–8). The ball bearings use silver plating as a high-temperature lubricant between the cuff and the anode shaft. Liquids tend to produce gas at high temperatures and this would reduce the vacuum in the tube. When the rotor switch is depressed prior to an exposure, the sound that is heard from the tube is actually the sound of the ball bearings turning at high speed. A new tube rotor with fresh bearings should coast for about 60 seconds after a 3,000 rpm exposure before stopping. When the coasting time slows to less than 20 seconds, the bearings are usually near binding.

High-speed anodes have a particular problem that is caused by the tone produced by their rotating. At between 5,000 and 7,000 rpm the harmonics produced by the rotating cuff are at a frequency capable of shattering the glass envelope. Consequently, at the end of an exposure, the stator is run in reverse to quickly slow the rotor safely through the dangerous harmonic range. Another problem associated with high-speed anodes is the gyroscopic effect produced by the centrifugal force of the rotation. This force is great enough that if a high-speed anode tube housing is quickly rotated from one position to another (for example, from horizontal to perpendicular), the gyroscopic effect can cause trauma to the anode disk and bearing, causing the destruction of the tube. Usually the reversal of the stator prevents this problem but constant rough handling of this sort can cause undue wear on the rotor bearings. Any rough or extremely fast movement of the housing is not healthy for an x-ray tube and should be avoided.

A common cause of tube failure is bad bearings caused by long use at high temperatures. Although the molybdenum shaft that attaches the anode disk is designed to conduct a minimal amount of heat, the ball bearings eventually become imperfectly round. This leads to a grinding noise and wobbling of the rotor. Rotor wobble throws the focal track off center and tube efficiency drops dramatically.

Another effect of stator or rotor failure is that the electron stream overheats the target area of the anode focal track. When the temperature exceeds the melting point of tungsten, melting will occur. Superheated melted tungsten that drips onto the glass envelope will destroy the tube.

Any tube is dangerous to use when these events occur. A wobbling or melting anode disk can crack from the heat of exposure. A cracked anode can divert the electron and/or photon stream toward the glass envelope. Either instance will crack the envelope, permitting implosion of the vacuum, which can suck the insulating oil into contact with the superheated anode assembly. This can cause vaporization of the oil in a violent explosion that can blow out the rubber expansion seals of the housing, permitting hot oil to drop from the tube housing. Superheated oil is a severe hazard to the patient and the normal response should be emergency removal of the patient from under the tube. In nearly all instances, it is quicker to pull the patient from under the tube than to release the locks necessary to manipulate the tube away from the patient. In an angiographic laboratory or surgical situation, the breaking of sterile aseptic technique would be justified. A blown tube is a rare event and should never occur if proper tube loading, quality control and maintenance procedures are followed.

THE GLASS ENVELOPE

The entire cathode assembly and all of the anode assembly except the stator are enclosed within a glass envelope commonly called the tube (Figure 7–19). A common glass envelope is made by sculpting several different types of heat-resistant Pyrex glass together to form a tube about 10″ long, 6″ in diameter at the center and 2″ in diameter at the ends. The glass is joined to the metal of the cathode assembly at one end and the anode assembly at the other. The envelope is constructed around both the cathode and anode assemblies and must be sealed tight to maintain a high vacuum. At the point where the primary x-ray beam exits the glass envelope, a **window** segment is constructed. In some tubes this is simply a thinner section of the envelope to allow less absorption or scatter of the photons. Some special application tubes have other types of windows. For example, a molybdenum target tube for mammography uses a special metallic beryllium window to avoid attenuating the lower-energy photons, as discussed earlier.

The Vacuum The primary function of the glass envelope is to maintain the vacuum between the cathode and anode. After construction, the air is removed from the tube until a pressure of less than 10^{-5} mm mercury (Hg) is achieved. This is done by use of a vacuum pump through a special vent, which is then permanently sealed. **The removal of the air permits electrons to flow from cathode to anode without encountering the gas atoms of air** and greatly increases the efficiency of the tube's operation.

Historical Notes Röntgen discovered x-rays with a Crookes or Hittorf tube which did not enclose a vacuum but instead contained known volumes of various gasses. Specialized tubes were quickly developed to meet the increasing need for x-ray production and the vacuum tube was an early improvement. The x-

Figure 7–19.   A complete diagnostic x-ray tube with glass envelope,
cathode assembly, anode disk and rotor.

ray pioneers simply placed the glass envelope within a leaded glass bowl. This was convenient when tubes had to be changed manually during the era of cold cathodes. Rapidly increasing awareness of the biological effects of ionizing radiation led to the development of metallic housings for x-ray tubes.

PROTECTIVE HOUSING

Modern x-ray tubes must be mounted inside a protective housing (Figure 7–20). **The housing controls leakage and scatter radiation, isolates the high voltages and provides a means to cool the tube**.

Control of Leakage Radiation and Scatter Radiation
When x-ray photons are produced at the anode they are emitted isotropically (in all directions). The primary beam consists of photons emitted through the glass

window. The remaining photons are unwanted and the tube housing is designed to absorb them. The protective housing is composed of cast steel and is capable of absorbing most of the unwanted photons. The housing is usually lined with lead for additional absorption only at the cathode end because of the direction of the photons being emitted from the anode. The housing is equipped with a window to permit unrestricted exit for the useful photons from the glass envelope window. Any photons that escape from the housing except at the port are **leakage radiation. Leakage radiation must not exceed 100 mR/hr at 1 meter**. The housing also serves to cushion the x-ray tube from rough handling by operators.

High-Voltage Isolation and Tube Cooling
A special dielectric oil is used to fill the space between the glass envelope and the tube housing. The dielectric property of the oil

Figure 7–20.   A diagnostic x-ray tube housing.

insulates the high-voltage components from the tube housing, which is handled by the radiographer. In addition, the oil absorbs much of the heat that is produced by x-ray production. One end of the tube housing is sealed with an expandable gasket to permit the oil to expand as it is heated (see Figure 7–20). This gasket can be blown out by an imploded tube that has vaporized some of the insulating oil, thereby presenting a hazard to the patient. Many tube housings include a small air fan to remove heat from the housing itself. In tubes that are subjected to extremely high loads, such as computed tomography tubes, the oil may be routed through a recirculation system (heat exchanger) to further cool it. Under no circumstances should anyone be in contact with a tube housing during an exposure.

OFF-FOCUS RADIATION

An often overlooked factor that can cause serious degradation of radiographic image quality is **off-focus or extrafocal radiation. Off-focus radiation is composed of photons that were not produced at the focal spot.** It occurs when the high-voltage electrons striking the focal spot produce scattered electrons or photons. In some cases these scattered electrons or photons have sufficient energy remaining that when they strike another object in the tube (the cathode assembly, vaporized metal on the glass envelope, off-target sites on the anode, etc.) they produce photons. These photons are produced away from the focal spot and are therefore considered off-focus. The tube housing will absorb the majority of off-focus radiation but enough will be produced at a proper angle that they will exit through the tube window, housing port and collimator (Figure 7–21). These photons can cause "ghosting" of structures adjacent to the edge of the primary beam (Figure 7–22). This is not the result of scatter from the patient. Patient scatter is not capable of creating a diagnostic image of anatomical structures. Off-focus radiation may contribute as much as 25–30 percent of the total primary beam. However, all off-focus radiation is of significantly lower energy than the primary beam itself. X-ray tubes are available

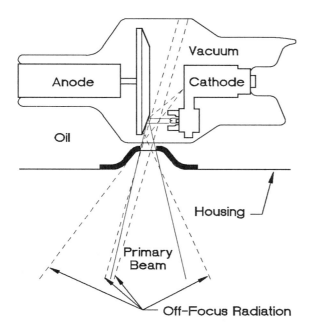

Figure 7–21. The production of off-focus radiation.

with a grounded metal and ceramic envelope to absorb off-focus radiation. These tubes may also use two sets of bearings to increase the heat-loading capacity. They have received limited acceptance because of their cost and the fact that they will not fit most existing tube housings. However, they can increase the total tube life by up to three times.

RATING CHARTS AND COOLING CURVES

Three types of heating charts are available to help radiographers avoid thermal damage to x-ray tubes: **radiographic tube rating charts, anode cooling charts and housing cooling charts**. Radiographic rating charts, sometimes called **tube rating charts**, are the most valuable because they provide a guide regarding the maximum technical factor combinations that can be used without overloading the tube. All radiographic tube rating charts plot

milliamperage, kilovoltage and time (the three most important factors set by the radiographer). Various manufacturers plot these factors in different ways (Figure 7–23). In most instances any combination of factors at or under the curve is safe. However, the radiographer should verify this fact by establishing that lower technical combinations lie under the curve. (If both the x and the y axes have lower values at the lower left corner of the chart, safe factors are under the curves.) **Each filament of each tube has a unique radiographic tube rating chart**. The radiographer must ascertain that the correct chart for the **tube and filament** is being used.

Example: Is an exposure of 80 kVp, 0.1 second and 200 mA within the limits of the 1φ, 0.6 mm focal-spot tube rating chart shown in Figure 7–23?

Answer: When the intersection of the 80 kVp and 0.1 second lines is located on the tube rating chart, it is below the 200 mA line. Since the lower technical combinations lie below the mA lines, this is within limits.

Example: Is an exposure of 90 kVp, 0.08 second and 600 mA within the limits of the 3φ, 1.2 mm focal-spot tube rating chart shown in Figure 7–24?

Answer: When the intersection of the 90 kVp and 0.08 second lines is located on the tube rating chart, it is above the 600 mA line. Since the lower technical combinations lie below the mA lines, it is not within limits.

Anode cooling charts permit the calculation of the time necessary for the anode to coole-nough for additional exposures to be made (Figure 7–25). All cooling charts are calculated in terms of radiographic heat units. **A heat unit is calculated as kVp × mAs × time × rectification constant**. The heat unit (HU) con-

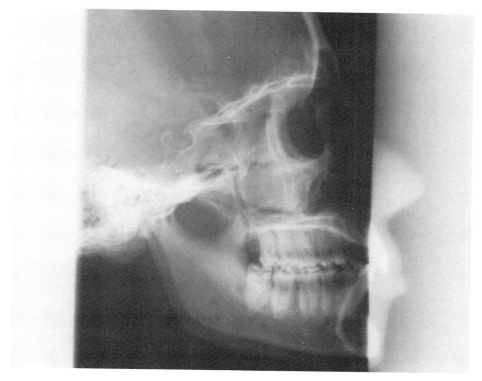

Figure 7–22. Off-focus radiation producing an image of the nose on a collimated sinus radiograph.

stants are given in Table 7–1. (Radiographic heat units are based on 1 kVp × 1 mA = 1 watt × 1 sec = 1 watt/sec × 0.71 rms voltage = 1 heat unit. Technically 1 radiographic heat unit = 0.78 joules.)

Example: How many heat units are generated by an exposure of 80 kVp, 200 mA and 0.2 second on a 1φ full-wave rectified unit?

Answer:

$$80 \text{ kVp} \times 200 \text{ mA} \times 0.2 \text{ sec}$$
$$\times 1.00 = 3,200 \text{ HU}$$

Example: How many heat units are generated by an exposure of 70 kVp, 300 mA and 0.15 sec on a 3φ 6 pulse unit?

Answer:

$$70 \text{ kVp} \times 300 \text{ mA} \times 0.15 \text{ sec}$$
$$\times 1.35 = 4,253 \text{ HU}$$

Example: How many heat units are generated by two exposures of 65 kVp, 400 mA and 0.05 sec on a 3φ 12 pulse unit?

Answer:

$$65 \text{ kVp} \times 400 \text{ mA} \times 0.05 \text{ sec}$$
$$\times 1.41 \times 2 \text{ exposures}$$
$$= 3,666 \text{ HU}$$

To use the chart, the exposure factors must first be calculated in heat units. The length of time for the anode to cool can then be calculated by the following steps:

Figure 7–23.   Tube rating chart for 1φ full-wave rectification. (Courtesy of Varian EIMAC.)

HEAT UNIT RECTIFICATION CONSTANTS	
Rectification	**Constant**
1φ 2 pulse (full wave)	1.00
3φ 6 pulse	1.35
3φ 12 pulse	1.41

TABLE 7–1

Figure 7–24.   Tube rating chart for 3φ full-wave rectification. (Courtesy of Varian EIMAC.)

Figure 7–25.   An anode cooling chart.

1. Find the total heat units applied on the vertical scale.

2. Read from the heat units over to the cooling curve and then down to read the corresponding time.

3. Calculate the time necessary for the anode to cool to any desired level and subtract the corresponding time of the initial exposure. (Or make the corresponding time of the initial exposure zero and calculate the time necessary for the anode to cool to any desired level from this point.)

For example, with the anode cooling chart in Figure 7–25, if a series of exposures produces 200,000 HU, the corresponding time is 2 minutes. The anode will cool to 150,000 HU in 2.5 minutes, so it will take 0.5 minute for the ane to cool from 200,000 HU to 150,000 HU. Similarly, the anode will cool to 100,000 HU in 1.5 minutes, to 50,000 HU in 4 minutes, and to room temperature (0) in 13 minutes.

Example: Use the anode cooling curve in Figure 7–25 to calculate the length of time necessary for the anode to cool to 50,000 HU after five exposures of 80 kVp, 500 mA and 0.5 second on a 1φ unit.

Answer:

$$80 \text{ kVp} \times 500 \text{ mA} \times 0.5 \text{ sec} \times 1.00 \times 5$$
$$= 100{,}000 \text{ HU}$$

50,000 HU = 6 minutes on cooling curve
100,000 HU = 3.5 minutes on cooling curve, so
6 min − 3.5 min = 2.5 min to cool from 100,000 to 50,000 HU

A more practical application of an anode cooling curve is to solve a problem regarding whether a desired exposure will overload the anode. For example, again using Figure 7–25, how long would it be after a load of 250,000 HU before a series of exposures equal to 150,000 HU could be made? Since the total HU capacity of

the anode is 350,000 HU, it must cool to 200,000 HU in order to take the additional 150,000 HU. The question becomes, "How long will it take the anode to cool from 250,000 to 200,000 HU?" It will take 0.75 minute (2 − 1.25 min), or 45 seconds, before the new series of exposures can be made because 250,000 HU corresponds to 1.25 minutes and 200,000 HU corresponds to 2 minutes.

Example: Use the anode cooling curve in Figure 7–25 to calculate the length of time necessary for the anode to cool sufficiently from 350,000 HU to accept a series of exposures totaling 150,000 HU on a 1φ unit.

Answer:
350,000 HU − 150,000 HU = 200,000 HU as level to which anode must cool
350,000 HU = 0 minutes
200,000 HU = 2 minutes
It will be 2 minutes (2 − 0 min) before the series of exposures can be made.

After working through several of these problems for most tube anodes, it becomes apparent that modern x-ray tubes are designed to withstand most exposures within the diagnostic range for average patients. It is when a series of exposures must be made (as occurs routinely in angiographic procedures) that most radiographic tube rating and anode cooling charts must be consulted.

Housing cooling charts permit the calculation of the time necessary for the housing to cool enough for additional exposures to be made (Figure 7–26). As with anode cooling charts, they are calculated in terms of radiographic heat units. They are used in exactly the same manner as an anode cooling chart. In actual practice the anode will usually reach its limits long before the housing. However, there are instances, as when the forced-air fan for the housing is not functioning, when these charts can be useful.

Figure 7–26. A housing cooling chart. (Courtesy of Varian EIMAC.)

RECOMMENDATIONS FOR EXTENDING TUBE LIFE

There are many things that the professional radiographer can do to extend the life of an x-ray tube. Warming up the anode according to the manufacturer's recommendations prevents thermal shock (cracking of a cold anode). Cracking can occur when the anode is unable to expand rapidly enough to absorb a room temperature-to-operating heat level exposure. Holding the rotor switch unnecessarily should be avoided. The rotor switch increases the filament's thermionic emission to exposure levels. Thermionic emission removes the electrons from the filament, deposits vaporized electrons on tube surfaces and decreases the tube vacuum, all of which can cause tube failure. In addition, the rotor switch causes stress to the rotor bearings, which can also decrease tube life. To avoid these problems, double-press switches should be completely depressed in one motion and dual switches should have the exposure switch depressed first, followed

by the rotor switch. Lower mA stations should be used when possible because high mA increases filament thermionic emission. The lower-speed rotor should be used when possible because the high-speed rotor increases rotor bearing wear. Repeated exposures near tube loading limits should not be made as total heat units may approach anode or housing loading limits. Rotating the tube housing rapidly from one position to another should be avoided because the gyroscopic effect may crack or otherwise damage the rotor. A tube should not be used when loud rotor bearings can be heard (unless it has been checked by a qualified service person) because a wobbling anode disk can cause tube failure. These recommendations are summarized in Table 7–2.

SUMMARY

X-ray production requires a source of electrons, an appropriate target material, a high voltage and a vacuum. The x-ray tube is the device that permits these conditions to exist. It consists of a cathode and an anode enclosed within a glass envelope and then encased in a protective housing.

The cathode is the negative side of the x-ray tube. The function of the cathode is to produce a thermionic cloud, conduct the high voltage to the gap between cathode and anode and focus the electron stream as it heads for the anode. The cathode assembly consists of the filament or filaments, focusing cup and associated wiring. The filament is a small coil of thin, thoriated tungsten wire. The focusing cup serves to narrow the thermionic cloud as it is driven to the anode.

The anode is the positive side of the x-ray tube. Anodes are divided into two types: stationary and rotating. Anodes are made using tungsten because of its high atomic number, high melting point and good heat-conducting

TABLE 7–2

RECOMMENDATIONS FOR EXTENDING TUBE LIFE

1. Warm up the anode following manufacturer's recommendations.
2. Do not hold the rotor switch unnecessarily. Double-press switches should be completely depressed in one motion.
   Dual switches should have exposure switch depressed first, followed by rotor switch.
3. Use lower mA stations when possible.
4. Use lower-speed rotor when possible.
5. Do not make repeated exposures near tube loading limits.
6. Do not rotate the tube housing rapidly from one position to another.
7. Do not use a tube when you can hear loud rotor bearings (unless it has been checked by a qualified service person).

ability. The anode assembly consists of the anode, the stator and the rotor. The portion of the anode where the high-voltage electron stream impacts is called the target, focus, focal point, focal spot or focal track. The term actual focal spot is used to describe the physical area of the focal track that is impacted. The term effective focal spot is used to describe the area of the focal spot that is projected out of the tube toward the object being radiographed.

The line-focus principle is used to reduce the effective area of the focal spot. This permits the best resolution of detail in as large an actual area as possible. The effective focal-spot size is controlled by the anode target angle. When the target angle is less than 45°, the effective focal spot is smaller than the actual focal spot.

The anode heel effect states that radiation intensity is greater on the cathode side than on the anode side.

An often overlooked factor that can cause serious degradation of radiographic image quality is off-focus or extrafocal radiation. Off-focus radiation is composed of photons that were not produced at the focal spot.

Three types of heating charts are available to help radiographers avoid thermal damage to x-ray tubes: radiographic tube rating charts, anode cooling charts and housing cooling charts. Radiographic rating charts, sometimes called tube rating charts, are the most valuable because they provide a guide regarding the maximum technical-factor combinations that can be used without overloading the tube. There are many things a radiographer can do to extend the life of an x-ray tube.

REVIEW QUESTIONS

1. What conditions must exist for x-rays to be produced?
2. What are the basic parts of a cathode assembly?
3. What is the purpose of the focusing cup?
4. Explain the space charge effect.
5. Why is tungsten the best metal for the x-ray source?
6. Explain the line-focus principle.
7. How does the anode heel effect affect radiation intensity?
8. What is the advantage of a high-speed rotor?
9. Why is it necessary for a vacuum to exist within the glass envelope?
10. Define leakage radiation.
11. How is off-focus radiation produced?
12. What is the function of rating charts and cooling curves?
13. Define a heat unit.
14. Name five things a radiographer can do to extend the life of an x-ray tube.

REFERENCES AND RECOMMENDED READING

Brookstein, Joseph J., and Walter Steck. Effective focal spot size. *Radiology* 98, 31–34, 1971.

Chesney, D. Noreen, and Muriel O. Chesney. *X-Ray Equipment for Student Radiographers.* 3rd ed. Oxford: Blackwell Scientific Publications, 1984.

Coolidge, W. D. Experiences with the Roentgen-ray tube. *American Journal of Roentgenology* 54, 583–589, 1945.

Coolidge, W. W. A powerful Röntgen ray tube with a pure electron discharge. *The Physical Review* 2:6, 1913.

Dendy, P. P., and B. Heaton. *Physics for Radiologists.* Oxford: Blackwell Scientific Publishers, 1987.

Dietz, D. *The X-ray Tube in Diagnostic Applications.* Erlangen, West Germany: Siemens Aktiengesellschaft, Medical Engineering Group. Publication MR A 5/1241.121.

Drew, Philip G. Lowly x-ray tube may be in for some big changes. *Diagnostic Imaging* Jan., 50, 1989.

Engel, Terry L. Effect of kilovoltage and milliamperage on focal spot size. *Radiologic Technology* 50:5, 559–561, 1979.

Everson, Jeffrey D., and Joel E. Gray. Focal-spot measurement: Comparison of slit, pinhole, and star resolution pattern techniques. *Radiology* 165:1, 261–264, 1987.

Fodor, Joseph III. Recent advances in x-ray tube design. *Radiologic Technology* 60:1, 33, 1988.

Gifford, Derek. *A Handbook of Physics for Radiologists and Radiographers.* New York: John Wiley and Sons, 1984.

Glasser, Otto. *Dr. W. C. Röntgen.* Springfield, IL: Charles C. Thomas, 1958.

Glasser, Otto. What kind of tube did Röntgen use when he discovered x-ray? *Radiology* 27, 138–140, 1936.

Grigg, E. R. N. *The Trail of the Invisible Light: From X-Strahlen to Radio(bio)logy.* Springfield, IL: Charles C. Thomas, 1965.

Harrison, R. M., and E. Forster. Performance characteristics of x-ray tubes and generators. *Radiography* 50:594, 245, 1984.

High and normal speed rotors: Effect on focal spot size, resolution and density. *Radiologic Technology* 53:1, 1981.

Machlett Laboratories, Inc. *"Trade-Offs" A Guide to the Selection of Diagnostic X-Ray Tubes.* Stamford, CT: The Raytheon Corporation. Publication ST–2859–1.

National Electrical Manufacturers Association. Measurements of dimensions and properties of focal spots of diagnostic x-ray tubes. NEMA Standards Publication No. XR–5–1984, 1985.

Seeram, Euclid. *X-Ray Imaging Equipment.* Springfield, IL: Charles C. Thomas, 1985.

Selman, Joseph. *The Fundamentals of X-Ray and Radium Physics.* 7th ed. Springfield, IL: Charles C. Thomas, 1985.

Sprawls, Perry. *Physical Principles of Medical Imaging.* Rockville, MD: Aspen Publications, 1987.

Stears, John G., Joel E. Gray, William E. Webbles, and Eugene D. Frank. Radiologic exchange (resolution according to focal spot size). *Radiologic Technology* 60:5, 429–430, 1989.

Stears, John G., Joel E. Gray, William E. Webbles, and Eugene D. Frank. Radiologic exchange (tube warm-up and leaving x-ray units on). *Radiologic Technology* 59:4, 325–326, 1988.

Stears, John G., Joel E. Gray, and Eugene D. Frank. The three limits to prevent x-ray tube damage. *Radiologic Technology* 58:5, 423, 1987.

Stears, John G., Joel P. Felmlee, and Joel E. Gray. Half-value layer increase owing to tungsten buildup in the x-ray tube: Fact or fiction? *Radiology*, 837, 1986.

Stears, John G., Joel E. Gray, and Eugene D. Frank. Overcoming tube failure in a special procedures room. *Radiologic Technology* 51:1, 89, 1979.

Stockley, Sybil M. *A Manual of Radiographic Equipment*. Edinburgh: Churchill Livingstone, 1986.

Thomas, Stephen R. Radiation physics—characteristics of extrafocal radiation and its potential significance in pediatric radiology. *Radiology* March, 793, 1983.

Thompson, Thomas T. *A Practical Approach to Modern Imaging Equipment*. 2nd ed. Boston, MA: Little, Brown, & Co., 1985.

Wallace, Rita J. Diagnostic x-ray tube failure and prevention. *Radiologic Technology* 48:5, 565, 1977.

Wilks, Robin J. *Principles of Radiological Physics*. Edinburgh: Churchill Livingstone, 1981.

THE CASE OF THE METAL FENCE

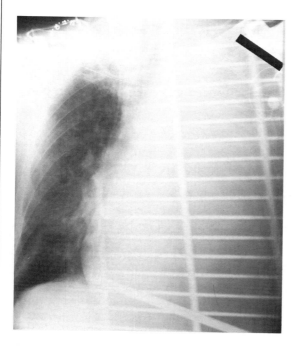

Can you determine what common object caused the metal fence artifact on this mobile chest radiograph? Hint: Try viewing the film sideways.

(Image courtesy of E. D. Frank and J. G. Stears, Mayo Foundation)

Answers to the case studies can be found in Appendix E.

8 X-RAY PRODUCTION

I did not think, I investigated.

Professor Wilhelm Röntgen to Sir James Mackenzie-Davidson during his only recorded interview, when asked what he thought when he discovered x-rays.

OUTLINE

CONDITIONS
TARGET INTERACTIONS
EMISSION SPECTRUM

OBJECTIVES

Upon completion of this chapter, the student should be able to:

1. State the percentage of electron energy that is converted to x-ray photon energy in the x-ray tube.
2. Describe a bremsstrahlung target interaction.
3. Describe a characteristic target interaction.
4. Identify factors affecting characteristic K-shell photon production.
5. Explain the shape of the x-ray photon emission spectrum curve.

CONDITIONS

X-ray photons are produced when the high-speed electrons from the cathode strike an anode target. The fact that they are man-made is the only difference between x-rays and gamma rays (which are products of nuclear radioactive decay). An understanding of how x-ray photons are created from the atoms of the target material permits the radiographer to assert full control over the production of the primary beam.

The electrons that form the thermionic cloud around the filament arrive at the anode target (2 cm distant) traveling at nearly half the speed of light. A true understanding of the force contained in a kilovoltage-level exposure can be obtained by realizing that these electrons were accelerated from zero to half the speed of light in about 2 cm. These incoming electrons are called **incident electrons** and are represented in drawings by a solid arrow. In contrast, photons are represented by a wave arrow.

When incident electrons strike the target, they convert their tremendous kinetic energy to the atoms of the target material and this interaction produces x-ray photons. The greater the mass or speed of the incident electrons, the greater the quality (energy) and quantity (number) of photons produced. This process occurs through two very different **target interactions**. All target interactions occur within 0.25 to 0.5 mm of the surface of the target. After giving up their energy to the target atoms, the electrons slow down enough to be conducted through the anode and the remainder of the high-voltage circuit. However, the incident electrons often experience 1,000 or more interactions before reaching this state.

TARGET INTERACTIONS

Heat Production

The target interactions that produce the x-ray photons consist of **less than one percent** of the total kinetic energy of the incident electrons. **Over 99** percent of the kinetic energy of the incident electrons is converted to heat. This is the reason why so much technical research has gone into the development of the thermal aspects of x-ray tubes. In spite of the cost and performance capabilities of modern x-ray tubes, they are tremendously inefficient because they waste over 99 percent of the energy they use. This is true only in the range of diagnostic x-rays. As the kinetic energy of the incident electrons increases, so does the efficiency of photon production. By the time the therapeutic MeV range is reached, the majority of the energy is producing photons instead of heat.

Because they have such high kinetic energy, incident electrons seldom transfer enough energy to the outer shells of target atoms to cause ionization. Instead, they transfer enough energy to excite the outer-shell electrons to the point where they will emit infrared radiation as heat. These electrons then return to their normal state—where they will be re-excited again and again, each time emitting infrared radiation as heat.

There are two types of target interactions that can produce diagnostic-range x-ray photons: **bremsstrahlung interactions and characteristic interactions**. The interaction which will occur depends on the **photon energy** and the **binding energy of the electron shells** of the atom. Tungsten and rhenium are used as target materials in an effort to provide appropriate atomic number atoms, and a maximum number of similar electron shell binding energies.

Bremsstrahlung Interactions

Bremsstrahlung interactions are named by the German word for braking or slowing. The abbreviation "brems" is also used. **Brems interactions may occur only when the incident electron interacts with the force field of the nucleus**. The incident electron must have enough energy to pass through the orbital shells and approach the nucleus of the atom. Because atomic nuclei have a positive charge and the incident electron has a negative charge, there is a mutual attraction between them. When the incident electron gets close to the nucleus, the powerful nuclear force field is much too great for the electron to penetrate. Instead, the force field causes the incident electron to slow down (or brake) and then it diverts the electron's course. As a result, the electron loses energy and changes direction. The energy that is lost during the braking (or bremsstrahlung) is emitted as an x-ray photon. **These emissions are called bremsstrahlung photons and their energy is exactly the difference between the entering and exiting kinetic energy of the electron** (Figure 8–1).

These energies are individually unpredictable and can range from the total value of

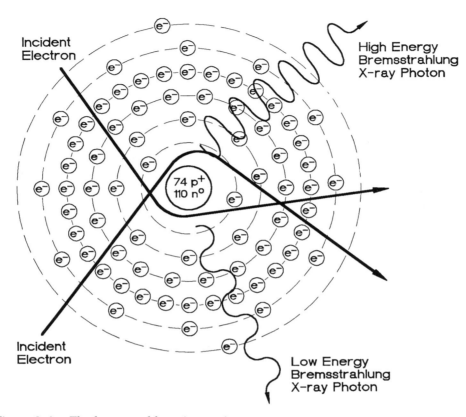

Figure 8–1.   The bremsstrahlung interaction.

the incident electron (which could be as high as the peak kilovoltage) to such a minimal amount of energy that it is immeasurable. Statistically, it is possible to predict their energies quite accurately, as will be discussed later in this chapter. Only when the incident electron loses all of its excess kinetic energy would the electron drift away to join the current flow. A single incident electron can cause numerous brems interactions in many different atoms before losing enough energy to become included in the current flow.

Characteristic Interactions

Characteristic interactions may occur only when the incident electron interacts with an **inner-shell electron** (Figure 8–2). The incident electron must have enough energy to knock an inner-shell electron from orbit, thereby ionizing the atom. The incident electron will usually continue but in a slightly different direction. More important is the fact that the electron "hole" that has been created in the inner shell makes the atom unstable. An electron from another shell will immediately drop into the "hole." This dropping of an electron from an outer, higher-energy state into an inner, lower-energy state results in the energy difference between the two shells being emitted as an x-ray photon. **These emissions are called characteristic photons because their energy is exactly the difference between the binding energy of the outer and inner shells between**

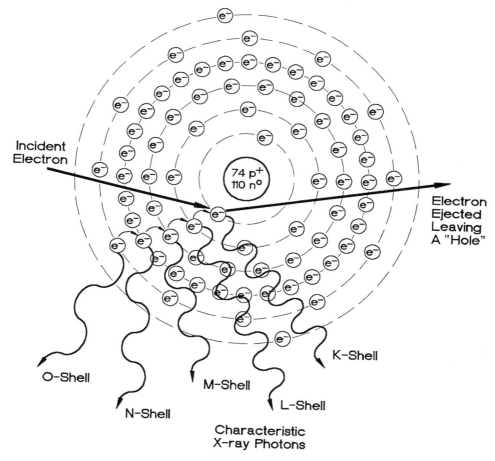

Figure 8–2. The characteristic interaction.

which the electron dropped. After an outer shell electron has dropped to fill the "hole," another electron will drop to fill the "hole" it left and so on until only the outermost shell is missing an electron. This process is called a **characteristic cascade** and it can produce numerous x-ray photons for each electron that leaves the atom.

The first electron that was knocked from position in an inner orbital shell often has sufficient energy that it, too, may cause further interactions before it loses enough energy to become part of the current flow. Of course this

will also contribute to the total number of photons created.

Unlike brems photons, characteristic photon energies are so predictable that the science of x-ray spectroscopy uses measurements of these photon energies to determine what types of atoms make up the sun, stars and other celestial bodies.

A tungsten atom, with its high atomic number of 74, has sufficient electron shells to produce relatively high-energy characteristic photons. Tungsten has a total of 74 electrons, with 2 electrons in the K-shell, 8 in L, 18 in M,

32 in N, 12 in O and 2 in the P-shell (see Figure 2–5). The binding energies of the electrons in these shells are 69.5 keV for the K-shell electrons, 21.1 keV for L-shell electrons, 2.8 keV for M, 0.6 keV for N and 0.08 keV for the O-shell electrons. The electron that drops into the "hole" may be from any shell further away from the nucleus. Of course the further out the dropping electron's original position, the greater the energy imparted to the characteristic photon.

Characteristic photons can be created from incident electron ionization of any shell and "hole" filling from any shell. For example, K-shell ionizations can result in characteristic photons from electron drops between shells L and K, M and K, N and K, etc. Characteristic photons can also result from L-shell ionizations with electron drops between shells M and L, N and L, and so on. A wide variety of characteristic photon energy levels are thus produced (Table 8–1). Note that only electron drops into the K-shell will produce characteristic photons within the diagnostic x-ray range.

A single incident electron can cause a variety of interactions in many different atoms before losing enough energy to become included in the current flow (Figure 8–3). Remember, most of these interactions will result in the production of heat.

EMISSION SPECTRUM

Within the diagnostic x-ray range most photons are produced by bremsstrahlung target interactions. Characteristic photons will not comprise any of the useful beam until the kVp is above 70 because removal of a K-shell electron from tungsten requires 69.5 keV. Between 80–100 kVp about 80–90 percent of the primary beam is produced by brems interactions and 10–20 percent by characteristic interactions.

As mentioned previously, the K-shell emissions are the only ones within the diag-

---

TABLE 8–1

CHARACTERISTIC PHOTON EMISSIONS FROM X-RAY TARGET MATERIALS

TUNGSTEN

K-Shell Characteristic Photons		L-Shell Characteristic Photons		M-Shell Characteristic Photons	
L to K	59.0 keV				
M to K	67.2 keV	M to L	9.6 keV		
N to K	69.1 keV	N to L	11.0 keV	N to M	2.5 keV
O to K	69.9 keV	O to L	12.3 keV	O to M	2.9 keV
P to K	70.1 keV	P to L	12.4 keV	P to M	3.0 keV
Effective energy	69.5 keV	Effective energy	12.0 keV	Effective energy	2.0 keV

MOLYBDENUM

K-Shell Characteristic Photons		
L to K	17	keV
M to K	20	keV
Effective energy	18	keV

nostic x-ray range, although the L-shell emissions form a similar group and the M- to P-shell emissions form a third group. Both brems and characteristic emissions combine to form the complete primary beam spectrum (Figure 8–4). The L-shell characteristic emissions are included within the total spectrum, but when filtration is added to the tube these photons do not have sufficient energy and are absorbed by the filter. The K-shell emissions form a **characteristic peak** at their effective energy range of 69 keV. This characteristic peak is worthy of special note as it can cause strange results for the radiographer who is operating the x-ray tube slightly above the K-shell peak and needs a slight decrease in radiation output. A slight decrease that sets the tube potential directly on the 69 keV K-shell peak would greatly increase the tube output instead of decrease it, as anticipated. Modern x-ray equipment is capable of somewhat overcoming these fluctuations by programmed switching and the use of tungsten alloys (such as molybdenum) in the target to smooth out characteristic peaking. However, characteristic peaks are a point of consider-

ation, not only in the target material but in the construction of x-ray tabletops, grids, cassettes, intensifying screens and any other object through which the primary beam must pass. **The kilovoltage peak of the exposure is the maximum possible energy for any photon that exits the x-ray tube.**

Example: At what kVp was the exposure made that produced the graph in Figure 8–4?

Answer: As the maximum brems photons were at 80 keV, the kVp was set at that level.

What is interesting about Figure 8–4 is that it clearly demonstrates an often overlooked fact about radiographic exposures. **The average primary beam photon has a keV energy of only about 30–40 percent of the kVp.**

The emission spectrum for a mammographic molybdenum target is quite different from that of a tungsten target. The K-shell characteristic peak is about 18 keV and the average photon energy range is between 20–40 keV, which is perfect for soft-tissue visualization.

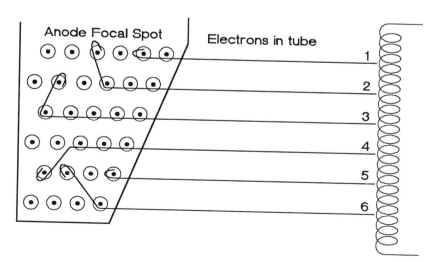

Figure 8–3. Sample paths of interactions for incident electrons striking the tube target.

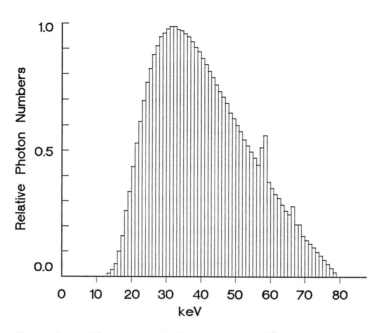

Figure 8–4.   The x-ray emission spectrum with a tungsten target. This graph is the result of an exposure made with 2.8 mm Al/Eq filtration at constant potential, producing 17.8 mR/mAs at 30" (75 cm). The effective photon energy was 31 keV. (Courtesy of Raymond P. Rossi, University of Colorado Health Science Center.)

It is very useful to examine the effect on the primary beam emission spectrum of various factors under the control of the radiographer. When **mA, time or mAs** is changed, all of which control the quantity (number) of electrons striking the target, the result is a change in the **amplitude** of the emission graph (Figure 8–5). Note that each point on the higher curve represents exactly twice the number of photons on the lower curve. When **kVp**, which controls the quality (energy) of electrons striking the target, is changed, the result is a change in the **number of higher-energy photons as well as in the amplitude** of the emission graph (Figure 8–6). Note that there are more higher-energy photons on the higher curve, as well as an increase in the number of photons (seen in the increased amplitude). There was no increase in

the total number of electrons striking the target. The increase in amplitude represents more emitted photons due to the higher energy of each incident electron striking the target.

The x-ray emission spectrum is affected by the quantity and composition of the materials through which it must pass to exit the x-ray tube and housing. This is the filtration, which is the subject of the next chapter. As the x-ray beam passes through the filtering materials, some of the lower-energy photons are absorbed. This **decreases** the intensity of the beam but at the same time **increases** the average photon energy. Increased filtration decreases image density, and vice versa.

The generator phasing also has an effect on the emission spectrum. As the efficiency of x-ray production increases—from 1φ 2 pulse to

Figure 8–5. The effect of mA changes on the x-ray emission spectrum.

3φ 6 pulse to 3φ 12 pulse to constant potential—the emission spectrum changes (Figure 8–7). As generator phasing efficiency increases, the x-ray beam **increases** in intensity and there is also an **increase** in the average photon energy. Decreased phasing efficiency decreases both intensity and average photon energy.

SUMMARY

X-ray photons are produced when the high-speed electrons from the cathode strike an anode target. When incident electrons strike the target, they convert their tremendous ki-

netic energy to the atoms of the target material and this interaction produces x-ray photons. The greater the mass or speed of the incident electrons, the greater the quality (energy) and quantity (number) of photons produced.

The two target interactions that produce x-ray photons are bremsstrahlung (brems) and characteristic interactions. Less than one percent of the total kinetic energy of the incident electrons produces these interactions. Over 99 percent of the kinetic energy of the incident electrons is converted to heat.

Brems interactions occur when the incident electron interacts with the force field of the nucleus. This force field causes the incident electron to slow down (or brake) and then it diverts the electron's course. As a result, the electron loses energy and changes direction. The energy that is lost during the braking is emitted as a bremsstrahlung photon and the photon energy is exactly the difference between the entering and exiting kinetic energy of the electron.

Characteristic interactions occur when the incident electron interacts with an inner-shell electron. The incident electron knocks out an inner-shell electron and continues in a slightly different direction. An electron "hole" is created in the inner shell, making the atom unstable. An electron from another shell will

Figure 8–6. The effect of kVp on the x-ray emission spectrum.

Figure 8–7. The effect of generator phase on the x-ray emission spectrum.

immediately drop into the "hole," which results in the emission of an x-ray photon. This emission is called a characteristic photon because the energy is exactly the difference between the binding energy of the outer and inner shells between which the electron dropped.

Within the diagnostic x-ray range most photons are produced by bremsstrahlung target interactions. An x-ray emission spectrum graph illustrates the relationship between the two target interactions within the primary beam. The average primary beam photon has a keV energy of only about 30 percent of the kVp.

When mA, time or mAs is changed, all of which control the quantity (number) of electrons striking the target, the result is a change in the amplitude of the emission spectrum graph. When kVp is changed, which controls the quality (energy) of electrons striking the target, the result is a change in the number of higher-energy photons, as well as in the amplitude of the emission spectrum graph.

REVIEW QUESTIONS

1. What is the approximate percentage of electron energy that is converted to x-ray photon energy in the x-ray tube?

2. The majority of the electron energy in the x-ray tube is converted to what form of energy?

3. Describe a bremsstrahlung target interaction.

4. Describe a characteristic target interaction.

5. What is a characteristic cascade?

6. What is the average keV of the primary beam as compared to the kilovoltage peak?

7. What effect does increasing mAs and kVp have on the total x-ray emission spectrum?

REFERENCES AND RECOMMENDED READING

Dendy, P. P., and B. Heaton. *Physics for Radiologists*. Oxford: Blackwell Scientific Publishers, 1987.

Erickson, Jon J., and Craig M. Coulam. Production of x-rays. *The Physical Basis of Medical Imaging*. 37–46. Editors: Coulam, Craig M., John J. Erickson, F. David Rollo, and A. Everette James, Jr. New York: Appleton-Century-Crofts, 1981.

Fewell, Thomas R., and Ralph E. Shuping. Photon energy distribution of some typical diagnostic x-ray beams. *Medical Physics* 5:3, 187–197, 1977.

Irfan, A. Y., V. I. Pugh, and C. D. Jeffery. Some practical aspects of peak kilovoltage measurements. *Radiography* 51:599, 251–254, 1985.

Johns, Harold E., and John R. Cunningham. *The Physics of Radiology.* 4th ed. Springfield, IL: Charles C. Thomas Publishers, 1983.

National Council on Radiation Protection and Measurements, NCRP Report No. 102: *Medical X-ray, Electron Beam and Gamma-Ray Protection of Energies up to 50 MeV.* (Equipment Design Performance and Use), Bethesda, MD: NCRP, 1989.

Sprawls, Perry. *Physical Principles of Medical Imaging.* Rockville, MD: Aspen Publishers, 1987.

Stears, John G., Joel E. Gray, William E. Webbles, and Eugene D. Frank. Radiologic

exchange (kVp measurements). *Radiologic Technology* 60:3, 233–236, 1989.

Storm, E., and H. I. Israel. Photon cross sections from 1 keV to 100 MeV. *Nuclear Data Tables,* 1970.

Ter-Pogossian, Michel. *The Physical Aspects of Diagnostic Radiology.* New York: Harper & Row, 1967.

van der Platts, G. J. *Medical X-Ray Techniques in Diagnostic Radiology: A Textbook for Radiographers and Radiological Technicians.* The Hague: Martinus Nijhoff Publishers, 1980.

Wilks, Robin J. *Principles of Radiological Physics.* Edinburgh: Churchill Livingstone, 1981.

Wilson, Peter. Theoretic basis of the nature and origin of x-radiation. *Canadian Journal of Radiography, Radiotherapy, and Nuclear Medicine* 8:1, 12–27, 1977.

THE CASE OF THE DOUBLE ROW OF CAPSULES

What could possibly produce this image? Special attention to the thin radiopaque lines is helpful.

Answers to the case studies can be found in Appendix E.

9 FILTRATION

the bones gleam
out of the dark.
like the ghost of a fern
in stone here
are spine and ribs.

Celia Gilbert, "X-Ray."

OUTLINE

MEASUREMENT
TYPES OF FILTRATION
EFFECT ON OUTPUT

OBJECTIVES

Upon completion of this chapter, the student should be able to:

1. Define filtration, inherent filtration, added filtration, compound filtration, compensating filtration, and total filtration.
2. Explain the concept of half-value layer equivalency measurements of filtration.
3. Appraise various types of filters for specific clinical situations.
4. Describe the effect of filtration on the entire x-ray beam.

Filtration is the process of eliminating undesirable low-energy x-ray photons by the insertion of absorbing materials into the primary beam. When inserted properly, filtration permits the radiographer to shape the photon emission spectrum into a more useful beam. Filtration is sometimes called **hardening** the beam because it removes the low-energy (soft) photons (Figure 9–1). The primary reason for filtration is the elimination of photons that would cause increased radiation dose to the patient but would not enhance the radiographic image.

At 20 keV, about 45 percent of the incident photons will penetrate 1 cm of soft tissue but only about 0.0006 percent will penetrate

Figure 9–1.   Effect of filtration on the x-ray beam.

15 cm. At 50 keV, 3.5 percent of the incident photons (a significant percentage) will penetrate 15 cm. Significant soft-tissue penetration occurs between 30 and 40 keV. Although they contribute to the patient dose, low-energy photons have insufficient energy to exit the patient and make any contribution to the image. Therefore their elimination is desirable.

MEASUREMENT

Any material designed to selectively absorb photons from the x-ray beam is called a filter. In diagnostic radiology, filtration is typically added between the source and the patient. Aluminum is the most common filter material used, although other materials, such as glass, oil, copper and tin are used or become filters in various instances. **Aluminum is considered the standard filtering material and all filtration can be expressed in terms of the thickness of aluminum equivalency (Al/Eq).** For example, the attachments, mirror and plastic of a collimator might be the equivalent of 0.5 mm of aluminum (Figure 9–2). This would be expressed as 0.5 mm Al/Eq. Filtration is also expressed in terms of half-value layer. **The half-value layer (HVL) is that amount of absorbing material that will reduce the intensity**

of the primary beam to one-half its original value. Half-value layers are usually expressed in terms of aluminum filtration equivalency; for example, HVL = 2.0 mm Al/Eq.

TYPES OF FILTRATION

Filtration occurs at various points between the x-ray tube and the image receptor. It is either **inherent** in the design of the tube or **added** between the tube and the image receptor.

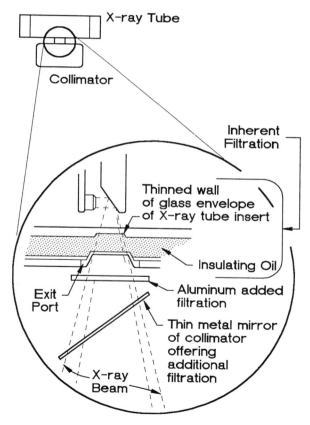

Figure 9–2.   Total filtration of the x-ray beam. (Adapted by permission from David Jenkins, *Radiographic Photography and Imaging Processes*, Lancaster, MTP Press, 1980.)

Inherent Filtration

Filtration that is a result of the composition of the **tube and housing** is often called **inherent filtration** because it is a part of these structures. The thickness of the glass envelope of the tube, the dielectric oil that surrounds the tube, and the glass window of the housing all contribute to the inherent filtration. A typical x-ray tube might have a total inherent filtration of 0.5–1.0 mm Al/Eq. Most of the inherent filtration comes from the window of the glass envelope.

Because of this, mammographic tubes with special molybdenum targets that are designed to produce lower photons for soft-tissue imaging often have special beryllium (atomic number 4) windows in the glass envelope to eliminate the majority of the inherent filtration. Beryllium windows can reduce the inherent filtration to 0.1 mm Al/Eq. As tubes age they become gassy, the anode begins to pit and the glass envelope may gain a mild coating of vaporized metal. All these factors will cause an increase in the inherent filtration, thus reducing the tube efficiency. This is the reason why HVL testing of tubes is a recommended quality control procedure for evaluation of tube efficiency and age.

Added Filtration

Any filtration that occurs outside the tube and housing and before the image receptor is considered added. Filtration materials are selected to absorb as many low-energy photons as possible while transmitting a maximum number of high-energy photons. Aluminum, with an atomic number of 13, functions very well as a low-energy absorber.

The collimator device also adds filtration to the beam and is considered to be added filtration. Collimators average 1.0 mm Al/Eq, most of which comes from the silver on the mirror situated in the beam. The mirror is de-signed to reflect the collimator light to simulate the primary beam field size for positioning purposes. This addition to the inherent filtration is why mammographic units often do not use collimators. The filtering effect would cause absorption of the low-energy photons that are desirable for soft-tissue imaging.

Compound Filtration

A compound filter uses two or more materials that complement one another in their absorbing abilities. Most compound filters are constructed so that each layer absorbs the characteristic photons created by the previous layer. For this reason, compound filters are also referred to as **K-edge filters**. Compound filters place the highest atomic number material closest to the tube and the lowest atomic number material closest to the patient. The final layer is usually aluminum, which has an atomic number of 13.

Although aluminum is the most common filtering material, copper, with an atomic number of 29, functions well for slightly higher energies. When a copper filter is used, it must be backed by an aluminum filter to absorb the 8 keV K-shell characteristic radiation produced by the copper. Copper filters should be at least 0.25 mm thick and backed with a minimum of 1 mm of aluminum.

A good example of a compensating filter is the **Thoreaus filter**, used in radiation therapy. This filter combines tin, copper, and aluminum, in that order. Tin has the highest atomic number (50) and is placed first in the beam. Next, a copper filter is added to absorb the 29.3 keV characteristic photons created by the tin. Finally, aluminum is added to the copper to absorb copper's characteristic photons, which would only contribute to increasing patient dose. The 1.5 keV K-shell characteristic radiation produced by the aluminum filter is absorbed in the air between the filter and the patient.

Compensation Filtration

A **compensating filter** is usually designed to solve a problem involving unequal subject densities. The goal is to add an absorber to compensate for unequal absorption within the subject, thus making the overall absorption of the primary beam more equal. This helps in producing a more uniform radiographic film density. Compensating filters can be made of aluminum, leaded plastic trademarked under the name ClearPb™ or plastic. Even an ordinary saline solution bag can be a useful compensating filter.

The two most popular compensating filters are the **wedge filter** and the **trough filter** (sometimes called a double wedge). The thicker portions of the filter are matched to the less dense patient body parts (Figure 9–3). A wedge filter can be useful for procedures on the thoracic spine, the feet (Figure 9–4) and the lower extremities, particularly during venography and femoral angiography. A trough filter is useful to even the density differences between the mediastinum and the lungs on a chest radiograph.

It is also possible to custom design filters by several methods. Aluminum, ClearPb™ or plastic pieces may be attached by magnets or rods underneath the collimator to permit movement into or out of the primary beam. The advantage of the ClearPb™ is its ability to use the collimator light to project the filter position onto the patient's body. Some plastic filters, such as the boomerang filter, are designed to be placed under the patient. Radiologists may object to the use of compensating filters on the justifiable grounds that they cast artifacts onto the radiographic image.

Explorations have been made into the use of various heavy elements, including some of the rare earths, to utilize K-shell characteristic production to enhance energy ranges that are especially useful. For example, studies have been done using rare earths to increase photon emissions at the energies needed by iodine contrast agents. Difficulties in making these filtration techniques practical have kept them from becoming popular. However, very good results have been obtained for mammography by using a 0.05 mm molybdenum filter and operating the tube at a constant 35 kVp.

Wedge Filter

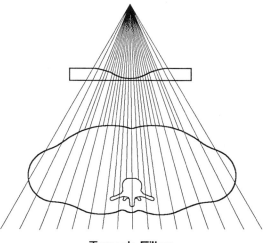

Trough Filter

Figure 9–3. Compensating filters.

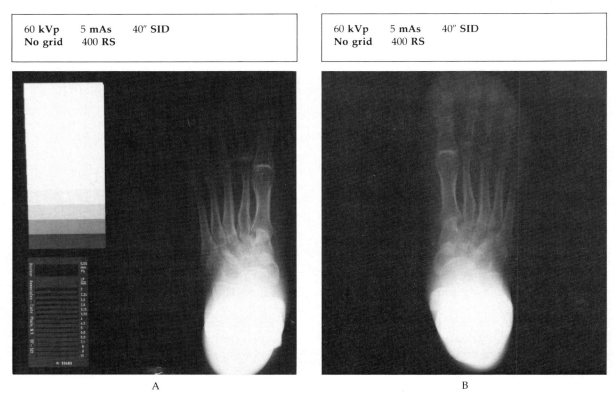

| 60 kVp | 5 mAs | 40″ SID |
| No grid | 400 RS | |

| 60 kVp | 5 mAs | 40″ SID |
| No grid | 400 RS | |

A   B

Figure 9–4A and B.   The use of a compensating wedge filter for an AP foot projection is shown in B.

Total Filtration

Total filtration is equal to the sum of inherent and added filtration and does not include any compound or compensating filters that may be added later. The thickness of the added filtration varies depending on the anticipated uses of the equipment. The percentage of photons attenuated decreases as photon energy increases, even when filtration is increased (Table 9–1). Note that aluminum filters of 1–3 mm absorb significant percentages of photons below the diagnostic range while permitting the vast majority to pass. The National Council on Radiation Protection (NCRP) recommends minimum total filtration levels for diagnostic radiography, as shown in Table 9–2.

These filtration levels are commonly used in the United States and correspond to International Council on Radiation Protection (ICRP) recommendations. The importance of the reduction in patient dose, as shown in Table 9–3, must not be overlooked.

EFFECT ON OUTPUT

Not only does filtration reduce the patient exposure dose by eliminating low-energy photons from the primary x-ray beam, it also removes a portion of the useful beam. This has a visible effect on radiographic film density. To compensate for the loss of film density **when filtration is increased, technical factors must be increased to maintain the same density.**

TABLE 9–1

Percent Attenuation of Monochromatic Radiation by Various Thicknesses of Aluminum Filtration

Photon Energy (keV)	Photons Attenuated (%)			
	1 mm	2 mm	3 mm	10 mm
10	100	100	100	100
20	58	82	92	100
30	24	42	56	93
40	12	23	32	73
50	8	16	22	57
60	6	12	18	48
80	5	10	14	39
100	4	8	12	35

Reproduced with permission from Curry, T., Dowdey, J. and Murry, R. *Christensen's Physics of Diagnostic Radiology*, 4th ed. Philadelphia: Lea and Febiger, 1990.

Note that in Table 9–3 the decrease in patient dose compares very favorably with the increase necessary to maintain radiographic film density. In other words, although the exposure needs to be increased to maintain density, there is a greater decrease in overall exposure to the patient.

SUMMARY

Filtration is the process of eliminating undesirable x-ray photons by the insertion of absorbing materials into the primary beam. Any material designed to selectively absorb photons from the x-ray beam is called a filter. Aluminum is the most common filter material used. It is considered the standard filter material and all filtering in diagnostic radiography can be expressed in terms of the thickness of aluminum equivalency (Al/Eq). The half-value layer (HVL) is that amount of absorbing mate-

TABLE 9–2

Operating kVp	Total Filtration
Below 50 kVp	0.5 mm aluminum
50 to 70 kVp	1.5 mm aluminum
Above 70 kVp	2.5 mm aluminum

Adapted by permission from Table 3–1, National Council on Radiation Protection and Measurements. *NCRP Report No. 102, Medical X-Ray, Electron Beam and Gamma-Ray Protection for Energies Up to 50 MeV (Equipment Design, Performance and Use)*. Bethesda, MD: NCRP, 1989.

rial that will reduce the intensity of the primary beam to one-half its original value.

Filtration occurs at various points between the x-ray tube and the image receptor. It is either inherent in the design of the x-ray tube or added between the tube and the image receptor. Filtration that is the result of the composition of the tube and housing is often called inherent filtration because it is a part of these structures. Any filtration that occurs outside the tube and housing and before the image receptor is considered added. The collimator device adds approximately 1.0 Al/Eq to the beam.

The compound filter uses two or more materials that complement one another in their absorbing ability. A compensating filter is usually designed to solve a problem involving unequal subject density. Two common compensating filters are the wedge and the trough. Total filtration is equal to the sum of inherent and added filtration.

Not only does filtration reduce the patient exposure dose by eliminating low-energy photons, it also removes a portion of the useful beam and can therefore affect image density.

REVIEW QUESTIONS

1. What is filtration?

2. What is the standard filter material used in diagnostic radiography?

TABLE 9–3

COMPARISON OF PATIENT DOSE WITH FILTRATION

Aluminum Filtration in mm	Entrance Skin Dose in mR	Decrease in Exposure Dose	Increase in Exposure Required to Maintain Same Film Density
60 KVP, 18 CM PELVIS			
none	2,380		
0.5	1,850	22%	14%
1.0	1,270	47%	17%
3.0	465	80%	52%
85 KVP, 18 CM PELVIS			
none	1,225		
0.5	860	30%	0%
1.0	684	44%	12%
3.0	287	77%	34%

From E. Dale Trout, J. P. Kelley, and G. A. Cathey. The Use of Filters to Control Radiation Exposure to the Patient in Diagnostic Roentgenology. *American Journal of Roentgenology* 67:942, 1952.

3. Define half-value layer.

4. What is inherent filtration?

5. When more than one filtering material is used, as in a compound filter, how are the materials arranged in relationship to the x-ray source?

6. What are the two most common compensating filters?

7. What is total filtration?

8. How does filtration affect patient exposure dose and beam intensity?

REFERENCES AND RECOMMENDED READING

Bernier, Peter. Clinical application of gadolinium filters in neonatal radiography. *The Canadian Journal of Medical Radiation Technology* 13:6, 273, 1982.

Croft, Melanie J. Filtration, the answer to the automatic exposure control response problem. *Radiologic Technology* 57:5, 447, 1986.

Cullinan, Angeline. *Producing Quality Radiographs.* Philadelphia, PA: J. B. Lippincott Co., 1987.

Curry, Thomas S., James E. Dowdey, and Robert C. Murry. *Christensen's Introduction to the Physics of Diagnostic Radiology.* 3rd ed. Philadelphia, PA: Lea & Febiger, 1984.

Dendy, P. P., and B. Heaton. *Physics for Radiologists.* Oxford: Blackwell Scientific Publishers, 1987.

Feczko, Peter J. Compensation filtration for decubitus radiography during double-contrast barium enema examination. *Radiology* Dec., 848, 1983.

Geissberger, Hans. Wedge-shaped filters for improved radiography of the thoracic vertebrae and the foot. *Medical Radiography and Photography* 42:1, 6, 1966.

Gray, Joel E., John G. Stears, and Eugene D. Frank. Shaped, lead-loaded acrylic filters for patient exposure reduction and image-quality improvement. *Radiology* 146, 825–828, 1983.

Johns, Harold E., and John R. Cunningham. *The Physics of Radiology.* 4th ed. Springfield, IL: Charles C. Thomas Publishers, 1983.

Jones, Robin, and Arlene McKenna Adler. The use of saline as a compensating filter. *Radiologic Technology.* 61:3, 1990.

Kassebaum, Mary Kathryn. The use of compensating filters. *Radiologic Technology* 20:4, 209, 1949.

Kohn, Mark L., Adrian W. Gooch, Jr., and Warren S. Keller. Filters for radiation reduction: A comparison. *Radiology,* 255, 1988.

Smith, Douglas C., and John Tidwell. Adjustable sliding aluminum wedge filter: Device for angiographic enhancement. *Radiologic Technology* 49:4, 459, 1978.

Sprawls, Perry. *Physical Principles of Medical Imaging.* Rockville, MD: Aspen Publishers, 1987.

Stears, John G., Joel E. Gray, William E. Webbles, and Eugene D. Frank. Radiologic exchange (added filtration). *Radiologic Technology* 59:3, 245–246, 1988.

Stears, John G., Joel E. Gray, and Eugene D. Frank. The variable filter dial. *Radiologic Technology* 57:6, 542, 1986.

Trout, E. Dale, John P. Kelley, and George A. Cathey. The use of filters to control radiation exposure to the patient in diagnostic roentgenology. *American Journal of Roentgenology* 67, 946–963, 1952.

Villagran, J. E., B. B. Hobbs, and K. W. Taylor. Reduction of patient exposure by use of heavy elements as radiation filters in diagnostic radiology. *Radiology* 127, 249, 1978.

Wilks, Robin J. *Principles of Radiological Physics.* Edinburgh: Churchill Livingstone, 1981.

10 THE PRIME FACTORS

X-ray technic, like x-ray equipment, has passed through an evolutionary stage from the beginning, in 1896, to the present time, and the end is not yet in sight.

E. C. Jerman, 1926.

OUTLINE

THE PRIME FACTORS
MILLIAMPERAGE-SECOND (mAs)
KILOVOLTAGE (kVp)
DISTANCE

OBJECTIVES

Upon completion of this chapter, the student should be able to:

1. Explain the relationships between milliamperage (mA), exposure time, mAs and x-ray emission.
2. State the reciprocity law.
3. Calculate mAs when given mA and exposure time, mA when given mAs and exposure time, and exposure time when given mAs and mA.
4. Explain the relationship between kVp and x-ray emission.
5. State the 15 percent rule.
6. Calculate the new kVp value needed to maintain density when changes are made in mAs, using the 15 percent rule.
7. Explain the relationship between distance and x-ray emission.
8. State the inverse square law.
9. Calculate x-ray emission (mR) when distance is changed.
10. Calculate the mAs needed to maintain density when changes are made in distance, using the density maintenance formula.

THE PRIME FACTORS

The emission of x-ray photons from an x-ray tube is controlled by a number of factors. Those factors related to tube design and construction have been covered in previous chapters and include tube housing, target material, filtration and voltage waveform. Three factors that affect x-ray emission are under the direct control of the radiographer. These are called the **prime factors**. They are milliamperage-second (mAs), kilovoltage (kVp) and distance (d).

The x-ray beam can be described in terms of both its quantity and its quality. **X-ray quantity** is a measure of the number of x-ray photons in the useful beam. It is also called x-ray output, intensity or exposure. Recall that the unit of measurement of x-ray quantity is the **roentgen (R)**. The factors that directly affect x-ray quantity are milliamperage-second (mAs), kilovoltage (kVp), distance (d) and filtration. **X-ray quality** is a measurement of the penetrating ability of the x-ray beam. Penetrability describes the distance an x-ray beam travels in matter. High-energy x-ray photons travel farther in matter than low-energy photons and are therefore more penetrating. Highly penetrating x-rays are termed hard x-rays and low penetrating x-rays are called soft x-rays. X-ray quality is numerically represented by the **half-value layer (HVL)**. The half-value layer of an x-ray beam is that thickness of absorbing material needed to reduce the x-ray intensity (quantity) to half its original value. The factors that directly affect x-ray quality are kilovoltage and filtration.

The factors that control the quantity and/or quality of x-ray emission are the prime factors and filtration (Table 10–1). Filtration is not something the radiographer controls from exposure to exposure.

MILLIAMPERAGE-SECOND (mAs)

Milliamperage (mA) is a measurement of x-ray tube current—the number of electrons crossing the tube from cathode to anode per second. Recall that an ampere is equal to an electric charge of one coulomb flowing through a conductor per second. The coulomb is equal to 6.3×10^{18} electron charges. Therefore, an ampere equals a flow of 6.3×10^{18} electrons per second and a milliampere would equal 6.3×10^{15} electrons per second. As mA increases so does the number of electrons which are able to cross the tube to reach the x-ray target. **Milliamperage is directly proportional to tube current**. As the mA doubles so does the number of electrons able to cross the tube. The number of electrons reaching the target is also controlled by the length of time the tube is energized. Remember that mA is the number of electrons **per second**. This means that changes in the length of time of exposure will affect the total number of electrons flowing from cathode to anode. X-ray exposure time is measured in **seconds**. Like mA, **exposure time is directly proportional to the number of electrons crossing the tube and is therefore directly proportional to the number of x-rays created**. This is the x-ray quantity.

The number of x-rays that will be created at the target is a product of the number of electrons crossing the tube (tube current) and how long the electrons are allowed to cross (exposure time). **Milliamperage-second (mAs)** is the unit used to describe the product of tube cur-

TABLE 10–1
FACTORS AFFECTING X-RAY EMISSION

Quantitative Factors	Qualitative Factors
Milliamperage-second	Kilovoltage
Kilovoltage	Filtration
Distance	
Filtration	

60 kVp	1.3 mAs	40" SID
No grid	**400 RS**	**2.46 mR**

A

60 kVp	1.3 mAs	40" SID
No grid	**400 RS**	**2.54 mR**

B

60 kVp	2.6 mAs	40" SID
No grid	**400 RS**	**5.72 mR**

C

Figure 10–1. These three radiographs demonstrate the effect of mAs on radiographic density. Although the mA and time may vary, if mAs = mAs, then radiographic density will be the same. A and B have the same mAs although A was exposed at 100 mA and 0.013 sec, while B was exposed at 400 mA and 0.003 sec. When the mAs is doubled, the radiographic density doubles (C).

70 kVp	0.65 mAs	40″ SID
No grid	400 RS	2.16 mR

60 kVp	0.65 mAs	40″ SID
No grid	400 RS	1.40 mR

A

B

60 kVp	1.3 mAs	40″ SID
No grid	400 RS	2.66 mR

C

Figure 10–2. These three radiographs demonstrate the effect of kVp on radiographic density. A & B show the effect of increasing kVp on density. In C, density is maintained by applying the 15 percent rule.

rent and exposure time. This simple relationship is described by the equation mA × s = mAs. Milliamperage-second (mAs) is the primary controller of x-ray quantity. X-ray quantity is directly proportional to mAs. This means that as mAs doubles, x-ray exposure (measured in roentgens) doubles; as mAs triples, x-ray exposure triples and so forth.

If an x-ray control panel is set at 100 mA and 0.05 (1/20) second, the mAs would be 100 × 0.05 or 5 mAs. If either the mA or the exposure time is doubled, the mAs will double, i.e., 200 mA at 0.05 second equals 10 mAs, as does 100 mA at 0.1 (1/10) second. This means that a number of possible settings on the x-ray control can all yield the same x-ray exposure. For example, 10 mAs can be set using any of the following technical factors:

$$50 \text{ mA} \times 0.2 \text{ (1/5) second} = 10 \text{ mAs}$$
$$100 \text{ mA} \times 0.1 \text{ (1/10) second} = 10 \text{ mAs}$$
$$200 \text{ mA} \times 0.05 \text{ (1/20) second} = 10 \text{ mAs}$$

Obviously, a number of other possibilities exist as well. This relationship can be described in the equation $mA_1 s_1 = mA_2 s_2$. Because mA and exposure time can be manipulated to achieve the same mAs, **it is best to think in terms of mAs when establishing technical factors**. It is important, for technical factor conversions, that the technologist be able to manipulate the mA and time to arrive at the proper mAs for a particular examination.

Examples: Given the following mA and exposure time values, calculate the mAs.
200 mA × 0.083 second = _____ mAs
100 mA × 2/5 second = _____ mAs

Answers:
200 mA × 0.083 second = 16.6 mAs
100 mA × 2/5 second = 40 mAs

Examples: Given the following mAs and mA values, calculate the exposure time.

75 mAs = 100 mA × _____ second
15 mAs = 300 mA × _____ second

Answers:
75 mAs = 100 mA × 0.75 (3/4) second
15 mAs = 300 mA × 0.05 (1/20) second

Examples: Given the following mAs and exposure time values, calculate the mA.
60 mAs = 0.3 (3/10) second × _____ mA
75 mAs = 0.15 (3/20) second × _____ mA

Answers:
60 mAs = 0.3 (3/10) second × 200 mA
75 mAs = 0.15 (3/20) second × 500 mA

Density Relationship to mAs

Radiographic density is the degree of blackening of an x-ray film. Density is created by deposits of black metallic silver on an x-ray film that has been exposed to light or x-ray and then processed. On the radiographic image, the densities are the result of an x-ray exposure to the film and intensifying screens. Recall that as mAs is increased, x-ray exposure will increase proportionally. This means that mAs is therefore a primary controller of radiographic density as well. As mAs increases, x-ray exposure increases proportionally, and radiographic density increases proportionally. This relationship holds true throughout the diagnostic x-ray range provided the x-ray equipment is properly calibrated and maintained.

The relationship of a film's reaction to exposure was described in 1875 by Bunsen and Roscoe, who studied the reaction of photographic film to light and stated that the reaction of a photographic film to light is equal to the product of the intensity of the light and the duration of the exposure. This concept is known as the **reciprocity law**. When applied to x-rays, the reciprocity law can be restated to say that the density on an x-ray film is proportional to the intensity and duration of the x-ray exposure (controlled by mAs). This law is true for x-ray films exposed using intensifying screens, because most of the film's exposure is from light and not x-rays. The reciprocity law fails for exposures made at extremely short exposure times (less than 1/100 second) or extremely long exposure times (more than 10 seconds). Under these circumstances, densities will be somewhat less than the exposures. Reciprocity law failure is not very significant in diagnostic radiology because exposure times are seldom at those extremes.

Radiographic density should remain unchanged as long as the total exposure to the film remains unchanged. If the mAs used to create one image is the same as the mAs used to create a second image of the same structure, then both images should have the same radiographic density. As long as mAs is constant, any combination of mA and exposure time values will create the same density. The radiographs in Figures 10–1A and 10–1B illustrate this point. Remember, accurate results will depend on using equipment that is properly calibrated. Equipment testing is an important part of a quality control program for the radiology department.

Radiographic density will increase proportionally when mAs increases and will decrease proportionally when mAs decreases. Either the mA or the exposure time or both may be increased or decreased to cause an increase or decrease in the mAs. The radiographs in Figure 10–1B and Figure 10–1C illustrate this point. When mAs is doubled, the radiographic density on the film is doubled. The resulting film is twice as dark as the original. If the mAs is reduced by half, the resulting film will be twice as light as the original image. If the mAs is increased by a factor of five, then the resulting image will be five times darker.

Milliamperage-second (mAs) is the primary controlling factor which will affect the x-ray quantity and radiographic density. The appropriate mAs should be selected to achieve an acceptable radiograph. The technologist is usually in control of the mAs selection. However, the equipment may be in control when the technologist is using an automatic exposure control system, a computerized exposure system, or falling load generators.

KILOVOLTAGE (kVp)

Kilovoltage (kVp) controls both the quantity and quality of the x-ray beam. **Increasing the kilovoltage on an x-ray control panel will cause an increase in the speed and energy of the electrons applied across the x-ray tube.** If the electrons move more quickly from cathode to anode, more electrons will reach the target per second, resulting in an increase in x-ray production. In addition, the energy of the electrons is greater, resulting in the production of x-ray photons with greater energy. As x-ray photon energy increases, the penetrating ability of the photon increases. Kilovoltage affects the **quantity** of the x-ray beam because **more** electrons will reach the target as kVp increases, and it affects the **quality** of the x-ray beam because each electron has more energy, resulting in a beam with greater **penetrability**.

The quantity (intensity) of x-ray photons increases very quickly with increases in kVp. X-ray quantity is **approximately** directly proportional to the square of the ratio of the change in kVp. This means that as kVp is doubled, the amount of x-ray photons increases approximately four times. Although this can be mathematically expressed, this formula would have no practical application because it does not take into account the fact that changes in kVp have a significant effect on the penetrability of the beam.

Density Relationship to kVp

Both the quantity and quality of the x-ray beam will vary significantly with changes in the kilovoltage applied across the x-ray tube. As a result, kVp has a tremendous impact on radiographic density (Figures 10–2A and 10–2B). In addition, because changes in kilovoltage create changes in beam penetrability, kVp is the primary controller of the differences in radiographic densities. This is known as contrast. An increase in kVp causes an increase in penetrability, which will result in an image with less contrast. For the present discussion, the effect of kVp on density will be detailed. Contrast is discussed in Chapter 24.

Research was done to determine a practical formula to take into account kVp's effect on both x-ray quantity and quality. This resulted in the **15 percent rule**. The intent of this rule was to provide a guide for radiographers to maintain density. **The 15 percent rule states that an increase in kVp by 15 percent will cause a doubling in exposure, the same effect as doubling the mA or exposure time.** The reverse is also true. If kVp is decreased by 15 percent, exposure will be reduced by one half (Figure 10–2B and Figure 10–2C). Because both the amount and penetrability of x-ray photons increase with increases in kVp, the effect of changes in kVp will vary from low kVps to high kVps. In other words, a smaller change in kVp will have a greater impact on x-ray emission in the lower kVp ranges than in the higher kVp ranges. For example, 15 percent of 40 kVp is 6, while 15 percent of 80 kVp is 12. Radiographic density will nearly double when kVp is changed from 40 to 46 kVp. At 80 kVp, an increase in 12 kVp is needed to approximately double the radiographic density.

Example: A radiograph of the pelvis is produced using 25 mAs at 70 kVp. What kVp would be needed to double the radiographic density?

Answer:
15 percent of 70 kVp = 10.5 kVp
$$70 + 10.5 = 80.5 \text{ or } 81 \text{ kVp}$$

Since kVp is expressed as a whole number, answers should be rounded to the nearest whole number.

While kVp has a tremendous impact on radiographic density, **kVp adjustments should not be used to control radiographic density**. The selection of a kVp range for specific radiographic procedures is determined by the desired contrast for the image. This will be discussed in Unit IV.

DISTANCE

The intensity of x-rays varies greatly with changes in distance. Just as the intensity of light from a light bulb will decrease the further one moves from the source, so will x-ray photons spread out from their source at the x-ray tube target. As a result, the x-ray intensity will decrease as the distance from the tube is increased. The measurement of the x-ray intensity is obtained using a dosimeter. X-ray intensity is measured in roentgens (R) or, more commonly in diagnostic radiology, in milliroentgens (mR).

From the point of origin of the x-ray beam at the tube target, the beam begins to diverge. The x-ray photons are most concentrated at the target and from there they spread out in all directions. Those photons that exit the tube port constitute the primary, useful beam. As the useful beam spreads and widens, x-ray intensity or quantity begins to diminish. The actual number of photons created remains unchanged but the distribution of the photons varies with the distance. The further from their source, the lower will be the quantity of photons within a given area.

The relationship of x-ray quantity to distance is described in the inverse square law. **The inverse square law states that the intensity of radiation at a given distance from the point source is inversely proportional to the square of the distance.** The inverse square law requires an understanding of some basic rules of geometry. In Figure 10–3 the diverging lines represent the x-ray beam diverging from a col-

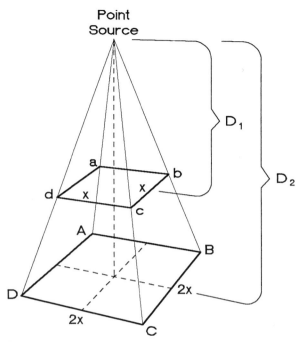

Point
Source

D_1

D_2

a

b

d

x

x

c

A

B

D

2x

2x

C

Figure 10–3. The inverse square law states that the intensity of radiation at a given distance from a point source is inversely proportional to the square of the distance. The lower surface area (ABCD) is twice as far from the source of radiation and is four times (2^2) the surface area of the upper surface area (abcd).

meter in square abcd would measure four times more than a dosimeter in square ABCD. For example, if a dosimeter in square abcd measures 100 mR, a dosimeter in square ABCD would measure 25 mR, or four times less.

Thus the intensity or quantity of photons decreases with increased distance, which is an inverse relationship. More specifically, the relationship is inversely proportional to the square of the distance change. If the distance increases by a factor of three, the intensity would decrease by a factor of 3^2, or nine times.

The inverse square law can be used to calculate changes in intensity that occur as a result of changes in distance. The mathematical expression of the law is:

$$\frac{I_1}{I_2} = \frac{D_2^2}{D_1^2}$$

where: I_1 = original intensity
I_2 = new intensity
D_1 = original distance
D_2 = new distance

The formula can also be expressed as:

$$I_1 D_1^2 = I_2 D_2^2$$

In order to calculate any of the four factors, three of the four must be known. The equation can then be rearranged to place the unknown factor alone on one side of the equal sign.

Example: An x-ray exposure of 240 mR is recorded at a distance of 20 inches. If the same technical factors are used, what will the exposure dose be if the distance is increased to 40 inches?

Answer:

$$\frac{240}{I_2} = \frac{40^2}{20^2}$$

$$I_2 = \frac{240 \times 20^2}{40^2}$$

limated source. At a distance of 36 inches (D_1), the x-ray beam covers a square area (abcd). Each side has a given dimension (x) so the area of square abcd would equal x times x or x^2. If the distance is increased to 72 inches (D_2), the sides of the second square (ABCD) are now twice as long, or 2x. The area of square ABCD would be 2x times 2x or $4x^2$. A doubling of the distance has increased the area of the square by four times.

X-ray photons falling in square abcd are spread out over an area four times as large by the time it reaches square ABCD. The number of photons remains the same, but they are now spread over an area four times larger. A dosi-

$$I_2 = \frac{240 \times 400}{1,600}$$

$$I_2 = 60 \text{ mR}$$

Example: An x-ray exposure of 400 mR is recorded at a distance of 72 inches. If the same technical factors are used, what will the exposure dose be if the distance is decreased to 40 inches?

Answer:

$$\frac{400}{I_2} = \frac{40^2}{72^2}$$

$$I_2 = \frac{400 \times 72^2}{40^2}$$

$$I_2 = \frac{400 \times 5,184}{1,600}$$

$$I_2 = 1,296 \text{ mR}$$

The inverse square law should be used when calculating the relationships between distance and x-ray intensity (mR).

Density Relationship to Distance

Since distance has an effect on x-ray intensity, it will in turn affect radiographic density. **As the distance increases, intensity decreases, which causes a decrease in density on the film** (Figures 10–4A and 10–4B). The reverse is also true. As the distance decreases, intensity increases, which in turn causes an increase in radiographic density. Radiographic density is also inversely proportional to the square of the distance. If the distance is doubled, radiographic density will decrease by a factor of four.

A practical application of the inverse square law is found in a formula which is used to compensate for the density changes that occur when distance is changed. The formula is sometimes known as the **density maintenance**

formula and is **based on** the principle of the inverse square law. The density maintenance formula is a **direct square law.** A direct relationship is necessary to compensate for the changes in intensity and density.

Since mAs is the primary controller of x-ray intensity and radiographic density, mAs can be adjusted to compensate for changes in distance. For example, an acceptable chest film results from an exposure taken using four mAs at 100 kVp at a 72-inch distance. A second film must be taken supine at a 36-inch distance. If the same technical factors are used, the inverse square law tells us that when the distance is decreased by a factor of two, the intensity and film density will increase by a factor of four. The second film will be four times too dark if the technical factors are not adjusted. The mAs can be adjusted to compensate for the distance change. The density maintenance formula can be used to determine the exact compensation necessary for any change in distance (Figure 10–4B and Figure 10–4C). It is a direct square law because mAs should increase proportionally to the square of the change when distance increases, and mAs should decrease proportionally to the square of the change when distance in decreased. In the example above, if the distance decreases by a factor of two (72 inches to 36 inches), the mAs should be reduced by a factor of 2^2, or four. The new mAs would be 1/4th the original, or one mAs. Four mAs at 72 inches will produce the same density as one mAs at 36 inches, provided all other factors remain the same.

The density maintenance formula is:

$$\frac{mAs_1}{mAs_2} = \frac{D_1^2}{D_2^2}$$

where: mAs_1 = original mAs
mAs_2 = new mAs
D_1 = original distance
D_2 = new distance

60 kVp	1 mAs	36″ SID
No grid	400 RS	2.56 mR

A

60 kVp	1 mAs	72″ SID
No grid	400 RS	0.76 mR

B

60 kVp	4 mAs	72″ SID
No grid	400 RS	2.40 mR

C

Figure 10–4. These three radiographs demonstrate the effect of distance on radiographic density. A and B show the effect of increasing distance on density. In C, density is maintained by applying the density maintenance direct square law

The same formula can be expressed as:

$$mAs_2 = \frac{mAs_1 \times D_2^2}{D_1^2}$$

These formulas have very direct applications to radiography because they provide the radiographer with a means for adjusting mAs to maintain density when changes are made in distance for a given radiographic procedure.

Example: An acceptable radiograph of the abdomen is taken using 25 mAs at 80 kVp at a distance of 40 inches. A second radiograph is requested to be taken at 56 inches. What mAs should be used to produce an acceptable radiograph if the distance is increased to 56 inches?

Answer:

$$mAs_2 = \frac{25 \times 56^2}{40^2}$$

$$mAs_2 = \frac{25 \times 3,136}{1,600}$$

$$mAs_2 = 49 \text{ mAs}$$

Changes in distance will create changes in the x-ray intensity and the radiographic density. The density maintenance formula can be used to compensate for the effect that changes in distance will have on the density of the radiographic image. The radiographs of Figures 10–4A and C demonstrate the application of the direct square law for density maintenance.

SUMMARY

Prime factors are under the direct control of the radiographer and have a significant impact on x-ray photon emission from the tube. The prime factors are milliamperage-second (mAs), kilovoltage (kVp) and distance (d). X-ray emission can be described in terms of both its quantity (amount) and quality (penetrability). X-ray quantity is affected by mAs, distance, kVp and filtration. X-ray quality is affected by kVp and filtration.

Milliamperage-second (mAs) is directly proportional to the number of x-ray photons created in the tube and is therefore directly proportional to radiographic density. Kilovoltage affects both quantity and quality and its relationship to x-ray emission is not as easily described. Kilovoltage is approximately proportional to the square of the ratio of the change in kVp. Therefore, if kVp is doubled, the x-ray quantity would increase by a factor of four. This does not, however, take into account the increased penetrability of the beam with increasing kVp. As a result, radiographic density is more significantly affected. To maintain density with changes in kVp, the 15 percent rule can be applied. The 15 percent rule states that an increase in kVp by 15 percent will cause an approximate doubling of the radiographic density. To maintain density, if kVp is increased by 15 percent, the mAs must be reduced to one half its original value. The distance from the actual focal spot to the image receptor is the third prime factor. The quantity of x-ray photons is inversely proportional to the square of the distance. As distance increases, radiographic density will decrease in an inverse proportion to the square of the change in the distance.

REVIEW QUESTIONS

1. What are the three prime factors that affect x-ray emission?

2. What is the unit of measurement for x-ray quantity?

3. Define an ampere.

4. What is the relationship between mAs and radiographic density?

5. What effect does increased kVp have on the speed and energy of the electrons in the x-ray tube?

6. What is the relationship between kVp and radiographic density?

7. State the inverse square law.

8. What is the relationship between distance and radiographic density?

REFERENCES AND RECOMMENDED READING

American Registry of Radiologic Technologists. Use of 'penumbra' studied. *Radiologic Technology* 58:1, 74, 1987.

Ball, J. L., and A. D. Moore. *Essential Physics for Radiographers*. 2nd ed. Oxford: Blackwell Scientific Publications, 1986.

Carroll, Quinn. *Fuchs's Principles of Radiographic Exposure, Processing and Quality Control*. 3rd ed. Springfield, IL: Charles C. Thomas Publishers, 1985.

Dendy, P. P., and B. Heaton. *Physics for Radiologists*. Oxford: Blackwell Scientific Publications, 1987.

De Vos, Dianne C. *Basic Principles of Radiographic Exposure*. Philadelphia, PA: Lea & Febiger, 1990.

Eastman Kodak Company, Health Sciences Markets Division. *The Fundamentals of Radiography*. 12th ed. Rochester, NY: Kodak Publication M1–18.

Fodor, Joseph, and Jack C. Malott. *The Art and Science of Medical Radiography*. 6th ed. St. Louis, MO: Catholic Health Association of the United States, 1987.

Fuchs, Arthur W. The rationale of radiographic exposure. *Radiologic Technology* 22:2, 62, 1950.

Gifford, Derek. *A Handbook of Physics for Radiologists and Radiographers*. New York: John Wiley & Sons, 1984.

Glasser, Otto, Edith H. Quimby, Lauriston S. Taylor, J. L. Weatherwax, and Russell H. Morgan. *Physical Foundations of Radiology*. 3rd ed. New York: Paul B. Hoeber Division of Harper & Brothers, 1961.

Hay, George A., and Donald Hughes. *First-Year Physics for Radiographers*. London: Bailliere Tindall, 1972.

Hiss, Stephen S. *Understanding Radiography*. Springfield, IL: Charles C. Thomas Publishers, 1978.

Jerman, E. C. An analysis of the end-result: The radiograph. *Radiology* 6, 59–62, 1926.

Selman, Joseph. *The Fundamentals of X-Ray and Radium Physics*. 7th ed. Springfield, IL: Charles C. Thomas Publishers, 1985.

Sprawls, Perry. *Principles of Radiography for Technologists*. Rockville, MD: Aspen Publishers, 1990.

Thompson, Thomas T. *Cahoon's Formulating X-Ray Techniques*. 9th ed. Durham, NC: Duke University Press, 1979.

11 X-RAY INTERACTIONS

Perhaps no single field of investigation has contributed more to our knowledge of atomic structure than has the study of x-rays.

Arthur H. Compton, preface to the first edition of *X-Rays and Electrons*.

OUTLINE

X-RAY INTERACTION WITH MATTER
PHOTOELECTRIC ABSORPTION
COHERENT SCATTERING
COMPTON SCATTERING
PAIR PRODUCTION
PHOTODISINTEGRATION
EFFECT ON TECHNICAL FACTOR SELECTION

OBJECTIVES

Upon completion of this chapter, the student should be able to:

1. Define attenuation.
2. Explain the interactions between x-rays and matter in the following:
   a. photoelectric absorption
   b. coherent scattering
   c. Compton scattering
   d. pair production
   e. photodisintegration
3. Describe the relationship between x-ray interactions and technical-factor selections.

X-RAY INTERACTION WITH MATTER

When an x-ray beam passes through matter, it undergoes a process called attenuation. Attenuation is the reduction in the number of x-ray photons in the beam as it passes through matter (Figure 11–1).

Attenuation is the result of x-ray photons interacting with matter and losing energy through these interactions. While some photons will pass through matter and not interact, an x-ray photon can interact with the whole atom, an orbital electron or directly with the nucleus. This will depend on the energy of the photon. Low-energy photons are most likely to interact with the whole atom, intermediate-energy photons generally interact with orbital electrons while very high-energy photons, such as those used for radiation therapy, are capable of interacting with the nucleus. In the diagnostic x-ray range, the interactions are most commonly with orbital electrons.

To fully understand x-ray interactions with matter, it is important to recall the structure of the atom. The center of the atom is a positively charged nucleus containing protons and neutrons. The negatively charged electrons are in orbital paths around the nucleus. The energy required to remove an electron from a shell is termed the binding energy of the shell. The K-shell electrons possess the highest binding energy for a given atom and binding energies decrease progressively for successive shells. Not only is the binding energy characteristic of a given shell, it is also specific to a given atom. K-shell electrons are more tightly bound to the nucleus in high atomic number elements. For example, the binding energy for the K-shell of tungsten (Z = 74) is approximately 70 keV while the binding energy for the K-shell of calcium

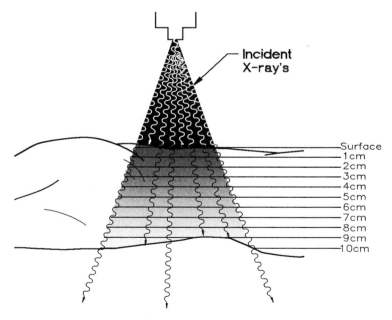

Figure 11–1. An x-ray beam undergoes attenuation as it passes through matter.

(Z = 20) is only about 4 keV. The average atom in the soft tissue of the body has an approximate K-shell binding energy of only 0.5 keV. Therefore, **the higher the atomic number of an element, the more energy will be required to remove a K-shell electron from the atom**.

Because electrons which are further from the nucleus are not held with as strong an electrical attraction, they possess a higher **energy level** than the inner-shell electrons. This means that outer-shell electrons possess more energy, in order to maintain their position around the atom, than inner-shell electrons. Recall the race car analogy discussed in Chapter 2. Race cars along the outside of the track need more speed to maintain the same position as the inner cars. As a result, a move closer to the center results in the ability to travel more slowly and still maintain the same position. When an outer-shell electron moves into an inner shell, it will release energy in the process because it will require less energy to maintain its new position. Therefore, **the further the electron is from the nucleus, the higher the energy level of the electron**.

Electrons in the K-shell have the lowest energy level with the highest binding energy, and with each successive shell, **energy levels increase and binding energies decrease**. These concepts are particularly important to the understanding of x-ray interactions with matter.

There are five basic interactions between x-rays and matter:

1. photoelectric absorption,
2. coherent scattering,
3. Compton scattering,
4. pair production and
5. photodisintegration.

With each of these interactions the x-ray photons either interact and change direction, a process called **scattering**, or are absorbed by the atom. When a photon is absorbed, all of the energy of the photon is transferred to the

matter and the photon no longer exists. If a photon interacts and scatters, the photon still exists but usually possesses less energy than before the interaction. Partial energy from the photon is transferred to the matter during the interaction and the lower-energy photon then continues along its new path until again it either interacts and scatters or is absorbed. One photon may scatter several times before it is finally absorbed completely by the matter. The likelihood of one interaction occurring over another varies, depending on the incident photon's energy and the atomic number of the matter. Certain interactions, pair production and photodisintegration, for example, occur only at very high photon energy ranges, while coherent scatter is most predominant in very low photon energy ranges.

PHOTOELECTRIC ABSORPTION

Photoelectric absorption results when an x-ray photon interacts with an inner-shell electron. This interaction is most likely to occur when the incident x-ray photon possesses a slightly greater energy than the binding energy of the electrons in the inner (K or L) shells. The incident photon ejects the electron from its inner shell and is totally absorbed in the interaction (Figure 11–2). The result is an ionized atom, because of the missing inner-shell electron, and an ejected electron, called a **photoelectron**. The photoelectron travels with kinetic energy, which is equal to the difference between the incident photon and the binding energy of the inner-shell electron. This is mathematically expressed in the equation:

$$E_i = E_b + E_{ke}$$

where: E_i = energy of the incident photon
E_b = binding energy of the electron
E_{ke} = kinetic energy of the photoelectron

The incident photon needs an energy which is slightly greater than the binding energy of

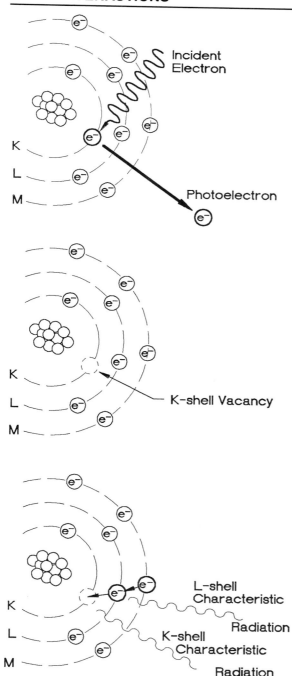

the electron for the interaction to occur. Since most of the atoms of the body are very low atomic number elements, the binding energies of the K-shell electrons are very low. For example, the K-shell binding energy for carbon is approximately 0.28 keV and oxygen is 0.53 keV. The K-shell binding energies of elements which are important in diagnostic radiology are listed in Table 11–1. Most photoelectric interactions in the body result in the majority of the incident photon energy being given to the kinetic energy of the photoelectron. The photoelectron is matter, not just energy, and therefore will not travel far. It is usually absorbed within 1 to 2 mm in soft tissue. Despite the localized absorption, this is still a significant way in which x-ray energy can create biological changes.

The ionized atom is in an unstable state with an inner-shell electron missing. The vacancy is instantly filled by an electron from the L-shell or, less commonly, from an M-shell or free electron. In the vast majority of cases the electron transfers from an outer shell to an in-

Figure 11–2. The photoelectric absorption interaction.

TABLE 11–1

K-SHELL BINDING ENERGIES OF RADIOLOGICALLY SIGNIFICANT ELEMENTS

Atom	Atomic Number	K-shell Binding Energies (keV)
Hydrogen	1	0.016
Carbon	6	0.284
Oxygen	8	0.53
Aluminum	13	1.56
Calcium	20	4.04
Molybdenum	42	20.0
Iodine	53	33.2
Barium	56	37.4
Tungsten	74	69.5
Lead	82	88.0

ner shell and, as it does, it releases energy in the form of a **characteristic photon**, known as **secondary radiation**. This secondary radiation is produced in the same manner as characteristic radiation is produced at the x-ray target— electron transfer from one shell to another. When it is created at the x-ray target it is considered primary radiation. When characteristic radiation is produced in irradiated matter outside of the x-ray target it is termed secondary radiation. Remember that outer-shell electrons possess a higher energy level than inner-shell electrons. Therefore when an outer-shell electron moves into an inner shell it has excess energy to release. This electron transfer process continues from shell to shell until the atom returns to a normal state and is no longer a positive ion. This process of each shell filling lower shells with a corresponding emission of photons is called a **characteristic cascade**. The energy of each photon of a characteristic cascade will be characteristic of the difference in energy in the two shells between which it dropped.

Because of the predominance of low atomic number elements comprising the human body, the secondary radiation produced is of extremely low energy. Secondary radiation energies are significantly higher for elements such as iodine and barium, which are commonly used as contrast agents in radiology.

There are three basic rules which govern the possibility of a photoelectric interaction:

1. **The incident x-ray photon energy must be greater than the binding energy of the inner-shell electron**. A 30 keV x-ray photon will not be able to remove the K-shell electron from an atom of iodine, which has a binding energy of 33.2 keV, or barium, which has a binding energy of 37.4 keV.

2. **A photoelectric interaction is more likely to occur when the x-ray photon energy and the electron binding energy are nearer to one another**. Of course, the x-ray photon

energy must always be greater, but a 40 keV photon is more likely to interact by way of the photoelectric effect with an atom of iodine (K-shell E_b = 33.2 keV) or barium (K-shell E_b = 37.4 keV) than would a 100 keV x-ray photon. As photon energy increases, the chance of a photoelectric interaction decreases dramatically. The actual relationship is expressed as an inverse proportion to approximately the third power of the photon energy (photoelectric effect = $1/(energy)^3$). A significant change is therefore seen in the percentage of photoelectric interactions that will occur when using low kVp techniques versus high kVp techniques (Table 11–2). This becomes very important to the radiographer when establishing appropriate technical factors for specific body tissues.

3. **A photoelectric interaction is more likely to occur with an electron which is more tightly bound in its orbit**. Binding energies of the electrons are greater in high atomic number elements than in low atomic number elements. In addition, inner-shell electrons have higher binding energies than outer- shell electrons in a given atom. With low atomic number elements, most interactions will occur with the K-shell electron. Because high atomic number elements bind their electrons more tightly, interactions will occur with the K-, L-, and M-shells. In fact, the incident x-ray photon often does not possess sufficient energy to remove a K-shell electron. For example, the K-shell binding energy for lead is 88 keV. X-ray photons below this level are incapable of removing the K-shell electrons but can be absorbed through photoelectric interactions with L- or M-shell electrons. The probability of a photoelectric interaction increases dramatically as the atomic number increases. The relationship is approximately proportional to the third power of the atomic number (photoelectric effect = $(atomic\ number)^3$). Since

TABLE 11–2

PERCENTAGE OF PHOTON INTERACTIONS, ATTENUATION, AND TRANSMISSION CHARACTERISTICS IN SOFT TISSUE BASED ON EFFECTIVE PHOTON ENERGIES

kVp	50	70	80	90	110	130
HVL(mm Al)	1.59	2.11	2.35	2.60	3.12	3.67
Mean Photon Energy(keV)	31.3	40.0	41.1	44.2	49.7	54.5
Effective Photon Energy(keV)	27.0	30.0	31.0	33.0	35.0	38.0
% of Photon Interactions by						
—Scattering (with coherent)	49.55%	62.70%	63.95%	66.70%	69.77%	75.22%
—Photoelectric	50.45%	37.30%	36.05%	33.30%	30.23%	24.78%
% Attenuation						
5 cm Tissue	91.45%	84.28%	83.45%	81.67%	79.70%	76.34%
10 cm Tissue	99.27%	97.53%	97.26%	96.64%	95.88%	94.40%
15 cm Tissue	99.94%	99.61%	99.55%	99.38%	99.16%	98.67%
20 cm Tissue	99.99%	99.94%	99.93%	99.89%	99.83%	99.69%
% Transmission						
5 cm Tissue	8.55%	15.72%	16.55%	18.33%	20.30%	23.66%
10 cm Tissue	0.73%	2.47%	2.74%	3.36%	4.12%	5.60%
15 cm Tissue	0.06%	0.39%	0.45%	0.62%	0.84%	1.33%
20 cm Tissue	0.01%	0.06%	0.07%	0.11%	0.17%	0.31%

Courtesy of Raymond P. Rossi, University of Colorado Health Science Center.

bone has an effective atomic number which is higher than that of soft tissue, photoelectric interactions are more likely to occur in bone than in soft tissue. **It is for this reason that radiography is so spectacularly useful in demonstrating the bones of the body**.

COHERENT SCATTERING

Coherent scatter is an interaction which occurs between very low-energy x-ray photons and matter. It is also called classical scatter or unmodified scatter. There are actually two types of coherent scattering: Thomson scattering and Rayleigh scattering. Thomson scattering involves a single electron in the interaction while Rayleigh scattering involves all of the electrons of the atom in the interaction. Both types have the same basic interaction results.

When a very low-energy photon, below approximately 10 keV, interacts with the electron(s) in an atom, it may cause the electron(s) to vibrate at the same frequency as the incident photon. The vibrating or excited atom immediately releases this excess energy by producing a secondary photon which has the same energy and wavelength as the incident photon but which travels in a direction different from the initial photon (Figure 11–3). The result is a scattered photon which possesses the same energy, frequency and wavelength as the initial photon but which is traveling in a different direction. Since there is no energy transferred in the interaction, the atom is not ionized in the process.

Coherent scattering occurs in a very low x-ray energy range which is generally outside

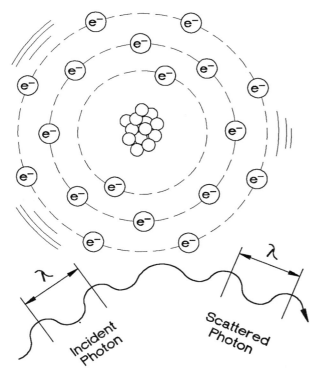

Figure 11–3.   The coherent scatter interaction.

the usual range for diagnostic imaging. A very small amount of the scatter radiation reaching the film is produced by this process and, as a result, this interaction has little significance to diagnostic imaging.

COMPTON SCATTERING

Compton scattering occurs when an incident x-ray photon interacts with a loosely bound outer-shell electron, removes the electron from its shell, and then proceeds in a different direction as a scattered photon (Figure 11–4). This interaction was described by the American Nobel laureate physicist Arthur H. Compton (1892–1962) in 1922 and is known as the **Compton effect** Part of the energy of the incident photon is used to remove the outer-shell electron and impart kinetic energy to it.

The dislodged electron is called a **Compton or recoil electron**. The photon which exits the atom in a different direction is called a **Compton scattered photon**. It possesses less energy than the incident photon and therefore has a lower frequency and longer wavelength.

The energy transfer in the Compton effect is mathematically expressed in the equation:

$$E_i = E_s + E_b + E_{ke}$$

where: E_i = energy of the incident photon
  E_s = energy of the Compton scattered photon
  E_b = electron binding energy of the Compton electron
  E_{ke} = kinetic energy given to the Compton electron

The incident photon energy is divided between the ejected electron and the scattered photon. The scattered photon retains most of the energy because little energy is needed to eject an outer-shell electron, due to its low binding energy. The scattered photon will continue to interact with atoms until it is eventually absorbed photoelectrically. The recoil electron is available as a free electron to fill a shell "hole" created by another ionizing interaction.

The amount of energy retained by the scattered photon is dependent on the initial energy of the photon and its angle of deflection from the recoil electron. The higher the initial energy of the photon, the greater the energy of the scattered photon. Scattered photons can be deflected at any angle from the recoil electron, just as a cue ball is deflected after it strikes a second ball in a game of billiards. At a deflection of 0° no energy is transferred because the photon is proceeding in its original direction. As the angle of deflection increases to 180° more energy is imparted to the recoil electron and less energy remains with the scattered photon (Figure 11–5).

When a scattered photon is deflected back toward the source, it is traveling in the di-

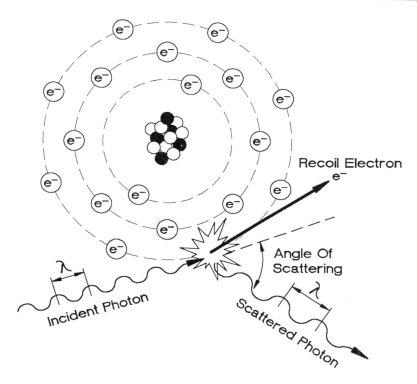

Figure 11–4.   The Compton scatter interaction.

rection opposite to the incident photon. These photons are called **backscatter radiation**. Most photons will scatter in a more forward direction, especially when incident photon energy increases.

Scattered Compton photons possess an energy high enough to create a radiation hazard, and to impair image quality. Scatter radiation is the primary cause of occupational radiation exposure to the radiographer and is therefore the primary reason for wearing protective devices, such as lead aprons and gloves, and for providing protective shielding for the x-ray room. Scatter also adds unwanted density to the radiographic image. These unwanted densities, caused predominantly by scattered photons and less commonly by secondary photons, are called **radiation fog**. Be-

cause scatter is coming from all directions, the scattered photons which strike the film place a density on the film which is unrelated to the patient's anatomy. Radiographic grids are devices designed to remove unwanted scatter and improve radiographic image quality.

PAIR PRODUCTION

In a pair production interaction the energy of the x-ray photon is converted to matter in the form of two electrons. For this interaction to occur, a very high-energy photon with an energy of at least 1.02 MeV is required. This is because the energy equivalent of the mass of one electron at rest is equal to 0.51 MeV. During this interaction, a high-energy incident photon comes close to the strong nuclear field and loses all its energy in the interaction. This

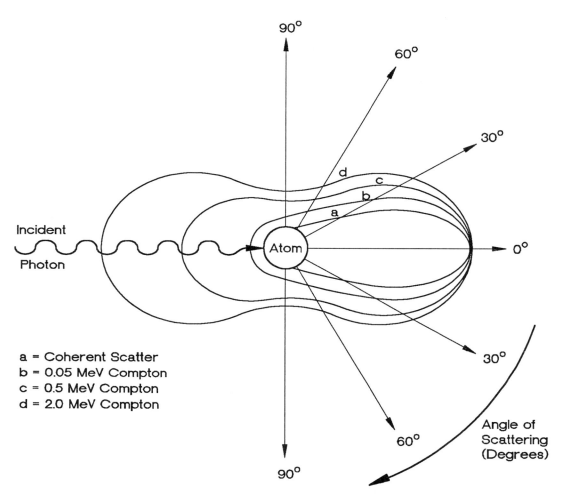

Figure 11–5. The distribution of photons in Compton scatter, along with various angles of deflection.

energy is used to create a pair of electrons, one with a negative charge, a **negatron**, and the other with a positive charge, a **positron** (Figure 11–6). Since a negative electron is common in nature it is quickly absorbed by other nearby atoms. A positron, because of its unique configuration, with some of the characteristics of a proton, is extremely volatile. It comes to rest and combines with a negative electron nearly instantaneously. When these two particles combine, they disappear and give rise to two photons moving in opposite directions and each possessing energies of 0.51 MeV. This process is called the **annihilation reaction** because matter is being converted back to energy. Pair production requires a minimum incident photon energy of 1.02 MeV but doesn't become a significant interaction until approximately 10 MeV. Therefore, it does not occur in the diagnostic x-ray imaging range.

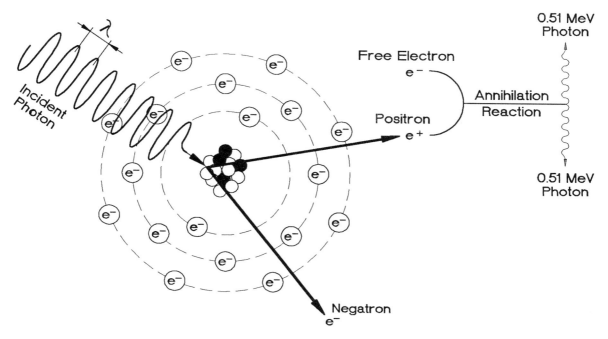

Figure 11–6. The pair production interaction.

PHOTODISINTEGRATION

Photodisintegration is an interaction between an extremely high-energy photon, above approximately 10 MeV, and the nucleus. In this interaction, the high-energy electron strikes the nucleus and all of its energy is absorbed by the nucleus, thereby exciting it. The excited nucleus responds by emitting a nuclear fragment (Figure 11–7). Because of the high energy level needed to cause this interaction, it is not relevant to diagnostic imaging.

EFFECT ON TECHNICAL FACTOR SELECTION

Of the five interactions between x-ray and matter, only two have a significant impact on an x-ray image. These two interactions, photoelectric absorption and Compton scattering, must be considered by the radiographer when technical factors are selected.

It is important to remember that in the diagnostic x-ray range the majority of the x-ray beam is attenuated and only a small percentage of photons exit to create the image (see Table 11–2). **As kVp increases, the total number of photons which are transmitted without interaction increases**. This means that the probability of photoelectric and Compton interactions decreases with increasing kVp. A shift does occur, however, in the percentages of photoelectric versus Compton interactions with increased kVp. **The percentage of photoelectric interactions decreases with increased kVp and the percentage of Compton interactions increases with increased kVp**. As a result, as kVp increases, there is an increased percentage of scatter and a decreased percentage of absorption of the primary beam.

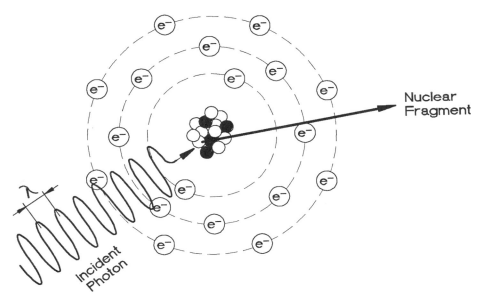

Figure 11–7.   The photodisintegration interaction.

In the human body, Compton scattering is the predominant interaction through most of the diagnostic x-ray range. Photoelectric interactions predominate in two circumstances: 1) in the lower-energy ranges (25–45 keV) produced by 40–70 kVp, and 2) when high atomic number elements are introduced, such as the contrast agents iodine and barium. Iodine and barium serve as useful contrast agents because they absorb a greater percentage of the photons through photoelectric interactions. These differences in absorption between the contrast agents and the soft tissues are responsible for creating the visible radiographic image (Figure 11–8).

When the photoelectric effect is more prevalent, the resulting radiographic image will possess high contrast. High-contrast images have great differences in densities from white to black, with fewer gray shades in between. This high contrast is the result of the complete absorption of the incident photons without the creation of undesirable scatter to fog the film. High-contrast images can be created by selecting low kVp/high mAs technical factors and through the introduction of contrast agents. In both of these instances, the photoelectric effect will be more predominant. Remember that as the percentage of photoelectric interactions increases so does the absorption of radiation by the patient. This increases the likelihood of biological effects. Therefore, high-contrast, low kVp/high mAs techniques tend to result in higher patient doses.

When Compton interactions prevail, the resulting radiographic image will possess lower contrast. Low-contrast images have very small differences between densities, with more gray shades in between. Low-contrast images can be created by using high kVp/low mAs techniques because Compton interactions predominate as kVp increases. Scatter from Compton interactions is a significant cause of the lower-contrast images. However, low-contrast, low kVp/high mAs techniques tend to reduce patient exposure dose.

Figure 11–8. The relative percentages of photoelectric absorption and Compton scatter in water and bone.

SUMMARY

As an x-ray beam passes through matter it undergoes attenuation, which is the reduction in the number of x-ray photons in the beam as it passes through a given thickness of matter. Attenuation is the result of x-rays interacting with matter by way of one of five types of interactions.

The five basic interactions between x-ray and matter are photoelectric absorption, coherent scattering, Compton scattering, pair production and photodisintegration. Only two are significant interactions within the diagnostic range of x-rays. These are the photoelectric effect and Compton scattering. Photoelectric absorption results when an x-ray photon interacts with an inner-shell electron. The incident photon is completely absorbed by the ejection of the electron, which then possesses kinetic energy and is called a photoelectron. The atom is ionized in the process and extremely unstable. The void in the inner shell is filled by the transfer of an electron from an outer shell. As

the electron moves into the inner shell it releases a photon, which is characteristic for a given atom. Characteristic photons created in irradiated material by way of the photoelectric effect are called secondary radiation.

Compton scattering is an interaction between an x-ray photon and an outer-shell electron. The incident photon ejects the outer-shell electron (Compton or recoil electron). The incident photon loses energy and as a result changes direction or scatters. The scattered photons have sufficient energy to interact again and again. Scatter radiation is the reason for wearing radiation protection devices and for shielding x-ray rooms. Scatter also adds unwanted densities to the film, which impairs image quality.

Image contrast is affected by the most predominant x-ray interaction. High-contrast images will result when the photoelectric effect is prevalent and low-contrast images will result when Compton scatter is more common. In addition, patient dose is increased when photoelectric interactions prevail. As kVp increases, more photons are transmitted without interaction and patient dose decreases as a result.

REVIEW QUESTIONS

1. Define attenuation.

2. Describe the photoelectric absorption interaction.

3. Describe the coherent scatter interaction.

4. Describe the Compton scatter interaction.

5. What is backscatter?

6. What are the two interactions which have a significant impact on the radiographic image?

7. What type of radiographic contrast will result if the prevalent interaction is photoelectric absorption?

8. What type of radiographic contrast will result if the prevalent interaction is Compton scatter?

REFERENCES AND RECOMMENDED READING

Ball, J. L., and A. D. Moore. *Essential Physics for Radiographers*. 2nd ed. Oxford: Blackwell Scientific Publications, 1986.

Bushong, Stewart C. *Radiologic Science for Technologists: Physics, Biology, and Protection*. 4th ed. St. Louis, MO: C. V. Mosby Company, 1988.

Compton, A. H., and H. K. Allison. *X-rays in Theory and Experiment*. 2nd ed. New York: Van Nostrand, 1935.

Curry, Thomas S. III, James E. Dowdey, and Robert C. Murry. *Christensen's Introduction to the Physics of Diagnostic Radiology*. 3rd ed. Philadelphia, PA: Lea and Febiger, 1984.

Dendy, P. P., and B. Heaton. *Physics for Radiologists*. Oxford: Blackwell Scientific Publications, 1987.

Fewell, Thomas R., and Ralph E. Shuping. Photon energy distribution of some typical diagnostic x-ray beams. *Medical Physics* 4:3, 187–197, 1977.

Gifford, Derek. *A Handbook of Physics for Radiologists and Radiographers*. New York: John Wiley & Sons, 1984.

Glasser, Otto, Edith H. Quimby, Lauriston S. Taylor, J. L. Weatherwax, and Russell H. Morgan. *Physical Foundations of Radiology*. 3rd ed. New York: Paul B. Hoeber Division of Harper & Brothers, 1961.

Hay, George A., and Donald Hughes. *First-Year Physics for Radiographers*. London: Bailliere Tindall, 1972.

Herman, Martin W. A comparative study of scattered radiation levels from 80 kVp and 240 kVp x-rays in the surgical ICU. *Radiology*, 552, 1980.

Johns, Harold E., and John R. Cunningham. *The Physics of Radiology*. Springfield, IL: Charles C. Thomas, 1974.

Meredith, W. J., and J. B. Massey. *Fundamental Physics of Radiology*. 3rd ed. Chicago, IL: Yearbook Medical Publishers, 1977.

Ridgway, Arthur, and Walter Thumm. *The Physics of Medical Radiography*. Reading, MA: Addison-Welsey Publishing Company, 1973.

Selman, Joseph. *The Fundamentals of x-ray and Radium Physics*. 7th ed. Springfield, IL: Charles C. Thomas, 1985.

Sprawls, Perry. *Physical Principles of Medical Imaging*. Rockville, MD: Aspen Publishers, 1987.

Ter-Pogossian, Michel M. *The Physical Aspects of Diagnostic Radiology*. New York: Hoeber Medical Division, Harper & Row, 1967.

Thompson, Thomas T. *A Practical Approach to Modern Imaging Equipment*. 2nd ed. Boston, MA: Little, Brown, & Co., 1985.

van der Plaats, G. J. *Medical X-ray Techniques in Diagnostic Radiology.* 4th ed. The Hague: Martinus Nijhoff Publishers, 1980.

Wilks, Robin J. *Principles of Radiological Physics.* Edinburgh: Churchill Livingstone, 1981.

Wilson, Peter. The interaction of x-radiation and matter. *Canadian Journal of Radiography, Radiotherapy, and Nuclear Medicine* 8:2, 76–95, 1977.

THE CASE OF THE DEEP SEA RODEO

This creature was radiographed after a sojourn in the deep. What is it?

(Reprinted by permission of the International Society of Radiographers and Radiological Technicians from the K. C. Clark Archives, Middlesex Hospital, London, England)

Answers to the case studies can be found in Appendix E.

UNIT II CREATING THE IMAGE

Creating the image that appears on the radiograph occupies the majority of the radiographer's time and requires a great deal of skill. The ability of the radiologist to make a diagnosis depends on the radiographer's ability to create a diagnostic quality image. This ability is predicated on a thorough knowledge of the scientific process by which the image was produced and on clinical experience.

This unit introduces the important aspects of **vision and image perception as the art of radiography**. Producing quality images requires knowledge of x-ray **beam restriction**, an understanding of **the concept of the patient as a beam emitter**, and of **the pathology problem** inherent in many examinations, proper use of the **grid**, **radiographic film** and **radiographic processing**.

Sensitometry is necessary to evaluate films and monitor their quality, while an understanding of **intensifying screens** and **film/screen combinations** is also required. The diagnostic image is created only when all of these factors are applied with professional skill.

12 VISION AND PERCEPTION: THE ART OF RADIOGRAPHY

She is so tall, so slender, and her bones—
Those frail phosphates, those carbonates of lime—
Are well produced by cathode rays sublime,
By oscillations, amperes and by ohms.
Her dorsal vertebrae are not concealed
By epidermis, but are well revealed.

Around her ribs, those beauteous twenty-four,
Her flesh a halo makes, misty in line,
Her noseless, eyeless face looks into mine,
And I but whisper, "Sweetheart, je t'adore."
Her white and gleaming teeth at me do laugh.
Ah! Lovely, cruel, sweet (radio)graph!

Lawrence K. Russell, *Life*, 1896.

OUTLINE

RADIOGRAPHY AS AN ART FORM
IMAGE PERCEPTION
CONTROLLING THE IMAGE IN SPACE

OBJECTIVES

Upon completion of this chapter, the student should be able to:

1. Identify numerous creative uses of radiography in medicine, technology and art.
2. Draw a cross-sectional image of a human eye with appropriate anatomical structures identified.
3. Explain the physiological function of the eye during photopic and scotopic vision.
4. Discuss the inefficiency of the medical imaging process.
5. Describe the boundary effect, Mach effect, eye motion, veil glare and the effect of viewing distance on visual perceptions.

6. State why pattern recognition is the domain of the radiologist.
7. Discuss the concept of controlling the radiographic image in space.
8. Apply the concept of three-dimensional thinking to clinical practice.

RADIOGRAPHY AS AN ART FORM

Radiography is an art form. In the century since its discovery it has been used to investigate an incredible variety of animals and objects. Examples of radiography as a technical and purely creative art form abound. Numerous radiographers have not only taken pride in the quality of their clinical abilities but have extended their technical skills into artistic expressions of creativity.

Artistic Radiography

William Conklin, a South Carolina radiographer artist, has achieved national acclaim for his radiography/photography of sea shells (Figure 12–1). Conklin's work has appeared in *National Geographic* and is in the permanent collection of the Smithsonian Institution. Radiography has often been used to produce a unique perspective of flowers, fruit and other plants, as well as of shells and fish.

Nondestructive Testing

The entire industrial radiography field, known as nondestructive testing (NDT) radiography, is unknown to many medical radiographers. The intent of NDT radiography is to assist in the examination and assessment of materials such as castings, welds, etc., through noninvasive techniques.

Biological Research

Radiography has proven an invaluable tool in biological research, not only in medical studies, but also in monitoring animal functions. For example, the study of birds and bats

in flight is greatly enhanced by high-speed radiography.

Veterinary Radiography

Veterinary medicine and dentistry also use radiography to accomplish many diagnoses. Figure 12–2, a canary with an egg, is an example of veterinary radiography. This type of radiography is also used in zoos. Radiographers have been called upon to examine all types of animals, from live venomous snakes to passive house pets.

Forensic Radiography

Forensic medicine uses radiography in a wide variety of ways. Grenz rays (5–30 kVp x-rays) are used, as are diagnostic x-rays. Grenz rays are emitted by specially designed tubes with minimal inherent filtration. They are useful for demonstrating objects as diverse as the ink on money when counterfeiting is suspected, the contents of envelopes and packages, fingerprints and art forgery.

Art Restoration

Grenz ray radiography has also proven useful during restoration of paintings and other art objects. Radiography can detect images under existing paint, frame and canvas construction and different types of paint and brush styles (Figure 12–3).

Archaeological Radiography

Radiography has become a useful archaeological tool, especially in the examination of fragile mummified remains. Numerous reports of such investigations have been published.

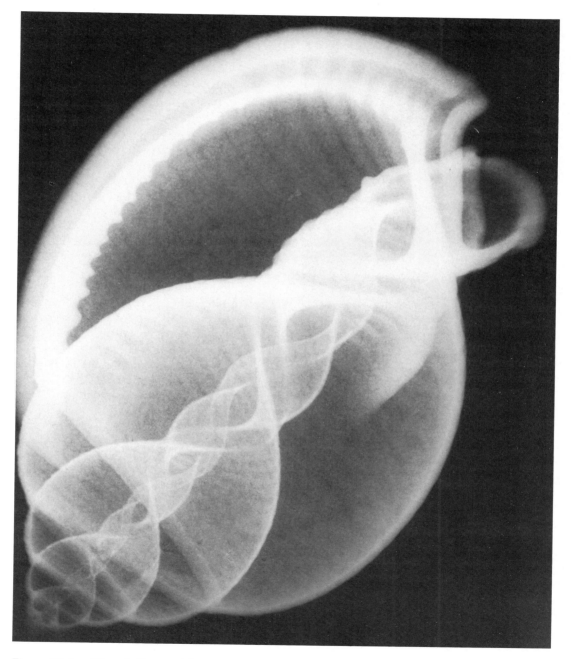

Figure 12–1. "Scotch Bonnet," by William A. Conklin, R.T., FASRT. (With permission of William A. Conklin, Inner Dimension, 1571 Marshall Ave., Orangeburg, S.C. 29115)

Figure 12–2. Canary with an egg. (Reprinted with permission of the International Society of Radiographers and Radiological Technicians from the K. C. Clark Archives, Middlesex Hospital, London, England.)

Most notable in this area is the book *X-Raying the Pharaohs*, in which University of Michigan researchers Harris and Weeks discuss their experiences radiographing the mummies at the National Museum in Cairo. Among their radiographic discoveries were jewelry, diseases, murders, dietary habits and the remains of a baboon that had been assumed to be a royal child (Figure 12–4).

Poetry

Radiographic images themselves inspire many of us. The physician poet Jack Coulehan was inspired by a chest radiograph to compose this poem:

The Old Man with Stars Inside Him

I look at the X-ray,
a shadow of pneumonia
deep in this old man's chest,
and watch Antonio shake
with a cough that traveled here
from the beginning of life.
As he pulls my hand to his lips
and kisses my hand,
Antonio tells me, for a man
whose death is gnawing at his spine,
pneumonia is a welcome friend
who reaches in between his ribs
without a sound and puff!
a cloud begins to squeeze
so delicately
the great white image of his heart.
The shadow advances
every time Antonio moves—
when a nurse positions his body,
when he takes a sip of ice,
when he shakes with a cough,
moist and diminished.

I see in that delicate shadow
a cloud of gas
at the galaxy's center,
a cloud of cold stunned nuclei
beginning to spin,
spinning and shooting
a hundred thousand
embryos of stars.
I listen to Antonio's chest
where stars crackle from the past
and hear the boom
of blue giants newly caught.
I hear the snap
of white dwarves coughing, shooting.
The second time Antonio
kisses my hand
I feel his dusky lips

Figure 12–3A.   A Grenz ray radiograph of a section of "Intemperance" by Hieronymus Bosch. (Courtesy of Gerald Conlogue, Gulf Coast Community College.)

Figure 12–3B.   "Intemperance" by Hieronymous Bosch. (Reprinted with permission from Yale University Art Gallery, The Rabinowitz Collection.)

reach out from everywhere in space.
I look at the place
his body was
and see inside Antonio, the stars.

Reprinted with permission from *Midwest Poetry Review,*© Jack Coulehan 1988

IMAGE PERCEPTION

At one time or another we have all been fooled by visual misperceptions. A common example is shown in Figure 12–5. Misperceptions of any type can be dangerous in clinical radiography. An important method of overcoming misperception is the elimination of preconceived ideas about an image. A mental erasing of these opinions is necessary to permit high-quality viewing of radiographic images. This is a skill that is cultivated by radiologists until it becomes part of their routine diagnostic procedure. Radiographers observe the diagnostic reporting of images by radiologists with amazement at first, but with increasing confidence as experience adds

knowledge about the potential pathological meaning of various radiologic signs. Radiographers should strive toward developing an understanding of the perceptual problems that radiologists encounter when attempting to interpret radiographic images. Through this understanding the radiographer can work toward producing images with patterns that provide maximum assistance to the radiologist in the diagnostic process.

Visual Anatomy

Because radiography depends entirely on images, it is helpful to be introduced to the complexities of visual perception. The mechanics of image perception are mostly unknown. It is little understood exactly how the eye perceives images and transmits them to the brain. Even less is known about how the brain neurologically processes the information.

The human eye is anatomically designed to gather light, focus it, convert it to nervous impulses and transmit it to the brain for processing. The aqueous humor, cornea, iris and

Figure 12–4.   A female hamadryas baboon mummy found buried with Makare, a member of an ancient Egyptian priesthood family, who was pregnant at the time of her death. (Reprinted with permission from ''X-Raying the Pharaohs,'' by James E. Harris and Kent R. Weeks.)

lens gather and focus the light (Figure 12–6). The specialized cells of the retina, especially the fovea centralis (or macula lutea), convert the image to nervous impulses, and the optic nerve transmits the impulses to the brain for processing. With corneal malfunction, such as myopia and hyperopia, the most common problems requiring corrective lenses, a distinct loss of detail is perceived because the incoming light is not properly focused on the retina. This is easily perceived and well-established means are available for correction. Image conversion and processing problems are not as easily perceived and these deserve some elementary study.

Visual Physiology

It is often uncertain whether conversion and processing problems are caused by the light-sensitive cells located in the retina or by mental misperceptions due to neurological processing. Sufficient research has been done at least to outline some of the factors that may cause misperceptions. Understanding that these factors exist and how they can prejudice perception can assist greatly in reducing visual problems.

An excellent example of misperception is the tendency to stare at an object that is difficult to see. Although this may be a good method of mental concentration, it does noth-

Figure 12–5. "The Lady and the Chalice" can be seen as either a pair of black faces in silhouette or as a white vase. This picture was devised by E. Rubin in 1915 and remains popular as a method of demonstrating perceptual differences.

does not provide enough information to be converted and processed in that time, the visual system will reset itself and reacquire information for the next 0.2 second. Therefore, when insufficient information is provided to the radiologist due to low illumination, excessive film density or distracting reflected light, only an improvement in the quality and quantity of light photons available will improve the visual image. The radiographic film does much to resolve the integration time problem. Because the film emulsion can integrate information for a considerable length of time and then hold that information until processed, it permits the human brain to integrate much more visual information than if the image were viewed as it was acquired from the patient.

Rod and Cone Cells

Human image conversion occurs in the **rod** and **cone** cells located in the retina. Both of these types of cells contain photosensitive pigments that will respond to light by sending an electrical potential to specialized nerve cells. These bipolar cells emit neurological im-

ing to improve the visual quality of the image. In fact, it does the opposite. The length of time the human visual system can integrate (acquire information) is only 0.2 second. If the image

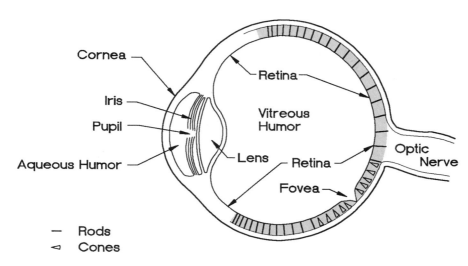

Figure 12–6. The human eye.

pulses when excited by light photons. The two types of cells are so different in their receiving and sending abilities that neurophysiologists tend to consider them as two separate visual systems. The cells are only about 1 μm in diameter and are concentrated to 100,000 per mm². There are approximately 7,000,000 cones, which are located only at the fovea centralis. There are approximately 120,000,000 rods covering the remainder of the retina.

Photopic Vision

Photopic (daylight) vision is controlled by the cones. Cone cells require relatively bright light to function (a minimum of approximately 100 light photons). Cone cells contain one of three different light-sensitive pigments, each of which is sensitive to a different range of photon wavelength (color of light). The cones are most sensitive to yellow light. Color blindness is a condition that occurs when there is a lack of cones sensitive to a particular color or colors.

Because most of the cones are located at the fovea centralis in high concentration, daylight vision is sharply focused. Therefore **visual acuity** is improved in daylight. The sparse

concentration of cones in the retina outside the fovea centralis accounts for poor peripheral vision in daylight. Cones are also able to detect changes in brightness far better than rod cells. This permits much greater recognition of density differences, or contrast, and results in what is called greater **contrast perception** (Figure 12–7).

Scotopic Vision

Scotopic (night) vision is controlled by the rods. Rod cells are sensitive to low light levels (they may respond to as few as fifteen photons) but cannot function in bright light. Rod cells cannot distinguish wavelength, although they are more sensitive to green light. As a result, humans are unable to perceive colors in extremely low light situations. Rod cells function by photosensitization of rhodopsin, also known as "visual purple," because it is most sensitive to blue-green wavelengths. When exposed to vast quantities of light photons, rhodopsin is oversensitized and becomes bleached out. The rod cells then regenerate rhodopsin at the rate of 50 percent each seven minutes. This is the reason a bright light causes temporary blindness in both humans

Figure 12–7. Human visual ability.

and animals. Because there are no rods in the fovea centralis, dim light vision is entirely peripheral and therefore difficult to bring into sharp focus. In addition, rods are not as concentrated because they are spread over a much greater area than cones. For these reasons, radiologists realize that dim objects are best viewed peripherally. Rods function better when the image information is changing. Slow scanning with an old fluoroscopic unit, night binoculars, or when walking in a dark room will increase visual acuity.

Inefficiency of the Medical Imaging Process

Few radiographers realize exactly how inefficient the entire imaging process is. An early fluoroscopic image study showed that although the x-ray tube was emitting 5,000,000 photons per second per mm^2 amplified over 5,000 times by the fluoroscopic intensification screen, only 65 photons contributed to the final impulses received by the brain. This is a conversion efficiency of 0.00005 percent (1 out of 2,000,000 photons) from the fluoroscopic screen and 0.001 percent (1 out of 100,000 photons) from the tube output.

Threshold Detection

Threshold detection is a visual phenomenon involving the perception of extremely small or faint details. This is more than an issue of the resolution, or fineness of the details, in the image. It also involves minimizing background density and other artifacts, known as visual noise.

Boundary Effect A boundary effect occurs because the visual system has difficulty perceiving contrast differences that are distant from one another. When a distinct boundary between various densities can be achieved (this

is actually contrast), adjacent differences as small as two percent can be perceived under high illumination (such as a radiographic view box). When the boundary is indistinct, a difference of up to 20 percent may be required. Less intense light levels also affect this perception ability.

There is a rule of thumb in radiography that density changes should be at least 25–33 percent to be visible. This is because two radiographs of differing densities are seen quite distant from one another. If a change of this magnitude formed an adjacent boundary, it would be strikingly apparent. Surrounding densities have an effect on the perception of nearby densities. This results in confusion when judging absolute and relative levels of density and contrast from one image to another.

Another aspect of the boundary effect concerns the length of the boundary line. A subtle density difference along the length of a long boundary may be perceived but when it is shortened the boundary may no longer be perceived. As yet there is no explanation for this phenomenon but radiologists can best observe extremely subtle density differences when they form a long boundary. They may fail to see diagnostic information when density differences are widely separated or form short boundaries. In these instances it is important for the radiographer to attempt to provide better perception through higher contrast.

Mach Effect Part of the boundary effect may be explained by a phenomenon called the **Mach effect**. The retina contains neural connections that inhibit impulses under certain conditions. One of these conditions is extremely bright light; another is a dramatic change in impulse intensity. The Mach effect occurs when the eye perceives a boundary. Each time there is a change in density there is a change in the intensity of the impulses sent

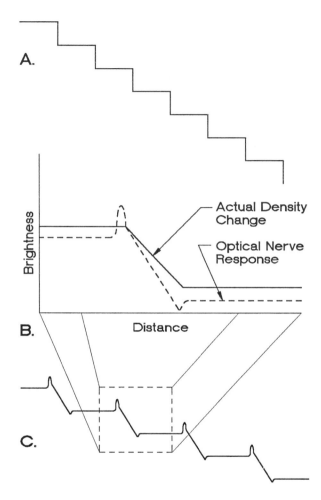

A.

B.

Brightness

Distance

Actual Density Change

Optical Nerve Response

C.

Figure 12–8. The Mach effect: (A) actual density differences, (B) comparison of actual density changes to optical nerve response, and (C) optical nerve response from A.

to the brain. When the beginning of the new intensity level is inhibited by the neural connectors, the impulses to the brain are transmitted as shown in the graph in Figure 12–8B. For density differences as shown in the step wedge in Figure 12–8A, the end result is a response as shown in Figure 12–8C. This creates an ef-

fect known as **edge enhancement**. Edge enhancement compresses the entire density scale while making the boundary appear more distinct than it really is. For example, in Figure 12–9 many of the lighter density steps appear to be lighter just before the edge of the next darker step. This perceptual illusion is the Mach effect. Although this makes it easier to perceive the edges, radiologists are concerned about the possibility of a small detail being lost because its density is overwritten by edge enhancement.

Eye Motion Contrast perception is dramatically increased when the eye uses a scanning motion, as when reading a book. Because the photosensitive cells in the eye can integrate a limited amount of information, eye movement maintains a constantly changing neurological signal, thus avoiding saturation of the optical nerves.

Veil Glare Veil glare occurs when the intensely bright light from a view box floods the eye directly. This occurs in unexposed areas of the image and between images. The bright light scatters inside the eye and reduces contrast perception, much as Compton scatter does within the patient.

Viewing Distance Data concerning threshold detection indicate that results change when the viewing distance is changed. This occurs because of the changes in intensity due to the inverse square law and because the physiological processing of the image changes when the angle of the incident light photons changes. In addition, the fovea centralis creates a blind spot at a viewing distance of about nine inches. Therefore, radiologists often vary their viewing distances when addressing areas of perceptual difficulty.

Figure 12–9.   Optical step wedges, each with twice the number of density differences. Note the prominent Mach effect through the lighter densities of the upper step wedges.

Pattern Recognition

Pattern recognition involves perceiving combinations of details that can be defined and classified toward a diagnosis. This is the area radiologists often study the hardest. Just as it is difficult to identify a picture of a familiar face when it is shown upside down, so it is important that radiologists be presented with images in a routine manner. For example, radiographs are universally viewed as if the viewer were facing the patient (the patient's left is on the viewer's right, etc.).

Pattern recognition involves comparing mental images of patterns—anatomical, physiological, pathological, and histological—to arrive at a diagnostic opinion. Because of the complexities between the visual system and the mental capability to store and recall image patterns from memory, and because of the lack of scientific knowledge about how the brain processes information, pattern recognition is a weak area of research and no data can be provided to help the radiographer assist the radiologist. Pattern recognition is the true domain of the radiologist, who has the requisite medical knowledge to be competent in this area.

CONTROLLING THE IMAGE IN SPACE

One of the challenges to the radiographer is to place the patient so that the area to be imaged is in a position that will enhance the quality of the image. It is helpful to visualize the object of radiographic interest (kidney, scapula, sinus, etc.) as floating in space within the body of the patient. The skill of the radiographer lies in manipulating the object to the correct position in relationship to the x-ray beam and image receptor (film). This is the art of controlling the image in space.

Thinking Three-Dimensionally

Artistic radiography is not limited to the creative endeavors described at the beginning of this chapter. The radiographer must be capable of controlling the image in space in an artistic manner. This is one of the critical elements of professionalism. In her book, *Fundamentals of Radiology,* radiologist Lucy Frank Squire encourages us with "An Invitation to Think Three-Dimensionally." This concept is extremely valuable in forming perceptual ability. The experienced radiographer can see an incredible amount of beauty in the radiographs that are produced every day. Just as the barium-coated finger (Figure 12–10) is easily perceived in three dimensions, so are most radiographs viewed in this manner by radiographers. The magnification of structures some distance from the film places them further away in perspective; finely detailed structures seem to move closer, and each image assumes a three-dimensionality usually not noticed by the novice.

Radiographic positioning requires a solid knowledge of the shape and location of skeletal and soft-tissue structures and an indepth understanding of their anatomical relationship to one another. For example, a diagnostic image of the maxillary sinuses can be obtained only after positioning the patient's head so the overlying structures of the cranium do not appear superimposed over the area of interest.

The human body is a three-dimensional object, but radiographic images possess only two dimensions—length and width. Consequently, all radiographic images are missing a critical diagnostic element—the dimension of depth. This can only be compensated for by never settling for a single radiographic view of any structure. **At least two images, as close to 90° angles to one another as possible, are required to view all three dimensions**.

The dimensional views required for all radiographic examinations are **anterior-posterior, medial-lateral and superior-inferior**. All radiographic images will demonstrate two, but never all three, of these perspectives. For example, a postero-anterior (PA) chest radio-

A   B   C

Figure 12–10.   A three-dimensional effect. (Reprinted with permission from the publishers of *Fundamentals of Radiology* by Lucy Frank Squire and Robert A Novelline, Harvard University Press, Cambridge, MA. First edition copyright 1964 by the Commonwealth Fund; second, third, and fourth editions copyright 1975, 1982, and 1988 by the President and Fellows of Harvard College.)

graph demonstrates the medial-lateral dimension and the superior-inferior dimension, but not the anterior-posterior dimension. The dimension that describes the entrance and exit of the central ray, which is used to describe the projection, is the dimension not visualized. In situations where superimposition makes PA and lateral projections useless, two oblique positions at 90° angles from one another can be used to achieve the same effect.

An important skill that must be developed by the radiographer is the ability to mentally visualize the changing and moving of overlying anatomical structures from any angle in order to provide an image free of superimposition. Artistic techniques should be understood, such as making exposures while the patient is breathing, thus using patient motion to blur superimposing structures from the image (i.e., to blur ribs from the lateral projection of the thoracic vertebral column).

Radiography as Art

Radiographers can become technically artistic; innovative adaptations of routine procedures should be considered technical artistry. For example, it is technically artistic to reverse routine angles to produce a diagnostic quality acanthio-parietal projection of the skull for a traumatized patient with anterior facial injuries, or to lower the tube and support a film cassette under a wheelchair patient's foot so that it is unnecessary to move a weak patient with a full leg cast onto a radiographic table.

SUMMARY

Radiography is an art form that has been used to investigate a wide array of animals and objects. It is used in nondestructive testing; biological research, veterinary and forensic radiography; art restoration; archaeological radiography; and has even been the subject of poetry.

Understanding visual perception is an important aspect of clinical radiography. This understanding helps to overcome misperceptions about an image.

The human eye is designed to gather light, focus it, convert it to nerve impulses and transmit it to the brain for processing. Image conversion occurs in the rod and cone cells, which contain photosensitive pigments that will respond to light. Photopic (daylight) vision is controlled by the cones and scotopic (night) vision is controlled by the rods.

Threshold detection is a visual phenomenon involving the perception of extremely small or faint details. The boundary effect occurs because the visual system has difficulty perceiving contrast differences that are distant from one another. When densities are adjacent, small differences can be perceived. Part of the boundary effect can be explained by the Mach effect. When the eye perceives a boundary, a change occurs in the intensity of the impulses sent to the brain. This change in intensity creates an effect known as edge enhancement, which makes the boundary appear distinct. Contrast perception is dramatically increased by eye motion or scanning the image. Veil glare occurs when bright lights, such as a view box, flood the eye. Viewing distance has an effect on threshold detection.

Pattern recognition involves perceiving combinations of details that can be defined and classified toward a diagnosis. It helps the radiologist compare mental images of patterns with medical knowledge.

Radiographers need to think three-dimensionally. Radiographic images possess two dimensions and, as a result, at least two images as close to 90° angles to one another as possible are required to view all three dimensions. It is considered technical artistry when radiographers use innovation to adapt a routine procedure.

REVIEW QUESTIONS

1. Name three examples of the use of radiography as an art form.

2. What is the human eye designed to do?

3. What is the difference between photopic and scotopic vision?

4. Explain the boundary effect.

5. What is the Mach effect?

6. How is pattern recognition used by the radiologist in making a diagnosis?

7. Why is it important for the radiographer to produce two images as close to 90° angles to one another as possible?

REFERENCES AND RECOMMENDED READING

Abgrall, Rene. La nature vue aux rayons x. *Le Manipulateur d'Electroradiologie Médicale* 91, 19–20, 1988.

Abgrall, Rene. Vingt ans déjà. *Le Manipulateur d'Electroradiologie Médicale* 81, 3, 1986.

Adrian-Harris, D. Aspects of visual perception in radiography. *Radiography* 45:539, 237–243, 1979.

Bridgman, Charles F., and Sheldon Keck. The radiography of paintings. *Medical Radiography and Photography* 37:3, 62–70, 1961.

Bruce, Vicki, and Patrick R. Green. *Visual Perception Physiology, Psychology, and Ecology.* London: Lawrence Erlbaum Associates, Publishers, 1985.

Chester, M. Susan. Perception and evaluation of images. *Scientific Basis of Medical Imaging.* Editor P. T. N. Wells. Edinburgh: Churchill Livingstone, 1982.

Conklin, William A. *Nature's Art: The Inner and Outer Dimensions of the Shell.* Columbia, SC: University of South Carolina Press.

Conlogue, Gerald, Michael Schlenk, Frank Cerrone, and John Ogden. Dr. Leidy's soap lady: Imaging the past. *Radiologic Technology* 60: 5, 411–415, 1989.

Conlogue, Gerald J., and John A. Ogden. The Grenz ray technique for painting analysis. *Radiologic Technology* 57:4, 338, 1986.

Conlogue, Gerald J., Eugene V. Warmoth, and James Wetmore. Microradiography using a noncommercially constructed Grenz ray unit. *Radiologic Technology* 56:2, 85, 1984.

Cornsweet, Tom N. *Visual Perception.* New York: Academic Press, 1970.

Coulehan, Jack. The old man with stars inside him. *Midwest Poetry Review,* 1988.

Cox, E. J. Flower radiography. *The X-Ray Technician* 25, 108–111, September 1953.

Curry, Thomas, James Dowdey, and Robert Murry. *Christensen's Introduction to the Physics of Diagnostic Radiology.* 3rd ed. Philadelphia, PA: Lea & Febiger, 1984.

Davson, Hugh. *Physiology of the Eye.* 4th ed. Edinburgh: Churchill Livingstone, 1980.

Flower radiography. *Radiography and Clinical Photography* 8, 12–13, 1932.

Fuchs, Arthur W. Radiography of the entire body employing one film and a single exposure. *Radiography and Clinical Photography* 10, 9–14, 1934.

Gibbs, S. Julian, Ronald R. Price, and A. Everette James, Jr. Image perception. *The Physical Basis of Medical Imaging.* 295–302. Editors: Coulam, Craig M., John J. Erickson, F. David Rollo, and A. Everette James, Jr. New York: Appleton-Century-Crofts, 1981.

Graham, Daniel, and John Thomson. *Grenz Rays: An Illustrated Guide to the Theory and Practical Applications of Soft X-Rays*. Oxford: Pergamon Press, 1980.

Gregg, Earle C. Image manipulation in radiology. *Physics of Diagnostic Radiology*. 282–334. Editor: Wright, D. John. Rockville, MD: U.S. Department of Health, Education, and Welfare, Public Health Service, Food and Drug Administration, Bureau of Radiological Health, USDHEW Publication No. (FDA) 74–8006.

Harris, James E., and Kent R. Weeks. *X-Raying the Pharaohs*. New York: Charles Scribner's Sons, 1973.

Hooker, Ellen Z. The perceptual domain: A taxonomy for allied health educators. *Journal of Allied Health* August, 198–206, 1981.

Jaffe, C. Carl. Medical imaging, vision, and visual psychophysics. *Medical Radiography and Photography* 60:1, 1–48, 1984.

James, A. Everette, S. Julian Gibbs, Ronald R. Price, Malcolm Sloan, Joseph Diggs, Richard M. Heller, Jr., and C. Leon Partain. Uncovering works of art. *Diagnostic Imaging* June, 40–44, 1981.

Mary Alice, Sister. Flowers under the x-ray—a new form of art. *Hospitals* 24, 53–56, November 1950.

Materials and Processes for NDT Technology. Editor: Harry D. Moore. Columbus, OH: American Society for Nondestructive Testing, 1981.

Myers, Bert. Radiography for art's sake. *Applied Radiology* 12:3, 23, 1983.

Neisser, Ulric. Visual search. *Scientific American* 210:6, 94–102, 1964.

Ott, Ted. Flower radiography: A portfolio. *Applied Radiology* 13:6, 103, 1984.

Randall, Patricia Ann. Mach bands in cine coronary arteriography. *Radiology* 129, 65–66, 1978.

Rose, Albert. The sensitivity performance of the human eye on an absolute scale. *Journal of the Optical Society of America* 38:2, 196–208, 1948.

Samji, Z. M. Radiography of live venomous snakes. *Radiography* 36:423, 57–59, March 1970.

Schnitzler, Alvin D. Image-detector model and parameters of the human visual system. *Journal of the Optical Society of America* 63:11, 1357–1368, 1973.

Squire, Lucy Frank and Robert A. Novelline. *Fundamentals of Radiology*. 4th ed. Cambridge, MA: Harvard University Press, 1988.

Sturm, R. E., and R. H. Morgan. Screen intensification systems and their limitations. *American Journal of Roentgenology* 62, 613, 1949.

Thompson, Gordon, and William S. Cornwell. An archeologic use of radiography. *Medical Radiography and Photography* 25:2, 43, 1949.

Tuddenham, William J. The visual physiology of roentgen diagnosis. *American Journal of Roentgenology* 78:1, 116–123, 1957.

van der Platts, G. J. *Medical X-Ray Techniques in Diagnostic Radiology: A Textbook for Radiographers and Radiological Technicians*. 4th ed., The Hague: Martinus Nijhoff Publishers, 1980.

13 BEAM RESTRICTION

Tell the world to wait
till we set the record straight
x-ray vision
baby, I can see thru you

Moon Martin, Pete Sinfield, and Terry Taylor, "X-Ray Vision," from *Mystery Ticket*.

OUTLINE

CONTROLLING SCATTER
BEAM RESTRICTORS
ANCILLARY DEVICES

OBJECTIVES

Upon completion of this chapter, the student should be able to:

1. Identify the factors that affect the amount of scatter radiation produced.
2. Discuss the primary methods used by radiographers to control the amount of scatter radiation reaching the film.
3. Explain the purpose and construction of beam-restricting devices.
4. Compare the advantages and disadvantages of the various beam-restricting devices.
5. Describe the effect of beam restriction on image quality and patient dose.

CONTROLLING SCATTER

Scatter radiation is produced during a Compton interaction. In this interaction, a primary photon interacts with an outer-shell electron and changes direction, thereby becoming a scattered photon. Scattered photons are not a part of the useful beam and will impair image quality by placing density on the film which is unrelated to patient anatomy. In order to provide the best possible image, the radiographer must try to minimize the amount of scatter radiation reaching the film. This can best be accomplished by restricting the x-ray beam and by using a grid. Proper beam restriction will keep the total amount of tissue irradiation to a minimum and has great importance in both improving image quality and reducing patient dose.

As the beam is restricted, fewer primary photons are emitted from the tube and collimator and fewer scattered photons are created. Additionally, the decrease in the number of primary photons results in a decrease in the dose to the patient. The only way to improve image quality once scattered photons have been created is to try to decrease the number that are allowed to interact with the film. Grids are devices which are placed between the patient and the film to absorb scatter radiation.

The principle factors that affect the amount of scatter produced are 1) kilovoltage and 2) the irradiated material. In order to control the amount of scatter produced, it is important to understand how kilovoltage and the irradiated material affect scatter production.

Kilovoltage

Kilovoltage affects the penetrability of the beam. As kVp increases, fewer photons undergo interaction with matter and more pass through the patient to interact with the film. For the photons that undergo an interaction, photoelectric absorption and Compton interactions are predominant in the diagnostic x-ray range. Although the total number of photons that undergo interaction decreases with increased kVp, a shift is seen in the percentage of photoelectric versus Compton interactions as kVp increases. As the kilovoltage increases, the percentage of x-rays that undergo a Compton interaction increases and the percentage of photons that undergo photoelectric absorption decreases. Because Compton interactions create scatter, as kilovoltage increases the percentage of primary photons that will undergo scattering also increases. At the same time, the percentage of primary photons that are absorbed photoelectrically decreases, resulting in a reduction in patient dose.

An x-ray image is created when some photons pass through the patient unaffected and others are absorbed photoelectrically. This difference is the basis for varying shades of radiographic density. When more photons pass through unaffected, the resulting image has greater density. When more photons are absorbed photoelectrically, the resulting image has less density. Scattered photons from Compton interactions are of no use in demonstrating the structures of interest. They merely add unwanted densities to the film that do not correspond to any particular structure. Much of the overall radiographic density on a film is created by scattered photons. Image quality is improved when the amount of scatter reaching the film is reduced.

Irradiated Material

The amount of scatter created during an interaction is affected by the volume and atomic number of the material being irradiated. The volume of irradiated material is controlled by field size and patient thickness (Figure 13–1).

As the volume of irradiated tissue increases, the amount of scatter increases. Volume increases as the field size increases or as the patient thickness increases. Larger field sizes, such as with 14″×17″ (35×43 cm) film, allow for more photons to interact with tissue, thereby creating more scatter. Larger body parts have more tissue to interact with the photons, resulting in greater scatter production. In order to decrease scatter, the smallest possible field size should be used. It is for this reason that beam restriction is an important part of scatter reduction and, of course, of patient protection. Patient thickness cannot be significantly altered by the radiographer, but certain techniques, such as the use of compression bands, can be useful in slightly reducing patient thickness.

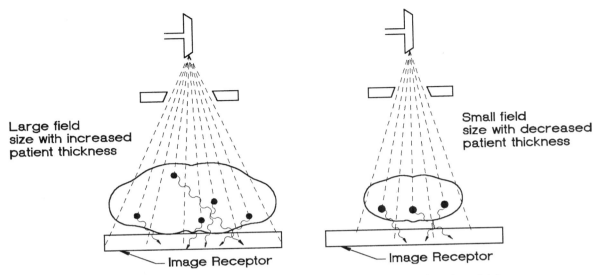

Figure 13–1.   The amount of scatter increases with increased field size and patient thickness.

The atomic number of the irradiated material also has an impact on the amount of scatter produced because higher atomic number materials have a greater number of electrons within each atom and photons have a greater chance of striking an electron, creating an interaction. More scatter is created in bone than in soft tissue for this reason. This is also the reason high atomic number materials, such as lead, absorb more radiation than low atomic number materials.

Of the factors affecting the amount of scatter produced, the kilovoltage and the field size are under the direct control of the radiographer. Kilovoltage levels must be selected based on the area being radiographed, and the smallest possible field size should always be used. Beam restriction is, therefore, important to image quality. Remember, however, that **when the beam is restricted, less scatter radiation will reach the film and, as a result, technical factors may need to be increased to compensate for the reduction in the overall film density**. For example, the technical factors

used for an AP projection of the abdomen using a 14"×17" (35×43 cm) film would be insufficient to produce a good image of the same patient's gallbladder imaged on an 8"×10" (18×24 cm) film. Technical factors would need to be increased 50–100 percent to compensate for the reduction in the field size.

BEAM RESTRICTORS

There are three basic types of beam-restricting devices used to control scatter and reduce patient dose: **aperture diaphragms, cones/cylinders** and **collimators**. Each of these devices has advantages and disadvantages which determine how and when they are used in radiography.

Aperture Diaphragm The aperture diaphragm is a flat sheet of metal, usually lead, with a hole cut in the center and attached to the x-ray tube port. This is the simplest of all beam-restricting devices both in design and in application. Different diaphragms are needed to accommodate different film sizes and different distances. The opening can be made in any size or shape but most are rectangular, square or round. Rectangular diaphragms are most common, to correspond to x-ray film sizes. The size of the opening depends on the desired exposure field, the source to image receptor distance (SID) and the distance from the aperture to the focal spot.

The main advantages in using an aperture diaphragm are its simple design, low cost and ease of use. The principle disadvantage is the increase in **penumbra**, a geometric unsharpness around the periphery of the image. This is the result of the diaphragm's close proximity to the tube port. Penumbra is reduced when the beam restrictor is at an increased distance from the port.

Penumbra is the result of x-ray photons being created in all areas of the focal spot rather than at just a single point. Primary photons diverge from the tube port at varying angles and intersect with the structures of interest at varying angles when creating the image. Reducing penumbra will improve the sharpness of the recorded image (Figure 13–2).

Another problem when using an aperture diaphragm is the increase in **off-focus (stem) radiation** reaching the film. This occurs because of the aperture's close proximity to the tube port. Off-focus radiation originates within the x-ray tube but not at the focal spot. Off-focus radiation can result in images, similar to shadows of the patient, beyond the exposed field of radiation (see figure 7–22). These shad-

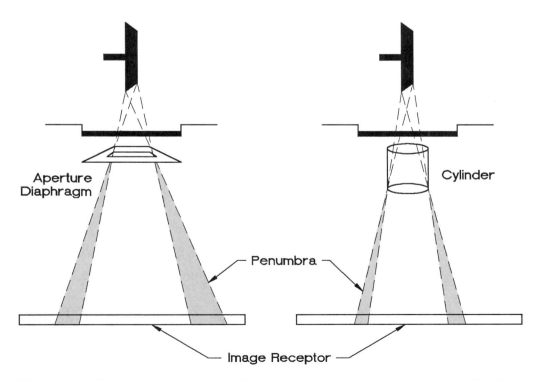

Figure 13–2.   Penumbra increases as the beam restrictor moves closer to the port. Use of an aperture diaphragm results in greater penumbra than does use of a cylinder.

ows are often believed to be caused by scatter radiation. However, scatter will never create an image of a specific anatomical structure.

The aperture diaphragm was the original type of beam restrictor, but its use is somewhat limited today. Since it is merely a flat sheet of metal with a hole cut in it, no light field is available for use as an aid in positioning. Its primary application is in dedicated equipment, such as for chest radiography, where the field size and the SID do not vary.

Determining the Diaphragm Field Size

When using an aperture diaphragm it may be necessary for the radiographer to determine the size of the projected image on the film. Aperture diaphragms, when used alone, do not provide the radiographer with a light field for viewing the projected image size. To avoid exposing an area larger than necessary, selection of the correct diaphragm and proper SID is critical. The following formula is used to determine the size of the projected image when using a specific aperture diaphragm. This formula is especially useful when a given diaphragm is used at varying distances.

projected image size =

$$\frac{\text{SID} \times \text{diameter of diaphragm}}{\text{distance from focal spot to diaphragm}}$$

Example: A diaphragm is placed 5 inches from the focal spot. The diameter of the opening in the aperature is a 2-inch circle. What would be the projected image size if the SID is 40 inches?

Answer: projected image size =

$$\frac{40 \times 2}{5} = \frac{80}{5} = 16\text{-inch circle}$$

Cones/Cylinders

Cones and cylinders are essentially circular aperture diaphragms with metal extensions (Figure 13–3). A cone has an extension which flares or diverges, with the upper diameter smaller than the bottom flared end. A cylinder does not flare. Instead, it has the same diameter at the bottom of the extension as it has at the top. A cylinder may be equipped with an extension sleeve which can expand or collapse to vary the degree of beam restriction.

Cones and cylinders are also relatively inexpensive and simple to use. They are most commonly employed in radiography of the skull, spine, gallbladder and breast. The physical weight of a cone sometimes makes it difficult to handle and, when used with a horizontal beam, the weight of the cone may cause the tube to angle slightly, causing cone cutting if the central ray is not checked carefully just prior to the exposure.

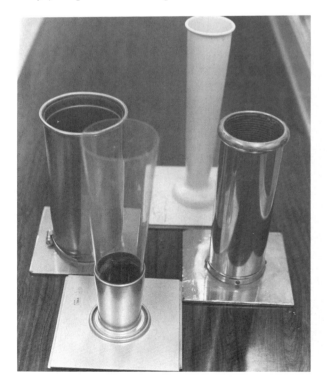

Figure 13–3.   Cones and cylinders.

Cones, like aperture diaphragms, have the disadvantage of a fixed field size unless they are equipped with an extension sleeve. In addition, flared cones are no better at reducing penumbra than are aperture diaphragms.

Cylinders, however, do reduce penumbra and off-focus radiation because they provide better beam restriction at a greater distance from the focal spot (see Figure 13–2). This is especially true when they are used in conjunction with a collimator, as is most often the case.

Determining the Cone Field Size

Determining the field size for a cone/cylinder involves a method similar to that used with an aperture diaphragm. The following formula can be used to calculate the size of the projected image when using a cone/cylinder.

$$\text{projected image size} = \frac{\text{SID} \times \text{lower diameter of cone}}{\text{distance from focal spot to bottom of cone}}$$

Example: The diameter of the lower rim of a cone is 3 inches. The bottom of the cone is placed at a distance 16 inches from the focal spot. What will be the size of the projected image at a 40-inch SID?

Answer: projected image size =

$$\frac{40 \times 3}{16} = \frac{120}{16} = 7.5\text{-inch circle}$$

Collimator

The collimator is the most commonly employed beam restrictor in radiography. Although it is more complex and expensive, the collimator permits an infinite number of field sizes using only one device (Figure 13–4). It also has the advantage of providing a light source for the radiographer as an aid in properly placing the tube and central ray.

A collimator consists of two sets of lead shutters at right angles to one another which

Collimator Assembly

Added Filtration

Light Field

Light Source

Mirror

Lower Lead Shutters

Upper Lead Shutters

Top View Of Lead Shutters

Figure 13–4. A typical collimator assembly.

move in opposing pairs. Each set moves symmetrically from the center of the field. These lead shutters can be adjusted to correspond to an infinite number of square or rectangular field sizes.

The two sets of shutters serve to regulate the field size and, in addition, have two other-purposes. The bottom shutters reduce penumbra along the periphery of the beam because of their greater distance from the focal spot. The upper shutters help in reducing the amount of off-focus (stem) radiation reaching the film by absorbing this radiation before it exits the tube.

The collimator offers the radiographer a light field which outlines the exposure field and provides a cross hair to identify the center of the beam. Some units also provide an outline of the automatic exposure control (AEC) chambers' size and location. The light field is provided by mounting a mirror in the path of the x-ray beam at a 45° angle. A light source is then placed opposite the mirror and the light is projected through the collimator. The light source and the x-ray source must be equidistant from one another to ensure that the light field and the x-ray field are the same size. Improper positioning of the mirror or the light can result in improper alignment of the light field to the exposure field. Collimator accuracy should be checked on a regular basis as a part of the department's quality control program.

In the United States it has been required by law since 1974 for all fixed radiographic equipment to be equipped with automatic collimators. These devices are known as **positive beam limitation (PBL) devices**. When a cassette is placed in the Bucky tray and secured in position, sensing devices determine the size and placement of the cassette. The sensing devices activate an electric motor which drives the collimator lead shutters into proper position. When operating properly, automatic collimators should leave a small unexposed border on all four sides of the exposed film. However, it is possible to override the PBL devices so that the field size can be controlled by the radiographer.

The use of a collimator results in some filtration of the x-ray beam because the primary beam is passing through the mirror in the collimator. The added filtration is equivalent to approximately 1 mm of aluminum. Because collimators result in increased filtration of the x-ray beam, their use during low-kVp radiography (such as mammography) is restricted.

Proper collimation is the responsibility of the radiographer. Under no circumstances should the exposure field exceed the size of the image receptor. Automatic collimation helps to ensure that the exposure field does not exceed the size of the image receptor, but the radiographer should always limit the field to the part being examined. By so doing, image quality can be improved and patient dose can be minimized.

ANCILLARY DEVICES

Beam restrictors may be made for a very specific purpose. Ancillary devices are generally designed with a special need in mind. Examples include lead blockers and lead masks. These devices are tailored for a specific use during a given procedure. They are designed to restrict the beam to a specific shape for a particular examination.

A lead blocker is simply a sheet of lead-impregnated rubber that can be cut to any size or shape. Placement of a lead blocker on the radiographic table during radiography of the lower spine in the lateral position will help to absorb the scatter that is produced in the soft tissue of the patient's back (Figure 13–5). A lead blocker may also be helpful when placed on the radiographic table above the level of the shoulder during positioning for AP projections of the shoulder joint. Lead blockers are most helpful when examining large patients, because the amount of scatter increases with increases in the size of the patient.

A lead mask is usually cut to correspond to the particular field size desired and is then secured to the end of the collimator. The most common use of a lead mask is during cerebral angiography. The lead mask helps improve image quality by reducing scatter (Figure 13–6 A & B).

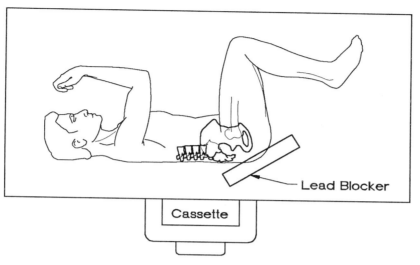

Figure 13–5. The use of a lead blocker for radiography of the lower spine (bird's eye view).

Figure 13–6A & B. Two radiographs of an AP cerebral angiogram—with and without a lead mask.

SUMMARY

In order to provide the best possible image, the radiographer must try to control the amount of scatter radiation reaching the film. The principle factors that affect the amount of scatter produced are: 1) kilovoltage and 2) the irradiated material. As kilovoltage increases, the percentage of primary photons that will undergo scattering also increases. As the volume of irradiated tissue increases, the amount of scatter produced is increased. Volume will increase as the field size increases or as the patient thickness increases. The atomic number of the irradiated material also has an impact on the amount of scatter produced. Higher atomic number materials have a greater number of electrons within each atom. Photons have a greater chance of interacting with these materials.

There are three basic types of beam-restricting devices that are used to control scatter and reduce patient dose: aperture diaphragms, cones/cylinders and collimators. Each of these devices has advantages and disadvantages which determine how and when they are used in radiography. The collimator is the most commonly employed beam restrictor in radiography because it permits an infinite number of field sizes using only one device. It also has the advantage of providing a light source for the radiographer as an aid in properly placing the tube.

Proper collimation is the responsibility of the radiographer. Under no circumstances should the exposure field ever exceed the size of the image receptor. In addition, the radiographer should always limit the field to the part being examined. By so doing, image quality will be improved and patient dose will be minimized.

REVIEW QUESTIONS

1. Why does beam restriction reduce scatter radiation production?

2. What are the two principle factors that affect the amount of scatter produced?

3. How does the atomic number of a material affect the amount of scatter produced?

4. What are the three basic types of beam-restricting devices?

5. What is penumbra and how can it be minimized?

6. What is the formula for determining the size of the projected image when using a cone?

7. How is a collimator constructed?

8. What is PBL?

9. How does beam restriction affect patient dose?

REFERENCES AND RECOMMENDED READING

Carroll, Quinn. *Fuchs's Principles of Radiographic Exposure, Processing and Quality Control.* 3rd ed. Springfield, IL: Charles C. Thomas Publisher, 1985.

Crooks, H. E., and G. M. Ardran. Checking x-ray beam field size. *Radiography* 42:503, 239, 1976.

Curry, Thomas S., James E. Dowdey, and Robert C. Murry. *Christensen's Introduction to the Physics of Diagnostic Radiology.* 4th ed. Philadelphia, PA: Lea and Febiger, 1990.

De Vos, Dianne C. *Basic Principles of Radiographic Exposure.* Philadelphia, PA: Lea & Febiger, 1990.

Rogers, K. D., and I. P. Matthers. X-ray field collimation in diagnostic radiology. *Radiography* 52:604, 161, 1986.

Seeram, Euclid. *X-ray Imaging Equipment: An Introduction.* Springfield, IL: Charles C. Thomas, 1985.

Thomas, Stephen R., John E. Freshcorn, Kent B. Krugh, Gary C. Henry, James G. Kereiakes, and Robert A. Kaufman. Characteristics of extrafocal radiation and its potential significance in pediatric radiology. *Radiology* 146, 793–799, 1983.

Thompson, Thomas. *Cahoon's Formulating X-ray Techniques*. 9th ed. Durham, NC: Duke University Press, 1979.

THE CASE OF THE GHOSTLY PLANTS

Can you identify this plant?

(Reprinted by permission of the International Society of Radiographers and Radiological Technicians from the K. C. Clark Archives, Middlesex Hospital, London, England)

Answers to the case studies can be found in Appendix E.

14 THE PATIENT AS A BEAM EMITTER

. . . the patient . . . would shape up into something that called for attention, his peculiarities, her reticences or candors. And though I might be attracted or repelled, the professional attitude . . . would steady me and dictate the terms on which I was to proceed.

—William Carlos Williams, *The Autobiography*.

OUTLINE

ATTENUATION
THE HUMAN BODY AS AN ATTENUATOR
THE PATIENT'S RELATIONSHIP TO IMAGE QUALITY

OBJECTIVES

Upon completion of this chapter, the student should be able to:

1. Explain the process of attenuation.
2. Describe the basic composition of the human body.
3. Describe the effect of the human body on the attenuation of the x-ray beam.
4. Explain the relationship of the subject (patient) to the density, contrast, recorded detail and distortion of the recorded image.

ATTENUATION

Attenuation is the reduction in the total number of x-ray photons remaining in the beam after passing through a given thickness of material (see Figure 11–1). It is the result of x-rays interacting with matter and being absorbed or scattered. The amount of attenuation is determined by the amount and type of irradiated material. X-rays are attenuated exponentially. This means that they are reduced by a certain percentage for each given thickness of material they pass through. Theoretically, then, the number of x-rays passing through an absorber will never reach zero. This is because each succeeding thickness of material reduces the number of photons by only a fraction of the previous amount.

As an x-ray beam passes through a patient, the beam is attenuated. The thicker the body part being radiographed, the greater the attenuation. In order to provide a sufficient number of x-ray photons for interaction with the film, the original quantity and quality of the photons must be increased with increased body part thickness. The incident beam is significantly altered as it passes through the patient. **The beam emitted from the patient contains the radiologically significant information needed by the radiologist to make a diagnosis.**

Attenuation is also affected by the type of absorber. **Higher atomic number materials** (such as lead and barium) **attenuate a greater percentage of the beam than low atomic number materials** (such as hydrogen, carbon and oxygen). This is due to the presence of a greater number of electrons with which photons may interact. Bone produces less radiographic density because it attenuates the x-ray beam more than soft tissue. This is predominantly because of the presence of calcium in bone, which has a higher atomic number than the majority of the elements found in the human body. The effective atomic number of the important materials comprising the human body are listed in Table 14–1.

The density of the absorbing material also has an impact on attenuation. **Density is the quantity of matter per unit of volume measured in kilograms per cubic meter.** It describes how tightly the atoms of a given substance are packed together. For example,

the molecules in an ice cube are less tightly packed than the same molecules when they are in their liquid state. Bone tissue is a denser substance than lung tissue. Table 14–1 lists the densities of the important materials comprising the human body. Because density and atomic number affect attenuation, it is important to understand the basic composition of the human body, particularly in terms of the average atomic number and density of the major substances.

THE HUMAN BODY AS AN ATTENUATOR

The patient is the greatest variable the radiographer faces when performing a radiographic procedure. The human body is comprised of a variety of organic and inorganic substances. At the atomic level, the body consists primarily of hydrogen, carbon, nitrogen and oxygen. These elements have atomic numbers of 1, 6, 7 and 8 respectively. Calcium, found in concentrated amounts in bones and teeth, has an atomic number of 20.

The composition of the human body determines its radiographic appearance (Figure 14–1). Although human anatomy and physiology are quite complex, when studying the absorption characteristics of the body, four major substances account for most of the variations in x-ray absorption: air, fat, muscle and bone (Figure 14–2).

Air

Air has an effective atomic number of 7.78, which is greater than either fat or muscle. Despite the slightly higher effective atomic number, air has a significantly lower tissue density. As a result, air will absorb fewer photons as they pass through it. Because air absorbs fewer photons than other body substances, more photons reach the x-ray film, thus producing a greater radiographic density.

TABLE 14–1		
Basic Substances Comprising the Human Body		
Substance	Effective Atomic Number	Density (kg/cm³)
Air	7.78	1.29
Fat	6.46	916
Water	7.51	1000
Muscle	7.64	1040
Bone	12.31	1650

Figure 14–1.   An antique full-body radiograph. (Reprinted with permission of the International Society of Radiographers and Radiological Technicians from the K.C. Clark Archives, Middlesex Hospital, London, England.)

Air is naturally present in the lungs, the sinuses and, in small amounts, in the gastrointestinal tract. On a typical radiograph of the abdomen, air can usually be seen in the stomach and colon.

Fat

Fat is similar to muscle in that they are both among the soft-tissue structures in the body. The soft-tissue structures have effective atomic numbers and tissue densities which are very similar to water's. For this reason, water is sometimes used to simulate soft tissue for experimental purposes. Fat has an effective atomic number which is slightly less than muscle's. In addition, fat has less tissue density than muscle. Muscle cells are more closely packed than fat cells. The amount of fatty tissue varies considerably between patients. While this is also true of muscle tissue, the variations are generally less pronounced and therefore have less effect on the overall attenuation of the beam. On a radiograph of the abdomen, the kidneys can often be outlined because of the perirenal fat capsule that surrounds them.

Muscle

Like fat, muscle is a soft tissue. Muscle, however, has a slightly higher effective atomic number and a greater tissue density than fat. As a result, muscle is a greater attenuator of the beam. On a radiograph of the abdomen, it is often easy to distinguish the psoas muscle on each side of the spine because of the increased absorption of radiation by these muscles.

Bone

The skeletal anatomy is easily seen radiographically because of the calcium content of bone. Calcium has a higher atomic number than most of the elements found in the human body. As a result, bone has the highest effective atomic number of the four basic substances. It also has the greatest tissue density and, as a result, absorbs radiation at a greater rate than any of the soft tissues or air-filled structures. This absorption means that fewer photons will reach the x-ray film and less radiographic density will be produced. On a radiograph of the abdomen, the lower ribs, spine and pelvis are all very easily distinguished because of the increased x-ray absorption that occurs in bone.

Figure 14–2. A radiograph of the abdomen demonstrating (1) air in the stomach and colon, (2) fat around the kidneys, (3) muscle to the right and left of the spine (psoas muscles) and (4) ribs, spine and pelvis.

THE PATIENT'S RELATIONSHIP TO IMAGE QUALITY

The patient has an impact on all properties affecting radiographic quality: density, contrast, recorded detail and distortion. These are described in detail in Chapters 23–26. The relationships between these factors and the patient (subject) are termed subject density, subject contrast, subject detail and subject distortion.

Subject Density

The various tissues in the human body are responsible for the specific radiographic densities that occur on the film. **Radiographic density will be altered by changes in the amount or type of tissue being irradiated**. In other words, thicker and denser body parts absorb more radiation, thus producing less radiographic density, and vice versa.

Subject Contrast

Radiographic contrast is the difference in densities of a recorded image. The differences in radiographic density are the result of differences in the absorption of the x-ray beam as it passes through the patient. **Subject contrast is the degree of differential absorption resulting from the differing absorption characteristics of the tissues in the body**. Subject contrast is dependent on the specific characteristics of an individual patient's tissues.

Subject Detail

One of the primary factors that affects the sharpness or detail of an image is the distance between the structure of interest and the film. Because anatomical structures are located at varying distances from the x-ray film, **the recorded detail of the structures is dependent on their position within the body and also on the body's placement in relationship to the film**.

The overall size and placement of the patient has a great impact on the recorded detail. The larger the patient, the greater the distance between the anatomical structures and the film. This results in less sharpness in the recorded details on the film. Conversely, greater sharpness will result when the anatomical part is closer to the film, as is the case with thinner patients. Specific positions have been established to place the anatomical structures of interest in as close proximity to the film as possible. For example, chest radiography is typically performed in the PA projection and in the left lateral position to place the heart closer to the film.

Subject Distortion

Distortion is the misrepresentation of the size or shape of the structure of interest. Because of the way in which certain structures lie within the body, **unless the patient is positioned specifically to demonstrate a particular structure, it may not be accurately represented on the film**. For example, to properly demonstrate the apophyseal joints of the lumbar spine, the patient should be in the oblique position. In the AP projection of the lumbar spine, these joints will be distorted. Distortion, in the form of magnification, also occurs because various anatomical structures sit at varying levels.

SUMMARY

Attenuation is the reduction in the total number of x-ray photons remaining in the beam after passing through a given thickness of material. It is the result of x-rays interacting with matter and being absorbed or scattered. The amount of attenuation will be determined by the amount and type of irradiated material.

The patient is the greatest variable that the radiographer faces when performing a radiographic procedure. The composition of the human body determines its radiographic appearance. When studying the absorption characteristics of the body, four major substances account for most of the variations in x-ray absorption: air, fat, muscle and bone.

The patient has an impact on all the properties that affect radiographic quality: density, contrast, recorded detail and distortion. The relationships between these factors and the patient (subject) are termed subject density, subject contrast, subject detail and subject distortion.

REVIEW QUESTIONS

1. How does atomic number affect attenuation?

2. How does tissue density affect attenuation?

3. What elements comprise the majority of those found in the human body?

4. What are the differences between air, fat, muscle and bone with respect to their attenuation and the resultant radiographic density?

5. How does the patient affect each of the factors of image quality?

REFERENCES AND RECOMMENDED READING

Bower, Richard. Stripes in the abdomen. *Radiologic Technology* 60:6, 511, 1989.

Carroll, Quinn. *Fuchs's Principles of Radiographic Exposure, Processing and Quality Control.* 3rd ed. Springfield, IL: Charles C. Thomas Publisher, 1985.

Cohen, M. Attenuation of x-rays in the human body. *Radiography* 37:436, 88–90, 1971.

Fuchs, Arthur W. Relationship of tissue thickness to kilovoltage. *Radiologic Technology* 19:6, 287, 1948.

Handbook of Chemistry and Physics. 69th ed. Boca Raton, FL: C.R.C. Press, 1989.

Hiss, Stephen S. *Understanding Radiography.* Springfield, IL: Charles C. Thomas Publisher, 1978.

Lindsay, R., and J.B. Anderson. Radiological determination of changes in bone mineral content. *Radiography* 44:517, 21–26, 1978.

Seeram, Euclid. *X-ray Imaging Equipment: An Introduction.* Springfield, IL: Charles C. Thomas, 1985.

Thompson, Thomas. *Cahoon's Formulating X-ray Techniques.* 9th ed. Durham, NC: Duke University Press, 1979.

15 THE PATHOLOGY PROBLEM

You don't look different
but you have changed
I'm looking through you
you're not the same

John Lennon and Paul McCartney "I'm Looking Through You," from *Rubber Soul.*

OUTLINE

PATHOLOGY AND RADIATION ABSORPTION
INCREASED ATTENUATION (ADDITIVE) CONDITIONS
DECREASED ATTENUATION (DESTRUCTIVE) CONDITIONS

OBJECTIVES

Upon completion of this chapter, the student should be able to:

1. Explain the effect that a pathological condition can have on radiation absorption.
2. Describe the effect of pathology on the radiographic image.
3. Differentiate between pathological conditions which result in increased attenuation versus those which result in decreased attenuation of the x-ray beam.
4. Identify pathological conditions which result in an increased attenuation of the x-ray beam.
5. Identify pathological conditions which result in a decreased attenuation of the x-ray beam.

PATHOLOGY AND RADIATION ABSORPTION

As radiation passes through the patient it undergoes attenuation or absorption of the x-ray photons. The patient is the greatest variable the radiographer faces when trying to select adequate exposure factors for a specific procedure. Attenuation will vary, depending on the thickness and the composition of the patient's tissues. As an added dilemma, the radiographer must also realize that pathological conditions can affect the overall thickness and composition of the patient's tissues. The radiographer must first be aware of the variations between normal body tissues and then be concerned about possible additional variations as a result of a specific disease process.

Pathology is the medical science that is concerned with all aspects of disease, including the structural and functional changes caused by a disease process. Disease will often bring about changes in body tissues that can be viewed radiographically and interpreted by the radiologist. If this were not true, radiography would be of no use in diagnosing disease. These changes may be structural and/or functional in nature and they may or may not have an impact on the degree of radiation absorbed by the patient. Certain diseases can increase or decrease tissue thickness or alter tissue composition (change the effective atomic number or density). When this occurs, the disease will affect the degree of radiation absorption for that specific body tissue. Two common pathologies of the chest demonstrate the differences in radiation absorption (Figure 15–1 A & B). In Figure 15–1A the patient has pneumonia, which causes air-filled lung tissue to fill with fluid. Fluid will absorb more radiation than air. In Figure 15–1B the patient has emphysema. With emphysema, normal lung tissue is destroyed and the air sacs become enlarged. A greater amount of air is then present in the lungs, which results in less attenuation of radiation.

Radiographers must have an understanding of pathology in order to properly select the technical factors for a procedure. Properly reading the x-ray requisition, taking an adequate patient history and close observation of the patient are the essential responsibilities of the radiographer. Fulfilling these responsibilities reduces the need to repeat a film, due to the patient's condition. For example, it may be necessary to adjust the technical factors if a chest x-ray is requested for a patient with emphysema. By taking a good history, the radiographer can determine how long the patient has had the condition and what signs and symptoms the patient has exhibited. By observing signs, such as shortness of breath or prolonged exhalation, the radiographer can assess the extent of the disease. Of course, disease conditions are not always known prior to performing the examination. This is one of the primary reasons a repeat film may be necessary, even though there was no error in judgment on the part of the radiographer. As an individual gains clinical experience, his assessment skills improve and he is able to make better judgments concerning the presence and extent of disease.

If a disease causes the affected body tissue to increase in thickness, effective atomic number and/or density, there will be a greater attenuation of the x-ray beam. As more photons are absorbed by the body tissues, fewer will be available to reach the film to create adequate radiographic density. These diseases are harder to penetrate and are called additive conditions because they require adding to the exposure to achieve the proper density on the film. There is an inverse relationship between additive conditions and radiographic density. This means that when additive conditions are present, radiographic density will decrease as the extent of the disease increases.

If a disease causes the affected body tissue to decrease in thickness, effective atomic number and/or density, there will be less attenuation of the x-ray beam. As more photons are able to pass through the body tissues, more will be available to reach the film to create the radiographic density. These diseases are easier to penetrate and are called **destructive conditions**. They require decreasing the exposure to achieve the proper density on the film. There is a direct relationship between destructive conditions and radiographic density. This means that when destructive conditions are present, the radiographic density will increase as the extent of the disease increases.

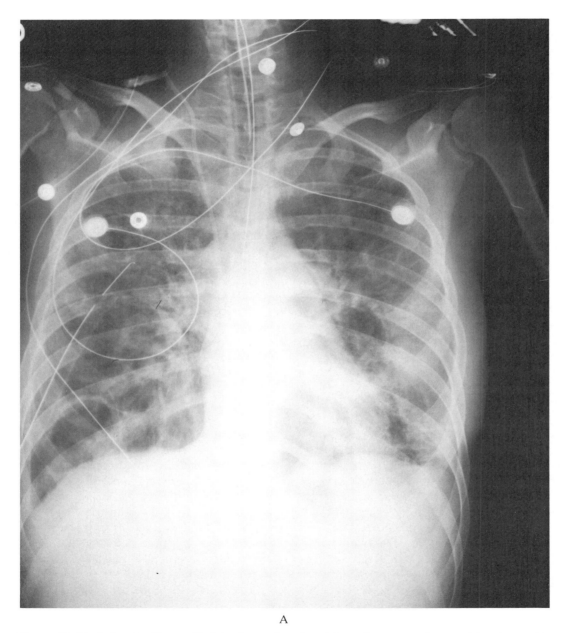

A

Figure 15–1A & B.   In Figure 15–1A, the patient has bilateral pneumonia, resulting in an increase in radiation absorption. In Figure 15–1B, the patient has severe emphysema, resulting in a decrease in radiation absorption.

B

A disease influences radiation absorption when it alters the overall number or types of atoms comprising the affected tissue. For example, if a person sprains an ankle, one of the body's responses to the injury is swelling or edema at the site. The ankle becomes enlarged because there is an increase in blood and serous fluid around the ankle joint. The body tissue increases in thickness, but, in this example, the opacity of the tissue is generally the same. Blood and serous fluid have approximately the same opacity as the soft tissue around the ankle. What is occurring at the molecular and atomic level is an increase, primarily in the number of water molecules (hydrogen and oxygen atoms), which comprise most of blood and serous fluid. If there are more water molecules present around the ankle, a greater number of x-ray photons will interact with that tissue, resulting in increased radiation absorption and decreased exposure to the x-ray film. Technical factors must be increased to compensate for an increase in the thickness of the part. Proper measurement of the body part and the use of technique charts will ensure that the correct technical factors are selected.

The extent to which a body part is affected by disease will determine if technical factors must be adjusted. For example, no change in technical factors is necessary to visualize a small, localized tumor in the lung, or a small kidney stone. If, however, the tumor is large and diffuse, or the kidney stone causes severe hydronephrosis, adjustments in the technical factors may be required to adequately visualize the pathology (Figure 15–2 A & B). It is important to remember that the degree or extent of the pathology is critical in determining the technical factor adjustments. If the technical factors must be adjusted, the change must be enough to make a visible difference in radiographic density. **To produce a visible difference requires a minimal change of 25–50 percent in the overall density of the image**.

Many diseases do not affect the thickness or opacity of body tissues but can be diagnosed by way of radiography simply because of the structural or functional changes that they produce. These diseases generally do not require an adjustment in the selected technical factors. Examples include ulcers, diverticula and simple fractures (provided there is minimal swelling). There are many diseases that do not affect the thickness or alter the composition of the body tissues and therefore cause no radiographically evident structural or functional changes. These conditions generally do not require radiography; they are usually diagnosed through laboratory testing. Diseases such as diabetes mellitus, anemia and meningitis are examples.

INCREASED ATTENUATION (ADDITIVE) CONDITIONS

Many disease processes will result in an increase in thickness, effective atomic number and/or density of the body tissue. Recall that the body tissues vary in thickness (the femur is thicker than the humerus) and in composition (bone has a higher effective atomic number and greater tissue density than muscle). These diseases absorb more radiation and require the radiographer to increase technical factors to compensate for the changes in the body tissues. The extent of the disease also plays an important role in technical factor adjustment. The technical factor adjustments will vary, depending upon the degree to which the body tissues are affected. Because of this, each patient will be different and must be examined individually.

No magic formula exists to adjust technical factors to compensate for a pathologic problem. The radiographer must carefully review the requisition, obtain a patient history and then examine the patient. By following these steps, the radiographer can make a judgment concerning the necessary technical adjustment to be made. Experience is particularly valuable in determining the proper changes to be made. As a general rule, additive conditions will require an increase in kilovoltage to adequately penetrate the thicker, more opaque body parts. Remember that an increase of 15 percent in kVp will approximately double the exposure to the film. An increase of 5–15 percent in kilovoltage will compensate for most additive pathologic conditions. Automatic exposure control (AEC) systems will compensate for most pathological changes by adjusting the exposure automatically. However, the compensation will be the result of increased mAs rather than increased kVp.

Some of the common conditions that cause an increase in attenuation and may therefore require an increase in technical factors are outlined. A summary of the conditions is provided in Table 15–1.

Conditions Affecting Multiple Systems

Certain diseases can occur in a wide variety of body systems and, as a result, they may be present in various sites. Whenever an x-ray requisition indicates the presence of any of the following conditions, it may be necessary to increase technical factors for the procedure.

Abscess—an encapsulated infection increases tissue thickness and may alter composition, particularly in the lungs.

Edema—swelling causes an increase in tissue thickness and may alter composition if it occurs in the lungs.

Tumors—an abnormal new growth in tissue results in an increase in tissue thickness and may alter composition, particularly in the lungs or bones or when calcification results.

TABLE 15–1

Summary of Pathology Problems

Increased Attenuation Conditions	Decreased Attenuation Conditions
Multiple Sites	**Multiple Sites**
Abscess	Anorexia Nervosa
Edema	Atrophy
Tumors	Emaciation
The Chest	**The Chest**
Atelectasis	Emphysema
Bronchiectasis	Pneumothorax
Cardiomegaly	
Congestive Heart Failure	
Empyema	
Pleural Effusions	
Pneumoconioses	
Pneumonia	
Pneumonectomy	
Tuberculosis (advanced/miliary)	
The Abdomen	**The Abdomen**
Aortic Aneurysm	Aerophagia
Ascites	Bowel Obstruction
Cirrhosis	
Calcified Stones	
The Extremities and Skull	**The Extremities and Skull**
Acromegaly	Active Osteomyelitis
Chronic Osteomyelitis	Aseptic Necrosis
Hydrocephalus	Carcinoma
Osteoblastic Metastases	Degenerative Arthritis
Osteochondroma	Fibrosarcoma
Paget's Disease	Gout
Sclerosis	Hyperparathyroidism
	Multiple Myeloma
	Osteolytic Metastases
	Osteomalacia
	Osteoporosis

A

Figure 15–2A & B.   When a tumor is smaller and more localized, as in Figure 15–2A, there is less need for technical factor adjustments. Tumors that are larger and more diffuse throughout both lungs, as in Figure 15–2B, require greater technical factor adjustments.

Conditions of the Chest

The chest is a common site for pathologic conditions and chest radiography is a common diagnostic procedure. It may be necessary to increase technical factors for a procedure whenever an x-ray requisition indicates the presence of any of the following conditions.

Atelectasis—a collapse of the lung results in airlessness of all or part of the lung tissue. This causes lung tissue density to increase.

Bronchiectasis—the chronic dilatation of the bronchi can result in peribronchial thickening and small areas of atelectasis. This causes an increase in lung tissue density.

Cardiomegaly—an enlargement of the heart causes an increase in thickness of the part.

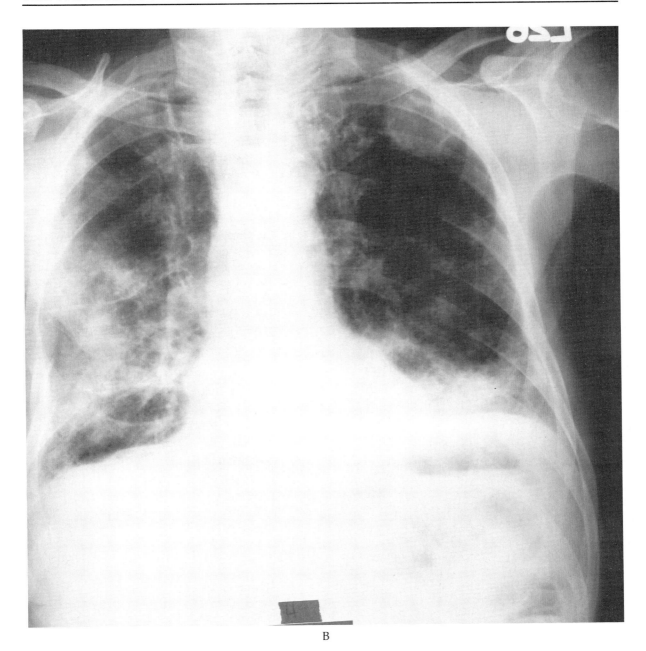

B

Congestive Heart Failure—when the heart is in failure, the cardiac output is diminished. This results in backward fail- ure, or increased venous congestion in the lungs. Lung tissue density is in- creased and the heart is enlarged as well.

Empyema—pus in the thoracic cavity causes an increase in tissue density.

Pleural Effusions (Hemothorax, Hydrothorax)—when the pleural cavity fills with either blood or serous fluid, it displaces normal lung tissue. This results in an increased tissue density within the thoracic cavity.

Pneumoconioses—the inhalation of dust particles can cause fibrotic (scarring) changes. When healthy lung tissue becomes fibrotic, density of the tissue increases.

Pneumonia (pneumonitis)—inflammation of the lung tissues causes fluid to fill in the alveolar spaces. Fluid has much greater tissue density than the air normally present.

Pneumonectomy—the removal of a lung will cause the affected side to demonstrate an increase in density since normal air-filled lung tissue is removed.

Pulmonary Edema—when fluid fills the interstitial lung tissues and the alveoli, tissue density increases. This is a typical complication of congestive heart failure.

Tuberculosis (advanced and miliary)—an infection by a mycobacteria causes the inflammatory response, which results in an increase in fluid in the lungs. If the mycobacteria was inhaled, it generally begins as a localized lesion (usually upper lobes), which can spread to a more advanced stage. If the infection reaches the lungs by the bloodstream, it has a more diffuse spread (miliary TB). Increased tissue density results in both advanced and miliary TB (Figure 15–3).

Conditions of the Abdomen

Abdominal conditions usually cause the abdomen to distend. It may be necessary to increase technical factors for a procedure when an x-ray requisition indicates the presence of any of the following conditions. Most technical factor changes, however, will be the natural result of the noted increase in abdominal size when measuring patient thickness.

Aortic Aneurysm—a large dilatation of the aorta will result in increased thickness of the affected part.

Ascites—fluid accumulation within the peritoneal cavity causes an increase in tissue thickness. The free fluid has a unique "ground glass" appearance radiographically.

Cirrhosis—fibrotic changes in the liver cause the liver to enlarge and ascites can result. The result is an increase in the thickness of the liver and the entire abdomen.

Calcified stones—stones are most commonly found throughout the abdomen in such organs as the gallbladder and the kidney. Calcium may be deposited, which causes an increase in the effective atomic number of the tissue.

Conditions of the Extremities and Skull

Conditions which result in new bone growth are termed osteoblastic. These conditions generally require an increase in technical factors. It may be necessary to increase technical factors for a procedure whenever an x-ray requisition indicates the presence of any of the following conditions.

Acromegaly—an overgrowth of the hands, feet, face and jaw as a result of hypersecretion of growth hormones in the adult will result in an increase in bone mass.

Chronic Osteomyelitis—a chronic bone infection results in new bone growth at the infected site.

Figure 15–3. This patient has miliary tuberculosis with bronchopneumonia. These are both additive conditions, resulting in increased radiation absorption.

Hydrocephalus—a dilatation of the fluid-filled cerebral ventricles causes an enlargement of the head, resulting in an increased thickness.

Osteoblastic Metastases—the spread of cancer to bone can result in uncontrolled new bone growth.

Osteochondroma—a tumor arising in the bone and cartilage will result in an increased thickness of the bone.

Paget's Disease (osteitis deformans)—an increase occurs in bone cell activity which leads to new bone growth. The result is increased bone thickness, with the pelvis, spine and skull most often affected (Figure 15–4).

Sclerosis—an increase in hardening as a result of a chronic inflammation in bone. This increases the density of the bone tissue.

DECREASED ATTENUATION (DESTRUCTIVE) CONDITIONS

Various disease processes can result in a decrease in thickness, effective atomic number and/or density of the body tissue. These conditions cause the absorption of less radiation and require the radiographer to decrease technical factors to compensate for the changes in the body tissues. Recall also that the extent of the disease plays an important role in technical factor adjustment. As a general rule, compensations for destructive conditions can be made by decreasing the mAs. Remember that a decrease of 50 percent in mAs will reduce the exposure to the film by half. A decrease of 25–50 percent in mAs will compensate for most of these pathologic conditions. Automatic exposure control (AEC) systems will compensate for most pathological changes by adjusting the exposure automatically.

Some of the common conditions that cause a decrease in attenuation and may there-

Figure 15–4. Paget's disease is an additive condition, resulting in increased radiation absorption.

fore require a decrease in technical factors are outlined. A summary of the conditions is provided in Table 15–1 above.

Conditions Affecting Multiple Sites

Certain diseases can occur in a wide variety of body systems and, as a result, they may be present in various sites. Whenever an x-ray requisition indicates the presence of any of the following conditions, it may be necessary to decrease technical factors for the procedure.

Anorexia Nervosa—a psychological eating disorder which results in an extreme weight loss. Overall body thickness is reduced.

Atrophy—a wasting away of body tissue with diminished cell proliferation, resulting in reduced thickness of a specific part or the entire body.

Emaciation—a generalized wasting away of body tissue, resulting in reduced thickness of the body.

Conditions of the Chest

The chest is a common site for pathologic conditions and chest radiography is a common diagnostic procedure. It may be necessary to decrease technical factors for a procedure when an x-ray requisition indicates the presence of the following conditions.

Emphysema—the overdistention of the lung tissues by air will result in a decrease in lung tissue density.

Pneumothorax—free air in the pleural cavity displaces normal lung tissue and results in decreased density within the thoracic cavity (Figure 15–5).

Conditions of the Abdomen

Abdominal conditions usually cause the abdomen to distend. This distention may be the result of the accumulation of fluid (in which case technical factors need to be increased) or air. Distention of the abdomen from air will require a decrease in technical factors. Whenever an x-ray requisition indicates the presence of the following conditions, it may be necessary to decrease technical factors for the procedure because of the presence of air.

Aerophagia—a psychological disorder resulting in abnormal swallowing of air. The stomach becomes dilated from the air and overall tissue density decreases.

Bowel Obstruction—an obstruction in the bowel results in the abnormal accumulation of air and fluid. If a large amount of air is trapped in the bowel, the overall density of the tissues is decreased (Figure 15–6).

Conditions of the Extremities and Skull

Conditions which result in the destruction of bone tissue are termed osteolytic. These conditions result in a loss of bone mass or calcium within the bone. They alter the composition of the bone by decreasing the effective atomic number and/or the tissue density. The result is areas of radiolucency which are easier to penetrate than normal bone. Approximately 50 percent of the bone substance must be lost before changes can be seen radiographically. As a result, these conditions must generally be extensive before technical factor changes are necessary.

Active Osteomyelitis—with a bone infection there is initially a loss of bone tissue (containing calcium), resulting in a decrease in the thickness and composition of the part.

Aseptic necrosis—death of bone tissue results in a decrease in composition and thickness of the part.

Carcinoma—malignancies in bone can cause an osteolytic process, resulting in decreased thickness and composition of the part.

Degenerative Arthritis—inflammation of the joints results in a destruction of adjoining bone tissue, which decreases the composition of the part.

Fibrosarcoma—this malignant tumor of the metaphysis of bone causes an osteolytic lesion with a "moth-eaten" appearance. The result is reduced bone composition.

Gout—during the chronic stages of this metabolic disease, areas of bone destruc-

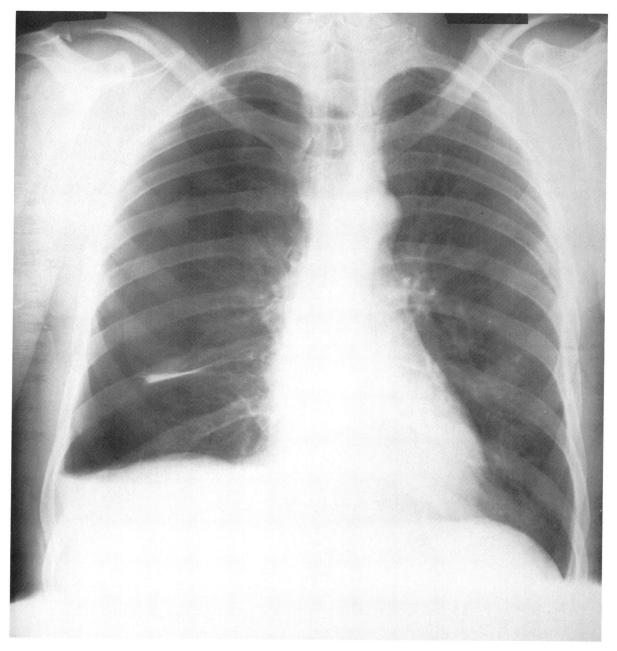

Figure 15–5. A large, right-sided pneumothorax is a destructive condition, resulting in decreased radiation absorption.

Figure 15–6.   An obstruction of the large bowel is a destructive condition, resulting in decreased radiation absorption.

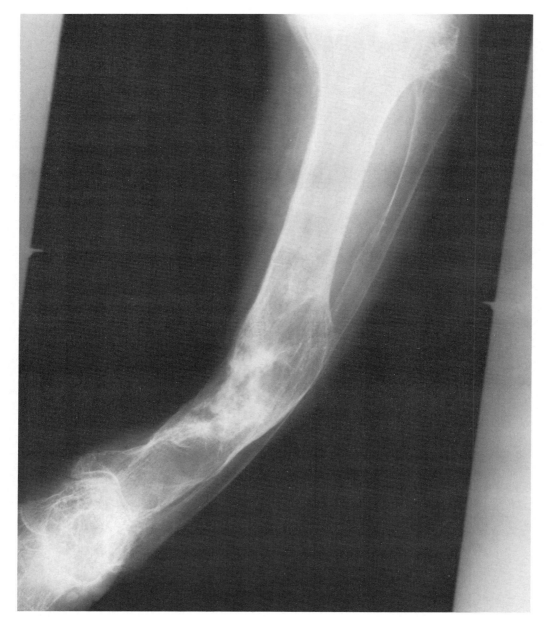

Figure 15–7. This patient has a severe bone deformity from a fracture which resulted in chronic osteomyelitis and diffuse osteoporosis. The chronic osteomyelitis is an additive condition (seen around the fracture site) and the osteoporosis is a destructive condition, resulting in a decrease in radiation absorption throughout the remaining bone.

tion result in punched-out lesions that reduce the bone composition.

Hyperparathyroidism—oversecretion of the parathyroid hormone causes calcium to leave bone and enter the bloodstream. The bone becomes demineralized and composition is decreased.

Multiple Myeloma—this malignant tumor arises from plasma cells of bone marrow and causes punched-out osteolytic areas on the bone. Often many sites are affected and reduced bone tissue composition results.

Osteolytic Metastases—when some malignancies spread to bone they produce destruction of the bone, resulting in reduced composition.

Osteomalacia—a defect in bone mineralization results in decreased composition of the affected bone.

Osteoporosis—a defect in bone production due to the failure of osteoblasts to lay down bone matrix results in decreased composition of the affected bone (Figure 15–7).

SUMMARY

The presence of a pathologic condition can greatly affect the degree of radiation absorption. Radiographers must have an understanding of pathology in order to properly select the technical factors for a procedure. Properly reading the x-ray requisition and taking an adequate patient history are essential responsibilities of the radiographer. Fulfilling these responsibilities reduces the need to repeat a film, due to the patient's condition.

If a disease causes the affected body tissue to increase in thickness, effective atomic number and/or density, that disease will result in a greater attenuation of the x-ray beam. As more photons are absorbed by the body tissues, fewer will be available to reach the film to create adequate radiographic density. These diseases are harder to penetrate and are called additive conditions because they require adding to the exposure to achieve the proper density on the film.

If a disease causes the affected body tissue to decrease in thickness, effective atomic number and/or density, that disease will result in less attenuation of the x-ray beam. As more photons are able to pass through the body tissues, more will be available to reach the film to create the required radiographic density. These diseases are easier to penetrate and are called destructive conditions. They require decreasing the exposure to achieve the proper density on the film.

REVIEW QUESTIONS

1. Why do some pathological conditions affect the attenuation of the x-ray beam?

2. Why is it important that radiographers have an understanding of pathological conditions?

3. What is the relationship between additive conditions and attenuation? destructive conditions and attenuation?

4. Why should the radiographer take a good clinical history and closely observe the patient?

5. Describe how the following additive conditions may affect the radiographic image:
   a) edema
   b) congestive heart failure
   c) pneumonia
   d) ascites
   e) Paget's disease

6. Describe how the following destructive conditions may affect the radiographic image:

a) atrophy
b) emphysema
c) pneumothorax
d) degenerative arthritis
e) osteoporosis

REFERENCES AND RECOMMENDED READING

Eisenberg, Ronald L., and Cynthia A. Dennis. *Comprehensive Radiographic Pathology*. St. Louis, MO: C.V. Mosby, 1990.

Hiss, Stephen C. *Understanding Radiography*. Springfield, IL: Charles C. Thomas, 1978.

Laudicina, Paul F. *Applied Pathology for Radiographers*. Philadelphia, PA: W.B. Saunders Company, 1989.

Mace, James D., and Nina M. Kowalczyk. *Radiographic Pathology for Technologists*. St. Louis, MO: C. V. Mosby Company, 1988.

Sheldon, Huntington. *Boyd's Introduction to the Study of Disease*. 10th ed. Philadelphia, PA: Lea and Febiger, 1988.

Thompson, Thomas T., M.D. *Cahoon's Formulating X-ray Techniques*. 9th ed. Durham, NC: Duke University Press, 1979.

THE CASE OF THE DARK LINE IN THE ABDOMEN

What is the most likely cause of this strange dark line running transversely through the patient's abdomen?

Answers to the case studies can be found in Appendix E.

16 THE GRID

We . . . hope that roentgenologists . . . may become convinced of the serious role played by object-secondary rays, to the end that it will soon be practicable for every roentgenologist to rid himself of their nuisance in his every-day work.

Hollis E. Potter, "The Bucky diaphram principle applied to roentgenography."

OUTLINE

**PURPOSE OF THE GRID
GRID CONSTRUCTION
GRID PATTERNS
GRID TYPES
GRID USES
GRID SELECTION/CONVERSIONS
GRID PERFORMANCE EVALUATION
GRID ERRORS
OTHER SCATTER REDUCTION METHODS**

OBJECTIVES

Upon completion of this chapter, the student should be able to:

1. Describe the purpose of the grid.
2. Explain the construction of a grid, including grid materials, grid ratio, grid frequency and lead content.
3. Describe the various grid patterns.
4. Differentiate between parallel and focused grids.
5. Differentiate between the uses of a stationary and a moving grid.
6. Explain the process of grid selection for specific radiographic procedures.
7. Explain the relationship of grid selection to patient dose and radiographic density.
8. Calculate changes in technical factors to compensate for changes in grid selection.
9. Describe methods for evaluating the performance of a grid.

259

10. Discuss common errors that are made when using a grid and the effects of these errors on the radiographic image.
11. Describe other scatter reduction methods.

PURPOSE OF THE GRID

A grid is a device which is used to improve the contrast of the radiographic image. It does this by absorbing scatter radiation before it can reach the film. When an x-ray beam passes through the body, one of three things will occur with the primary photons that originated at the target. They will: 1) pass through the body unaffected, 2) be absorbed by the body or 3) interact and change direction (Figure 16–1).

The photons that pass through the body unaffected will interact with the film to create the image. These are the photons responsible for creating the contrast (differences in the

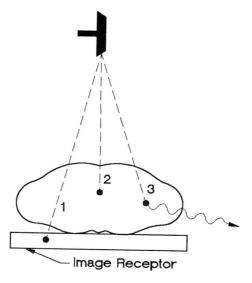

Figure 16–1. When x-rays interact with the patient, they will either 1. pass through unaffected, 2. be absorbed or 3. interact and change direction (scatter).

densities) on the radiograph. These differences exist because some photons pass through the body while others are absorbed. Absorption of photons occurs as the result of photoelectric interaction. This interaction results in the complete absorption of the primary photon and the production of a secondary photon. The secondary radiation created by this interaction is, with few exceptions, very weak and is quickly absorbed in the surrounding tissues.

Primary radiation that interacts and, as a result of this interaction, changes direction is known as scatter radiation. The interaction that produces scatter radiation is known as a Compton interaction. These interactions can result in photons which are strong enough to be emitted by the patient and interact with the film. Since these photons have changed direction they are no longer able to record densities on the film that relate to the patient's anatomy. The densities that they add to the film are of no diagnostic value. Scattered photons add an overall density to the film and, as a result of this overall graying of the image, contrast is lowered. An important point to remember is that the percentage of Compton interactions increases with increased kVp. Therefore, **scatter increases and contrast is further impaired as kVp increases**.

Since the patient is the source of the scatter that is degrading the image, it is logical to assume that the patient will also control the quantity of scatter produced. Scatter increases with increases in the volume and density of the tissue irradiated. The volume of tissue that is irradiated is controlled by the thickness of the patient and the exposure field size. While thickness of the patient is predetermined (although it can sometimes be reduced by compression), the field size can be kept to a minimum by collimation. The tissue type will also affect the quantity of scatter. The greater the density of the tissue, the greater will be the quantity of scatter created. For example, more scatter is produced in bone than in soft tissue, and more in soft tissue than in air. This is the result of changes in the number and types of atoms that are present for interaction. In summary, **the amount of scatter radiation increases with increases in patient thickness, increases in tissue density and with larger field sizes**.

Since a grid is designed to absorb the unwanted scatter radiation, it is necessary to use a grid with thicker, denser body parts and with procedures that require higher kVp techniques. As a general rule, a grid is employed when:

1. body part thickness exceeds 10 cm and tissue density is primarily soft tissue and bone, and

2. kVp is above 60.

A grid is a thin, flat, rectangular device which is made by placing a series of radiopaque lead strips side by side and separating the strips by an interspace material which is radiolucent. The lead strips are of very thin foil and the interspace material is thicker and usually made of aluminum. These strips are then encased in an aluminum cover to protect them from damage.

The very first grid was made in 1913 by the American radiologist Gustav Bucky (1880–1963). Dr. Bucky's first grid consisted of wide strips of lead spaced 2 cm apart and running in two directions, along the length of the film and across the film (Figure 16–2). This crude design created an image of the grid that was superimposed on the patient's image. Despite having to view the anatomy through this checkerboard pattern, the original grid did remove scatter and improve contrast.

Figure 16–2. Dr. Bucky's original grid. (Reprinted with permission, Smithsonian Institute Photo No. 47022.)

In 1920 Hollis Potter (1880–1963), a Chicago radiologist, improved Dr. Bucky's grid design. Dr. Potter realigned the lead strips so they would run in only one direction, made the lead strips thinner and therefore less obvious on the image, and then designed a device (now known as the Potter-Bucky diaphragm) which allowed the grid to move during the exposure. By moving the grid, the lead strips became blurred and were no longer visible on the film. All these improvements resulted in a practical grid device which significantly improved contrast without impairing the view of the patient's anatomy.

GRID CONSTRUCTION

A wide variety of grids are available today (Table 16–1). The choice of the proper grid for a particular clinical procedure requires an understanding of a grid's function. Grid construction involves the selection of materials, grid ratio and grid frequency.

TABLE 16–1	TYPICAL GRID SPECIFICATIONS					
Ratio	Linear/ Crosshatch	Focused/ Parallel	Interspace	Lines/Inch	Weight (g/cm^2)	Thickness (mm)
15:1	L	F	AI	103	1.74	3.7
15:1	L	F	AI	85	1.64	4.4
12:1	L	F	FIBER	80	1.45	4.4
12:1	L	F	AI	152		1.86
12:1	L	F	AI	103	1.21	3.2
12:1	L	F	AI	85	1.35	3.8
8:1	L	F	FIBER	80	0.96	3.4
8:1	L	F	AI	152		1.34
8:1	L	F	AI	103	0.87	2.3
8:1	L	F	AI	85	0.96	2.8
6:1	L	F	AI	103	0.67	1.9
6:1	L	F	AI	85	0.77	2.3
6:1	L	P	AI	85	0.77	2.3
6:1	C	F	AI	85	1.40	3.8
Specialty Low-ratio Grids					**Purpose**	
4:1	L	F	FIBER	60	Image intensification/Spot filming	
3.5:1	L	P	AI	196	Mammography	
2:1	L	P	AI	196	Mammography	

Adapted with permission from product catalogs of the Liebel-Flarsheim division of Sybron Corporation, Cincinnati, Ohio.

Grid Materials

A grid is a series of radiopaque strips which alternate with radiolucent interspace strips. These strips are bonded firmly together and then sliced into flat sheets. The radiopaque strips are needed to absorb the scatter radiation and must therefore be made of a dense material with a high atomic number. Lead is the material of choice because it is relatively inexpensive and is easy to shape into very thin foil.

The interspace material must be radiolucent. In other words, it allows radiation to pass easily through it. Several organic and inorganic materials have been tried but only two are commercially available—aluminum and plastic fiber. Ideally, this material should not absorb any radiation. However, in reality, it does absorb a small amount. Aluminum is more com-

monly used than fiber because it is easier to use in manufacturing and is more durable. Also, because it has a higher atomic number than fiber, it can provide additional absorption of low-energy scatter. With its higher atomic number, aluminum also increases the absorption of primary photons. This can be a disadvantage, especially with low kVp techniques where this absorption would be greater. Fiber interspace grids are preferred when using low kVp techniques where their application can contribute to lower patient dose, such as in pediatric radiography.

Grid Ratio

Grid ratio has a major influence on the ability of the grid to improve contrast. It is defined as the ratio of the height of the lead

Figure 16–3. Grid ratio is the height of the grid strips divided by the width of the interspace.

strips to the distance between the strips (Figure 16–3). This is expressed in the formula:

$$\text{Grid ratio} = \frac{h}{D} \text{ where}$$

$$h = \text{lead strip height}$$
$$D = \text{interspace width}$$

Example: If the lead strips are 3.0 mm high and are separated by an interspace of 0.25 mm, what is the grid ratio?

Answer:

$$\text{grid ratio} = \frac{3.0}{0.25}$$

$$\text{grid ratio} = 12\!:\!1$$

If the height of the grid is a constant, decreasing the distance between the lead strips would result in an increase in the grid ratio. Conversely, if the height of the grid is a constant, increasing the distance between the lead strips would result in a decrease in grid ratio. **An inverse relationship exists between the distance between the lead strips and grid ratio when the height of the grid strips remains the same.**

Higher grid ratios allow less scatter radiation to pass through their interspace material to reach the film. Figure 16–4 demonstrates the effect of grid ratio on the maximum angle possible for a scattered photon to pass through the grid. The higher the grid ratio, the straighter the scattered photon has to be in order to pass

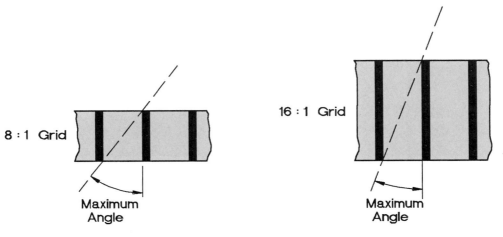

Figure 16–4. Grid ratio affects the amount of scatter absorbed by determining the maximum angle of a scattered ray that can get through the grid. The smaller the angle, the less scatter reaches the film.

through the interspace material. Scattered photons, therefore, have to be more closely aligned to the direction of the primary photons in order to reach the film. This means that higher grid ratios are more effective at removing scatter. For the same reason, higher-ratio grids require greater accuracy in their positioning and are more prone to grid errors.

Grid Frequency

Grid frequency is defined as the number of grid lines per inch or centimeter. Grids are made with a range in frequency from 60–196 lines/inch (25–78 lines/cm). Most commonly used grids have a frequency of 85–103 lines/inch (33–41 lines/cm). In general, grids with higher grid frequencies have thinner lead strips (Figure 16–5). Very high-frequency grids of approximately 200 lines/inch (80 lines/cm) with very low grid ratios of 2:1 or 3:1 are used in mammography because of the low kVp techniques and the desire to minimize the possibility of seeing the grid lines on the film.

By combining information about grid ratio and frequency, one can determine the total quantity of lead in the grid. It is the grid's lead content that is most important in determining the grid's efficiency at cleaning up scatter. Lead content is measured in mass per unit area, or grams per square centimeter. In general, the lead content is greater in a grid that has a higher grid ratio and lower grid frequency. **As the lead content of a grid increases, the ability of the grid to remove scatter and improve contrast increases**.

GRID PATTERNS

Grid strips can be made to run in one or two directions. Grids with lead strips running in only one direction are called linear grids. Grids are also made by placing two linear grids on top of one another so the grid lines are running at right angles. These grids are termed **criss-cross** or **cross-hatched** (Figure 16–6). Dr. Bucky's original grid was made using this pattern.

Linear grids are more commonly used in clinical practice because they can be used when performing procedures that require tube angulation. Linear grids allow the technologist to angle the tube only *along* the long axis of the grid. Angulation *across* the long axis would re-

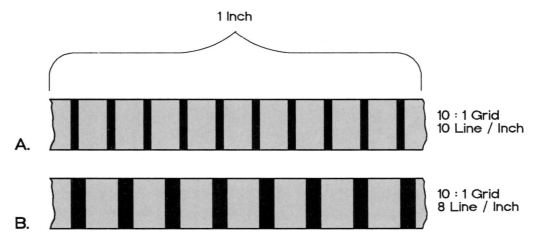

Figure 16–5. Grid frequency is the number of grid lines per inch or centimeter. Grids A and B have the same grid ratio but A has a lower grid frequency than B.

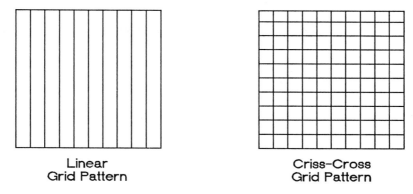

Linear
Grid Pattern

Criss-Cross
Grid Pattern

Figure 16–6. A linear vs. a criss-cross grid pattern.

sult in the primary beam being directed into the lead strips. If the primary beam is angled into the lead, the lead will absorb an undesirable amount of primary radiation, resulting in a problem known as grid cut-off. When criss-cross grids are used, no tube tilt is permitted since any angulation would result in grid cut-off because lead strips are running in both directions.

GRID TYPES

Grids are manufactured with either a parallel or a focused design. Parallel grids are made with the lead and interspace strips running parallel to one another. This means that if the grid lines were extended into space they would never intersect. Focused grids are designed so that the central grid strips are parallel and as the strips move away from the central axis they become more and more inclined (Figure 16–7).

The focused design results in a grid with lead strips designed to match the divergence of the x-ray beam. If these lead strips were extended, the strips would intersect along a line in space known as the convergence line. The distance from the face of the grid to the points of convergence of the lead strips is called the grid radius. **For the grid to be properly fo-**

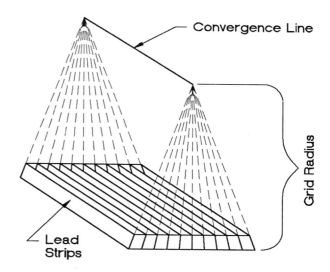

Figure 16–7. A focused grid is designed to match the divergence of the x-ray beam. The grid ratio is the distance from the face of the grid to the points of convergence of the lead strips.

cused, the x-ray tube must be located along the convergence line. Each focused grid will identify the focal range within which the tube should be located. For example, grids are made with short, medium or long focal ranges, depending on the distance for which they are designed. Short focal range grids (14–18 inches or 36–46 cm) are made for use in mammography; long focal range grids (60–72 inches or 152–183 cm) are used for chest radiography. Focused grids with lower grid ratios allow for greater latitude in the alignment of the tube with the grid. With higher grid ratios, proper alignment of the grid with the tube is more critical.

Parallel grids are less commonly employed than focused grids and are only available in lower ratios. Because the strips do not try to coincide with the divergence of the x-ray beam, some grid cut-off will occur along the lateral edges, especially when the grid is employed at short SIDs. The parallel grid is best employed at long SIDs because the beam will be a straighter, more perpendicular one (Figure 16–8).

GRID USES

A grid is used either in a stationary position or mounted in a Potter-Bucky diaphragm to move it during exposure. Most radiology departments have a supply of stationary grids, in various sizes, which can be mounted to the front of a cassette. These are generally made approximately one inch larger than the film size they are intended to cover. Stationary grids are used primarily in portable procedures or for upright or horizontal beam views. Some departments may also purchase a special cassette with a grid built into it. This design, called a grid cassette, requires reloading the film between exposures using the grid. This may be an inconvenience in situations where multiple films are needed. When grids are used in a stationary fashion, grid lines on the film will usually be noticed on close inspection of the image. This is especially true with low-frequency grids. High-frequency grids, like those used for mammography, have a minimal visual effect.

The most common use of the grid is for procedures using the Potter-Bucky diaphragm (usually called the bucky). This device is mounted below the tabletop of radiographic and radiographic/fluoroscopic tables and holds

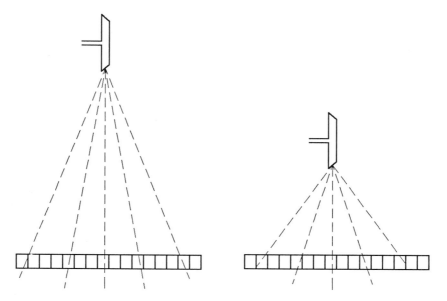

Figure 16–8.   Parallel grids function best at long, as opposed to short, SID.

the cassette in place below the grid. It can move the grid during the exposure so that grid lines will be blurred and therefore not evident on the film. These grids are 17"×17" (43× 43 cm), large enough to cover a 14"×17" (35×43 cm) cassette placed either lengthwise or crosswise in the cassette tray.

The direction in which the grid moves is important if it is to accomplish the job of blurring the grid lines. The lead strips of the grid run along the long axis of the table. To blur the lead lines, the grid must move at a right angle to the direction of the lines. This means that it will be moving back and forth across the table and not from top to bottom.

There are two movement mechanisms used today. The movements are described as reciprocating and oscillating. With the reciprocating grid, a motor drives the grid back and forth during the exposure for a total distance of no more than 2–3 cm. With the oscillating grid, an electromagnet pulls the grid to one side and then releases it during exposure. The grid oscillates in a circular motion within the grid frame.

GRID SELECTION/ CONVERSIONS

Selecting the best grid to use for a specific radiographic procedure is a complex process. Most procedures which are done with a grid use a moving grid mounted in a table or upright holder. Grid choice must be made in the equipment purchase phase of quality control. Once a grid is selected and mounted in the Potter-Bucky diaphragm, it is not easily changed. Purchase decisions are generally made by the department administrator in collaboration with the radiologist.

Grids absorb scatter and scatter adds density to the film. The more efficient a grid is at absorbing scatter, the less density will be seen on the film. Therefore compensations must be

made to increase density. This is generally accomplished by increasing mAs, which in turn results in greater patient dose. The better the grid cleans up scatter, the greater will be the dose given to the patient to achieve adequate density. The amount of mAs needed can be calculated using the following formula:

$$\text{Grid Conversion Factor (GCF)} = \frac{\text{mAs with the grid}}{\text{mAs without the grid}}$$

This formula is referred to as the Bucky factor as well as the grid conversion factor. **Grid-conversion factors (GCF) increase with higher grid ratios and increasing kVp.** Since grids vary in respect to their ratio, frequency and lead content, it would be useful to check the grid conversion factor for each of the common grids used in a department. Table 16–2 offers a guide of grid conversion factors for commonly purchased grids.

Example: A satisfactory chest radiograph is produced using 5 mAs at 85 kVp without a grid. A second film is requested using a 12:1 grid. Using Table 16–2, what mAs is needed to produce a second satisfactory radiograph?

TABLE 16–2

GRID CONVERSION FACTORS

Grid Ratio	60 kVp	85 kVp	110 kVp
No grid	1	1	1
5:1	3	3	3
8:1	3.75	4	4.25
12:1	4.75	5.5	6.25
16:1	5.75	6.75	8

Adapted with permission from *Characteristics and Applications of X-Ray Grids,* Liebel-Flarsheim division of Sybron Corporation, Cincinnati, Ohio.
Approximate values based on clinical tests of pelvis and skull.

Answer:

$$GCF = \frac{\text{mAs with the grid}}{\text{mAs without the grid}}$$

$$5.5 = \frac{X}{5} \text{ mAs}$$

$$X = 5.5 \times 5 \text{ mAs}$$
$$X = 27.5 \text{ mAs}$$

When converting from one grid ratio to another, the following formula is used:

$$\frac{\text{mAs}_1}{\text{mAs}_2} = \frac{GCF_1}{GCF_2}$$

where: mAs_1 = original mAs

          mAs_2 = new mAs

          GCF_1 = original grid conversion factor

          GCF_2 = new grid conversion factor

Example: A satisfactory abdominal radiograph is produced using an 8:1 grid, 35 mAs and 85 kVp. A second film is requested using a 12:1 grid. Using Table 16–2, what mAs is needed to produce a second satisfactory radiograph?

Answer:

$$\frac{\text{mAs}_1}{\text{mAs}_2} = \frac{GCF_1}{GCF_2}$$

$$\frac{35}{X} = \frac{4}{5.5}$$

$$4X = 192.5$$
$$X = 48 \text{ mAs}$$

GRID PERFORMANCE EVALUATION

The efficiency of a grid in cleaning up or removing scatter can be quantitatively measured. The International Commission on Radiologic Units and Measurements (ICRU)

Handbook 89 defines two criteria for measuring a grid's performance: selectivity and contrast improvement ability.

Selectivity

Although grids are designed to absorb scatter, they also absorb some primary radiation. Grids that absorb a greater percentage of scatter than primary radiation are described as having a greater degree of selectivity. Selectivity is identified by the Greek sigma (Σ) and is measured by using the following formula:

$$\text{Selectivity} = \frac{\% \text{ primary radiation transmitted}}{\% \text{ scatter radiation transmitted}}$$

The better a grid is at removing scatter, the greater will be the selectivity of the grid. **This means that a grid with a higher lead content would have a greater selectivity**.

Contrast Improvement Ability

The best measure of how well a grid functions is its ability to improve contrast in the clinical setting. The contrast improvement factor is dependent on the amount of scatter produced, which is controlled by the kVp and volume of irradiated tissue (see Chapter 24). As the amount of scatter radiation increases, the poorer the contrast and the lower the contrast improvement factor. The contrast improvement factor (K) can be measured using the following formula:

$$K = \frac{\text{Radiographic contrast with the grid}}{\text{Radiographic contrast without the grid}}$$

If K = 1, then no improvement in contrast has occurred. Most grids have contrast improvement factors between 1.5 and 3.5. This means that contrast is 1.5–3.5 times better when using the grid. **The higher the K factor, the greater the contrast improvement**.

GRID ERRORS

Poor radiographs can result from improper use of the grid. Errors in the use of the grid occur mainly with grids that have a focused design. This is because focused grids are made to coincide with the divergence of the x-ray beam. The tube must be centered to the focused grid and aligned at the correct distance. Additionally, a focused grid has a tube side and a film side based on the angulation of the grid strips. Proper tube/grid alignment is essential to prevent the undesirable absorption of primary radiation known as grid cut-off.

Off-Level

An off-level grid error occurs when the tube is angled across the long axis of the grid strips. This can be the result of improper tube or grid positioning (Figure 16–9). Improper tube positioning results if the central ray is directed across the long axis of the radiographic table. Recall that it is only possible to angle along the long axis of the table with a linear grid and it is not possible to angle at all with a criss-cross grid. Improper grid positioning most commonly occurs with stationary grids being used for mobile procedures or decubitus views. If, for example, a patient is lying on a grid for a mobile abdominal procedure and the patient's weight is unevenly distributed on the grid, the grid may not be properly aligned to the tube.

An off-level grid error can occur with a focused grid and it is the only positioning error possible with a parallel grid. Care must always be taken when aligning the tube to the grid, especially when using stationary grids, to avoid this error. When this error occurs,

Convergence Point

X-ray Beam

Grid

Image Receptor

A.

Convergence Point

X-ray Beam

Grid

Image Receptor

B.

Figure 16–9. An off-level grid error can occur with a parallel or a focused grid. A linear grid can be off-level in one direction while a criss-cross grid can be off-level in both directions (across and along the grid).

there is an undesirable absorption of primary radiation which results in a radiograph with a decrease in density across the entire image (Figure 16–10).

Off-Center

The x-ray tube must be centered along the central axis of a focused grid to prevent an off-center (off-axis or lateral decentering) grid error (Figure 16–11). The center grid strips are perpendicular and become more and more inclined away from the center. This design coincides with the divergence of the x-ray beam from the tube. If the central ray is off-center, the most perpendicular portion of the x-ray beam will not correspond to the most perpendicular portion of the grid. The result is a decrease in film density across the entire film (Figure 16– 12). The greater the degree of lateral decentering, the greater the grid cut-off.

Figure 16–11. An off-center grid error.

75 **kVp**	15 **mAs**	40″ **SID**	
15:l **grid**	400 **RS**	63.4 **mR**	

75 **kVp**	15 **mAs**	40″ **SID**	
15:1 **grid**	400 **RS**	66.1 **mR**	

Figure 16–10. A radiograph illustrating an off-level grid error.

Figure 16–12. A radiograph illustrating an off-center grid error.

Off-Focus

A focused grid is made to be used at very specific distances identified as the focal range labeled on the front of the grid. When a grid is used at a distance other than that specified as the focal range, an off-focus error results (Figure 16–13). For example, if a grid has a focal range of 36–44 inches (91–112 cm) and it is used at 72 inches, severe grid cut-off will occur. Off-focus errors result in grid cut-off along the peripheral edges of the film (Figure 16–14). Higher grid ratios require greater positioning accuracy to prevent grid cut-off.

Upside-Down

A focused grid has an identified tube side based on the way the grid strips are angled. If the grid is used upside-down, severe peripheral grid cut-off will occur (Figure 16–15). Radiation will pass through the grid along the central axis where the grid strips are most perpendicular and radiation will be increasingly absorbed away from the center (Figure 16–16). It is important that the technologist check the tube side prior to using a focused grid.

OTHER SCATTER REDUCTION METHODS

In addition to the use of a grid, there are a number of other methods that can be employed to reduce the amount of scatter reaching the film. Remember, the most important way to improve image quality is to decrease the amount of scatter initially being created. This is best done by restricting the primary beam. Collimating to the size of the area being examined is critical to image quality. Even with the use of close collimation, it is still necessary to reduce scatter reaching the film when radio-

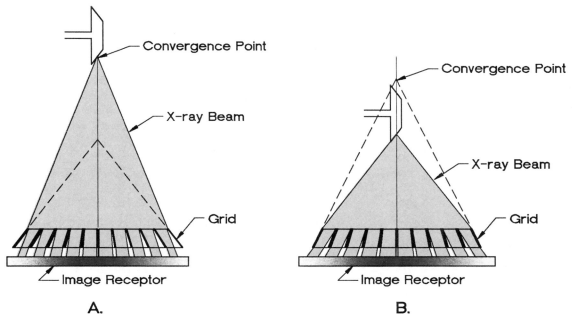

A.   B.

Figure 16–13.   An off-focus grid error occurs when the grid is used at distances less than or greater than the focal range.

75 **kVp**   60 **mAs**   72″ **SID**
15:1 **grid**   400 **RS**   69.3 **mR**

75 **kVp**   15 **mAs**   40″ **SID**
15:1 **grid**   400 **RS**   64.2 **mR**

Figure 16–14.   A radiograph illustrating an off-focus grid error taken at less than the recommended focal range distance.

Figure 16–16.   A radiograph illustrating an upside-down grid error.

graphing larger body parts or when using higher kVps. The grid is the primary device employed to reduce scatter. The body part may also be compressed to decrease the amount of scatter created. Two other methods that can be used to decrease scatter reaching the film are the air-gap technique and the reverse Kodak X-Omatic™ cassette technique.

Air-Gap Technique

The air-gap technique is an alternative to the use of a grid. It has primary applications in magnification radiography and, to a lesser extent, in chest radiography. The technique involves placing the patient at a greater object image receptor (OID) distance, thus creating an air gap between the patient and the film. By moving the patient away from the film, the amount of scatter reaching the film will be reduced. As stated earlier, the patient is the source of the majority of scatter. While the

Figure 16–15.   An upside-down grid error.

same amount of scatter will be created during the exposure, less of the scatter will reach the film if the patient is moved farther away (Figure 16–17). The result is improved contrast without the use of the grid. The primary disadvantage of the air-gap technique is the loss of sharpness that results from increased OID.

Gould and Hale evaluated contrast improvement between the use of a grid and the air-gap technique, showing that a 10-inch (25-cm) air gap has the same degree of clean-up of scatter as a 15:1 grid for a 10-cm body part. This same grid was shown to be more effective at eliminating scatter than the air gap with a thicker (20-cm) body part.

Figure 16–17. The air-gap technique reduces the amount of scatter reaching the film.

Reverse-Cassette Technique

When performing a procedure that borders between the use of a grid or a nongrid technique, it may be helpful to use an inverted cassette. The Kodak X-Omatic™ cassette may be used in a reverse fashion because the back of the cassette does not contain hinges which would interfere with the image. These cassettes are designed with the front and back made from the same radiolucent material. The only difference between the back and the front of the cassette is a thin sheet of lead foil approximately 0.0006 inches thick, which is located behind the back intensifying screen. This lead is intended to absorb backscatter radiation, which could fog the image.

When the cassette is used in an inverted position, the lead foil will serve as a filter to absorb low energy scattered photons. It functions much like a very low ratio grid. As a result, image contrast can be improved. It should be noted, however, that an increase in technical factors is necessary to compensate for the reduction in radiation reaching the film.

SUMMARY

A grid is a tool used by the radiographer to improve image contrast. Grids are made of lead strips alternating with an interspace material which is usually made of aluminum. Grids are constructed with a specific grid ratio and frequency. The grid ratio and frequency are important in determining the total lead content of the grid. Generally, grids with higher grid ratios and lead content are more efficient at improving contrast. This can be quantitatively studied by measuring the selectivity and contrast improvement ability of the grid.

Grids absorb scatter and scatter adds density to the film. The more efficient a grid is at absorbing scatter, the less density on the film. Therefore compensation must be made to increase density. This is generally accomplished by increasing the mAs, which in turn results in greater patient dose. The better the grid is at cleaning up scatter, the greater is the dose given to the patient to achieve adequate density.

Grids are manufactured in either a linear or criss-cross pattern, with either a parallel or focused design. They can be used in either a stationary manner or may be placed in a device which moves the grid and thereby blurs the grid lines.

Alternatives to the use of a grid are the air-gap technique and the reverse-cassette technique.

REVIEW QUESTIONS

1. Why does a grid improve contrast?

2. As a general rule, when should a grid be used?

3. How is a grid constructed?

4. Define grid ratio.

5. What type of grid pattern has lead strips running in only one direction?

6. How is a focused grid designed?

7. As the ability of a grid to clean up scatter increases, what is the effect on patient exposure and radiographic density?

8. How is the contrast improvement of a grid measured?

9. How does an off-level grid error occur?

10. How does the air-gap technique improve contrast?

REFERENCES AND RECOMMENDED READING

Bednarek, Daniel P., Stephen Rudin, and Ronald Wong. Artifacts produced by moving grids. *Radiology* April, 255, 1983.

Cullinan, Angeline. *Producing Quality Radiographs*. Philadelphia, PA: J. B. Lippincott Co., 1987.

Curry, Thomas S., James E. Dowdey, and Robert C. Murry. *Christensen's Introduction to the Physics of Diagnostic Radiology*. 3rd ed. Philadelphia, PA: Lea and Febiger, 1984.

Fry, Orvis E., and Cesare Gianturco. Bedside radiography reduction of patient exposure and orientation of grid cassettes. *Radiologic Technology*. 31:4, 387, 1960.

Gould, R. G., and J. Hale. Control of scattered radiation by air gap techniques: Applications to chest radiography. *American Journal of Roentgenology* 122, 109, 1974.

Hufton, A. P., C. M. Crosthwaite, J. M. Davies, and L. A. Robinson. Low attenuation material for table tops, cassettes, and grids: A review. *Radiography* 53:607, 17, 1987.

Jensen, Gerald, and Carl Scheid. The performance of radiographic grids. *Optimization of Chest Radiography*. Rockville, MD: U.S. Department of Health and Human Services, HHS Publication (FDA) 80–8124, 1980.

Lauer, O. Gary, John B. Mayes, and Rosemary P. Thurston. *Evaluating Radiographic Quality: The Variables and Their Effects*. Mankato, MN: The Burnell Company Publishers, Inc., 1990.

Potter, Hollis E. History of diaphragming roentgen rays by the use of the Bucky principle. *The American Journal of Roentgenology* 25, 396, 1931.

Potter, Hollis E. The Bucky diaphragm principle applied to roentgenology. *The American Journal of Roentgenology* 7, 292, 1920.

Seeman, H. E., and H. R. Splettstosser. The effect of kilovoltage and grid ratio on subject contrast in radiography. *Radiology* 64:572–580, 1955.

Seeman, H. E., and H. R. Splettstosser. The physical characteristics of Potter-Bucky diaphragms. *Radiology* 62, 575–583, 1954.

Seeram, Euclid. *X-ray Imaging Equipment - An Introduction*. Springfield, IL: Charles C. Thomas, 1985.

Stanford, R. W., R. D. Moore, and T. H. Hills. Comparative performance of grids in relation to their stated ratio. *British Journal of Radiology* 32:374, 106–113, 1959.

Stears, John G., Joel E. Gray, and Eugene D. Frank. Grids are not created equal. *Radiologic Technology* 57:4, 345, 1986.

Sweeney, Richard J. The use of an inverted Kodak X-Omatic cassette as an improvised grid. *Radiologic Technology* 49:3, 257–261, 1977.

Thompson, Thomas T. *Cahoon's Formulating X-ray Techniques*. 9th ed. Durham, NC: Duke University Press, 1979.

THE CASE OF THE INJURED ANIMAL

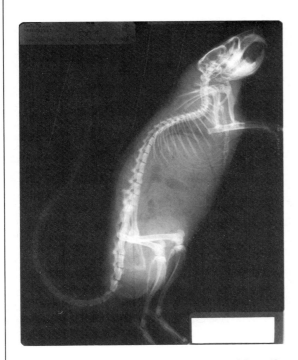

This animal was brought to the radiographic laboratory, dead on arrival. What type of animal is it and what was the cause of death?

(Radiograph courtesy of Ron Cramer, Mary Rutan Hospital, Bellefontaine, Ohio)

Answers to the case studies can be found in Appendix E.

17 RADIOGRAPHIC FILM

Any discussion relating to the rationale of radiographic exposure should begin with the understanding that the characteristics and the exposure response of x-ray film are the foundations of an exposure system.

Arthur W. Fuchs, from the Jerman Memorial Lecture at the 1950 Annual Meeting of the American Society of X-Ray Technicians.

OUTLINE

CONSTRUCTION
LATENT-IMAGE FORMATION
TYPES OF FILM
FILM STORAGE AND HANDLING
FILM IDENTIFICATION

OBJECTIVES

Upon completion of this chapter, the student should be able to:

1. Describe the components of radiographic film.
2. Explain the production of silver halide crystals.
3. State the purpose of various additives to radiographic film.
4. Describe latent image formation.
5. Discuss the differences between direct exposure film, screen film and films for various special applications.
6. Explain the fundamentals of proper film storage and handling.
7. Discuss automated and daylight loading film systems.
8. Explain the responsibilities involved in proper radiograph identification.

Photosensitive film remains the most common radiographic image receptor, although modern imaging technology has developed many other receptors (e.g., fluoroscopic screens, computer-linked detectors, scintillation and piezoelectric crystals and selenium plates). Film was the first image receptor chosen by Röntgen, and it has remained the primary means of recording radiographic images to the present day.

Radiographic and photographic film are very similar in nature and both derive from early experiments in recording light images. The discovery of photography cannot be assigned to one person. A permanent photographic process was discovered about 1816 by the French inventor Joseph Nièpce (1765–1833). Nièpce eventually collaborated with the French artist Louis Daguerre (1787–1851), who improved the process and sold it to the French government, which released it to the public in 1839. Simultaneously, between 1835 and 1840, the English photographer William Fox Talbot (1800–1877) developed the now common negative-to-positive process that was given the name photography. Many photographers contributed to the scientific understanding of the process and by the 1850s the process was similar to, although more primitive than, that used today.

Photographic materials are photosensitive, or capable of responding to exposure by photons. Both are sensitive to the wavelengths and energies that comprise most of the electromagnetic spectrum of both light and x-rays (Figure 2–10), although it is possible to manufacture film that is insensitive to portions of the spectrum. Proper use of photosensitive materials requires an understanding of how film is constructed and how the image is formed.

CONSTRUCTION

Diagnostic radiographic film is manufactured by coating both sides of a base material with an emulsion containing photosensitive crystals. Several other materials are also used to improve the performance and permanence of the film. The complete construction of diagnostic radiographic film includes the **base, adhesive, emulsion with crystals and supercoat** (Figure 17–1). The total thickness of the film varies with the manufacturer, from 175 to 300 μm (0.007″ to 0.012″).

Base

The film base was originally composed of a glass plate. Glass plates coated with emulsion were used in photography from soon after its discovery until World War I (circa 1914) (Figure 17–2). Modern radiography has re-

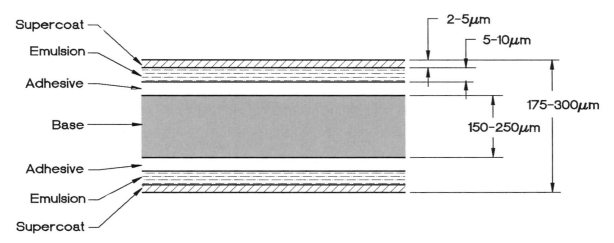

Figure 17–1.   Cross-sectional view of diagnostic radiographic film.

Figure 17–2. Glass plate radiograph of Theodore Roosevelt taken at Mercy Hospital in Chicago on October 15, 1912, after he was shot in the chest during an assassination attempt in Milwaukee. (Reprinted with permission from the American College of Surgeons, Chicago, IL.)

tained in the professional jargon an old-fashioned term, "flat plate of the abdomen," from this period. Of course, the physician requesting such an image intends the film base to be of polyester plastic, not a glass plate. Modern plastic bases solved problems such as cut fingers from broken films and strained backs from carrying and filing stacks of heavy radiographs.

During World War I a shortage of the good, optical quality glass needed for the film base caused film manufacturers to switch to cellulose nitrate. Because of its flammable nature (which caused several tragic hospital fires), nonflammable cellulose triacetate was introduced in the 1920s. Modern radiographic film base is polyester, which was introduced in the 1960s by DuPont. It is usually 150–200 μm (0.006″–0.008″) thick.

The film base must be flexible yet tough, stable, rigid and uniformly lucent. It must be flexible to permit easy handling in the darkroom and to make good contact with the cassette pressure pads. It must be stable so that it does not change its dimensions during the heating and immersion in chemicals required for processing. It must be rigid enough to be conveniently placed onto a view box (radiographic illuminator). Most important, it must be uniformly lucent so that it permits the transmission of light without adding artifacts to the diagnostic image.

Adhesive

A thin coating of adhesive is applied to the base material before it is coated with the emulsion. This substratum coating is designed to glue the emulsion to the base and prevent bubbles or other distortion when the film is bent during processing or handling, or when it is wet and heated during development.

Emulsion

The emulsion is composed of gelatin in which photosensitive silver halide crystals are suspended. It is spread in an extremely even coating that, depending on the manufacturer, ranges from 5–10 μm (0.0002″–0.0004″) of thickness on each side of the base. The purpose of the gelatin is to act as a neutral lucent suspension medium for the silver halide crystals that must be separated from one another to permit processing chemicals to reach them. Gelatin serves as a nonreactive medium through which chemicals can diffuse to reach the silver halides. The gelatin also distributes the crystals evenly over the surface of the film, thus preventing clumping of silver halides that would make one area of the film more photosensitive than another. Additionally, the gelatin must be clear, to permit light to travel through it uniformly, and flexible enough to permit bending without distorting the recorded image. The gelatin that is used for film is of extremely high quality.

The photosensitive agents suspended in the emulsion are silver halide crystals (or grains). The silver halides used in radiographic film are **silver bromide**, **silver iodide** and **silver chloride**. Although the exact formula of each company is a closely guarded trade secret, film manufacturers agree that modern silver halides are 95–98 percent silver bromide, with the remainder usually consisting of silver iodide. This has led to the term **silver iodobromide** as a generic specification of the silver halide crystals.

Because photographic film normally has emulsion on a single side, diagnostic radiographic film is sometimes called **duplitized**, double emulsion or double coated film. Not all radiographic film is duplitized, though. There are special radiographic films (such as duplication, mammography and fine detail extremity films) that are coated on a single side.

Supercoat

The supercoat is a layer of hard, protective gelatin designed to prevent the soft emulsion underneath from being physically or chemically abused by scratches, abrasions from stacking and skin oils from handling. It is usually designed to be antistatic as well. The supercoat is extremely strong and, when combined with the tough base material, makes it nearly impossible to tear a radiograph. A Chicago phone book would be easier to tear in half than a radiograph unless an edge is cut first.

The only items routinely used during film handling that are capable of permanently damaging the surface of a radiograph are a paper clip and a staple. For this reason, plastic holders or paper film envelopes should always be used to keep radiographs together. Radiographs should not be paper-clipped to reports or requisition orders, and stapled medical records should not be filed in the same envelope with radiographs. To avoid this problem, a properly designed radiograph envelope has a separate compartment for the consultation report.

The film base usually includes a blue dye to tint the film and reduce eyestrain for the interpreting radiologist, thereby increasing the diagnostic accuracy available from the image. The film base is also often coated with a special substance to prevent light from one screen crossing over to the other, causing blurring of the image. This reflection of light is called the **crossover effect**. **Halation** is a different effect caused by light being reflected from the air interface on the back of the base material (Figure 17–3). An **antihalation coating** is applied to the back of single-emulsion film. This coating is

Light Beam

Primary Image

Secondary Image
By Reflection

Film Emulsion

Film Base

Reflection At Film
Base–Air Interface

Figure 17–3. The halation effect. (Reprinted with permission of David Jenkins from *Radiographic Photography and Imaging Processes*, MTP Press, Lancaster, England.)

designed to absorb the light coming from the emulsion and prevent backscatter, visible light or reflected light from degrading the image. The coating is removed by the processing chemicals to permit light to be transmitted through the film for viewing.

If a single emulsion film is loaded into a cassette with the antihalation coating toward the intensifying screen (the source of the light photons), most of the light will be absorbed. **Single emulsion film must be loaded with the emulsion toward the intensifying screen**. The emulsion side of the film always appears dull, the nonemulsion side shiny. In addition, single emulsion films have an identifying notch cut in the lower left corner. The mnemonic double L (LL) for the lower left corner makes this easy to remember.

Manufacturing

Radiographic film is manufactured in four stages: **crystal production**, **ripening**, **mixing** and **coating**.

Crystal Production Silver-bromide crystal production is accomplished, in total darkness, by combining silver nitrate and potassium bromide in the presence of gelatin. The silver bromide will precipitate out and the potassium nitrate can be washed away as a waste product. The gelatin must be present as a medium to permit the crystals to form. The gelatin functions to limit oxidation and reduce crystal surface energy tension, as well as to facilitate other chemical reactions. This process is described by the formula:

$$AgNo_3 + KBr \rightarrow AgBr\downarrow + KNO_3$$

silver + potassium → silver + potassium
nitrate   bromide   bromide   nitrate
                      (precipitate)

The silver halide crystals are flat and roughly triangular in shape (Figure 17–4). Although different types of film emulsions require different size crystals, they are all very small, about 1 μm (0.00004″) on each side. A cubic millimeter contains over half a billion (>500,000,000) crystals. The new tabular grain process develops flat, tabular crystals two to four times larger that can be more evenly dispersed throughout the emulsion. The advantages of tabular grains include the absorption of a greater portion of the exposing photons, reduced light crossover from one emulsion to the other and reduced silver coating requirements. Tabular grains may also permit 45-second processing.

Each crystal is a cubic lattice (or matrix) of silver, bromide and iodine atoms (Figure 17–5). A conventional crystal contains approximately 10^{10} (100,000,000,000) atoms. They are bound together by moderately strong ionic bonds

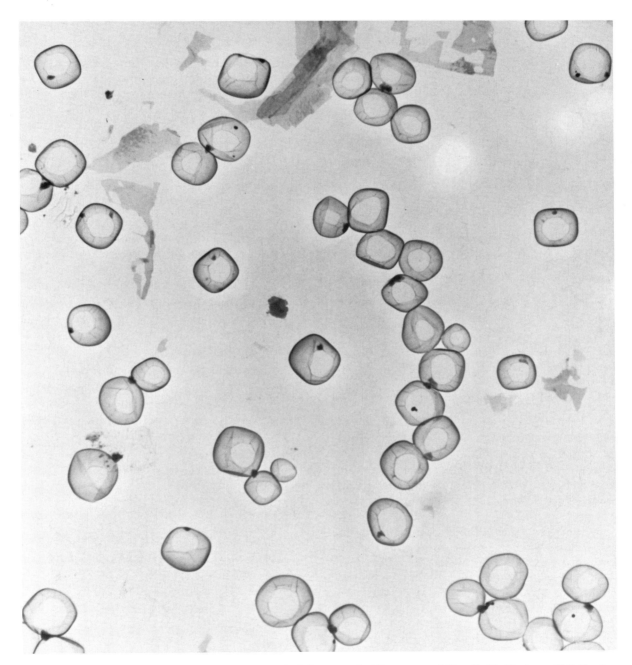

Figure 17–4. A photomicrograph of a silver halide crystal. (Courtesy of Dr. C. G. Barlow, 3M Center, St. Paul, MN.)

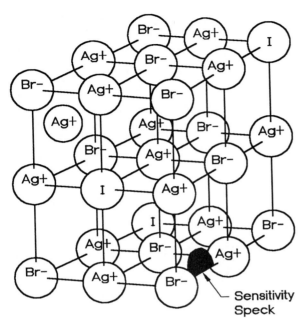

Figure 17–5.   Cubic lattice arrangement of ions in a silver halide crystal. The surfaces are primarily positive bromine and iodine halides while the interior is primarily negative silver. Note the free silver atom and the sensitivity speck.

with the silver positive (Ag^+) and the bromine or iodine negative (Br^- or I^-). The crystal structure permits both free silver atoms and free electrons to drift through the lattice. This ability is the key to the formation of the latent image.

It is thought that the halide ions (bromine and iodine) tend to cluster on or near the surface of the crystal while the silver ions form the center. This results in silver halide crystals having negatively charged surfaces and positively charged interiors.

The silver halide crystals must have an impurity added, usually silver sulfide, to form **sensitivity specks**. The silver sulfide may adhere to the surface of the crystal or even be partially incorporated into its structure. There can be a few or many specks, but they must be present to provide film sensitivity.

Ripening Ripening is the period during which silver halides are allowed to grow. The size of the crystals determines their total photosensitivity, so the longer the ripening period, the larger the crystals (or grains) and the more sensitive the emulsion. The relationship of crystal size and emulsion thickness to various film factors is shown in Table 17–1. At the proper time, the emulsion is cooled, shredded and washed to remove the potassium nitrate.

Mixing The mixing process follows ripening. The shredded emulsion is melted at a precise temperature to properly sensitize the crystals. A number of additives are then mixed into the emulsion. Usually included among these are:

— colored dyes that improve the sensitivity of the silver halides to match the wavelengths of photons that will be striking the emulsion during exposure,

— hardeners to prevent physical trauma,

— bactericides and fungicides to inhibit the growth of these organisms (especially in warmer climates or where water supplies are not chemically treated) and

— antifogging agents to decrease sensitivity to environmental factors, such as heat.

TABLE 17–1				
RELATIONSHIP OF FILM CRYSTAL AND EMULSION TO FILM FACTORS				
	Crystal Size		Emulsion Layer	
	Small	Large	Thin	Thick
Resolution	high	low	high	low
Speed	low	high	low	high
Contrast	low	high	low	high
Latitude	wide	narrow	wide	narrow

Films are often classified as **panchromatic** or **orthochromatic**, according to their sensitivity to the color of light. **Panchromatic** films are sensitive to all colors while **orthochromatic** films are not sensitive to the red spectrum. This sensitivity is controlled by the dyes that are added during this stage.

Coating The coating process requires extremely precise and expensive coating equipment. There are only a few factories in the world that can coat emulsions. First the adhesive layer is applied to the base, then the emulsion and finally the supercoat. The emulsion is applied to 40-inch-wide (102-cm) sheets of film which are stored on rolls, cut to size and packaged for the consumer. Standard film sizes are shown in Table 17–2. All film manufacture, packaging, transport, exposure and processing must be accomplished in total darkness.

LATENT IMAGE FORMATION

The photons that reach the emulsion are primarily light photons from the intensifying screens that are in contact with the film. However, x-ray photons are also involved in the production of the image. This deposits energy from the photon within the lattice of the silver halide crystals.

The latent image is the unseen change in the atomic structure of the crystal lattice that results in the production of a visible image. Although there is still much that is unknown about the exact mechanisms that control the formation of the latent image, the theory proposed by Gurney and Mott in 1938 remains almost unchallenged. Their theory accounts for sensitivity specks being essential to the image formation process.

The arrangement of the silver and halide ions, free silver atoms and sensitivity specks (Figure 17–5) has been simplified to illustrate the Gurney-Mott theory (Figure 17–6) of latent

TABLE 17–2	
STANDARD RADIOGRAPHIC FILM SIZES	
SI	U.S. Customary
35 × 91 cm	14 × 36 inches
40 × 40 cm	
35 × 43 cm	**14 × 17 inches**
35 × 35 cm	**14 × 14 inches**
30 × 40 cm	
30 × 35 cm	
28 × 35 cm	**11 × 14 inches**
25 × 30 cm	**10 × 12 inches**
24 × 30 cm	
24 × 24 cm	9.5 × 9.5 inches
20 × 40 cm	
20 × 25 cm	**8 × 10 inches**
18 × 24 cm	
18 × 43 cm	**7 × 17 inches**
	5 × 12 inches
15 × 30 cm	6 × 12 inches
	6.5 × 8.5 inches

Bold sizes are in routine use at most institutions.
NOTE: In most cases the metric and English sizes are **not** equivalent; they are similar but not exactly interchangeable.

image formation. The process begins when an incident photon (light or x-ray) interacts with one of the halides (bromine or iodine). The ejected electron is freed to wander and may eventually be attracted and trapped by a sensitivity speck, giving the speck a negative charge. The negatively charged sensitivity speck attracts a free silver atom. The silver atom neutralizes the sensitivity speck (thus resetting the "trap"). This process is known as the ionic stage and is repeated several times until a clump of silver atoms rests at the sensitivity speck. A single incident photon may free thousands of silver atoms for deposition at sensitivity specks. However, not all freed silver is deposited at sensitivity specks. At least

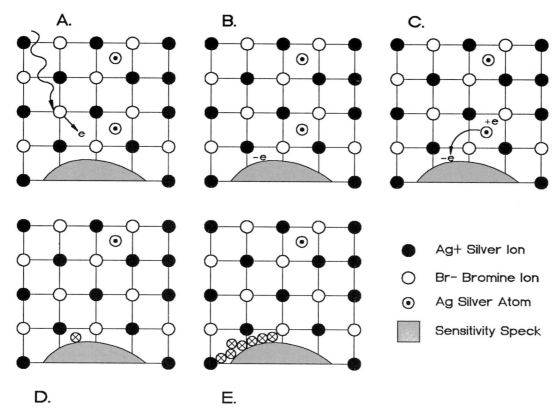

Figure 17–6.   Latent image formation according to the Gurney-Mott theory.
A–A bromine ion absorbs an incident photon and ejects an electron.
B–The ejected electron is trapped at the sensitivity speck, giving it a negative charge.
C–The negatively charged sensitivity speck attracts a free silver atom.
D–The silver atom neutralizes the sensitivity speck.
E–Repetition of the process deposits several silver atoms at the sensitivity speck.

three silver atoms must be deposited for a visible clump of black metallic silver to be formed by chemical development of the image.

TYPES OF FILM

The first radiographs were exposed to x-ray photons only. Film is still manufactured for direct exposure, but because it requires a much greater radiation dose, its use is severely limited for medical applications. Once the technology had been developed to use the x-rays to produce light at the intensifying screen, the dose reduction resulted in intensifying screen film (usually called screen film) becoming predominant in medical radiography. In addition, numerous special application films have been developed, such as mammography, detail extremity, contact surgical, computer-driven cathode ray tube (CRT), laser exposed, duplication, subtraction, cine and fluoroscopic films.

Direct Exposure or Nonscreen Film

Although used primarily for industrial nondestructive testing (NDT) radiography (Figure 17–7), occasional use of direct exposure film can be justified when extremely fine detail is critical to the diagnostic quality of the image. Dental radiography, reconstructive surgery of the hands, monitoring of degenerative bone diseases, healed fracture surveys on suspected battered children and intra-abdominal surgical needs are examples of appropriate applications. Direct exposure film has a single emulsion, extremely fine grain silver halide crystals and a much greater silver content. It also requires a much thicker emulsion layer (two or three times that of medical screen film) in order to achieve sufficient sensitivity and still maintain a fine grain. Because of the emulsion

Figure 17–7. Industrial nondestructive testing radiograph of a welded joint with a fracture line.

thickness, many brands of direct exposure film cannot be processed in automatic radiographic processors and require manual processing.

Intensifying Screen Film

Commonly called screen film, this type of film is available in a wide variety of speeds, contrast ranges, latitudes and resolutions. Each manufacturer has developed specific characteristics for its particular films. Table 17–3 lists the major manufacturers and their trade names to permit identification in clinical situations.

The primary differences are in speed (sensitivity of the silver halides), which is controlled by the size of the crystals and the thickness of the emulsion layer. Contrast, latitude and resolution tend to be linked to speed. Smaller crystals and thinner emulsions are slower but usually provide greater contrast, narrower latitude and better resolution. Larger crystals and thicker emulsions usually provide lower contrast, wider latitude and less resolution. Screen films are made faster through their double emulsion while a reduction in the silver content has been achieved through more efficient distribution of the silver.

Special Application Films

Most special applications require single emulsion films, although some have a pure gelatin coating on one side to avoid shrinking and curling during processing. **Mammography** and **detail extremity radiography** films have developed as fine-grain films sensitive to a single screen. **Contact surgical radiography** is accomplished with nonscreen film in sterilized plastic packages. **Cathode ray tube (CRT) imaging**, also called video imaging, requires a film that is sensitive to the light emitted by the CRT. Films for CRT are available in blue and green sensitivities as well as orthochromatic for either. They are usually fine grain because

TABLE 17–3	
MAJOR MANUFACTURERS OF RADIOGRAPHIC FILM AND THEIR TRADE NAMES	
Manufacturer	**Trade Names**
Eastman Kodak	X-Omat, X-Omatic, Lanex, T-Mat
E.I. Du Pont de Nemours	Cronex, Quanta
Agfa Matrix	Curix, Scopix
3M	Trimax, Trilite
Fuji	
Konica	
Ilford	Rapide

Note: All trade names are registered trademarks of the manufacturers.

patient dose is not a factor when recording CRT images. **Laser-exposed** films are sensitive to the red laser light used in laser multi-format cameras.

Duplication film is designed to provide an exact image of the original film. Diagnostic radiographs are actually negatives because they reverse the blacks and whites of the subject (white-bone). Fluroscopy produces a positive image (black-bone). If an unexposed diagnostic film is laid under a processed film with a good image, a light is turned on for a brief moment and the exposed film is processed, the duplicate film will have densities opposite from the original (i.e., the white-bone image will be converted to black-bone). Duplicating film is pre-exposed to permit it to duplicate the original image (i.e., a white-bone image is recorded as a white-bone image). It is sensitive to the ultraviolet light used in duplicating machines.

Subtraction film is available in two types: **subtraction mask film** and **subtraction film**. Subtraction mask film is a fine grain, clear (nontinted) base film designed to reverse the image of a preliminary scout angiogram film. It produces a black-bone image from a white-bone original. It is used during the subtraction process to produce a mask of the scout film. The subtraction film is a different type of film, also fine grain with a clear base, that duplicates the original scout film superimposed over the mask film.

Cineradiography film is 35 mm roll film, exactly like the film used in most single-lens reflex cameras (16 mm roll film is seldom used). It is sensitive to the green light emitted by the fluoroscopic unit. Its primary application is for cardiac catherization angiography where fine detail is often critical to diagnosis. Cineradiography is an extremely high patient dose technique and therefore should be limited to critical diagnostic areas such as cardiac catherization.

Fluoroscopic spot filming can be accomplished with screen film but is often done with 70 mm roll film or 105 mm film chips. These films are similar to cineradiography film in that they are sensitive to the green light from the fluoroscope.

Special minimum sensitivity films have been developed for verifying the radiation field during MeV radiation therapy treatments. These films are exposed to massive amounts of radiation.

FILM STORAGE AND HANDLING

Although often overlooked, the proper storage and handling of film is an important part of radiography. It is not uncommon for a hospital diagnostic radiography department to have an annual film budget of over $1,000,000, and any unit performing radiography quickly discovers that film cost is a considerable budget item. Improper storage and handling of film can be very expensive.

Basic Storage and Handling

Attention must be given to the **age** of the film, **heat, humidity, light, radiation and handling**. All film is sold with an expiration date stamped on the box. Photosensitive materials are constantly absorbing photons of both heat and background radiation and, over time, this exposure can reach a level where the fog on the film interferes with image quality. Rotation of new stock must be established to observe expiration dates.

Film should be stored at a temperature of 20°C (68°F) or lower at all times. Professional photographers refrigerate all film, and radiography departments should follow this recommendation. Most radiography departments avoid the problem by arranging film shipments to keep film in storage for only 45 to 60 days. Special application films that must be stored for long periods of time should be frozen. All refrigeration and freezing must be done with the film sealed in moisture-proof containers, as sold by the manufacturer. This essentially arrests the aging process. **Film must be brought to room temperature in advance of use** and before breaking the moisture-proof seal. Failure to do this will destroy the film when atmospheric moisture condenses on the cool film surface, creating waterspot artifacts.

The humidity must be maintained between 30 and 60 percent. Static discharge artifacts are a danger at low humidity, and high humidity causes condensation. A basement area that contains steam, cold water or other fluid pipes and is not included in the building's heating and cooling system is a poor choice for film storage.

All photosensitive materials must be protected from unfiltered light. Because film is sold in light- and moisture-proof packaging, this becomes a problem only with damaged or opened packages. Darkroom safelighting permits film handling with the convenience of limited visibility. All film must be protected from exposure to ionizing radiation. Lead lining of film storage areas will eliminate this problem. Handling of film is often overlooked as a source of problems. **Film should be stored on end**, not flat. Film boxes should be opened carefully, and under no circumstances should a film, paper interleaf or cardboard insert be removed quickly. Abrasion artifacts can occur from quick movement over film and under pressure. Even at the proper humidity, quick movement can cause static discharge with artifact exposure from the resulting light (Figure 4–5). Chemical fumes can also cause film fog. Film should not be stored near cleaning solutions, formaldehyde or other strong chemicals.

Automated Systems

Automatic film handling systems involve a transport mechanism that feeds a single film from a storage unit, transports it into position for exposure between a pair of intensifying screens and then transports it into a processor after exposure. Automatic feed diagnostic units have been marketed successfully. However, in spite of the fact that they save the expense of cassettes, they have not been extremely popular, but automatic feed dedicated chest units have become a standard fixture in high volume departments.

Daylight Systems

Daylight cassette loading systems that can be operated in full light have been available since the 1960s. These systems utilize light-proof loading units, cassettes with light-proof loading slots or doors and a light-proof unloading unit connected to a processor.

FILM IDENTIFICATION

All radiographs should be permanently identified with medical record information. This includes the date of the exposure, the full name of the patient, the institution where the exposure was made, the referring physician, the patient identification number, the examination ordered and any other important information. The identification information is usually added to the film by a light exposure after the radiographic exposure and can be accomplished with a special daylight identification camera and cassette system. It can also be done in the darkroom after the film has been removed from the cassette but before it is processed. Most radiographic cassettes have a lead blocker space in one corner to prevent the film from being exposed to x-rays in that small area. This reserves the space for identification information to be "flashed" by light. This information, like the radiograph, becomes part of the legal medical record and should be treated as such. Additionally, a method of identifying right and left sides of the patient should be required. Many institutions use lead markers, although film punches and blocker placement systems can also be used. The radiographer performing the examination is usually identified through some means; initials or number on a lead marker and signature of accompanying paperwork are common.

Depending upon institutional policy, it may or may not be acceptable to change the identification information if it is recorded incorrectly. Some institutions permit changes to be made with wax pencil, stickers or punches while others require that the radiograph be repeated. The radiographer is nearly always held responsible for recording the identification information correctly.

SUMMARY

Photographic materials are photosensitive, or capable of responding to exposure by photons. Diagnostic radiographic film is duplitized; in other words, the base is coated on both sides with an adhesive, an emulsion with crystals and a supercoat.

The film base is polyester, the adhesive glues the emulsion to the base to prevent distortion during processing or handling, the emulsion is gelatin in which photosensitive silver halide crystals are suspended and the supercoat is a protective layer. An antihalation coating is used to decrease light reflections within the base itself.

Radiographic film is manufactured in four stages: crystal production, ripening, mixing and coating. The silver halides used are silver bromide, silver iodide and silver chloride. The term silver iodo-bromide best describes the silver halides used in radiographic film. They are produced in total darkness by combining silver nitrate and potassium bromide in the presence of gelatin. The silver halide crystals that are produced are flat and roughly triangular in shape. Each crystal is a cubic lattice of silver, bromide and iodine atoms with sensitivity specks. Ripening time determines crystal size and sensitivity. During mixing, additives are included in the emulsion. Panchromatic films are sensitive to all colors while orthochromatic films are not sensitive to red. Coating is the final stage before the film is cut and packaged.

The latent image is the unseen change in the atomic structure of the crystal lattice that results in the production of a visible image. At least three silver atoms must be deposited to form a visible clump of black metallic silver.

Direct exposure or nonscreen film is used when extremely fine detail is critical. Intensifying screen film is the most common radiographic film. Films vary in speed, contrast, latitude and resolution. Special application films have been developed for mammography, detail extremity, contact surgical, cathode ray tube (CRT), laser-exposed, duplication, subtraction, cine and fluoroscopic films.

Care must be taken in storing and handling film because it is affected by age, heat, humidity, light, radiation and handling. Some of the handling is avoided by automated and daylight systems. All radiographs should be permanently identified with the appropriate medical record information.

REVIEW QUESTIONS

1. What are the primary components of radiographic film?

2. Explain the production of silver halide crystals.

3. What is the purpose of various additives to radiographic film?

4. How is the latent image produced?

5. What are the primary differences between direct exposure film and screen film?

6. Describe common problems due to improper film storage and handling.

7. What are the radiographer's responsibilities concerning proper radiograph identification?

REFERENCES AND RECOMMENDED READING

Carroll, Quinn. *Fuchs's Principles of Radiographic Exposure, Processing, and Quality Control.* 3rd ed. Springfield, IL: Charles C. Thomas Publisher, 1985.

Chow, Mai F. The effect of a film's sensitivity to its speed, contrast, and latitude. *The Canadian Journal of Medical Radiation Technology* 19:4, 147, 1988.

Cullinan, Angeline M. *Producing Quality Radiographs.* Philadelphia, PA: J. B. Lippincott, 1987.

Curry, Thomas S., James E. Dowdey, and Robert C. Murry. *Christensen's Introduction to the Physics of Diagnostic Radiology.* 4th ed. Philadelphia, PA: Lea & Febiger, 1990.

Daniels, Cupido, and Arthur F. Halloway. Comparison and variations of the speed of radiographic film. *Radiology* Jan., 203, 1983.

Davis, Loyal. *J. B. Murphy: Stormy Petrel of Surgery.* New York: G. P. Putnam's Sons, 266–268, 1938.

Doi, Kunio. Effect of crossover exposure on radiographic image quality of screen-film systems. *Radiology* June, 707, 1981.

Egyed, Mark, and Douglas R. Shearer. A comparative physical evaluation of four x-ray films. *Radiology Management* 3:4, 11–20, 1981.

Frantzell, Arne. The practical roentgenographic importance of reciprocity law failure. *Acta Radiologica* 34, 6–16, 1950.

Fuchs, Arthur. Evolution of Roentgen film. *American Journal of Roentgenology* 75, 30–48, 1956.

Huda, W., A. M. Sourkes, M. Loutatzis, G. B. Watkins, C. Ross, H. Halabuza, and D. Rutledge. An intercomparison of Kodak Ortho-G and TMG x-ray film. *The Canadian Journal of Medical Radiation Technology* 18:3, 105, 1987.

James, T. H. *The Theory of the Photographic Process.* 4th ed. New York: Macmillan Publishing Co., Inc., 1977.

Jenkins, David. *Radiographic Photography and Imaging Processes.* Lancaster, England: MTP Press Limited, 1980.

McKinney, William. *Radiographic Processing and Quality Control.* Philadelphia, PA: J. B. Lippincott, 1988.

Morgan, Russell H. Reciprocity law failure in x-ray films. *Radiology* 42, 471–479, 1944.

Morgan, Russell H. An analysis of the physical factors controlling the diagnostic quality of roentgen images: Part IV. Contrast and the film contrast factor. *American Journal of Roentgenology and Radiation Therapy* 55:5, 627–633, 1946.

Neblette, C. B. *Photography: Its Materials and Processes.* 6th ed. Princeton, NJ: Van Nostrand Co., 1962.

Newhall, Beaumont. *The History of Photography.* New York: The Museum of Modern Art, 1964.

Rao, Gopala U. V., William Witt, Michael C. Beachley, Herman A. Bosch, Panos P. Fatouros, and Philip T. Kan. Radiographic films and screen-film systems. *The Physical Basis of Medical Imaging.* Editors: Coulam, Craig M., John J. Erickson, F. David Rollo, and A. Everette James, Jr. New York: Appleton-Century-Crofts, 1981.

Roberts, Derrick P., and Nigel L. Smith. *Radiographic Imaging: A Practical Approach.* Edinburgh: Churchill Livingstone, 1988.

Rossi, R. P., W. R. Hendee, and C. R. Aherns. An evaluation of rare-earth screen-film combinations. *Radiology* 121, 465, 1976.

Seeram, Euclid. *X-Ray Imaging Equipment: An Introduction.* Springfield, IL: Charles C. Thomas, 1985.

Stephenson, George W. American College of Surgeons archivist, personal communication. Feb. 8, 1990.

Sweeney, Richard J. *Radiographic Artifacts: Their Cause and Control.* Philadelphia, PA: J. B. Lippincott, 1983.

Wilson, Peter. Principles of formation of the latent and developed images. *Canadian Journal of Radiography, Radiotherapy, and Nuclear Medicine* 7:6, 268–278, 1976.

18 RADIOGRAPHIC PROCESSING

At first it seems to be
a smeared
print: blurred lines and grey flecks
blended with the paper

Margaret Atwood, "This Is A Photograph Of Me."

OUTLINE

DEVELOPING
FIXING
ARCHIVING
AUTOMATIC PROCESSING
DARKROOM
SILVER RECOVERY SYSTEMS

OBJECTIVES

Upon completion of this chapter, the student should be able to:

1. Explain the process of film development.
2. Describe the synergistic properties of automatic processor reducing agents.
3. Identify the primary chemical and its function for each of the developer and fixer agents.
4. Explain the process of film fixation.
5. Explain the washing and drying processes of film archiving.
6. Describe the functions of the subsystems of an automatic processor.
7. Discuss the design of a radiographic darkroom, including entrances, pass boxes, centralized and decentralized plans.
8. Explain the rationale for the use of silver recovery systems.
9. Compare the advantages and disadvantages of metallic replacement, electrolytic, chemical precipitation and resin silver recovery units.

The primary purpose of radiographic processing is to deposit enough black metallic silver at the latent image sites to permit a permanent visible image to form. The development of the latent image can be accomplished manually or with automatic processing equipment. Due to the predominance of automatic processors in radiography, manual processing will not be discussed. The process is very similar to automatic processing and any radiographer can apply his knowledge of automatic processing to manual processing with the modifications provided by the manufacturer's information inserts that are packed with the chemicals.

Quality control experts agree that the radiographic film processor is the most sensitive and variable factor in the production of a radiograph. A high percentage of radiographic quality problems can be traced to processor variations or malfunctions. It is the role of the radiographer to monitor the performance of the processor, troubleshoot problems and repair minor malfunctions.

Automatic processing of a radiograph involves four primary steps: **developing**, **fixing** and two **archiving** steps—**washing** and **drying**. Developing and fixing are accomplished in solutions of numerous chemicals. Archiving involves a two-step process of washing and drying the radiograph for use as a medical record.

DEVELOPING

Developing is the first step in processing the film. At this stage silver is deposited at the latent image sites and an image becomes visible. The silver ions of the latent image are stabilized and more silver is added to the site until a visible silver clump is formed. The primary agents of the developer are two **reducing agents**, although automatic radiographic developer solutions also include an **activator, re-**strainer, preservative, hardener** and water as a **solvent** (Table 18–1). The action of the developer is controlled by the immersion **time**, solution **temperature** and chemical **activity**.

Reducing Agents

Reducing agents provide electrons to the silver ions attached to the sensitivity specks of the silver halide crystals (the latent image). Silver halides have negative exteriors (where bromine and iodine atoms are located) and positive interiors (where silver atoms are located). This arrangement effectively prohibits the reducing agent from supplying electrons to the silver atoms because the bromine and iodine repel electrons. However, when a sensitivity speck has attracted silver ions, a gate exists through which the interior of the crystal can be supplied with electrons. When a silver ion obtains an extra electron, it is converted to a stable black metallic silver atom. Reduction is actually the process of the reducing agents giving up electrons to neutralize the positive silver ions. This reduction process is illustrated in Figure 18–1.

The secret to the production of the various densities is that the sensitivity speck gate will be larger when more silver ions are deposited at the speck during exposure. A larger gate permits faster reduction of the internal silver atoms. When the reduction process is stopped at the appropriate time, the silver halides have accumulated black metallic silver in proportion to the size of the sensitivity speck gate. This produces a film with varying degrees of blackness. Of course, all silver halides with gates will become totally reduced, and the entire film will appear black if the reducing agents are permitted to work for too long a time, if they work too fast due to high **temperature** or if the solution has too high a **concentration**. The term **chemical fog** is used to describe development when these factors cause unexposed silver halides to be reduced.

TABLE 18–1

AUTOMATIC RADIOGRAPHIC PROCESSING CHEMICALS AND THEIR FUNCTIONS

Solution	Time in 90-second Processor	Chemical	Function
DEVELOPER	20–25 sec		reduces latent image to visible black metallic silver
reducing agent		phenidone	rapidly produces fine detail shades of gray
reducing agent		hydroquinone	slowly produces heavy densities
activator		sodium carbonate	produces alkaline pH, swells gelatin
restrainer		potassium bromide	decreases reducing agent activity, antifogging agent
preservative		sodium sulfite	controls oxidation, buffer agent
hardener		glutaraldehyde	hardens emulsion, reduces gelatin swelling
solvent		water	dissolves chemicals
FIXER	20 sec		stops reduction and removes undeveloped silver halides from emulsion
clearing agent		ammonium thiosulfate	removes undeveloped silver halides from emulsion
activator		acetic acid	provides acidic pH, stops reduction
hardener		potassium alum	hardens emulsion
preservative		sodium sulfite	maintains pH
solvent		water	dissolves chemicals
WASH	20 sec		removes developing and fixing chemicals
solvent		water	removes excess chemicals
DRY	25–30 sec		removes water and seals emulsion
		hot air	evaporates water and hardens emulsion

Those silver halide crystals that have fewer than three silver ions on their sensitivity specks are unable to open a gate and remain unreduced (undeveloped). Each reduced silver atom is accompanied by a liberated bromine atom with a negative charge. A bromide ion barrier is created when too many liberated bromine atoms are permitted to accumulate. They may produce sufficient charge to repel reducing agents and effectively stop silver-halide development. This is the same effect that is achieved by using potassium bromide as a "starter" solution to slow down the hyperactivity of newly mixed developer replenisher solutions. The problem is overcome by replenishment of the developer strength at regular

Latent Image   Reduction (development)   Fixation

Figure 18–1. The reduction of a silver halide crystal through a sensitivity speck gate.

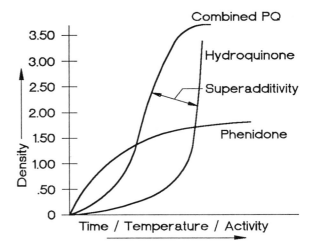

Figure 18–2. The superadditivity or synergistic effect of phenidone and hydroquinone combined, as compared to their independent reducing abilities.

intervals. A freshly cleaned processor may require seasoning by running for 20–30 minutes to thoroughly mix the starter solution.

The **reducing agents** used in automatic radiographic processors are **phenidone** (known as P developer) and **hydroquinone** (known as Q developer). **Phenidone quickly reduces silver, producing fine detail and subtle shades of gray and works only in areas of light exposure. It cannot reduce heavily exposed areas.** Phenidone replaces the function of metol (often known by the Kodak brand name Elon) in manual processing. **Hydroquinone slowly reduces silver and produces heavy density. Hydroquinone is ineffective at first but then rapidly increases in action. When the two reducing agents are combined**, forming a PQ developer, **their reducing ability is greater than the sum of their independent abilities.** This is a synergistic phenomenon known as **superadditivity** (Figure 18–2). As can be seen from the graph, phenidone controls the lower part of the curve (the toe) while hydroquinone controls the upper portion (the shoulder).

Oxidation and reduction are opposite processes. When the reducing agent is oxidized, it produces electrons. Reduction occurs when a silver halide crystal takes one of the electrons and is changed to black metallic silver. The oxidation/reduction process reduces the strength of the developer solution. As developer oxidizes, it changes color, first to a deep amber, then to brown, and finally to a thick, rust red.

Activator

The action of the reducing agents is enhanced by maintaining the developer solution in an alkaline state (around pH 10.0) by using an activator, usually sodium carbonate. Potassium carbonate, sodium hydroxide and potassium hydroxide may also be used. The activator also assists the reducers in reaching the silver halides by causing the gelatin to swell and become more permeable. The activator is caustic and therefore rubber gloves and an apron should be worn when handling developer solutions. Developer solution that is splashed onto clothing and walls is corrosive and should be neutralized with fixer solution or diluted with water.

Restrainer

A **restrainer**, usually potassium bromide, is also added to the developer to restrict the reducing action to those crystals with sensitivity speck gates. It does this by permitting overactive reducers to attack it, instead of unexposed silver halides.

Preservative

Sodium sulfite is used as a **preservative** agent to help decrease the oxidation of the reducing agents when they are combined with air. The attraction of air for the reducers is so strong that developer solutions remain effective for only a few weeks after mixing. Common techniques to assist with this problem include floating plastic lids and styrofoam balls to reduce the air-developer interface. This is also a consideration when buying developer solution tanks. Tall, narrow tanks reduce the surface and the oxidation effect. They are more desirable than low, wide tanks. A floating plastic cover or balls (i.e., ping-pong balls) will also reduce the surface area. The tank should not hold more than a two-week supply of solution.

Hardener

Glutaraldehyde is the most common developer solution **hardener**. It controls the swelling of the gelatin to prevent scratches and abrasions to the emulsion during processing. It also maintains uniform film thickness to assist in transport through an automatic processor. Insufficient hardener will cause films to deposit gelatin on processor rollers, which may cause transport and artifact problems for subsequent films. Insufficient hardener may also cause films to exit the processor with moist, softened surfaces. Hot-air drying alone cannot seal the emulsion. Excessive hardener may cause the emulsion to harden prematurely, preventing chemical interactions with the silver halides and trapping moisture in the gelatin.

Solvent

The chemicals are suspended in water as a **solvent**. The water used for mixing chemistry should be filtered to remove impurities (a 5– 10 μm filter is recommended). In tropical climates it should be treated to eliminate bacteria and fungus that may find the gelatin emulsion an attractive meal.

Contamination

The developer is the only solution that is dramatically affected by contamination. Only 0.1 percent fixer in a developer tank will destroy the ability of the reducing agents (10 ml in a 2.5 gallon [10 liter] tank). Films processed in contaminated developer appear extremely gray (they exhibit extremely low contrast). Because the fixer tank is adjacent to the developer, it is easy for splashing to occur during quality control and repair procedures. The most common cause of contamination is splashing, which occurs during lifting or replacing the fixer transport rack. Special splash guards are supplied with automatic processors and they should always be used. Developer contamination requires total dumping, washing, refilling and seasoning of the developer tank. Not only is this difficult and time consuming but it also wastes money. When cleaning a processor, the fixer tank should always be filled first. If splashing occurs, it is a simple matter to reclean the developer tank before it is filled.

Evaporation of solutions can also cause contamination. Due to the heat necessary for processing, solutions evaporate and condense on the processor lid. Contamination can occur if fixer condensation drips into the developer tank. Individual evaporation covers for both developer and fixer tanks should be in place at all times. When a processor is shut down, excessive condensation can occur as it cools. To prevent contamination, the processor lid should be propped open whenever the processor is not in use. Splashing or evaporation of developer into the fixer tank does not cause contamination. Developer is regularly carried into the fixer by the films being processed.

FIXING

If a film is exposed to light after development, the unreduced silver halides will open gates and be converted to black metallic silver. This is seen as a slow blackening of the film, which obscures the image. Undeveloped silver halides must be removed from the emulsion to permanently fix the image before exposure to light for viewing. (This was the last reaction to be discovered and delayed development of the photographic process by nearly 25 years.) This important step is accomplished by using a clearing agent that bonds with the unexposed silver halides and removes them from the emulsion. The primary agent of the fixer is the **clearing agent**, although automatic radiographic fixer solutions also include an **activator, preservative, hardener** and water as a solvent (see Table 18–1).

Clearing Agent

Nearly all fixer solutions use ammonium thiosulfate as the clearing (fixing) agent (also known by the old-fashioned term "hypo"). Ammonium thiosulfate uses silver in the emulsion to form ammonium thiosilversulfate. Within 5–10 seconds after the clearing agent has begun to function, the film can be exposed to full room light for inspection without damage to the image. If the fixer has not completely cleared the film of unexposed silver halides, the film will have a milky appearance. The **clearing time** is defined as twice the time necessary for the milky appearance to disappear. In a 90-second automatic processor, the clearing time is usually 15–20 seconds.

Activator

Acetic acid is used as the **activator** in the fixer. It maintains an acidic pH (4.0–4.5) to enhance the functioning of the clearing agent. It also serves as a stop bath to keep the reducing agents from continuing to function when the film is immersed in the fixer. Recall that reducing agents function in an alkaline solution. An acidic solution will neutralize and thereby stop the alkaline developing solution from continuing its reduction of the silver halides.

Preservative

The fixer uses the same **preservative** as the developer—sodium sulfite. It dissolves silver from the ammonium thiosilversulfate, thus permitting it to continue to remove silver from the emulsion.

Hardener

The **hardener** in the fixer must function in an acidic environment. Glutaraldehyde is effective only in an alkaline solution, so fixer hardeners are aluminum chloride, chromium alum or potassium alum. The hardener serves the same purpose as glutaraldehyde in the developer—prevention of scratches and abrasions to the emulsion during processing and maintenance of a uniform thickness of the film during transport. Insufficient hardener will cause films to exit the processor with moist, softened surfaces.

Solvent

Water (which should be filtered and treated) is used as the solvent.

Depletion

After a time the fixer solution will become saturated with silver ions from the emulsion. The solution slowly becomes unable to accept additional silver and requires a longer clearing time. Automatic processors constantly replenish the fixer solution to eliminate this problem. The silver ions in the fixer can be reclaimed through various silver recovery processes.

ARCHIVING

The archiving process is composed of two steps: washing and drying. Archiving prepares the film for long-term storage as a medical record by protecting it from deterioration by chemicals, fading and physical forces.

Washing

The **washing** process uses water to remove as much of the fixer and developer solutions as possible. The water temperature should be slightly lower than the other solutions (about 5°F or 3°C) because some processors use the water to help control temperature fluctuations in the developer and fixer. The emulsion may reticulate (crack into many pieces) if the temperature is changed too dramatically.

Both fixer and developer solutions contain chemicals that, even in weak concentrations, can damage the image over time. Because most of the developer action is stopped by the acidic pH of the fixer, the main concern is removing the fixer from the emulsion. Failure to provide sufficient agitation or wash time to clear fixer from the film may result in silver stains or a yellowing of the emulsion after a few years.

Warm water will increase the efficiency of the wash. Wash tanks, especially those not made of stainless steel, are susceptible to algae and bacteria growth during periods when the processor is turned off. To eliminate this problem the wash tank should be drained whenever the processor is shut down.

Drying

Drying is done by forcing hot air over both sides of the film as it begins its exit from the processor. The air temperature ranges from 110–150°F (43–65°C). The hot air sets a final hardening to the emulsion and seals the supercoat. Table 18–1 illustrates all of the automatic processing steps, the processing times and the functions of the component chemicals.

Storage

Proper storage is a critical part of the archiving process. The length of time an original radiograph is stored is usually 5–7 years, depending on institutional policies and applicable laws. Films taken of minors and cases involved in litigation may be retained much longer (sometimes permanently). Processed radiographs should be stored at about 70°F (23°C) and 60 percent humidity.

AUTOMATIC PROCESSING

Radiographic films were manually processed until Eastman Kodak introduced the first continuous roller automatic processor in 1957. This unit processed a film in 15 minutes and was so large that an overhead winch was required to lift the racks of rollers from the chemical tanks for cleaning. It was a great improvement over manual processing, which required an hour to process and dry a film, darkroom technicians and often produced erratic results. Modern processors are much more compact (their racks can easily be lifted by hand) and they process a film in 45–120 seconds (Figure 18–3A).

Automatic processors are complex and utilize several subsystems to completely process a radiograph: the **transport system, dryer system, replenishment system, circulation system and temperature control system.** Table 18–2 illustrates the processor systems and subsystems and their functions. The radiographer should understand the functions of automatic processing systems well enough to diagnose problems that affect image quality. The radiographer should also be capable of basic disassembly of a processor for cleaning or removal of lost or stuck films.

Transport System

The transport system is designed to move a film through the developer, fixer, wash

Figure 18–3.   (A) A modern automatic x-ray film processor. (B) A transport rack and crossover networks in a single tank.

and dryer sections of the processor. As it does this, it controls the length of time the radiograph is **immersed in each of the solutions and agitates the chemistry to ensure maximum reaction**. The transport system consists of three subsystems: **transport racks, crossover networks** and a **drive system**.

Transport Racks The **transport racks** consist of three series of rollers designed to move a film through a processing tank (Figure 18–3B). The offset of the three series of rollers provides constant tension to propel the film down into and up out of the processing tank. Note that the center series of rollers may handle films traveling down and up at the same time. The original processors had difficulty handling films due to shrinking and expansion of the emulsion. The solution temperature, quantity of hardeners and expandability of the emulsion

TABLE 18–2

AUTOMATIC RADIOGRAPHIC PROCESSOR SYSTEMS AND SUBSYSTEMS

System	Subsystem	Function
Transport		Move film through processor, control immersion time, agitate solutions
	Transport rack	Move film down into and up out of solution tanks
	Crossover network	Turn film down into next tank
	Drive system	Turn rollers
Dryer system		Remove excess water, shrink and seal emulsion
Replenishment system		Replace depleted chemicals in developer and fixer
Circulation system		Stabilize solution temperatures, agitate solutions, mix replenishment chemistry into tank
Temperature control		Maintain solution temperatures

are all designed specifically for automatic processing. Films without these characteristics may not transport through the processor and may even leave artifact causing emulsion deposits on rollers. Single emulsion films are especially difficult because the single emulsion tends to cause the film to curl as it expands and contracts.

Special turnaround equipment is needed to bend and turn a film at the bottom and top of the transport racks. This is accomplished at the bottom of the rack by a combination of master roller, planetary rollers and guide shoes (deflectors) (see Figure 18–3B). The master roller pushes the leading edge of the film against the guide shoes. The guide shoes then force the edge around the master roller with the help of the planetary rollers until it is pointed upwards and can be pulled by the offset rollers. Guide shoes are ribbed to prevent wet films from sticking to a smooth metallic surface. Each transport rack can be lifted from its tank for easy cleaning. The final set of rollers in a transport rack are special squeegee rollers that remove excess solution from the film as it is pulled from each tank.

Crossover Networks
A **crossover network** is used to bend and turn the film when it

reaches the top of the transport rack and must be directed down into the next tank or section (see Figure 18–3B). Each crossover network operates with a master roller and guide shoes system similar to that in the transport rack. Misaligned guide shoes will scratch the film emulsion as it is driven past. The most common cause of guide shoe misalignment is improper seating of transport racks and crossover networks.

The **entrance rollers** are a special crossover network designed to start the film traveling from the feed tray down into the developer section. These rollers are specially designed with ribs to grip the film and feed it evenly into the first rack. It is important that the entrance rollers grip the film so that it will feed straight through the entire processor. A film that is fed at a slight angle will be driven into the transport gears by the time it travels a distance into the processor.

Always use the guides at each side of the feed tray to align each film as it is fed into the entrance rollers. Films should be fed from alternate sides of the feed tray to avoid excess wear to one side of the transport rollers (i.e, first film right side, second film left side, etc.). **Films should always be fed with the short axis**

along the feed tray side guide (Figure 18–4). In some processors the entrance rollers also open a microswitch that activates the replenishment system.

Drive System The **drive system** consists of a series of mechanical devices designed to turn the numerous rollers in the processor from power supplied by a single motor. The speed of the drive system is usually set to move a film from the entrance rollers to the feed tray (dry to dry) in 45–120 seconds. This speed controls the time the film is immersed in each chemical solution, and slowing or speeding by as little as 2 percent can dramatically affect image quality.

Dryer System

The final stage of processing is drying the film with the **dryer system**. The emulsion of a wet film is sticky and may adhere permanently if brought into contact with another film. The dryer system begins with a series of squeegee crossover rollers removing excess wash water from the surface of the film. The film is then driven between a double row of slotted, hot forced-air tubes (see Figure 18–3A). A high-speed fan draws room air past electric heating coils, producing air at 120–150°F (50–65°C). The film emulsion shrinks and seals dry in a single pass and the film is ready for viewing and storing when it exits the processor. The excess air is returned to the room. This is the primary cause for uncomfortable temperatures in processing areas during hot weather. When damp films exit the processor, the cause is more likely to be in the fixer (depletion or lack of hardener) or wash tank (saturation or insufficient fresh water) than in the dryer section.

Replenishment System

The **replenishment system** replaces chemicals that are depleted through the chemical reactions of processing, oxidation and evaporation. The developer replenisher solution has a different composition than the solution in the processing tank. Because bromides build up in functioning developer, they tend to restrain the activity of the reducing agents on the silver halides. For this reason, developer replenisher lacks sufficient restrainer. A special

A.

CORRECT : Short side of film against feed tray guide

B.

WRONG : Long side of film and not against feed tray guide

Figure 18–4. (A) Proper film feeding. (B) Improper film feeding.

starter solution of acetic acid and potassium bromide (the restrainer) must be added to the replenisher solution when starting a fresh tank of developer.

Volume replenishment is used for high-volume and **flood replenishment** for low-volume units. A volume replenishment system is activated when films enter the processor. The entrance rollers may activate a microswitch or an infrared sensor. In this manner, replenishment of chemical solution strength begins when a film enters the processor and ends when it passes the entrance rollers. This permits replenishment according to the amount of film entering the processor. (A 14″ film would replenish solutions more than a 10″ film. This is appropriate since it would require more chemistry to process the longer film.) Infrared sensors provide more accurate replenishment as they are capable of sensing not only the length but also the width of the film. A microprocessor can then activate the replenishment pumps for an appropriate length of time. **Flood replenishment** (also called **timed** or **standby** replenishment) is designed for low-volume units where films enter the processor at irregular intervals. The replenishment unit is controlled by a timer that automatically floods the developer and fixer tanks with replenisher solution at a regular interval regardless of the number of films processed.

Although not a replenishment system, a **standby switch** is supplied on many processors. These processors are programmed to shut down some systems when two minutes pass without a film entering the unit. The standby switch must be manually activated to bring the entire unit to processing readiness. The standby mode inactivates the entrance rollers so films cannot be fed until the unit is activated.

The replenishment rate can be adjusted so that more fixer is replenished than developer. Although they must be adjusted for specific conditions, procedures and manufacturers' recommendations, developer replenishment rates often range from 4–5 ml per inch (1.5–2.0 ml per cm) of film feed. This is about 55–70 ml per 14-inch (36-cm) length of film. Fixer rates range from 6–8 ml per inch (2.5–3.0 ml per cm). This is about 85–110 ml per 14-inch (36-cm) length of film. Some processors provide a digital display of this information on the front panel.

A replenishment system is designed to pump replenisher solutions from separate storage tanks for the developer and fixer (Figure 18–5). Replenisher tubing usually includes a filter at the exit of the supply tank to collect dirt and sediment. Processors often use dual pumps operated by a single motor. The motor rotates a magnet, which in turn causes magnets in vanes inside the plastic pump bodies to rotate. This system isolates the solutions from each other and the pump motor and makes replacement of pump bodies easy and inexpensive. The replenishment system uses a metering pump, which is more complicated but operates on the same principle.

The storage tanks may be under or adjacent to the processor or, in the case of some large institutions, replenisher may be pumped great distances from a central mixing station. The tanks must be located at a site convenient for the mixing of chemical solutions. A clean area with a drain and corrosive-resistant floor and wall coverings is required.

All mixing should be done strictly according to the manufacturer's recommendations regarding temperature, the proper sequence of additives (for example, solution A, then B, then C), etc. Always mix additives to water. Adding water to additives will cause splashing of corrosives and a decrease in solution strength. There are occasions when the chemicals react in undesirable ways with one another, the water and air. For example, if hardener is added to fixer replenisher too rap-

Figure 18–5.   A typical processor replenishment and circulation system. (Adapted with permission of David Jenkins from *Radiographic Processing and Imaging Processes*, MTP Press, Lancaster, England.)

idly, it may precipitate sulfur and aluminum, leaving the solution with insufficient hardener.

Processing solutions are hazardous materials and are covered by several federal agencies in the United States. Since 1986 the Occupational Health and Safety Administration (OSHA), the Environmental Protection Agency (EPA) and the Department of Transportation have all implemented regulations affecting processing chemicals. Users of the chemicals are required to have material safety data sheets on hand, policies regarding handling, a teaching program and safety equipment, particularly an eyewash station.

Radiographic solutions are not available to the general public in the U.S. When developer solution is mixed on site, the concentrated solution containing hydroquinone and the preservative and activator (usually the first part mixed) has a pH of about 12.0, which is extremely destructive to the eyes if splashed. For this reason, protective eyeglasses should always be worn when mixing solutions. Additionally, hydroquinone can be absorbed through the skin, and glutaraldehyde is a tan-

ning agent that will work on human skin just as it works in leathermaking.

Circulation System

The **circulation system** is designed to **stabilize temperatures, agitate solutions, mix the chemistry and filter** the solutions. Temperatures are maintained in conjunction with the temperature control system. Constant mild agitation of the developer and fixer solutions is required so the chemicals will enter and exit the emulsion. The fresh chemistry added by the replenishment system must be constantly mixed throughout the tanks to avoid overdevelopment, underdevelopment and underfixation. Separate developer, fixer and wash tank circulation systems are required, although a single motor may drive all of the pumps.

Most circulation systems draw chemistry from the bottom ends of the developer and fixer tanks and pump it to the upper ends. Because old chemistry tends to rise in the tank, the excess solution is permitted to overflow from the top of the tank into a drain. In addition, the replenishment pumps usually add fresh chemistry to the upper or middle end of a tank. Some wash systems are made more efficient by the addition of a circulation pump (see Figure 18–5). The fixer circulation lines are usually fitted with a 100 μm-wire mesh filter to trap dirt or bits of gelatin that have been washed from films.

The fixer tank overflow has sufficient accumulated silver content to make it financially feasible to attempt to recover as much as possible. **Fixer overflow should be considered toxic and under no circumstances should it be dumped directly into an open drain**.

The wash tank uses a discard circulation system. Constantly recirculated water would quickly become saturated with fixer, which would set up an ionic barrier against additional fixer leaving the emulsion. To prevent this problem from occurring, the wash tank uses a constant flow of fresh water, which is pumped in at the bottom ends of the tank and overflows from the top to a drain. Most manufacturers recommend 4–8 liters per minute (1–2 gallons [US] per minute). **It is environmentally unsound to drain wash tank water into sewer lines**. Increasing concern over heavy metal pollution may place liability on persons or institutions responsible for dumping processing chemicals, especially silver. Although expensive, storage of processing overflow and disposal by hazardous materials professionals is advisable.

Temperature Control System

The **temperature control system** maintains all three solutions at compatible temperatures. This is accomplished in conjunction with the circulation system by various methods, depending on the model and manufacturer. A **heat exchanger** is the most common system. It uses a thermostat to heat the developer, since its temperature is the most critical. The developer is then routed through a circulation coil

in the bottom of the fixer or wash tank to permit exchange of heat to the fixer by conduction. Developer in a circulation coil does not mix with the fixer or wash water. A 90-second automatic processor will usually require a developer temperature of 92–96°F (33–35°C) while a two-minute processor will operate at 83–86°F (28–30°C).

Cold water processors accept incoming water at cold line temperatures and divert it to the wash tank, where it is heated and stabilized. Some systems require mixing of incoming hot and cold water within a set temperature range. The incoming water is then added to the wash tank, where the temperature stabilizes. Wash tank overflow is diverted to surround the developer and fixer tanks where heat can be conducted through the metal tank wall to maintain solution temperatures. These systems may also use circulation or heater coils in the developer and fixer tanks.

The developer temperature is especially critical. A difference is visible with a fluctuation of only 0.5° (F or C). Some processors provide a digital display of this information on the front panel. The optimal reducing agent temperature is 68°F (20°C) for an immersion time of 4–8 minutes. Much research has been devoted to the formulation of special developer solutions that will produce quality images at temperatures of 92–96°F (33–35°C). These high-temperature developers reduce immersion time to 20–22 seconds, thus permitting 90-second or less processing. Specific developing temperatures vary with manufacturer and can be adjusted with a thermostat. The thermostat is often not easily accessible (sometimes requiring a screwdriver or set screw) to remove the temptation for casual adjustment.

Periodic maintenance of an automatic processor is essential to obtain dependable performance. Since the processor affects the final image produced by nearly all radiographic equipment, and because the unit is often expected to operate 24 hours a day, nonstop, it should have a top maintenance priority.

DARKROOM

The darkroom is the light proof laboratory used for loading and unloading cassettes and feeding film into the automatic processor. Film is twice as sensitive after exposure and must be handled carefully to preserve a diagnostic quality image. An exposed film should be handled in the darkroom with the understanding that mishandling will require a double radiation dose to the patient.

Safelights

Radiographic film is designed to be insensitive to specific wavelengths of orange-red light. This permits the use of low level illumination within this wavelength to make work in the darkroom easier. The amount of light is controlled by the type of filter, wattage of the light source and distance from the working surface. Not all films are insensitive to the same wavelengths. For example, some films designed for rare-earth intensifying screen phosphors require shorter wavelengths (dark red), and some cathode ray tube (CRT) films are sensitive to all light and require total darkness.

Sodium vapor safelights emit an orange-yellow light but their intensity is too high for direct illumination. These safelights must be installed to indirectly illuminate the working area. Installation near the ceiling facing up makes certain that the light loses intensity as it reflects from the ceiling to the working area.

Direct illumination for most radiographic films is possible with a Kodak GBX filter (dark red) over a low intensity (7–15 watt) bulb that is 4 feet (1.25 meters) from the working area. Films that are sensitive only to calcium tungstate phosphor light (blue-violet) may be handled with a Kodak Wratten Series 6B filter (orange-brown) at the same intensity and distance.

Too many safelights may result in too great an intensity. A safelight test calculates how long a film may be handled before fogging becomes a problem. Darkroom walls and floor should be light-colored to increase the amount of light in the darkroom. If light is safe at its first reflection, it loses intensity and remains safe on additional reflections. When benches and flooring are light colored, it is much easier to locate films and other objects.

Entrance

The darkroom entrance may be of several types. A single door, double interlocking doors, revolving door or light-proof maze may be used. The disadvantage of the single door is that all film must be protected from light, film storage bins must be closed, processor feed tray must be empty, etc., each time the door is opened. The advantage is in space and cost savings. Single-door darkrooms should be equipped with an electric lock on the door that will not open when the film bin is open. This eliminates costly accidental exposure of the entire film bin. The electric lock must open automatically in the event of a power failure. Otherwise, another emergency entrance must be provided for the darkroom. Radiographers and darkroom aides should make it a habit to **always check all film bins before opening a single door entrance**. Double interlocking doors, revolving doors and light-proof mazes permit persons to enter and leave the darkroom without disrupting work in progress.

Pass Box

Film cassettes are passed into the darkroom through a **pass box**, or cassette hatch, which is a light-proof container set in the darkroom wall. Most pass boxes have two sides, one labeled "exposed," the other "unexposed," and both have interlocking light-proof doors. The interlocking doors are designed to prevent both doors from being opened at once, allowing light into the darkroom. A film cassette is taken from the "unexposed" side and the door is closed. The film is then exposed in a radiographic room and returned to the "exposed" side of the pass box. When the door is closed, the darkroom aide may remove the exposed cassette from the pass box, remove and process the film, refill the cassette and return it to the "unexposed" side of the pass box again. This system is very popular because of its speed and convenience.

Plan

A typical darkroom plan is shown in Figure 18–6. This plan has the automatic processor set in the wall between the darkroom and the viewing area. Only the feed tray of the processor extends into the darkroom. The processor is actually located in the viewing area to facilitate periodic maintenance.

When planning a darkroom, one should ensure that the pass boxes and film bins are located where the darkroom aide (who may often be the radiographer) does not have to take steps to reach the processor feed tray. A grounded loading bench should be located directly under each pass box. Grounding of the bench by connecting a wire between the bench top and a well-grounded object (such as a water pipe) reduces the possibility of electrostatic discharge. The film bin should be located under the loading bench.

Darkrooms should be small enough so the darkroom aide does not have to move more than 1–2 steps to perform any operation. A large darkroom is poorly designed and serves no purpose unless other light-proof procedures

Figure 18–6.   A typical darkroom plan.

are routinely performed there (i.e., manual subtraction or duplication, loading specialized cassettes or film holders, etc.).

The darkroom plan should also include a communication system, such as a light-proof speaking grill installed in the door or an intercom. Lighting should be controlled by two separate switches removed from one another. Both full white light illumination (for maintenance and repairs) and safelight illumination (for normal work) should be controlled by a switch. To avoid accidental exposure, the white-light switch should be located higher than the safelight switch (5–6 feet [1.5–1.75 meters] from the floor).

Darkroom ventilation should be a primary concern. Chemical fumes must be vented directly to the outside of the building. Failure to do so can result in toxic fumes being picked up by ventilation systems and delivered to critical areas within a hospital. Most automatic processors have special connections to assist in venting. Good circulation of air from outside the darkroom should also be maintained. Darkrooms in colder climates may also require humidifiers to assure humidity of 40–60 percent during winter months so electrostatic discharge conditions are reduced.

Floor drains are required both inside the darkroom and near the automatic processor outside the darkroom to facilitate maintenance, repairs and daily clean-up. Drains are also a safety precaution against leaks and overflow. They must not be made of copper because processing chemicals will react with copper.

Large departments may use a central processing plan where all films are routed through one or more central darkrooms. These darkrooms are often equipped with two processors. In a compact, well-designed darkroom, an experienced, full time darkroom aide can feed a steady stream of films faster than a single 90-second processor can handle them. Dual processors also permit the darkroom to

function even if one is inoperable or undergoing maintenance. Central processing saves the cost of numerous processors and economizes space usage, staffing, etc.

Because of the time required in carrying exposed films to a central darkroom, many large departments utilize a satellite darkroom plan, where single processor darkrooms are placed throughout the department and institution. If a processor is inoperable or undergoing maintenance, the radiographer uses the next nearest darkroom. Satellite processing saves time but is more expensive in equipment, maintenance, facilities and staffing.

Regardless of the plan selected, the area where the processors deposit the finished radiographs should be equipped with benches for handling films and illumination view boxes for viewing them. This area becomes the natural gathering point for the entire radiology department and it is often equipped with computers, telephones, log books, seats, etc., to make it a convenient place to do paperwork and data entry while waiting for radiographs to be processed.

SILVER RECOVERY SYSTEMS

As mentioned in the fixer and circulation system sections, sufficient silver is dissolved in the fixer solution to make recovery before discarding feasible from a financial standpoint and to prevent toxic heavy metal pollution of the environment. In the United States the Water Control Act of 1972, Resources Conservation-Hazardous Waste Act of 1976, Clean Water Act of 1984 and Resource Conservation and Recovery Act of 1986 all affect the disposal of heavy metals into the public environment. In essence, these laws require that the best available methods be used to clear silver from fixer overflow solutions prior to disposal. In addition, they limit liquid waste to a toxic level of 5 parts per million (ppm). A permit is required for dumping more than 27 gallons (US) per month into a public sewer and any amount into the ground. Even shipping the waste to a treatment plant requires a permit. Compliance with these regulations is the reason commercial firms are usually employed to handle silver recovery.

The fixer may accumulate silver at the rate of as much as 100 mg/m^2 of film processed. This is well above the dumping limits allowed by law in the United States. In fact, **the fixer is as valuable, if not more valuable, after processing than before**.

About half of the silver in the film remains in the emulsion after processing. The other half is dissolved into the fixer solution. Much of this silver may be removed from the fixer by diverting the overflow through a silver recovery system before discarding. About 5 percent of the silver is carried into the wash tank which, in extremely high-volume circumstances, may also be worth recovery. It is estimated that about 10 percent of the purchase price of film may be recovered, depending on the type of recovery system used and the market price for silver. The cost of recovery will almost always pay for the processing and handling and usually provides a modest financial return to help offset film costs. Silver mining and refining is expensive, and as a result, about half of all silver on the market worldwide comes from recycling.

There are several types of silver recovery units. The most common fixer recovery units are **metallic replacement, electrolytic, chemical precipitation** and **resin**. All of these units operate by providing electrons that can be used by the silver in the fixer solution to form black metallic silver. They differ in the method by which the electrons are provided and by the process used to refine the metallic silver.

All silver recovery methods require that the fixer sit within the unit for some time to permit the chemical interactions to occur. This **dwell time** is the single most important factor in unit effectiveness. **Agitation** of the fixer solution during this time is also important because it enhances the ability of electrons and silver to contact each other. Finally, the surface area controls the region from which electrons are available or where silver can be deposited.

Metallic Replacement

Metallic replacement units are also called metallic displacement because in these units the fixer acid breaks down the iron in a steel screen or in steel wool and displaces or replaces it with silver. The iron oxides give up electrons for the silver. The metallic silver is precipitated onto the steel. These units are sometimes called silver buckets or cartridges (Figure 18–7). They operate by having the fixer drain into the top, filter through the steel wool or screen, and overflow through a tube connected to the bottom of the container. Metallic replacement buckets are designed for low-volume situations only. They are inefficient as they age and processing is expensive. Fixer overflow from metallic replacement buckets should not be sent to the same drain as the developer overflow. As the steel wool or screen reacts with the fixer, it produces iron oxide, which can form drain-clogging fibers when it reacts with developer.

Electrolytic

Electrolytic units pass a current from a cathode to an anode through the fixer. The ionized silver in the fixer solution is attracted to the negatively charged cathode. It then plates onto the cathode as metallic silver (Figure 18–8). These units are sometimes called cells because they function like a cell in a battery. They are rated according to their recovery capacity (i.e., troy ounces per gallon). They are also classified by their method of agitation, rotating anode, rotating cathode and pumped so-

Figure 18–7. A metallic replacement silver recovery unit. (Reprinted courtesy of Eastman Kodak Company.)

lution. Electrolytic units are available that will recirculate the fixer for reuse in the processor. Electrolytically processed fixer is deficient in sodium sulfite (the preservative) and this can lead to incomplete fixing. A method of replenishing sodium sulfite must be added when a recirculating fixer system is used. If no silver is present in the fixer, the current will cause the thiosulfate to form sulfur, a smelly process that degrades the quality of the silver plating. This problem can be avoided by using an automatic electrolytic unit that is programmed to increase the current during high volume operation and to reduce it during other periods. **Electrolytic units should not be run when the processor has not been used for a long period of time (such as overnight)**. Electrolytic units are designed for moderate and high volume situations and produce easily processed silver flakes (which are chipped from the coated cathode). Most units require regular mainte-

nance because they are an electrical hazard. Their electrical components are exposed to moisture, they are prone to short-circuiting and their failure, overuse or underuse may cause hazardous fumes.

Chemical Precipitation

Chemical precipitation units use chemicals (such as zinc chloride and sodium sulfite) that break down in the fixer and release electrons. The metallic silver is heavy enough to precipitate out and fall to the bottom of the tank, where it forms silver sludge. The chemical reactions produce hazardous gasses that are both toxic and explosive. New reagents are available for precipitating extremely large volumes of fixer. Because of the complexity of the process, they are currently used only by commercial silver dealers.

Resin

Resin units use acid to form resin ions. The silver in the solution is attracted to the resin and forms black metallic silver. The resin is then processed to remove the silver.

Monitoring

All silver recovery units must be properly sized for the amount of silver in the fixer. If undersizing is suspected, a second (**tailing**) unit may be added to process the solution exiting from the first unit. Various types of test strips are available to determine the silver content remaining in the solution as it exits the silver recovery unit. A copper test can be done by dropping a copper penny into the exiting solution. A very light gray coating after 10 seconds is acceptable. A heavy coating indicates too much silver is not being recovered. Correction should begin by checking the function of the existing recovery unit. If it is functioning within acceptable limits, either a larger-capacity recovery unit is needed or a tailing unit should be installed.

Figure 18–8.   An electrolytic silver recovery unit.

Film

The film itself retains half the silver (about 0.1 troy ounce per pound [0.45 kg]) and this can also be recovered. Unexposed (green) film has twice the amount of silver as processed film. However, recycling firms will not pay more for unexposed film. To reclaim the silver, it is recommended that unexposed film be run through a processor to permit the fixer to reclaim half the silver. All scrap film should be saved for recycling, as should all original film when medical files are purged. Because of the weight, space required and value of the silver in radiographs, storage is expensive in hospitals, clinics and physician's offices. When original films are discarded, recycling is a very profitable undertaking.

SUMMARY

The primary purpose of radiographic processing is to deposit enough black metallic silver at the latent image sites to permit a permanent visible image to form. Quality control experts agree that the radiographic film

processor is the most sensitive and variable factor in the production of a radiograph. Automatic processing of a radiograph involves developing, fixing, washing and drying.

During development, silver is deposited at the latent image sites and an image becomes visible. The primary agents of the developer are: the two reducing agents, phenidone and hydroquinone; an activator, sodium carbonate; a restrainer, potassium bromide; a preservative, sodium sulfite; a hardener, glutaraldehyde; and water as the solvent. The action of the developer is controlled by immersion time, solution temperature and chemical activity.

Fixing removes the undeveloped silver halides from the emulsion. This is necessary before exposure to light for viewing. The primary agent is the clearing agent, ammonium thiosulfate. Fixer solutions also include an activator, acetic acid; a preservative, sodium sulfite; a hardener, aluminum chloride; and water as the solvent.

The archiving process prepares the film for long-term storage as a medical record. Archiving involves washing the film with water to remove the processing chemicals and drying to harden and seal the radiograph.

Automatic processors utilize several subsystems to completely process a radiograph: 1) the transport system to move a film through the developer, fixer, wash and dryer at a controlled speed; 2) the dryer system to force hot air across the film for drying; 3) the replenishment system to replace chemicals which are depleted through the chemical reactions of processing, oxidation and evaporation; 4) the circulation system to stabilize temperature, agitate solutions, mix the chemistry and filter the solutions and 5) the temperature control system to maintain all three solutions at compatible temperatures.

The darkroom is the light-proof laboratory used for loading and unloading cassettes and feeding them into the automatic processor. Radiographic film is designed to be insensitive to specific wavelengths of orange-red light. Safelights use low-level illumination within this wavelength to make work in the darkroom easier.

Sufficient silver is dissolved into the fixer solution to make recovery before discarding feasible from a financial standpoint and desirable for environmental reasons. The most common types of silver recovery units are metallic replacement, electrolytic, chemical precipitation and resin.

REVIEW QUESTIONS

1. What are the four primary steps in automatic processing?

2. How do the reducing agents, phenidone and hydroquinone, differ in their functions?

3. What is the chemical name and function of the hardener in the developer?

4. What is the purpose of fixing?

5. What are the two steps of the archiving process?

6. How should a film be fed into the automatic processor?

7. Differentiate between volume replenishment and flood replenishment.

8. What is the function of the circulation system in an automatic processor?

9. Under what conditions is direct illumination of a radiographic film safe?

10. How does an electrolytic silver recovery unit operate?

REFERENCES AND RECOMMENDED READING

Bruce, Geoffrey. Darkroom safelighting and its effects. *Radiography* 46:542, 45, 1980.

Carroll, Quinn. *Fuchs's Principles of Radiographic Exposure, Processing, and Quality Control.* 3rd ed. Springfield, IL: Charles C. Thomas Publisher, 1985.

Cullinan, Angeline M. *Producing Quality Radiographs.* Philadelphia, PA: J. B. Lippincott, 1987.

Curry, Thomas S., James E. Dowdey, and Robert C. Murry. *Christensen's Introduction to the Physics of Diagnostic Radiology.* 4th ed. Philadelphia, PA: Lea & Febiger, 1990.

Eastman Kodak Company. *Recovering Silver from Photographic Materials.* Rochester, NY: Eastman Kodak Company, Publication No. J–10, 1980.

Gordon, Marjorie. Chemical hazards in film processing. *International Society of Radiographers and Radiological Technicians Newsletter* 24:1, 9–12, 1988.

Green, A., and G. I. P. Levenson. Silver recovery and fixer management: A new approach. *Radiography* 47:562, 225, 1981.

Gray, Joel, Norlin Winkler, John Stears, and Eugene Frank. *Quality Control in Diagnostic Imaging: A Quality Control Cookbook.* Baltimore, MD: University Park Press, 1983.

Jenkins, David. *Radiographic Photography and Imaging Processes.* Lancaster, England: MTP Press Limited, 1980.

McKinney, William. *Radiographic Processing and Quality Control.* Philadelphia, PA: J. B. Lippincott, 1988.

Neblette, C. B. *Photography: Its Materials and Processes.* 6th ed. Princeton, NJ: Van Nostrand Co., 1962.

Newhall, Beaumont. *The History of Photography.* New York: The Museum of Modern Art, 1964.

Nusbaum, Ronald C. Silver reclamation: Management controls maximize yields. *Radiology Management* 9:3, 42, 1987.

Roberts, Derrick P., and Nigel L. Smith. *Radiographic Imaging: A Practical Approach.* Edinburgh: Churchill Livingstone, 1988.

Smith, H. Sharon. Silver recovery trail. *Radiography* 53:609 125, 1987.

Sprawls, Perry. *Principles of Radiography for Technologists.* Rockville, MD: Aspen Publishers, 1990.

Sprawls, Perry. *Physical Principles of Medical Imaging.* Rockville, MD: Aspen Publishers, 1987.

Sweeney, Richard J. *Radiographic Artifacts: Their Cause and Control.* Philadelphia, PA: J. B. Lippincott, 1983.

van der Plaats, G. J. *Medical X-Ray Techniques in Diagnostic Radiology: A Textbook for Radiographers and Radiological Technicians.* 4th ed. The Hague: Martinus Nijhoff Publishers, 1980.

White, John. Silver recovery—departmental management approach. *Radiography* 46:542, 35, 1980.

Wilson, Peter. Principles of formation of the latent and developed images. *Canadian Journal of Radiography, Radiotherapy, and Nuclear Medicine* 7:6, 268–278, 1977.

19 SENSITOMETRY

You lie on a turning table cold as snow.
Down press the camera's praying-mantis arms,
Avid to embrace your negative below;
Your inner organs light their secret farms
Not even lovers come close enough to know.

Howard Moss, "In the X-Ray Room."

OUTLINE

SENSITOMETRIC EQUIPMENT
THE D LOG E CURVE
FILM CHARACTERISTICS

OBJECTIVES

Upon completion of this chapter, the student should be able to:

1. Define sensitometry as it is applied to radiography.
2. Describe the production of a step wedge on radiographic film through the use of a penetrometer and a sensitometer.
3. Explain the function of a densitometer.
4. Estimate the percentage of light transmitted by a radiograph according to optical density logarithms.
5. Construct a D log E curve from sensitometric data.
6. State acceptable base-plus-fog and diagnostic range optical density numbers.
7. Describe the effect of automatic-processor reducing agents on the shape of a D log E curve, especially with relation to speed and contrast.
8. Define resolution, speed, contrast and latitude.
9. Explain the effect of silver halide crystal size on image resolution.
10. Discuss the physical and processing factors that affect film speed.
11. Calculate speed points, speed exposure points and relative speeds from D log E curves.

12. Calculate gamma, gradient point, average gradient and latitude from D log E curves.
13. Analyze D log E curves to determine speed, contrast and latitude relationships.
14. Discuss the relationships between resolution, speed, contrast and latitude.

Sensitometry is the measurement of the characteristic responses of film to exposure and processing and is accomplished by exposing and processing a film and then measuring and evaluating the resulting densities. It is primarily the responsibility of the radiographer to use sensitometric methods to evaluate technical factor exposure systems, films, intensifying screens and processing equipment. In addition, sensitometric methods are useful in establishing, evaluating and maintaining technical exposure factor charts and systems, a duty that can be done only by a qualified radiographer.

SENSITOMETRIC EQUIPMENT

A variety of equipment is necessary to carry out sensitometric procedures. Either a **penetrometer** or a **sensitometer** is required to produce a uniform range of densities on a film. A **densitometer** is required to provide an accurate reading of the amount of light transmitted through the film.

Penetrometer

A **penetrometer** is a series of increasingly thick, uniform absorbers. They are usually made of aluminum steps, although tissue-equivalent plastic is sometimes used (Figure 19–1). A penetrometer is referred to as a **step wedge** because of its shape. It is used to produce a step wedge on radiographic film by exposure to x-rays (Figure 19–2). Because of the vast number of variables in x-ray-generating equipment, the use of a penetrometer is not recommended for quality control monitoring of film processors. However, it is an excellent method for monitoring both x-ray equipment

Figure 19–1. Two types of penetrometers (step wedges)—aluminum and tissue-equivalent plastic.

and film/intensifying screen combinations because it reproduces the variables associated with a clinical situation.

Sensitometer

A **sensitometer** is designed to expose a reproducible, uniform, optical step wedge onto a film (Figure 19–3). It contains a controlled intensity light source (a pulsed stroboscopic light is best) and a piece of film with a standardized optical step wedge image (a step tablet). The controlled light source reproduces the same amount of light each time it is triggered. Voltage fluctuations and other factors that might cause the intensity to vary are controlled by

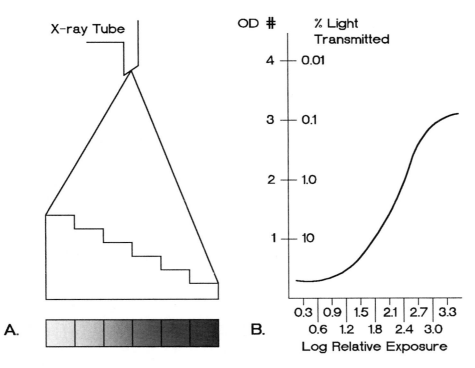

Figure 19–2.   A density curve produced from graphing the exposures of a pene-trometer exposure. (A) The exposure. (B) The graph.

circuits that supply an exact quantity of power to a capacitor that discharges to the strobo-scopic light when triggered. The optical step wedge absorbs a calibrated amount of this light, leaving a uniform and reproducible "light penetrometer" to expose any film placed in the sensitometer over the optical step wedge. The optical step wedge should not be touched because hands leave a film of oil that interferes with the light intensity.

Optical step wedges (step tablets) are available in 11- and 21-step versions. The 11-step wedges usually increase density 100 per-cent (by a factor of two) per step. The 21-step wedges usually increase density 41 percent (by a factor of 1.41 times [which is $\sqrt{2}$]) per step. cause the rigid control of the densities pro-duced on the film eliminates other variables,

sensitometer produced step wedges are perfect for processor quality control monitoring. Very

Figure 19–3.   A sensitometer.

slight density differences can be detected by sensitometric equipment. When a film is processed, there is a tendency for exhausted reducing agents and bromine ions to be carried backwards on the emulsion as it is driven through the rollers of an automatic processor. For this reason, sensitometric film strips should be fed into automatic processors with either the long axis of the step wedge parallel to the entrance rollers or with the light edge entering the processor first.

Densitometer

A **densitometer** is an instrument that provides a readout of the amount of blackening (density) on a film. A densitometer consists of a calibrated uniform light source, a stage for placing the film to be measured, a light aperture to control the amount of light from the source, a sensor arm with an optical sensor, a readout display and a calibration control (Figure 19–4). Density readings are accomplished by comparing the amount of light emitted by the light source with the amount of light transmitted through the film. To do this, the densi-

tometer must be calibrated before each reading by recording the amount of light the light source is emitting. This is done by pushing the sensor arm so that the sensor is in contact with the light source (this eliminates the inverse square law factor) and by using the calibration control to set the readout display at zero. This **calibrates** or **zeroes** the densitometer and prepares it for a reading. When a film is placed on the stage and the sensor arm is pushed down into contact with the film, the densitometer can calculate the difference between the calibration intensity and the intensity of light the film is transmitting. Some densitometers include a filter to negate the blue tint in the film base.

Because films are sensitive to a wide range of exposures, their densities are best visualized if the range is compressed into a logarithmic scale. When using a logarithmic scale with a base of 10, an increment of 0.3 represents a doubling of exposure. This is because the log of 2 is 0.3. The numbers that are displayed by a densitometer are known as **optical density numbers**. They can be expressed with the term OD in front of the number (i.e., OD 1.5). They are calculated using the following formula:

$$OD = \frac{\log_{10} I_i}{I_t}$$

where: OD = optical density number
I_i = intensity of the incident light source as calibrated to zero
I_t = intensity of the light transmitted through the film

This formula can be stated as the log of the intensity of the incident light divided by the intensity of the light transmitted through the film. Radiographic film densities range from OD 0.0 to 4.0. Table 19–1 shows the percentage

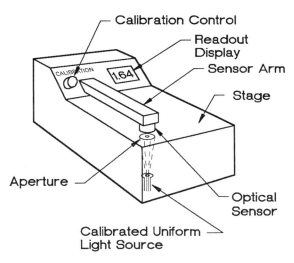

Figure 19–4.   A densitometer.

TABLE 19–1	

COMMON OPTICAL DENSITY NUMBER LIGHT TRANSMISSION PERCENTAGES

OD Number	Percentage of Light Transmitted Through Film
0.0	100
0.3	50
0.6	25
0.9	12.5
1.0	10
1.3	5
1.6	2.5
1.9	1.25
2.0	1
2.3	0.5
2.6	0.25
2.9	0.125
3.0	0.1
3.3	0.05
3.6	0.025
3.9	0.0125
4.0	0.01

of light transmitted for optical density numbers in this range.

THE D LOG E CURVE

Sensitometry is normally shown as a graphic relationship between the amount of exposure and the resultant density on the film (Figure 19–5). The horizontal exposure axis (x axis) is compressed into a logarithmic scale (because of the wide range of densities possible) and the vertical density axis (y axis) is shown as a linear scale. Consequently, the curves are known as Density log Exposure, or **D log E curves**. They are also called **characteristic, sensitometric and Hurter and Driffield**

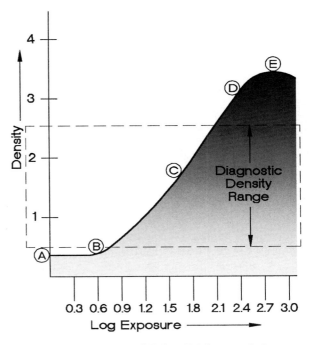

Figure 19–5.   A typical D log E (characteristic, sensitometric or H&D) curve. (A) base plus fog; (B) toe; (C) straight line portion; (D) shoulder; (E) D_{max}.

(H&D) curves after the two photographers who first described the relationships in 1890. The important elements of a typical D log E curve are the base plus fog, toe, straight line portion (gamma), shoulder and maximum density (D_{max}).

The **base plus fog** (b+f) (Figure 19–5A) is the density at no exposure, or the density that is inherent in the film. It includes the density of the film base, including its tints and dyes, plus any fog the film has experienced. Radiographic film base density ranges around OD 0.05–0.10. Processing the film usually adds about OD 0.05–0.10 in fog density. The total base plus fog is seldom below OD 0.10 but should not exceed OD 0.22. Fog may be caused by heat, chemical fumes, light and x-radiation. Over time, the natural amounts of these radiations will produce a slight density that is sometimes called age fog. Most of the fog level will be produced by the processing system. This includes the hyperactivity of the developer solution, primarily caused by the high temperature at which automatic processors operate.

Phenidone is the reducing agent that controls the subtle gray tones early in the development process. This region of the curve is known as the toe (see Figure 19–5B) and is predominantly controlled by phenidone.

The **straight line portion** of the curve is that portion between the toe and shoulder (see Figure 19–5C). It is usually fairly straight because the film is reacting in a linear fashion to exposure in the range of its primary sensitivity, which is in this region. The range of diagnostic densities varies from a low of OD 0.25–0.50 to a high of OD 2.0–3.0. The majority of diagnostic quality information on a radiograph will measure between OD 0.5–1.25. These densities are within the straight line portion of the curve.

Hydroquinone is the reducing agent that controls the heavy black tone later in the development process. This region of the curve is known as the **shoulder** (see Figure 19–5D) and is entirely controlled by hydroquinone.

D_{max} is the maximum density of which the film is capable (see Figure 19–5E). It is the highest point on the D log E curve. It represents the point where all the silver halides have a full complement of silver atoms and cannot accept more. Additional exposure beyond D_{max} will result in less density because silver atoms attached to sensitivity specks will be ionized again, reversing their charge and causing them to be repelled from the speck. This process of **reversal**, or **solarization**, reduces the intensity of the latent image and will produce less density. The true D log E curve is bell-shaped (Figure 19–6). Duplication film is actually film that is preexposed to D_{max} so that additional exposure will cause a reversed, duplicated image instead of a negative one.

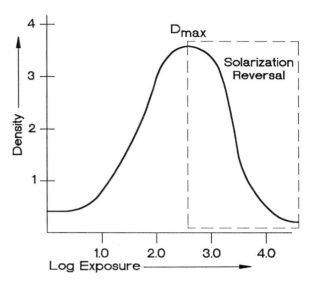

Figure 19–6. Solarization or reversal of duplicating film.

FILM CHARACTERISTICS

The primary characteristics of film are classified as **resolution, speed, contrast and latitude**. Sensitometry permits analysis of these characteristics within the normal exposure ranges of the film. Extremely long or high-intensity exposure can overload the silver halide crystals and cause a phenomenon known as reciprocity failure. Although films are designed to handle a wide range of exposures, when unusual circumstances require large exposures, films may deviate from their expected performance.

Resolution

Resolution is the ability to accurately image an object. It is also called **detail, sharpness, definition and resolving power**. Resolution is measured by the ability to see pairs of lines. The unit of resolution is line pairs per millimeter, expressed as lp/mm.

Film resolution is determined by the **size of the silver halide crystals**. Smaller crystals will darken a smaller area of the film while larger ones will darken larger areas. Information that is smaller than an individual silver halide crystal cannot be visualized. **An inverse relationship exists between film resolution and crystal size** (the smaller the crystals, the higher the resolution; the larger the crystals, the lower the resolution). Silver halide crystals are sometimes called grains, thus the term graininess for poor resolution. Although film graininess can sometimes be seen, radiographic film/screen system resolution is generally controlled by the size of the intensifying screen crystals, not the size of the silver halide crystals in the film emulsion.

Speed

The amount of density (degree of blackening) a film produces for a given amount of exposure is the film **speed**. It is determined by its sensitivity to exposure. Speed is controlled by the activity of the phenidone because it affects the toe of the D log E curve. The position of the toe determines how soon the straight line portion will begin, and this indicates the overall speed of the film. Figure 19–7 illustrates the effect of the toe and shoulder on the overall position of the curve.

Film sensitivity is determined primarily by the **size of the silver halide crystals**. However, **the number of sensitivity specks and the thickness of the emulsion layer** also have an effect. Larger crystals will receive more photons because of the greater area they cover. They will also produce more photons than smaller crystals for the same reason. Larger crystals will darken a greater area of the film than smaller crystals with the same exposure. Therefore, **film speed and crystal size are directly proportional** (the larger the crystals, the faster the film speed; the smaller the crystals, the slower the film speed).

Film speed and the number of sensitivity specks are also directly proportional for the

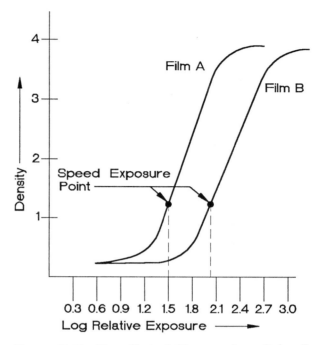

Figure 19–7. The effect of film speed on D log E curves.

same reason. A thicker emulsion layer will place more crystals in a given area. Each incoming photon may interact with more than one crystal, so when more crystals are stacked on top of one another in the same area, the same number of photons will produce more film density. Therefore, **film speed and thickness of emulsion layer are directly proportional** (the thicker the emulsion, the faster the film speed; the thinner the emulsion, the slower the film speed).

Screen films are capable of responding to (producing visible densities for) exposures as low as 1 mR and as high as 1,000 mR. In Figure 19–7, film A produces all density levels with less exposure than film B requires for the same density. This demonstrates that film A is more sensitive to exposure, or faster. Film B is less sensitive, or slower.

The **speed point** of a film is that point on the D log E curve where a density of OD 1.0 + b+f is achieved. The American National Standards Institute (ANSI) specifies x-ray film speed as the exposure required to reach OD 1.00. However, many users add base plus fog to this standard. The **speed exposure point** is the log exposure that will produce the speed point for a given film. Film A in Figure 19–7 has a speed exposure point of 1.5, while film B has a speed exposure point of 2.0.

In clinical radiography is it important to be able to adjust technical factors from one film to another. The radiographer must be able to calculate the difference in exposure that will produce a diagnostic quality image on a new film when the proper factors are known for a previous one. In Figure 19–7, film B would require a log exposure of 1.9 to produce OD 1.0. Film A would require a log exposure of 1.4 to produce the same density. The difference in film speed is calculated as:

$$\left| \frac{\log E_1 - \log E_2}{0.3} \right|$$

where: $\log E_1$ = log exposure of 1st film

$\log E_2$ = log exposure of 2nd film

0.3 = $\log_{10}$ percent doubling

| | = absolute value

Example: What is the difference in speed between film A and film B in Figure 19–7?

Answer:

$$\left| \frac{\log E_1 - \log E_2}{0.3} \right| =$$

$$\left| \frac{1.9 - 1.4}{0.3} \right| =$$

$$\left| \frac{0.5}{0.3} \right| = 1.66$$

Film A is 66 percent faster than film B.

Relative speeds have been assigned by film manufacturers to assist radiographers in relating films to one another as they are used in film and intensifying screen combinations (film/screen combinations). Relative film/screen speed can be determined by using the reciprocal of the exposure required to produce a given density:

relative speed =

$$\frac{1}{\text{exposure in R needed to produce the speed point density (OD 1.0 + b+f)}}$$

Example: What is the relative speed for a film that requires an exposure of 5 mR to produce the speed point density?

Answer:

relative speed =

$$\frac{1}{\text{exposure in R needed to produce the speed point density (OD 1.0 + b+f)}}$$

Relative speed = $\frac{1}{5 \text{ mR}}$

Relative speed = $\frac{1}{0.005 \text{ R}}$ = 200

Film speed is affected by immersion **time**, solution **temperature** and chemical **activity**. The immersion **time** in a high-speed automatic processor may be as short as 20–25 seconds. The longer the film is subjected to the chemical action of the developer solution, the greater is the amount of black metallic silver deposited on the latent image sites through the reduction process (Figure 19–8). Film speed is most affected by developer solution **temperature** (Figure 19–9). Only 0.5° will cause a visible change in film density. Higher temperature increases the activity level of the reducing agents in the developer and this produces greater density on the film. High speed automatic processors use high temperatures to permit sufficient development to occur in the 20–25 seconds the film is

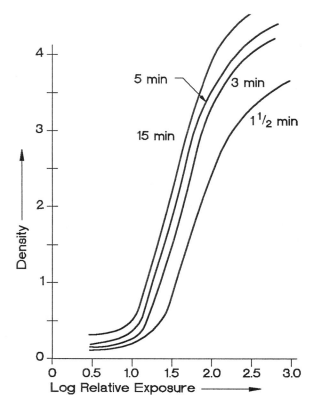

Figure 19–8.   The effect of developer solution immersion time on film speed.

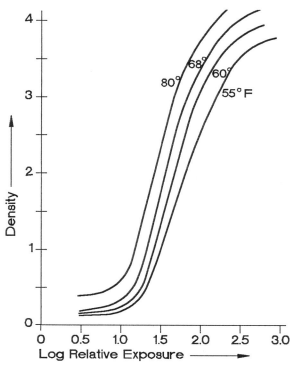

Figure 19–9.   The effect of developer solution temperature on film speed.

immersed in the developer. The chemical **activity** of the developer solution will also increase the development of density. Film speed is affected when the bromide ion barrier has not formed properly (due to insufficient restrainer or overreplenishment) or when it is too strong (due to excess restrainer or underreplenishment). Determination of the proper time, temperature and activity for a particular developer and film is done by graphing speed, contrast and base plus fog levels for various activity concentrations (Figure 19–10). This is how the manufacturer arrives at the recommended time and temperature for optimal results.

Contrast

Contrast is the difference between adjacent densities. This concept can be confusing when one tries to understand the difference between density and contrast. There is a relationship between contrast and density because contrast consists of the difference between adjacent densities. For the same film type, **a change in density will affect contrast**.

When slight increases in the number of photons reaching the film cause visible density differences, higher contrast exists. This makes it easier to see differences in the tissues of the subject. However, the contrast must exist within the diagnostic range of the film if it is to be visualized. Contrast is controlled by the

Figure 19–10. Determination of optimal development time and temperature for a particular film by
comparison of contrast, speed and base+fog for a
particular developer solution concentration.

Figure 19–11.   Comparison of film contrast.

level of activity of the hydroquinone. Hydroquinone establishes the shoulder of the D log E
curve and the position of the shoulder affects
the slope of the straight line portion of the
curve (Figure 19–11).

Contrast is defined by the slope of the
straight-line portion of the D log E curve, but,
because the straight line portion is actually a
curve, it is important to define the point at
which the slope is measured. **Gamma** is simply a measure of the slope of the straight line
portion of the curve at the speed point (OD
1.0). In practice, a gamma may be read with
the speed point in the center, top end or bottom end, as long as all comparative readings
are done from the same reference point. Contrast differences cannot be appreciated unless
they are measured from identical reference
points.

The slope can be read as "rise over run"
(Figure 19–12). More sophisticated measurements, such as the trigonometric tangent of
the slope, are also used. The slope of any portion of the D log E curve can be calculated and
this is known as a **gradient point**. Gradient
points must have their OD values stated, e.g.,
a gradient of 1.75 at OD 0.80. Gradient points
are sometimes known by their location: toe
gradient, middle gradient and upper gradient.
The toe gradient is calculated between OD 0.25

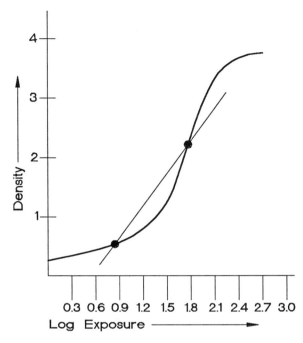

Figure 19–12. Average gradient calculations from a D log E curve.

and OD 1.00. The middle gradient is calculated between OD 1.00 and OD 2.00. The upper gradient is calculated between OD 2.00 and OD 2.50. Overall radiographic film contrast is more commonly defined by the **average gradient** of the straight line portion of the D log E curve between OD 0.25 + b+f and OD 2.50 + b+f. Opinions differ on whether b+f should be added to average gradient calculations. The average gradient is calculated as:

$$\text{average gradient} = \frac{\Delta D}{\Delta E} \text{ or}$$

$$\text{average gradient} = \frac{D_2 - D_1}{E_2 - E_1}$$

where: D_1 = OD 0.25 + b+f,
         D_2 = OD 2.50 + b+f,
         E_1 = exposure that produces D_1

E_2 = exposure that produces D_2

Note: ΔD is a constant of OD 2.25 (OD 2.50–0.25).

Figure 19–13 illustrates the difference between various gradient points and the average gradient and calculates the average gradient. Most radiographic film average gradients are between 2.5 and 3.5. If the average gradient were 1.0, the film would be reproducing contrast equivalent to the actual contrast of the subject. Because radiographic film average gradients are higher than 1.0, **radiographic film amplifies subject contrast**.

Toe and shoulder gradients are less than a 45° angle and therefore not only fail to amplify the subject contrast, but actually decrease it. This is why extremely light or dark areas on radiographs are not acceptable for diagnosis.

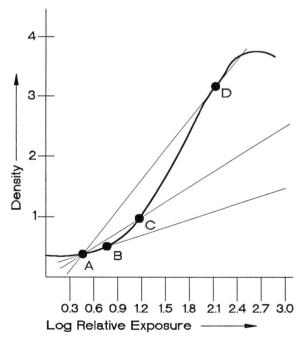

Figure 19–13. Average gradient and gradient point calculations from a D log E curve. The slopes of points A-B, A-C and A-D are quite different.

Latitude

For clinical radiographic purposes, **latitude** is the range of exposures that will produce densities within the diagnostic range (Figure 19–14). Latitude can be recorded as the width of the range of exposures that will produce diagnostic range densities according to the following formula:

$$latitude = E_h - E_l$$

where E_h = OD 2.50 exposure point
E_l = OD 0.25 exposure point

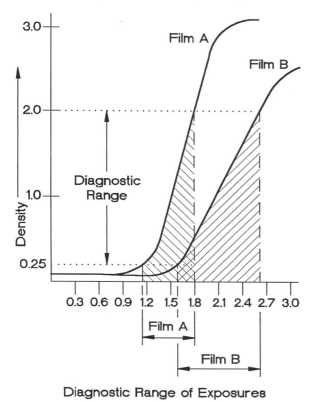

Figure 19–14. Comparison of film latitude. The range of relative exposures is indicated for each film.

when E_h = high exposure point
E_l = low exposure point

Example: What is the latitude for film A in Figure 19–14?

Answer:
latitude = $E_h - E_l$
latitude = $1.8 - 1.1$
latitude = 0.7

The latitude for film B can be calculated to be 1.0. Film A has a narrow latitude while film B has a wider latitude. Because a wide latitude film permits considerable variation in the exposure while still exhibiting densities within the diagnostic range, it is sometimes called a forgiving film. The use of a narrow latitude film for routine radiography requires greater exposure accuracy.

Latitude and contrast are inversely related. As contrast increases, latitude tends to decrease. This affects the overall shape of the D log E curve. Latitude changes whenever there is a change in the average gradient of the D log E curve. Speed could change without altering the average gradient and latitude. A difference in film speed usually results in different contrast and latitude because it is rare for the entire D log E curve to shift the same degree. Usually the toe and shoulder will not shift exactly the same amount and this causes a change in the slope of the straight line portion of the curve (which changes contrast and latitude). The relationships of resolution, speed, contrast and latitude to one another are listed in Table 19–2.

SUMMARY

Sensitometry is the measurement of the characteristic responses of a film to exposure and processing. It is accomplished by exposing and processing a film and then measuring and evaluating the resulting densities. Either a

TABLE 19–2				
COMMON RELATIONSHIPS BETWEEN RESOLUTION, SPEED, CONTRAST, LATITUDE AND PATIENT DOSE				
Resolution	**Speed**	**Contrast**	**Latitude**	**Patient Dose**
high	slow	high	narrow	high
low	fast	low	wide	low

NOTE: Resolution and speed affect one another. Patient dose is a function of the speed. Contrast and latitude affect one another. However, the relationship between resolution/speed and contrast/latitude may not be as shown in every circumstance.

penetrometer or a sensitometer is required to produce a uniform range of densities on the film. A densitometer is required to provide an accurate reading of the amount of light transmitted through the film.

Because films are sensitive to a wide range of exposures, their densities are best visualized if the range is compressed into a logarithmic scale. When using a logarithmic scale with a base of 10, an increment of 0.3 represents a doubling of exposure. This is because the log of 2 is 0.3.

Sensitometry is normally shown as a graphic relationship between the amount of exposure and the resultant density on the film. The horizontal axis (exposure) of the graph is compressed into a logarithmic scale and the vertical axis (density) is a linear scale. Consequently, the curves are known as Density log Exposure or D log E curves. They are also called characteristic, sensitometric and Hurter and Driffield (H&D) curves. The important elements of the D log E curve are the base plus fog, toe, straight-line portion (gamma), shoulder and maximum density (D max).

The primary characteristics of film are resolution, speed, contrast and latitude. Resolution is the ability to accurately image an object and is measured by the ability to see line pairs. The amount of density a film produces for a given amount of exposure is the film speed. The film speed is determined by the size of the silver halide crystals, the number of sensitivity specks and the thickness of the emulsion. Relative speeds have been assigned by film manufacturers to assist radiographers in relating films to one another as they are used in film/screen combinations. Contrast is the difference between adjacent densities. It is defined as the slope of the straight line portion of the D log E curve. Latitude is the range of exposures that will produce densities within the diagnostic range. As contrast increases, latitude tends to decrease.

REVIEW QUESTIONS

1. What is the purpose of sensitometry?

2. Explain the design of a penetrometer.

3. Why is a logarithmic scale used for describing optical densities?

4. Describe the five important elements of the D log E curve.

5. What is the relationship between film resolution and the size of the silver halide crystals?

6. What is the relationship between film speed and emulsion layer thickness?

7. State the formula for relative speed.

8. How is the average gradient calculated?

9. What is the relationship between contrast and latitude?

REFERENCES AND RECOMMENDED READING

Carroll, Quinn. *Fuchs's Principles of Radiographic Exposure, Processing, and Quality Control.* 3rd ed. Springfield, IL: Charles C. Thomas Publisher, 1985.

Chow, Mai F. The effect of a film's sensitivity to its speed, contrast, and latitude. *The Canadian Journal of Medical Radiation Technology* 19:4, 147, 1988.

Eastman Kodak Co. *Sensitometric Properties of X-Ray Films.* Rochester, NY: Eastman Kodak Company Radiography Markets Division.

Gray, Joel, Norlin Winkler, John Stears, and Eugene Frank. *Quality Control in Diagnostic Imaging: A Quality Control Cookbook.* Baltimore, MD: University Park Press, 1983.

Jenkins, David. *Radiographic Photography and Imaging Processes.* Lancaster, England: MTP Press Limited, 1980.

McKinney, William. *Radiographic Processing and Quality Control.* Philadelphia, PA: J. B. Lippincott, 1988.

Rao, Gopala U. V., William Witt, Michael C. Beachley, Herman A. Bosch, Panos P. Fatouros, and Philip T. Kan. Radiographic films and screen-film systems. *The Physical Basis of Medical Imaging.* Editors: Coulam, Craig M., John J. Erickson, F. David Rollo, and A. Everette James, Jr. New York: Appleton-Century-Crofts, 1981.

Roberts, Derrick P., and Nigel L. Smith. *Radiographic Imaging: A Practical Approach.* Edinburgh: Churchill Livingstone, 1988.

Rossi, R. P., W. R. Hendee, and C R. Aherns. An evaluation of rare-earth screen-film combinations. *Radiology* 121, 465, 1976.

Sprawls, Perry. *Principles of Radiography for Technologists.* Rockville, MD: Aspen Publishers, 1990.

Sprawls, Perry. *Physical Principles of Medical Imaging.* Rockville, MD: Aspen Publishers, 1987.

20 INTENSIFYING SCREENS

I decided to try a combination of Edison's fluorescent screen and the photographic plate. . . . The combination succeeded even better than I had expected. A beautiful photograph was obtained with an exposure of a few seconds. That was the first x-ray picture obtained by that process during the first part of February 1896.

Autobiography of M. Pupin, *From Immigrant to Inventor.*

OUTLINE

CONSTRUCTION
PHOSPHORS
CHARACTERISTICS
CASSETTES AND HOLDERS
CARE

OBJECTIVES

Upon completion of this chapter, the student should be able to:

1. Explain the purpose of radiographic intensifying screens.
2. Describe the function of each layer of an intensifying screen.
3. Evaluate the desirability of phosphor materials according to atomic number, conversion efficiency, spectral emission and fluorescence.
4. Describe luminescence.
5. Analyze the effect of phosphor crystal size, layer thickness and concentration on intensifying screen resolution.
6. Explain the effect of film/screen contact on resolution.
7. Describe how to remedy quantum mottle.
8. Classify intensifying screens according to intensification factor, descriptive rating and relative speed number.
9. Describe the effect of K-shell absorption edges on intensifying screen efficiency.
10. Describe the components of a radiographic cassette.
11. Describe the proper cleaning and care of radiographic cassettes and screens.
12. Evaluate film/screen combinations for specific clinical uses.

Intensifying screens are used to amplify the incoming x-ray beam and reduce patient radiation dose. Introduced in 1896 by the American inventor Thomas Edison (1847–1931), intensifying screens produce large quantities of light photons when struck by x-rays. In this manner they intensify the latent imaging power of the beam, even though less than 33 percent of the x-ray photons that strike the cassette interact with the intensifying screen. Over 99 percent of the latent image is formed by this light, with less than one percent contributed by x-ray photons. This permits a great reduction in the amount of radiation necessary to produce a diagnostic quality image. Intensifying screens are normally used in pairs with duplitized film, although there are specialized cassettes that are designed for a single screen with single emulsion film.

CONSTRUCTION

Intensifying screens are composed of radiolucent plastic, coated with phosphors that will emit light when struck by x-ray photons. They are designed to be mounted in pairs inside the top and bottom of a light proof cassette so that a sheet of radiographic film can be sandwiched tightly between them. A screen consists of **a base, a reflective layer, a phosphor layer and a protective coat** (Figure 20–1).

Base

The **base** is usually made of polyester plastic 1 mm thick, although cardboard and metal have been used. Its requirements are similar to those for a film base. It must be flexible yet **tough**, rigid, chemically **inert** and uniformly radiolucent. It **must be flexible** to permit it to achieve good contact with the film. It must be rigid enough to stay in place in the top and bottom of a cassette. It must be chemically inert so that it does not react with the phosphor and interfere with the conversion of x-ray photons to light. It also must not react with air or chemicals in a manner that would cause discoloration. Discoloration filters and changes the wavelengths of the light emitted by the screen by absorbing wavelengths that could be used to create the radiographic image. Because films are designed to be most sensitive to the particular wavelength of light emitted by the screen, discoloration may require more light, and consequently more patient radiation dose, to form the latent image. Most important, base material must be uniformly radiolucent so that it permits the transmission of x-ray photons without adding artifacts to the diagnostic image.

Reflective Layer

The base material is not transparent to light. In fact, a special layer of reflective mate-

Figure 20–1. Cross-sectional view of a typical radiographic intensifying screen.

rial, such as magnesium oxide or titanium dioxide, about 25 μm thick, is used to reflect light toward the film. When a phosphor is struck by an x-ray photon, it will emit light isotropically (in all directions) (Figure 20–2A). When a reflective layer is added (Figure 20–2B) nearly twice as much light is reflected toward the film. This increase in light striking the film assists in creating the latent image and decreases the radiation dose to the patient.

Light that is emitted at a large angle from the direction of the incident x-ray photon will have a slightly longer wavelength. Some intensifying screens use dyes in the reflective layer to selectively absorb this longer-wavelength light. This assists in reducing the scattering of light that would decrease the resolving ability of the screen. Scattered light of this type causes a large area of penumbra, which reduces the sharpness of the image.

Phosphor Layer

The active layer of the intensifying screen is the **phosphor** layer. Phosphors are materials that are capable of absorbing the energy of an incident x-ray photon and then emitting light photons. Röntgen discovered x-rays when he observed the luminescence of the phosphor

Figure 20–2.   Intensifying screen reflective layer redirection of isotropic light emission to film.

barium platinocyanide from a piece of cardboard in his laboratory. This phosphor layer varies from 150–300 μm, depending on the speed and resolving power of the screen.

Protective Coat

A coating of protective plastic about 25 μm thick is applied on top of the phosphor layer. The coating protects the phosphor layer from abrasions and stains during the loading and unloading of films. Fingernails and jewelry are the prime trauma to screens in the darkroom. Although the protective coating will prevent scratching of the phosphor layer during normal handling, repeated trauma can remove the coating. When intensifying screens are scratched, phosphor crystals may be removed, creating unexposed white line artifacts on the radiographic image.

PHOSPHORS

Phosphors must have a high **atomic number**, high **conversion efficiency**, **appropriate spectral emission and minimal fluorescence**.

Atomic Number

A high **atomic number** is desirable to increase the probability of an incident x-ray photon interaction. Because x-ray photons are of high energy, a high atomic number is required to permit photoelectric and Compton interactions.

Conversion Efficiency

The ability of the phosphor to emit as much light per x-ray photon interaction as possible is a measurement of the screen speed. As this **conversion efficiency** increases, the radiation exposure dose to the patient decreases. A typical conversion efficiency would produce 1×10^3 light photons per incident 50 keV x-ray photon for a rare-earth screen.

Spectral Emission

The **spectral emission** is an indication of the precise wavelength of light emitted by the phosphor. It is important that the spectral emission match the sensitivity of the film to ensure maximum latent image formation.

Luminescence

Luminescence is the ability of a material to emit light in response to excitation (usually by increased outer-electron-shell energy levels). Because of the narrow energy band within which these interactions occur, luminescent materials emit light with wavelengths that are characteristic of the particular luminescent material. This results in light emissions of a characteristic color. **Fluorescence and phosphorescence are the two types of luminescence.** Fluorescence occurs when the light is emitted within the time it takes an electron to complete one orbit of the affected shell electrons (within one nanosecond). Phosphorescence occurs when the light is emitted for a period longer than that necessary for one orbit of the affected shell electrons. In other words, **fluorescence is instantaneous emission while phosphorescence is delayed emission**, sometimes considerably delayed. Phosphorescence occurs when the phosphor continues to emit light after the incident x-ray photon energy has dissipated. Maximum fluorescence and minimal phosphorescence are desirable because delayed emission of light may permit the film to be removed from the cassette before the maximum latent image formation has occurred. Additionally, if another film is loaded into the cassette it may be faintly exposed to a previous image.

Delayed phosphorescent emission is called **screen lag or afterglow** and is common in older intensifying screens with exhausted phosphors. The normal life of intensifying screen phosphors is five to seven years. All intensifying screens must be replaced routinely. As screens age, their phosphors decrease in activity. Because of this, it is highly recommended that all screens in a particular working area be replaced simultaneously. For example, all radiographic rooms serviced by a single darkroom should have the screens replaced at the same time. This assures the radiographer that all cassettes contain intensifying screens of approximately the same activity level.

A simple demonstration of phosphor activity is achieved by darkening an x-ray room and observing the light emitted by intensifying screen phosphors when an exposure is made. Observations of this type can be made through leaded glass and from behind leaded walls. The light emissions can be varied by using screens of different phosphors, different ages and exposures of different mAs and kVp levels. Roughly 50,000 photons per mm^2 must exit the object being examined to produce a radiographic image. The intensifying screens must produce enough light from these photons to create the latent image in the film emulsion.

Several phosphors have been used in radiography since Röntgen's discovery: zinc sulfide, barium lead sulfate, calcium tungstate ($CaWO_4$) and a family of hybrid rare earths including gadolinium, lanthanum and yttrium. Calcium tungstate was used by Edison and it predominated as the best phosphor until the late 1970s, when the rare earths were introduced. Rare earths are now beginning to predominate.

Rare Earths

Rare earths have become popular as phosphor materials because they have greater absorption abilities, intensification factors and conversion efficiency. Calcium tungstate screens have an x-ray-to-light conversion efficiency of about five percent, as compared to rare-earth conversion efficiencies of 15–20 percent. The rare-earth screens use phosphors with atomic numbers of 57–71. These elements are known as rare earths because they are infrequently found in nature. Currently, gadolinium and lanthanum are being used in compounds with activators and other chemicals (Table 20–1). The primary reason rare-earth phosphors have gained widespread acceptance is because they offer increased speed while maintaining resolution, when compared to similar speed calcium-tungstate screens. Their cost is greater but radiographers are increasingly choosing the expense over the patient dose required when using calcium tungstate screens. Phosphor technology has outstripped advancements in other radiographic equipment. Some of the rare earths are so fast that tubes cannot emit sufficient mAs to prevent quantum mottle, automatic exposure control minimum reaction times are too long to avoid erratic densities, and reciprocating grids are not fast enough to prevent grid lines from being imaged. These factors must be considered when using extremely fast rare-earth screens (film/screen combinations above RS 500).

CHARACTERISTICS

Intensifying screens exhibit the same types of characteristics as films. Consideration must be given to screen **resolution, speed, contrast and latitude**.

Resolution

Resolution is the ability to accurately image an object. Intensifying-screen resolution is controlled by the size of the phosphor crystals, the thickness of the layer and the concentration of the crystals, exactly as silver halide size and distribution affect film resolution (Figure 20–3). Smaller crystals and a thinner layer increase resolution but decrease screen speed. Larger crystals and a thicker layer decrease resolution but increase screen speed (Figure 20–4). **Phosphor crystal size and layer thickness are both inversely proportional to resolution and directly proportional to screen speed**. A greater concentration of crystals will increase both resolution and screen speed. Phosphor concentration is directly proportional to resolution and screen speed. Intensifying screen phosphor crystals are much larger than the silver-halide crystals in the film emulsion. In radiographic film and intensifying screen combinations **the screen resolution always predominates over the film resolution**.

Measurement

The naked eye can resolve about 10–20 lp/mm. Direct exposure nonscreen radiographic film can resolve up to 100 lp/mm, detail speed screens about 15 lp/mm, par

TABLE 20–1			
RARE-EARTH INTENSIFYING SCREEN PHOSPHORS WITH MANUFACTURER AND TRADE NAME			
Rare Earth	**Primary Emission Color**	**Manufacturer**	**Trade Name**
gadolinium oxysulfide	green	Kodak	Lanex
gadolinium oxysulfide	green	3M	Trimax
gadolinium oxysulfide	green	Fuji	
lanthanum oxybromide	blue	Agfa-Matrix	
lanthanum oxybromide	blue	Du Pont	Quanta III
lanthanum oxybromide	blue	Ilford	Rapide

Note: All trade names are registered trademarks of the manufacturers.

60 kVp	5 mAs	40″ SID
No grid	100 RS	10.7 mR

60 kVp	0.8 mAs	40″ SID
No grid	600 RS	1.74 mR

Figure 20–3A & B.   The effect of intensifying screen resolution on image quality: (A) fine detail intensifying screens; (B) high speed intensifying screens.

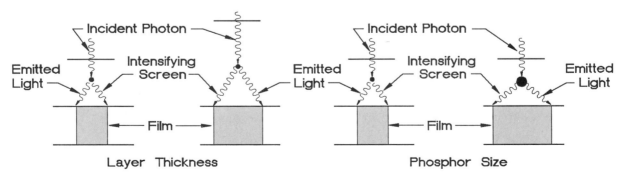

Figure 20–4.   The effect of intensifying screen phosphor layer thickness and crystal size on film resolution.

speed screens about 10 lp/mm and high speed screens about 7 lp/mm.

Film/Screen Contact One of the most common screen resolution problems is caused by poor contact between the film and the intensifying screen in the cassette (Figure 20–5). Poor film/screen contact also increases the image density. There are numerous possible causes of poor film/screen contact, including foreign objects in the cassette and warped or damaged cassettes.

Quantum Mottle Each phosphor crystal emits light that exposes a corresponding area of silver-halide crystals in the film emulsion. When insufficient phosphor crystals emit light to expose a coherent expanse of film, the resulting image will appear grainy (Figure 20–6). As can be seen, quantum mottle is caused by an insufficient quantity of photons striking the intensifying screen. Although film graininess may appear mottled, radiographic mottle is nearly always a result of intensifying screen quantum mottle. The radiographer controls the quantity of photons with the mAs setting, so an increase in this factor will eliminate quantum mottle. Fluoroscopic tubes normally operate at very low mA levels. For this reason, quantum mottle is more commonly seen in fluoroscopy.

Speed

The speed or sensitivity of the intensifying screen is determined by the same factors that control resolution. The phosphor size, thickness and concentration have the same effect on speed as on resolution. **Screen resolution and speed are directly proportional and are, in fact, related to each other**. However, there are additional factors that affect speed but not resolution. As kVp is increased, the efficiency of the intensifying screen will also increase. **An increase in kVp will cause an increase in screen speed**. Intensifying screen phosphors have relatively high atomic numbers, so higher kVp will increase the probability of light producing interactions within the phosphors. **Temperature** increases (over 100°F [38°C]) will decrease screen speed significantly. This is usually of concern only in extremely hot climates or during outdoor radiography.

Screen Speed Classifications Three casual systems of classifying intensifying-screen speed have developed: **the intensification factor, descriptive rating and relative-speed number**.

The most accurate factor that measures the speed or sensitivity of an intensifying screen is the **intensification factor**. It is a measurement of the amplification of the image that occurs due to the screen's ability to convert x-ray photons to light. It is directly related to

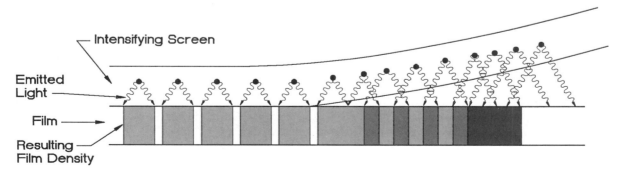

Figure 20–5.   Poor resolution and increased image density due to loss of film/screen contact.

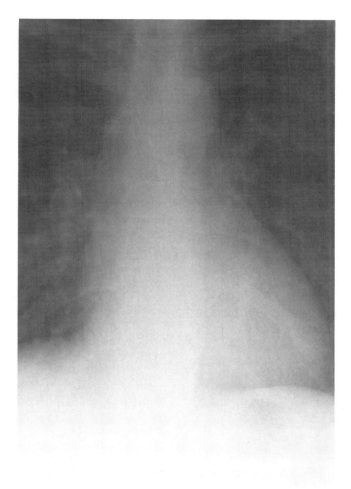

Figure 20–6. Quantum mottle.

the conversion efficiency of the phosphor. It is calculated as:

$$\text{intensification factor} = \frac{D_n}{D_s}$$

where: D_n = exposure in mR nonscreen
D_s = exposure in mR with screens

Most radiographic intensifying screens are also classified with a **descriptive rating** of either **high speed, par speed (also called universal or medium speed)** and **fine detail (high resolution)**. Some manufacturers use their own descriptive terms and many of these are trademarks.

The most useful rating of intensifying screens is the **relative speed**. Relative speed is expressed with par speed screens and film being arbitrarily assigned a relative speed (RS) number of 100 as a control point. High speed screens are usually rated RS 200–1,200 while fine detail screens are usually rated RS 20–80.

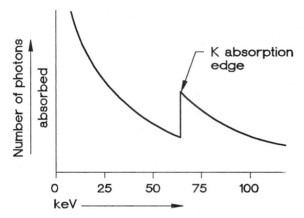

Figure 20–7. The K-shell edge effect for calcium tungstate phosphors.

K-shell Absorption Edge

Calcium tungstate screens will absorb about 20–40 percent and rare-earth screens will absorb about 50–60 percent of the incident beam. These percentages vary depending upon the keV level of the incident photons. Nearly 100 percent of the absorption occurs through photoelectric interactions. Because photoelectric interactions produce characteristic photons, when the incident x-ray photons match the K-shell binding energy of the phosphor, there is a dramatic increase in characteristic scatter within the screen. This is the **K-shell absorption edge** (Figure 20–7). The K-shell edges for screen phosphors can result in a dramatic increase in light emission. This causes problems for the radiographer who uses a variable kVp technical factor system. If the kVp selected happens to be on or slightly above the K-shell edge, a slight decrease in kVp can cause a tremendous decrease in light emission, greatly reducing film density, instead of the slight decrease intended. In the reverse situation, if the original kVp happens to be slightly below the K-shell edge and a slight increase is desired, if the increase activated the K-shell peak, the resulting increase in density might be excessive. On a

K-SHELL EDGES FOR INTENSIFYING SCREEN PHOSPHORS		
Phosphor	K-shell Edge	Atomic Number
lanthanum	39 keV	57
gadolinium	50 keV	64
tungsten	70 keV	74

TABLE 20–2

repeated examination, these situations could require third exposures. Table 20–2 provides the K-shell edges for the most common phosphors. **The kVp level should not be varied around screen-phosphor K-shell edges**. Note that the K-shell edges are stated in keV levels. About 5 to 6 percent higher kVp levels would be required to produce the maximum number of K-shell edge-level photons for single-phase generators.

The reason rare-earth phosphors are more efficient is because they take advantage of the increased absorption of x-ray photons after the K-shell edge. Figure 20–8 compares the absorption of both calcium tungstate and rare-earth phosphors. The range of increased efficiency due to the K-shell edge is highlighted. This increased efficiency range is approximately 35–70 keV (roughly equivalent to 40–75 kVp). However, there is not a linear relationship when comparing the speed of calcium-tungstate and rare-earth phosphors (Figure 20–9). Therefore it is important not to assume that one set of intensifying screens is twice or half as fast as another **across the entire kVp range**. Especially at lower kVps, this relationship may not hold true.

Asymmetrical Screens

Extremely efficient intensifying screens may require that they be used as matched pairs. When the conversion efficiency is very high, significantly

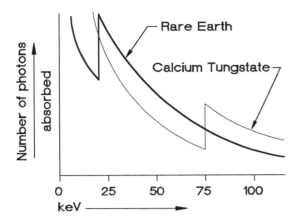

Figure 20–8. The increased efficiency range of rare-earth phosphors due to the K-shell edge effect.

Figure 20–9. The approximate kVp dependence of the relative speed of calcium tungstate and gadolinium-oxysulfide intensifying screens. (By permission of John Stears, Joel Gray, and Eugene Frank, Mayo Foundation, Rochester, MN.)

more light is emitted by the top screen than the bottom one. To compensate for the top side of the film being overexposed and the bottom underexposed, the top screen may be thinner to equalize the light emission between the screens. These types of screens are provided with labels for top and bottom. If they are in-

stalled improperly, a significant loss of screen speed results.

Contrast and Latitude

Intensifying screen contrast and latitude are insignificant factors because most phosphors have a relatively linear conversion efficiency except for their K-shell edges. Film contrast and latitude are much more critical because of the nonlinear shape of the D log E curve. A slight improvement in screen contrast is achieved by the use of antihalation crossover dyes in the screens, but their use remains primarily with film base and emulsion. However, the effect of intensifying screens on image contrast is so slight as to be negligible.

CASSETTES AND HOLDERS

Cassettes and holders are designed to create a portable, light proof case for film, to utilize the intensifying screens to best advantage and to attenuate the residual x-ray beam as much as possible (Figure 20–10). A wide variety of sizes and types of cassettes are available. Originally, direct exposure film was exposed in a cardboard holder, which is simply a light proof container. Today there are numerous specialty cassettes available, such as curved cassettes and cassettes designed for specialty equipment, such as panoramic facial units.

Characteristics

The front of the cassette must be uniformly radiolucent to eliminate artifacts, rigid to provide good support for body parts and lightweight. The intensifying screens are attached to the inside of the front and back of the cassette. At least one must be mounted on a foam pressure pad to provide good contact between the screens and the film. The back must be rigid and lightweight and may also include a sheet of lead foil to reduce the residual beam

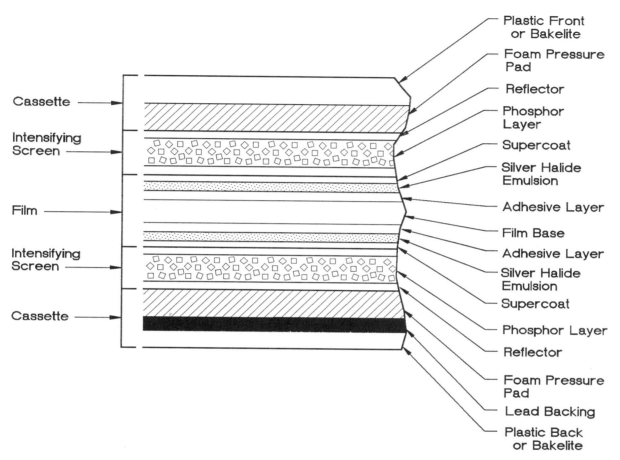

Figure 20–10. A typical radiographic cassette.

and absorb backscatter. Backscatter is a significant problem with large body parts, especially in hypersthenic chest and abdomen examinations. It is caused when the incident beam is of such magnitude that enough backscatter is produced from behind the cassette to form a second image (Figure 20–11). The lead sheet must be minimal in cassettes designed to be used with automatic exposure controls (AECs).

Extremely low-attenuation graphite carbon fiber materials are sometimes used for cassettes, grid interspaces and tables when low-energy photons may be carrying critical information. Computed tomography and angiography tables, grids and cassettes are examples. Although expensive, graphite can reduce attenuation by up to 50 percent and permit a corresponding reduction in patient exposure dose.

Eastman Kodak introduced the X-Omatic™ cassette (Figure 20–12) in the 1970s. This cassette was a significant improvement in film-screen contact, beam attenuation and weight. X-Omatic™ cassettes are manufactured

Figure 20–11. Backscatter forming an image of a cassette hinge. This resulted from lack of collimation, which permitted the remnant beam to strike a wall and backscatter through the back of the cassette onto the film (Courtesy of Eugene Frank, Mayo Foundation, Rochester, MN.)

with a slight curve, thus causing squeegeeing of air as they are closed and eliminating the air pockets that cause poor film/screen contact. The cassettes are made of lightweight plastic with excellent radiolucent qualities. A thin sheet of lead foil in the back of the cassette is designed to eliminate residual scatter. The lead foil absorbs sufficient scatter to permit the cassette to be used backwards as a no-line grid. Specialized mammography cassettes are available with polystyrene fronts for low attenuation and thin sides to permit film edges to demonstrate chest wall tissues.

CARE

Loading and Storage

When loading cassettes, the tops should never be fully open in order to prevent dust and condensation from accumulating and to prevent the formation of the artifacts they cause on the radiograph. The cassette top should be opened slightly; 2–3 inches or 6–8 cm is enough for the experienced darkroom technician to unload and load any cassette.

Cassettes should be stored on end like a book and empty of film. Because of the frequency of cassette use, nearly all radiography departments observe the first recommendation, but not the second.

Cleaning

Intensifying screens and cassettes should be cleaned regularly. They must not be cleaned with tap water or any cleaning solution not specifically designed for intensifying screens. Most commercial firms offer an electrostatic cleaning solution that will not leave mineral stains, will not become sticky (resulting in damage when screens stick to film or to one another after cleaning) and discourages static electricity that could discharge and expose film.

SUMMARY

Intensifying screens produce large quantities of light photons when struck by x-rays, thereby amplifying the incoming x-ray beam and reducing patient radiation dose. Over 99 percent of the latent image is formed by light from the screens, with less than one percent being contributed by x-ray photons.

An intensifying screen consists of a base, reflective layer, phosphor layer and protective coat. The base is usually made of polyester plastic and serves to hold the phosphor layer. The reflective layer is added to increase the amount of light reaching the film. The phosphor layer is the active, light emitting layer of the screen and the protective coat protects the phosphor layer from abrasions.

The phosphors used in intensifying screens must have a high atomic number,

Figure 20–12.   The Eastman Kodak X-Omatic™ cassette.

high conversion efficiency, appropriate spectral emission and minimal fluorescence. Luminescence is the ability of a material to emit light in response to excitation. The two types of luminescence are fluorescence and phosphorescence.

A variety of phosphor materials have been used in radiography. The most popular of the phosphors are the rare earths.

Intensifying screens exhibit the same characteristics as film: resolution, speed, contrast and latitude. Resolution and speed are affected by phosphor crystal size, layer thickness and the concentration of the crystals. Contrast and latitude are relatively insignificant factors.

Cassettes and holders are designed to create a portable, light proof case for the film, to utilize the intensifying screens to best advantage and to attenuate the residual x-ray beam as much as possible. Cassettes should never be fully open when loading and unloading film. Both cassettes and intensifying screens should be cleaned regularly.

REVIEW QUESTIONS

1. How do intensifying screens reduce patient dose?

2. What are the four basic components of an intensifying screen?

3. What characteristics should an intensifying screen phosphor possess?

4. What is the difference between fluorescence and phosphorescence?

5. What is the relationship between resolution and phosphor crystal size, layer thickness and phosphor concentration?

6. What is quantum mottle?

7. What is the difference between calcium tungstate screens and rare-earth screens in terms of x-ray beam absorption?

8. What is the purpose of a cassette?

REFERENCES AND RECOMMENDED READING

A cassette problem. *Radiologic Technology* 57:3, 247, 1986.

Ardran, G. M., H. E. Crooks, and V. James. Testing x-ray cassettes for film-intensifying screen contact. *Radiography* 35:414, 143, 1969.

Burgess, A. E., and P. Hicken. Comparative performance of x-ray intensifying screens. *Radiology* May, 55, 1982.

Carroll, Quinn. *Fuchs's Principles of Radiographic Exposure, Processing, and Quality Control*. 3rd ed. Springfield, IL: Charles C. Thomas Publisher, 1985.

Cullinan, Angeline M. *Producing Quality Radiographs*. Philadelphia, PA: J. B. Lippincott, 1987.

Curry, Thomas S., James E. Dowdey, and Robert C. Murry. *Christensen's Introduction to the Physics of Diagnostic Radiology*. 3rd ed. Philadelphia, PA: Lea & Febiger, 1984.

Davies, Jackie, and J. G. B. Russell. Carbon fibre faced cassettes in neonatal radiography: Their use and cost effectiveness. *Radiography* 52:603, 113, 1986.

Doi, Kunio, Len-Nien Loo, T. McDowell Anderson, and Paul H. Frank. Effect of cross-over exposure on radiographic image quality of screen-film systems. *Radiology* 139, 707–714, 1981.

Fuchs, Arthur W. Evolution of Roentgen film. *The American Journal of Roentgenology and Radium Therapy* 75:1, 30–48, 1956.

Fuchs, Arthur W. Edison and roentgenology. *The American Journal of Roentgenology and Radium Therapy* 57:2, 145–156, 1947.

Gray, Joel, Norlin Winkler, John Stears, and Eugene Frank. *Quality Control in Diagnostic Imaging: A Quality Control Cookbook*. Baltimore, MD: University Park Press, 1983.

Hiss, Stephen S. What we should know about x-ray intensifying screens. *Radiologic Technology* 43:3, 117, 1971.

Hufton, A. P., C. M. Crosthwaite, J. M. Davies, and L. A. Robinson. Low attenuation material for table tops, cassettes, and grids: A review. *Radiography* 53:607, 17, 1987.

Jenkins, David. *Radiographic Photography and Imaging Processes*. Lancaster, England: MTP Press Limited, 1980.

Kodera, Yoshie, Kunio Doi, and Hwang-Ping Chan. Absolute speeds of screen-film systems and their absorbed-energy constants. *Radiology* 151 229–236, 1984.

McKinney, William. *Radiographic Processing and Quality Control*. Philadelphia, PA: J. B. Lippincott, 1988.

Morgan, Russell H. Roentgenoscopic screen intensification. *Radiologic Technology* 25:2, 80, 1953.

Ritter, Ethel M. Use of gradient intensifying screen for scoliosis radiography. *Radiology* April, 230, 1980.

Roberts, Derrick P., and Nigel L. Smith. *Radiographic Imaging: A Practical Approach*. Edinburgh: Churchill Livingstone, 1988.

Roehrig, Hans, Sol Nudelman, and Tao-Yi Fu. Electro-optical devices for use in photo-electronic-digital radiology. *Electronic Imaging in Medicine*. 82–129. Editors: Fullerton, Gary D., William R. Hendee, John C. Lasher, William S. Properzio, and Stephan J. Riederer. New York: American Institute of Physics for the American Association of Physicists in Medicine, 1984.

Shearer, Douglas R., and Marleen M. Moore. Lag in radiographic imaging systems: Simple methods for evaluation. *Radiology* 159:1, 259–263, 1986.

Sklensky, A. F., R. A. Buchanan, T. G. Maple, and H. N. Bailey. Quantum utilization in x-ray intensifying screens. *The Institute of Electrical and Electronics Engineers Transactions on Nuclear Science* 21, 685–691, 1974.

Sprawls, Perry. *Principles of Radiography for Technologists*. Rockville, MD: Aspen Publishers, 1990.

Sprawls, Perry. *Physical Principles of Medical Imaging*. Rockville, MD: Aspen Publishers, 1987.

Stears, John G., Joel E. Gray, and Eugene D. Frank. New intensifying screens—twice the speed? *Radiologic Technology* 58:4, 345–346, 1987.

Sturm, Ralph E., and Russell H. Morgan. Screen intensification systems and their limitations. *The American Journal of Roentgenology and Radium Therapy* 62:5, 617–634, 1949.

Sweeney, Richard J. *Radiographic Artifacts: Their Cause and Control*. Philadelphia, PA: J. B. Lippincott, 1983.

Trout, E. Dale, and John P. Kelley. The effect of the temperature of intensifying screens on radiographic exposure. *Radiologic Technology* 45: 2, 70–72, 1973.

van der Plaats, G. J. *Medical X-Ray Techniques in Diagnostic Radiology: A Textbook for Radiographers and Radiological Technicians*. 4th ed. The Hague: Martinus Nijhoff Publishers, 1980.

Wilson, Peter. Principles of intensifying screens in image formation. *Canadian Journal of Radiography, Radiotherapy, and Nuclear Medicine* 8:3, 134–140, 1977.

THE CASE OF THE WHITE SNAKES

What is the most likely cause of these white snakelike structures circling the upper corner of the patient's abdomen?

Answers to the case studies can be found in Appendix E.

21 FILM/SCREEN COMBINATIONS

Mr. Edison has discovered . . . tungstate of calcium . . . [with which] you can see other people's bones with the naked eye. . . . On the revolting indecency of this there is no need to dwell. But what we seriously put before the attention of the Government is that the moment tungstate of calcium comes into anything like general use, it will call for legislative restriction of the severest kind.

Pall Mall Gazette, March 1896.

OUTLINE

EMISSION SPECTRA
CHARACTERISTICS
SELECTING FILM/SCREEN COMBINATIONS
CLINICAL CHOICES

OBJECTIVES

Upon completion of this chapter, the student should be able to:

1. Relate the emission spectra of various intensifying screens to specific types of radiographic film.
2. Explain radiographic film/screen combination relative speed numbering systems.
3. Calculate relative speed conversions from one film/screen combination to another.
4. Describe various methods of measuring resolution, including a basic description of line pairs per millimeter, line spread function and modulation transfer function.
5. Relate film/screen contrast to latitude.
6. Determine appropriate film/screen combinations for various clinical situations.

Radiographic film and intensifying screens are designed to complement each other and to produce the highest quality image with the lowest patient radiation dose. Film and screens must be matched to each other to achieve diagnostic quality images. If the screens have been designed to emit a specific wavelength, then the film must be designed to have enhanced sensitivity to the same wavelength. **Mismatching of film and screens often increases patient exposure dose.**

EMISSION SPECTRA

The spectral emissions of intensifying screen phosphors and radiographic films are shown in Figure 21–1. Note that blue sensitive film will not respond to most of the wavelengths emitted by the rare-earth phosphors. However, green sensitive film is more sensitive to the entire range of phosphor emissions, including the yellow-green wavelengths. Note also that green sensitive film is not quite as sensitive to the blue-violet wavelengths as the

blue sensitive film. The spectral emission colors for various brands of intensifying screens are shown in Table 20–1.

The appropriate film/screen combination for a specific clinical situation must be selected based on the combined qualities of the film and the screen. Clinical selection cannot be accomplished by evaluating film and intensifying screens separately. The qualities that must be considered are **speed, resolution, contrast and latitude**. Film/screen combination relationships are the same as the interrelationships of these factors for film (see Table 19–2). The most common decision that must be made when selecting film/screen combinations is image resolution versus patient exposure dose.

Figure 21–1. Light sensitivity of various films and intensifying screens. Note that blue sensitive films are not sensitive to the major rare-earth light emissions. (Reprinted with permission from Robert A. Buchanan, "An improved x-ray intensifying screen." *IEEE Transactions on Nuclear Science* © 1972 IEEE.)

CHARACTERISTICS

The important characteristics of film/screen combinations are **speed, resolution, contrast and latitude**.

Speed

The speed of an imaging system depends on the **thickness of the layer** of phosphor or silver halide, the crystal size and the **efficiency** of the crystal in emitting (in the case of intensifying screens) or capturing (in the case of silver halides) photons.

Commercial firms use relative speed (RS) numbers to rate film/screen combinations. The numbers are not quantitative and represent no units. They are based on a relative value of 100 for calcium tungstate intensifying screens used with a medium contrast and latitude blue sensitive film. This was the standard film/screen combination known as par or medium speed before the advent of rare-earth screens. Each manufacturer tends to calibrate film/screen combinations to its own brand of calcium tungstate medium-speed standard. However, it has been suggested that the base RS 100 be calibrated equal to 1.28 mR to produce the film speed point (OD 1.00 + base + fog). **Relative speed numbers are usually established at 70–80 kVp, with 80 kVp preferred**. When kVp values below 70 or above 100 are used, RS numbers may be less consistent. Therefore the relationship between the RS number and the sensitivity of the film/screen combination is established by the following formula:

$$\text{Sensitivity in mR} = \frac{1.28}{\text{RS}}$$

Table 21–1 shows the relationship of RS number to the sensitivity in mR to produce the film speed point.

Relative speed (RS) numbers are accurate enough to be used by radiographers to convert

TABLE 21–1
RELATIONSHIP BETWEEN RELATIVE SPEED NUMBER AND EXPOSURE SENSITIVITY

RS Number	Exposure Sensitivity in mR
1200	0.10
800	0.16
400	0.32
200	0.64
100	1.28
50	2.56
25	5.00
12	10.00

Reprinted with permission from *Physical Principles of Medical Imaging* by P. Sprawls, Aspen Publishers, Inc., © 1987, p. 198.

exposure technique settings from one situation to another. The formula for converting mAs from one relative speed to another is:

$$\frac{\text{mAs}_1}{\text{mAs}_2} = \frac{\text{RS}_2}{\text{RS}_1}$$

where mAs_1 = old mAs

mAs_2 = new mAs

RS_1 = old relative speed

RS_2 = new relative speed

The most common problem is to determine a new mAs for use with a relative speed that is different from the one for which an acceptable technique is known. To determine a new mAs, the following version is used:

$$\text{mAs}_2 = \frac{\text{RS}_1 \times \text{mAs}_1}{\text{RS}_2}$$

Example: What is the proper mAs for use with a 400 RS system when technical factors of 80 kVp and 50 mAs produce an acceptable image with a 200 RS system?

Answer:

$$\frac{mAs_1}{mAs_2} = \frac{RS_2}{RS_1}$$

$$\frac{50}{mAs_2} = \frac{400}{200}$$

$$mAs_2 \times 400 = 50 \text{ mAs} \times 200$$

$$mAs_2 \times 400 = 10,000 \text{ mAs}$$

$$mAs_2 = \frac{10,000 \text{ mAs}}{400}$$

$$mAs_2 = 25 \text{ mAs}$$

Example: What is the proper mAs for use with a 250 RS system when technical factors of 80 kVp and 50 mAs produce an acceptable image with an 800 RS system?

Answer:

$$\frac{mAs_1}{mAs_2} = \frac{RS_2}{RS_1}$$

$$\frac{50}{mAs_2} = \frac{250}{800}$$

$$mAs_2 \times 250 = 50 \text{ mAs} \times 800$$

$$mAs_2 \times 250 = 40,000 \text{ mAs}$$

$$mAs_2 = \frac{40,000 \text{ mAs}}{250}$$

$$mAs_2 = 160 \text{ mAs}$$

Film/screen combinations are available from RS 20 to RS 1,200, with an RS 400 combination the most common compromise between patient exposure dose and resolution. Although not an absolute relationship, for the most part higher RS numbers reduce patient exposure dose, decrease latitude and decrease resolution. Film/screen combinations to RS 1,800 have been produced but are not available due to unacceptable image quality.

Resolution

Recorded detail, sharpness and resolution are measured as **line pairs per millimeter** (**lp/mm** or cycles per mm), **line spread function** (**LSF**), and **modulation transfer function** (**MTF**).

Line Pairs Per Millimeter Line pairs per millimeter, or cycles per millimeter, measures the minimum size and space between objects that can be visualized on the final image.

Line Spread Function The line spread function (LSF) measures the ability of a film/screen system to accurately measure the boundaries of an image. It is calculated by using a microdensitometer to measure the ability of the image receptor to record a line from a 10 μm wide beam of radiation. A typical film/screen system might display density from a 10 μm line over 600–800 μm.

Modulation Transfer Function The modulation transfer function (MTF) provides the best measurement of the resolving ability of a film/screen combination. It measures the information lost between the subject and the image receptor. There are no units of MTF. The MTF is determined primarily by the amount of light diffusion that occurs between the screens and the film. The MTF is primarily controlled by the chemical composition of the screen, phosphor crystal size, thickness of the phosphor layer, absorbing dye and, most important, by film/screen contact. Therefore MTF is a function of the screens because the resolving power of film is far superior to that of the intensifying screens. The intensifying screens impose the resolution limitations on the film/screen system.

The MTF is sometimes presented as a formula:

$$MTF = \frac{\text{Recorded Detail (Resolution)}}{\text{Available Detail (Resolution)}}$$

A perfect MTF would be 1.0. Therefore MTFs are less than 1.0 because more information cannot be recorded than what is available. An MTF curve plots MTF against resolution (lp/mm) (Figure 21–2). Faster film/screen combinations

Figure 21–2. MTF versus lp/mm for several different film/screen combinations. (Reprinted from Kunio Doi, *MTF's and Wiener Spectra of Radiographic Screen-Film Systems*. HHS Publication FDA 82–8187.)

exhibit an obvious decrease in resolution when compared to the detail combinations.

Contrast

Contrast is primarily the contrast of the film, although intensifying screens, especially the rare earths, also exhibit contrast. The effect of higher contrast that is achieved when lower kVp can be used due to higher speed screens is often overlooked. In addition, the rare-earth phosphors often exhibit slightly higher contrast.

Latitude

The film/screen system latitude is primarily dependent upon the latitude of the film, which is directly related to the contrast. Higher speed film/screen systems often exhibit lower contrast and wider latitude.

SELECTING FILM/SCREEN COMBINATIONS

The selection of appropriate film/screen combinations requires consideration of the various film and screen characteristics. For exam-

ple, Figure 21–3 illustrates the differences between two types of screens and three types of film. The radiographs on the left were produced with detail screens while those on the right were produced with high speed screens. The top row of radiographs were produced with a general-purpose film, the middle row with a wide-latitude film and the bottom row with a high-contrast film. The exposure factors were adjusted to maintain a consistent density. Variations in resolution can be seen by comparing the resolution tools from the right column with those from the left. Variations in contrast can be seen by comparing the number of steps visible on the penetrometer from the top, middle and bottom rows.

CLINICAL CHOICES

Film and intensifying screen manufacturers publish film/screen combination charts that compare all possible combinations of their films and intensifying screens. These charts often highlight the RS numbers and provide commentary on appropriate clinical uses and the image quality factors (speed, resolution, contrast and latitude).

Figure 21–3. Differences between two types of screens and three types of film. The radiographs on the left were produced with detail screens while those on the right were produced with high speed screens. The top row of radiographs were produced with a general purpose film, the middle row with a wide latitude film and the bottom row with a high contrast film.

Figure 21–4. Absorption efficiency of various intensifying screen phosphors. Note that although rare earths are significantly more efficient between 40–70 keV, calcium tungstate is slightly more efficient above 70 keV. (Reprinted with permission from A. F. Sklensky, R. A. Buchanan, T. G. Maple, and H. N. Bailey, ''Quantum utilization in x-ray intensifying screens.'' *IEEE Transactions on Nuclear Science* © 1974 IEEE.)

Various types of intensifying screen phosphors are more efficient at various kVp levels (Figure 21–4). These factors must be considered when selecting combinations for various clinical situations. The primary advantages and disadvantages of rare-earth film/screen combinations are shown in Table 21–2.

The objectives of high-quality images and reduced patient exposure are well within the focus of modern film/screen combination technology. However, this depends considerably on the appropriate choice of film/screen combination for specific clinical situations.

Angiography

Rare-earth film/screen combinations were immediately recognized for their value in angiographic studies. The advantage of decreased patient exposure while maintaining image resolution is obvious when short exposure times are critical at the same time that numerous exposures are required, resulting in high total exposure. Because angiography produces high subject contrast between injected vessels and surrounding tissues, quantum mottle noise is less of a problem than in other studies.

Gastrointestinal and Urologic Radiography

Both gastrointestinal and urologic examinations are procedures in which high subject contrast permits the use of high speed rare-earth film/screen combinations. High subject contrast often permits higher quantum mottle noise ratios without objectionable interference with the diagnostic information of the image.

TABLE 21–2	
ADVANTAGES AND DISADVANTAGES OF RARE-EARTH FILM/SCREEN COMBINATIONS	
Advantages	**Disadvantages**
Reduced patient exposure dose	Increased quantum mottle noise
Reduced staff exposure dose	Increased cost
	kVp influences efficiency
Increased tube life	
Use of lower power generators	
Reduced patient motion	
Reduced kVp (while maintaining contrast)	
Reduced mA (while maintaining focal spot size)	

Abdominal Radiography

Faster calcium tungstate or slower rare-earth systems have been suggested for abdominal radiography because of low subject contrast, which requires reducing quantum mottle noise.

Skeletal Radiography

Skeletal examinations are usually divided into extremity examinations, in which detail film/screen combinations are very desirable due to the subtle differences that provide clues to some pathologies. Pelvic and lumbar examinations present totally different problems because of large subject thickness and the less subtle nature of regional pathologies.

Chest Radiography

High kVp chest radiography (>100 kVp) is achieved more efficiently with calcium tungstate film/screen combinations than with rare earths.

Pediatric Radiography

Pediatric examinations are also prime candidates for higher-speed film/screen combinations because large portions of the body are often included within the primary-beam field, effects of the radiation exposure will be carried longer and motion is the primary imaging problem for the radiographer.

SUMMARY

Radiographic film and intensifying screens are designed to complement each other and to produce the highest quality image with the lowest patient radiation dose. To accomplish this, film and screens must be matched to each other, especially with regard to their emission spectra. Mismatching of film and screens increases patient exposure dose.

The qualities that must be considered in a film/screen combination are speed, resolution, contrast and latitude. The most frequent decision that must be made when selecting film/screen combinations is image resolution versus patient exposure dose.

Commercial firms use relative speed (RS) numbers to rate film/screen combinations. The formula for converting mAs from one relative speed to another is:

$$\frac{mAs_1}{mAs_2} = \frac{RS_2}{RS_1}$$

Recorded detail, sharpness and resolution are measured as line pairs per millimeter (lp/mm or cycles per mm), line spread function (LSF), and modulation transfer function (MTF). Contrast is primarily the contrast of the film, although intensifying screens, especially the rare earths, also affect contrast. The film/screen system latitude is primarily dependent upon the latitude of the film. The selection of appropriate film/screen combinations requires consideration of the various film and screen characteristics and of the clinical situation for which they are to be used.

REVIEW QUESTIONS

1. What are the emission spectra of calcium tungstate and rare-earth intensifying screens?

2. What is the formula used to calculate a relative speed conversion from one film/screen combination to another?

3. What are the three methods of measuring resolution?

4. How is film/screen contrast related to latitude?

5. What clinical situation(s) would justify the use of a detail speed film/screen combination?

6. What clinical situation(s) would justify the use of a high-speed film/screen combination?

REFERENCES AND RECOMMENDED READING

Braun, Michael, and Brian C. Wilson. Comparative evaluation of several rare-earth film-screen systems. *Radiology* 144, 915, 1982.

Burgess, A. E., and P. Hicken. Comparative performance of x-ray intensifying screens. *Radiology* May, 55, 1982.

Curry, Thomas S., James E. Dowdey, and Robert C. Murry. *Christensen's Introduction to the Physics of Diagnostic Radiology.* 3rd ed. Philadelphia, PA: Lea & Febiger, 1984.

Doi, Kunio, Gunnila Holje, Leh-Nien Loo, and Heang-Ping Chan. *MTF's and Wiener Spectra of Radiographic Screen-Film Systems.* United States Department of Health and Human Services, Public Health Service, Food and Drug Administration, Bureau of Radiological Health: HHS Publication FDA 82-8187, 1982.

Gratal, Peter, Charles Burns, and Judy Murray. Advantages of a 400 speed image receptor system for cast radiography. *Radiologic Technology* 58:5, 401, 1987.

Haus, Arthur G., and John E. Cullinan. Screen film processing systems for medical radiography: A historical review. *Radiographics* 9:6, 1203–1224, 1989.

Higashida, Yoshiharu, Paul H. Frank, and Kunio Doi. High-speed, single-screen/single-emulsion film systems: Basic imaging properties and preliminary clinical applications. *Radiology* Nov., 571, 1983.

Jans, Ronald G. The status of film/screen mammography. *Radiology* July, 197, 1979.

Kodera, Yoshie, Kunio Doi, and Heang-Ping Chan. Absolute speeds of screen-film systems and their absorbed-energy constants. *Radiology* 151, 229–236, 1984.

New screen speed convention. *Radiologic Technology* 58:1, 73, 1986.

Rao, Gopala U. V., William Witt, Michael C. Beachley, Herman A. Bosch, Panos P. Fatouros, and Philip T. Kan. Radiographic films and screen-film systems. *The Physical Basis of Medical Imaging.* Editors: Coulam, Craig M., John J. Erickson, F. David Rollo, and A. Everette James, Jr. New York: Appleton-Century-Crofts, 1981.

Rossi, R. P., W. R. Hendee, and C. R. Aherns. An evaluation of rare-earth screen-film combinations. *Radiology* 121, 465, 1976.

Sprawls, Perry. *Principles of Radiography for Technologists.* Rockville, MD: Aspen, 1990.

Sprawls, Perry. *Physical Principles of Medical Imaging*. Rockville, MD: Aspen, 1987.

Taylor, K. W., B. P. McLeich, B. B. Hobbs, and T. J. Hughes. Selection of screen-film combinations. *The Canadian Journal of Medical Radiation Technology* 11:3, 154, 1980.

Thompson, Thomas T. Selecting medical x-ray film. *Applied Radiology* 3, 47–51, 1974.

U.S. Department of Health, Education, and Welfare, Food and Drug Administration. Bureau of Radiological Health. *First Image Receptor Conference: Film/Screen Combinations*. Washington, D.C.: HEW Publication FDA 77–8003, 1976.

Venema, Hank W. X-ray absorption speed and luminescent efficiency of rare-earth and other intensifying screens. *Radiology* March, 765, 1979.

Vyborny, Carl J. Relative efficiencies of energy to photographic density conversions in typical screen-film systems. *Radiology* 136, 465, 1980.

THE CASE OF LUMPY

(Reprinted by permission of the International Society of Radiographers and Radiological Technicians from the K. C. Clark Archives, Middlesex Hospital, London, England)

What is this lumpy object's name?

Answers to the case studies can be found in Appendix E.

UNIT III: ANALYZING THE IMAGE

The ability of the radiographer to analyze a radiographic image brings his or her professional skills to their highest level. The process of analyzing demands a thorough knowledge of the scientific basis by which the image was produced, as well as a significant amount of clinical experience. When these skills are applied to a problem solving technique, the result is the process of diagnosis. The radiographer diagnoses the image exactly as the physician diagnoses pathology. This unit is designed to provide the analytical abilities in both diagnosis and treatment that make the radiographer an image expert.

Before attempting to diagnose the quality of the image, it is important that the radiographer **establish imaging standards**, including a diagnostic problem-solving technique. It is then important to explore each of the properties which affect radiographic quality in depth to examine their controlling and influencing factors, their effect on the appearance of the image, and to determine how to assess them and how to make adjustment properly.

Separate chapters on **density, contrast, recorded detail and distortion** explore these elements. When a diagnostic process is applied to all of the properties together, an artistic skill in image evaluation results. A system that utilizes this process is presented as the **art of film critique**.

Finally, it is the responsibility of the radiographer to monitor and evaluate the performance of all radiographic equipment. This is accomplished through the process of **quality control**.

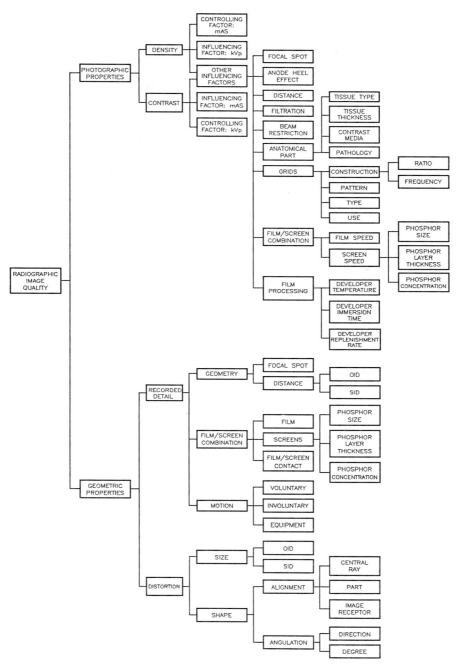

RADIOGRAPHIC IMAGE QUALITY FLOW CHART

22 ESTABLISHING IMAGING STANDARDS

[A] requirement of radiography when it is to be practiced as a personal art is the deliberate deviation from "average values." The practice of deviating from average values, settings, measurements, etc. is the mark of the successful professional man in almost any field, and is the principle reason for the esteem he enjoys in his community. His services are sought because he knows how and when to deviate from a standard solution of a problem.

Gerhart S. Schwarz, M.D., inventor of the XVS Unit-Step Radiography System.

OUTLINE

PROFESSIONAL IMAGING STANDARDS
THE ANALYTICAL PROCESS
ACCEPTANCE LIMITS

OBJECTIVES

Upon completion of this chapter, the student should be able to:

1. Describe the pyramid problem of geometrical progression as it relates to radiographic image quality.
2. Apply the four steps of the diagnostic process to a clinical imaging problem.
3. Explain how image acceptance limits may fluctuate due to various external factors.

PROFESSIONAL IMAGING STANDARDS

Just as all professionals are expected to adhere to the technical and ethical standards of their field, so radiographers are expected to establish personal imaging standards which satisfy the diagnostic needs of the radiologist and the quality needs of the supervisor. Additionally, they must not violate the personal ethical standards of radiation protection and patient care. Everyone makes mistakes, but professionals are able to correct their mistakes by using a careful analytical process to determine exactly what went wrong. In radiography, emphasis must be placed on learning how to look at images critically.

The Pyramid Problem

A major roadblock in overcoming complex problems such as establishing imaging standards is sometimes called the **pyramid**

353

problem. An acceptable radiograph is the result of a multitude of factors, including technical factor selection, subject density, contrast, pathology and film processing. Unfortunately, some factors can act upon each other, thus creating a pyramid of problems for the radiographer. When many factors are acting upon each other, the result is an astronomical number of possibilities.

THE ANALYTICAL PROCESS

Diagnosing and Treating the Image

Anyone working in a clinical setting quickly becomes acquainted with the process of medical diagnosis. Determining the cause of a problem is a fascinating process. Most medical professionals would welcome an opportunity to participate in this process but they are restricted by law. In fact, the *Scope of Practice of the American Registry of Radiologic Technologists* states "under no circumstances (shall a radiographer) give out oral or written diagnoses." However, the diagnosis of technical problems in the imaging process requires the same skills that a physician uses in medical diagnosis.

Physicians are experts in the science of anatomy and physiology. Radiologists are physicians who are expert in the art of diagnosing through anatomical images as well. But even radiologists are not trained in the finer points of creating and analyzing the image. In this area the radiographer is the true professional expert. The diagnosis and treatment of image quality is the domain of the radiography profession and radiographers are eminently qualified to practice this art and science.

The Diagnostic Process

A knowledge of the diagnostic process is necessary for the radiographer to diagnose and treat the image. The secret to solving any pyramid problem is a careful and meticulous breakdown of the whole into individual parts. The difference between being good and being great is often only a matter of attention to detail. Taking time to break down and analyze technical problems permits proper diagnosis to occur. When properly followed, the diagnostic process makes the treatment clear. Diagnosis involves the highest level of mental acuity. It requires the use of the skills of analysis, synthesis and evaluation to solve complex problems. A diagnostic problem-solving strategy includes four major steps.

Narrowing the Search Field The first phase involves **narrowing the search**. Experts begin with a review of the entire image to avoid premature narrowing. During this review a search is made for anything that is different from a diagnostic quality image. When differences are noticed a pattern is sought, especially when there is more than one cue. These cues focus attention on a suspicious area, thus narrowing the search. An example would be a film that looks light, gray and blurred. An inexperienced radiographer might jump to the conclusion that the image was too light and there was motion. However, an expert radiographer might notice additional cues, such as the loss of detail confined to a small region and proper film density in other areas.

Hypothesis Activation The second phase requires that the cues be used to **seek hypotheses**. An effort is made to formulate a hypothesis that will explain all the cues. Cues that do not fit the hypothesis should be held in reserve. In the example, the inexperienced radiographer might hypothesize that too little radiation was used and that the patient was breathing. The expert would realize that many hypotheses could account for the image, including several cases of "too little radiation," such as insufficient kVp, mA or time, excessive distance and improper film, screens or processing. They would also include several explanations for a blurred image, such as poor film/screen contact, increased object-to-image receptor distance and tube motion, as well as the patient motion hypothesis.

Information Seeking The next phase demands that the hypotheses be tested by **seeking more information**. When stumped, radiographers should use general questioning to produce more cue information. It may be necessary to shift focus to other possible solutions when new cues are discovered. In the example, the novice radiographer might ask the patient if she held her breath. When the patient answers "yes," the novice radiographer might not believe her, rather than reject the hypothesis of patient motion. The expert, on the other hand, might notice during the questioning of the patient that her breast was superimposed over the area of interest. This additional cue could be used to return to the image. A new look at the film might show that the light grayness was confined to the breast region.

Hypothesis Evaluation The last phase of the diagnostic process is the **evaluation of the final hypothesis**. It is critical that the hypothesis used resolves the greatest amount of cue data. At this point the radiographer should be able to predict the solution to the problem. The inexperienced radiographer would apply the "too little radiation and patient motion" hypothesis and reduce the mAs while watching the patient closely. The expert radiographer would conclude that the most likely hypothesis was increased subject density, decreased subject contrast and poor film/screen contact. The expert would then ask the patient to move the breast aside and use a different cassette with good film/screen contact. Of course, the expert

would produce a diagnostic quality image. The novice would be left with a darker film of even poorer quality than the first one.

Remember, however, data shows that novices often do surprisingly well when using the diagnostic process. Diagnosing ability can be improved by:

1. Remembering that cues are not a diagnosis;
2. Being careful to separate observations from inferences;
3. Not jumping to conclusions at the first cue;
4. Looking for competing hypotheses;
5. Trying each cue with each hypothesis;
6. Validating the hypothesis with questioning, when possible;
7. Ruling out hypotheses one by one;
8. Being cautious of premature closure;
9. Being tentative in the diagnosis until experienced; and, most important,
10. **Being confident in your expert knowledge**.

ACCEPTANCE LIMITS

Knowing how to diagnose an imaging problem is not helpful until the knowledge can be applied to radiographic quality analysis. This application involves establishing and adhering to quality imaging standards.

Graphing Acceptance Limits

The main goal must be to fix the limits of the radiographs that will be accepted against those that will not. This is much easier to understand by looking at the concept of acceptance limits graphically. The quality (in density and contrast) of all the radiographs produced by a technologist over a period have been graphed in Figure 22–1.

Although the radiographer's goal is to always produce a diagnostic quality image, sub-

Figure 22–1. Radiographic image quality distribution curve. Note that the curve is skewed to the dark side. Standard practice dictates that a dark or low contrast image is always preferable to one that is too light or high contrast.

Figure 22–2. Typical acceptance limits of radiographic quality.

optimal radiographs are often accepted for diagnosis. There are many reasons for this practice, the most important being the knowledge that the prime cause of increased patient radiation dose is repeated exposure. Radiologists do not expect textbook results on every patient. They do, however, have the right to expect the radiographer to provide an image that permits them to see all the structures critical to their diagnosis. Figure 22–2 shows where a typical radiologist might draw the line on dark or low and light or high films. The important thing to remember is that if the radiographer, supervisor, radiologist or other physician determines that an image is not acceptable, **it is outside the acceptance limits of quality**. When this occurs, the radiographer is obligated to analyze the image and make a proper decision on what factor or factors caused the error. The technique and procedure must then be adjusted to bring the unacceptable film back to the **perfect center** of diagnostic quality.

Striving for Perfection

Too often there is a tendency to correct only enough to obtain a passable image (Figure 22–3). **All corrections should strive for perfection**. Attempting to get by with minimal

Figure 22–3. Correcting image quality.

adjustments contributes to a negative image of the profession. The best radiographer can miscalculate and produce a poor image once, but competency is questioned when a radiographer is repeatedly unable to correct mistakes. The true professional completes the meticulous analysis by making a competent adjustment and achieves near perfection each time an exposure must be repeated.

Factors Affecting Acceptance Limit Curves

It is interesting to consider the factors that may affect the shape of the acceptance limit curve. Figure 22–1 is skewed to the dark or low contrast side because these errors are more acceptable than light or high contrast mistakes. A bright light is capable of revealing information that is obscured on a dark film. However, when a film is too light there is no method to see information that is not present in the emulsion. There are many other factors that can modify the shape of the acceptance curve. When acceptance limits are very narrow, a high repeat rate occurs (Figure 22–4).

However, if the radiographers are not producing many perfect films, the repeat rate will remain high (Figure 22–5) even when acceptance limits are very wide.

An interesting phenomenon has been observed over the years in many radiology departments. When a radiograph is hovering near the acceptance limits for the department, radiographers will often attempt to have it approved by a radiologist known to have wide acceptance limits. Departmental acceptance limits are simply a composite of the limits imposed by each radiologist, supervisor and radiographer in the department. Narrow acceptance limits may cause radiographers to produce more films near perfect center, thus changing the curve shape, as shown in Figure 22–6.

Conversely, wide limits may permit radiographers to become careless and produce fewer films near perfect center, thus changing the curve shape, as shown in Figure 22–5. Many factors can change the shape of the image quality curve. Among them are the positioning and technical abilities of the radiographer,

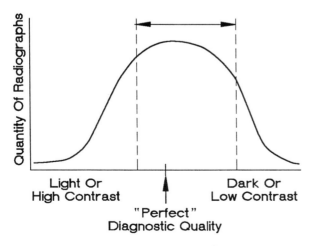

Figure 22–4. Narrow acceptance limits may produce a high repeat rate.

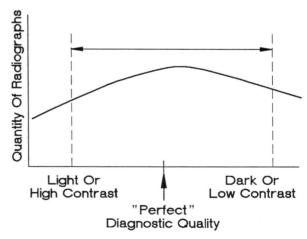

Figure 22–5. Wide acceptance limits may produce a high repeat rate by permitting radiographers to become careless and produce fewer films near perfect center.

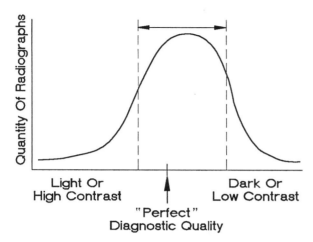

Figure 22–6. Narrow acceptance limits may cause radiographers to produce more films near perfect center.

the quality standards of everyone involved in the imaging chain, the condition of the equipment, the stress level of the department and on and on. Awareness of these factors, combined with high professional standards, can help one's personal curve appear as in Figure 22–7.

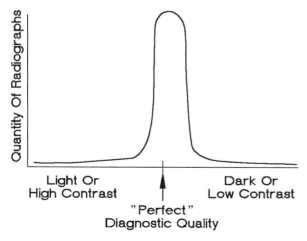

Figure 22–7. Ideal acceptance limits.

Practical Considerations

In actual clinical practice the achievement of a diagnostic quality image the first time is not as hard as it might at first appear. Each factor must be varied within set limits to see a noticeable change in the image. It is important not only to learn the rules pertaining to image quality but to be sure they are used in clinical practice. The real problem is in learning **to make large enough changes to cause visible differences** on the film. Radiographers who are unsure of their ability often make timid changes that cannot be seen in the repeat radiograph. When a decision is made to repeat a procedure (and doubly expose the patient), a change large enough to bring the image to the center of diagnostic quality must be made. Shifting the image from just outside the acceptance limits to just inside them is inexcusable. As professionals, radiographers must always strive toward perfection.

SUMMARY

Professional imaging standards can be established by overcoming the pyramid problem. Evaluating imaging problems is the true professional expertise of the radiographer. The analytical process of diagnosis is appropriate for use in solving these problems. The diagnostic process involves narrowing the search field, hypothesis activation, information seeking and hypothesis evaluation.

The concept of acceptance limits is helpful in understanding how repeated radiographs must be corrected. All repeated radiographs should strive for perfection by attempting to reach the "diagnostic quality" center of the acceptance limit curve. When a decision is made to repeat a procedure, a change large enough to bring the image to the center of diagnostic quality must be made.

REVIEW QUESTIONS

1. What is the pyramid problem?

2. What are the four steps in the diagnostic problem solving strategy?

3. What is the purpose of a cue in narrowing the search?

4. When is an image determined to be outside acceptance limits?

5. Why are acceptance limit curves skewed to the dark side?

REFERENCES AND RECOMMENDED READING

American Registry of Radiologic Technologists. Article I, Section D. *Rules and Regulations as Revised August 1987*. Minneapolis, MN: American Registry of Radiologic Technologists, 1987.

Carlton, Rick, and Arlene McKenna. Repeating radiographs: Setting imaging standards. *Postgraduate Advances in Radiologic Technology.* Berryville, VA: Forum Medicum, Inc., 1989.

Carlton, Richard. Quality Assurance in Radiology. *Introduction to Radiologic Technology.* 2nd ed. Chapter 15, 149–166. Editors: Gurley, LaVerne T., and William J. Callaway. St. Louis, MO: Multi-Media Publishing, Inc., 1986.

Carnevali, Doris L., Pamela H. Mitchell, Nancy F. Woods, and Christine A. Tanner. *Diagnostic Reasoning in Nursing*. Philadelphia, PA: J. B. Lippincott Co., 1984.

Cullinan, John E. A 'perfect' chest radiograph—or a compromise? *Radiologic Technology* 53:2, 121, 1981.

Goldman, Lee W. Effects of film processing variability on patient dose and image quality. *Second Image Receptor Conference: Radiographic Film Processing: Proceedings of a Conference Held in Washington, D.C., March 31–April 2, 1977.* 55–63. Rockville, MD.: U.S. Department of Health, Education, and Welfare, Public Health Service, Food and Drug Administration, Bureau of Radiological Health. HEW Publication FDA 77–8036, 1977.

Mumford, Linda C. Radiographic quality: 'A seminar.' *The Canadian Journal of Medical Radiation Technology* 11:1, 10, 1980.

Prior, John A., Jack S. Silberstein, and John M. Stang. *Physical Diagnosis: The History and Examination of the Patient.* St. Louis, MO: Mosby, 1981.

Singer, Barbara H. The aesthetic method in radiographic exposure. *Radiologic Technology* 42: 6, 411, 1971.

23 DENSITY

Radiographic density and contrast are closely related, but by a careful study of the radiograph they may be readily differentiated and each brought under control.

Ed. C. Jerman, The Father of Radiologic Technology.

OUTLINE

ASSESSING DENSITY
EFFECTS ON IMAGE APPEARANCE
FACTORS AFFECTING DENSITY

OBJECTIVES

Upon completion of this chapter, the student should be able to:

1. Identify density as a prime component of the photographic properties controlling visibility of detail of radiographic image quality.
2. Define density.
3. Describe the effects of density changes on image appearance.
4. Describe the process of evaluating image density.
5. Explain why mA and time are the controlling factors of density.
6. Explain how each influencing factor affects image density.
7. Assess radiographic density on various radiographic images.
8. Recommend appropriate adjustments to compensate for variation in the controlling and influencing factors that affect image density.

ASSESSING DENSITY

Density is one of the two photographic properties that comprise visibility of detail. Visibility of detail refers to the fact that the radiographic image is visible to the human eye only because sufficient density (and contrast) exists to permit the structural details to be perceived. **The density of the radiographic image is the degree of overall blackening from the black metallic silver deposited in the emulsion** and is the easiest of the prime technical factors to evaluate and adjust.

The physical concept of density has been discussed in detail in previous chapters. In this chapter the concept of density is approached in an artistically professional manner aimed at diagnosing the image. The art of radiography is a clinical one and must be practiced as such. It is extremely important that this information be used in a clinical setting concurrently with its study.

The major consideration in assessing density is verification that proper densities are visible throughout the anatomical area of interest on the radiograph. Of course, these densities must be well within the range of human

A

Figure 23–1. Clinical experience in assessing density. (A) Although this image is not acceptable for the clavicle, it is a diagnostic quality image of the acromio-clavicular joints. (B) Although this image is not acceptable for the thoracic spine, it is a diagnostic quality image of the chest.

B

visibility (usually OD 0.25–2.50). Much of this ability to verify proper densities is a result of clinical experience (Figure 23–1). It is obvious that the proper density for lung tissue is not as great as the proper density for the thoracic spine, even though they are both thoracic structures. Common sense and a trained professional eye are the primary tools of the radiographer when evaluating density. The ability to assess density is a result of continued conscientious evaluation of images during clinical experiences. The radiographer who becomes professionally interested in the process of diagnosing the image quickly gains and refines this ability.

Information is recorded on a radiograph that is too dark but may not exist at all on a radiograph that is too light. The dark radiograph has received too many photons and, as a result, has recorded too much information. A bright light or computerized optical scanner can eliminate the excess information and reveal details within the range of human visual ability. This is not the case with a radiograph that is too light. The light radiograph has not received the information in the first place and is not capable of being manipulated to reveal details that were never recorded. Consequently, **whenever a choice must be made between excess and insufficient density, the wise decision is always the choice that will produce the darker image**.

EFFECTS ON IMAGE APPEARANCE

When mAs is doubled, the radiographic density on the film image is roughly doubled. When mAs is reduced by half, the resulting film image is about twice as light as the original. If the mAs is increased by a factor of four, the resulting image is about four times darker, etc. The series of images shown in Figures 23–2A-D illustrate these effects.

The effects of mAs and the other influencing factors on image density are not exact because of the multiple variables that are part of the imaging system. Many of the variables affect the density of the image in a nonlinear fashion under some conditions. For example, the typical D log E curve is only somewhat linear in the straight line portion. If exposure conditions push into the toe or shoulder regions of the curve, dramatic density changes can be seen. Similarly, density changes can sometimes be seen from only a slight nonlinearity in the intensifying screen phosphor response curve, the film silver halide response, the thermionic emission of the x-ray tube filament, etc.

Fortunately, these variables have a statistical tendency to balance one another. But in cases where conditions cause a majority of the variables to increase or decrease a total of more than 30 percent, an unexpected change in image density may become visible. Even when unexpected density changes exceed the 30 percent necessary to become visible, they seldom place the image outside the acceptance limits.

FACTORS AFFECTING DENSITY

A wide variety of factors affect radiographic density (Figure 23–3). These factors are classified as either **controlling** or **influencing** factors. The controlling factor should be used as the principle method for adjusting for insufficient or excessive radiographic density.

Controlling Factor

Milliampere-Seconds   Milliampere-seconds (mAs) is the primary controller of density. The reciprocity law states that as mAs increases both x-ray exposure and radiographic density increase proportionally. Therefore **density is proportional to the intensity and duration of the x-ray exposure as controlled by mAs**. Remember that the reciprocity law fails for extremely short (less than 0.01 second) or

```
60 kVp   0.26 mAs   40″ SID
No grid   400 RS   0.58 mR
```

A

```
60 kVp   0.52 mAs   40″ SID
No grid   400 RS   1.12 mR
```

B

```
60 kVp   2.08 mAs   40″ SID
No grid   400 RS   3.5 mR
```

D

```
60 kVp   1.04 mAs   40″ SID
No grid   400 RS   2.16 mR
```

C

```
60 kVp   0.83 mAs   40″ SID
No grid   400 RS   1.68 mR
```

E

Figure 23–2. The effects of mAs changes on image density. Images A-D demonstrate the effect of increasing mAs. Each image is double the density of the previous one. Image E represents a 20 percent decrease in mAs from image C.

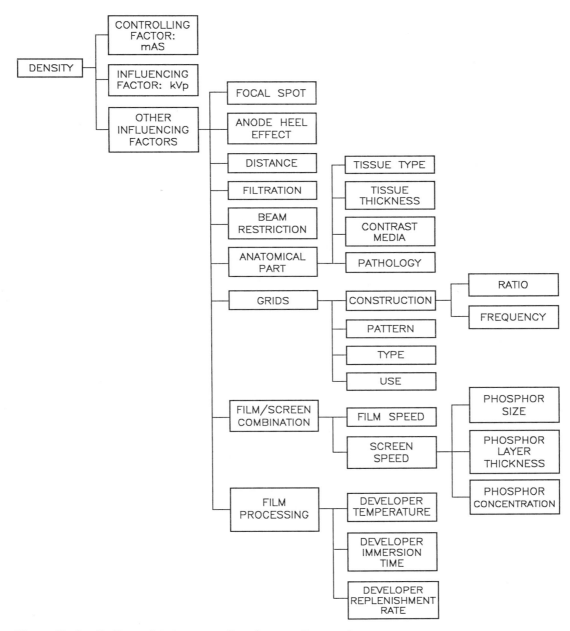

Figure 23–3. Radiographic image quality: factors affecting density.

long (more than 10 seconds) exposure times. within the range of normal radiographic exposures, it can become a factor in special situations (such as pediatric extremities or high-speed angiography).

Density should remain unchanged as long as the total exposure to the film and all other conditions remain unchanged. If the mAs used to create one image is the same as the mAs used to create a second image of the same structure, then both images should have the same radiographic density. As long as mAs is constant, any combinations of mA and exposure time values will create the same density. This was demonstrated previously by the radiographs in Figure 10–1. Of course, accurate results depend on using equipment that is properly calibrated and maintained through an effective quality control program.

The control of radiographic density in most instances rests with the radiographer. An appropriate mAs setting may be selected from a technique chart developed for the particular x-ray unit in use. An automatic exposure system will control the time but the mA and the exact density setting will be decided by the radiographer. Computerized exposure systems will provide a suggested technique setting which can then be modified. Other variables, such as generator phase or falling loads, may also affect the final decision. The experienced radiographer will adapt the suggested mAs setting for the individual patient. Experience and study of various body habitus, pathologies, positioning and equipment quickly provide the radiographer with clinical knowledge that can be used for these adjustments.

The minimum change necessary to cause a visible shift in density is 30 percent of mAs, or any other influencing factors that would equal this change. Various authors over the years have set the minimum for a visible density change at values between 25 and 35 percent of mAs. Although studies of vision have

demonstrated that some people can detect changes in density as small as one percent, this level of perception is not possible when viewing a complex clinical image with many widely separated densities. Some trained professionals, such as radiologists and radiographers, can perceive as small a change as 10 percent on a radiograph but this is extraordinary. In clinical practice a change as small as 30 percent is seldom justified. A comparison between Figures 23–2C and E illustrates a 20 percent change in mAs. This change is difficult to see and would not compensate for improper density.

A radiograph must be outside the acceptance limits to require repeating the exposure. All acceptance limits permit some degree of variation—at least 30 percent too light or too dark. In these instances the radiograph would have to be significantly more than 30 percent darker or lighter than a diagnostic quality image.

The rule for density changes is to make adjustments in increments of doubles or halves. For example, a repeated film that is too light at 10 mAs should be repeated at 20, 40 or 80 mAs, depending on the circumstances. Of course, determining which circumstances require 20 mAs, which require 40 mAs, and which require 80 mAs is something that is acquired only through experience and further study. Figures 23–2A-D illustrate the doubling and halving rule.

Regardless of variations in equipment output, anatomy, physiology or pathology, the idea is to adjust the intensity to permit the same amount of radiation to reach the film, thus creating the same density. From this perspective, the art of radiography does not look especially difficult. However, many other factors are yet to be added to the simple task of determining appropriate density.

One clinical practice that should be avoided is attempting to adjust density by increasing or decreasing "a step in time." Due to wide variation in x-ray unit controls, "a step in time" may be a 10 percent change on one unit but a 20 percent or even 30 percent change on another. In fact, time stations are often not linear on the same unit. This makes the "step in time" rule dangerous because of its inconsistency. In addition, in many instances "a step in time" will not even accomplish a visible density change.

Essentially, if the radiograph does not require doubling or halving of the density, it seldom requires repeating. Exceptions to this rule are special studies where a fine adjustment of barely 30 percent is crucial to demonstrating a small vessel or pathological condition. The radiographer will often adjust his or her technique chart by a 30 percent margin, but will seldom subject the patient to a second exposure for such a minor change. Making density adjustments should be a case of taking bold action (at least doubling or halving) or taking no action at all.

Influencing Factors

Kilovoltage Kilovoltage alters the intensity of the beam reaching the image receptor in two ways. Kilovoltage controls the energy and, therefore, the strength of the electrons striking the target of the x-ray tube for any given mAs. More important, kilovoltage controls the average energy of the x-ray photons produced at the anode target. Therefore, a change in kilovoltage alters the intensity of the beam when the mAs and other factors remain the same. Kilovoltage also controls the production of scatter radiation. Because of this, a change in kilovoltage alters the intensity of the beam after it enters the subject (or object) but before it forms the image.

Both the quantity and quality of the x-ray beam will vary significantly with changes in kilovoltage. As a result, kVp has a tremendous

impact on radiographic density. Research has been done to determine a practical formula which takes both the quantity and quality factors into account. The primary finding is that there are too many variables to be quantified into a reliable formula. A visible change in density can usually be detected with a 4–5 percent change in kVp in the lower ranges (30–50 kVp), but an 8–9 percent change is required in the middle ranges (50–90 kVp), and a 10–12 percent change in the higher ranges (90–130 kVp).

Because the radiographer must have a method of using kilovoltage to adjust and compensate for density changes, the rough guide known as the **15 percent rule** has been developed. The 15 percent rule is used as a guide to maintain the same density when kilovoltage changes, as follows:

> A 15 percent increase in kilovoltage causes a doubling of image density.
> A 15 percent decrease in kilovoltage causes a halving of image density.

Example: A radiograph of the elbow is produced using 4 mAs at 60 kVp. What kVp would be required to halve the density?

Answer:
60 kVp − (60 kVp × 15%)
60 kVp − (60 kVp × 0.15)
60 kVp − (9 kVp) = 51 kVp

The 15 percent rule is somewhat accurate within the range of 60 to 100 kVp. Of course, this does not include the entire diagnostic radiography range, which may run from 30 to 150 kVp. The percentage of kVp required to halve the image density is always greater as the kVp increases. This is primarily due to the increased scatter radiation produced at higher kilovoltages. However, the greatest variable in the production of scatter is the thickness of the part. Therefore, image density is increased when radiographing a thick subject (Figure 23–4). Consequently, a 20 percent rule may be more accurate when radiographing a 5 cm wrist, while a 15 percent rule may be more accurate when radiographing a 20 cm abdomen. Another factor which has a mathematical effect on the 15 percent rule is the starting kVp. The percentage change for doubling or halving decreases slightly as the starting kVp increases. In actual fact, the 15 percent rule may vary from a 15 percent rule to a 25 percent rule within the diagnostic radiography

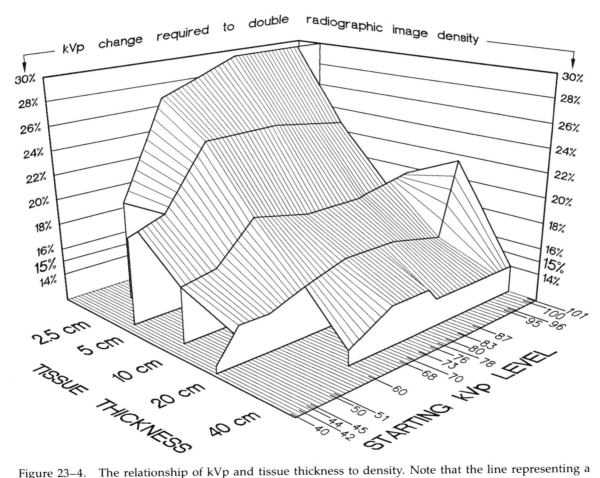

Figure 23–4. The relationship of kVp and tissue thickness to density. Note that the line representing a 15 percent increase in kVp is not within the range of some part thicknesses and kVps used in routine diagnostic radiography. It is apparent that the 15 percent rule is not a constant and must be applied with careful consideration of other factors, especially tissue thickness and starting kVp. (Data extracted from "Kilovoltage Conversion in Radiography" *The X-Ray Technician*, 31: 373–379, 436, 1960 by Gerhart S. Schwartz with permission of the American Society of Radiologic Technologists. Graphics courtesy of Chris Innskeep, Lima Technical College.)

range. The 15 percent rule is commonly applied by radiographers because it can be used without producing images outside the acceptance limits. However, understanding the variability of the rule will do much to increase awareness of potential problems when radiographing extremely large or small objects, or with unusually low or high kVp settings.

Changing kilovoltage is the primary method of changing image contrast. Consequently, the 15 percent rule will always change the contrast of the image. When a contrast change is desirable, the 15 percent rule is a useful method of maintaining image density. However, when only a density change is desired, the 15 percent rule should not be used because it causes a contrast change as well. When image density changes are desired, the method of choice is to vary the mAs because it is the controlling factor.

The configuration of the generator is another important consideration in how kVp affects image density. The total number of higher energy photons in the x-ray tube emission spectrum is controlled by the amount of ripple in the waveform. For example, a single-phase, two-pulse (1ϕ2p) waveform has a significantly lower average photon energy than a three-phase, twelve-pulse (3ϕ12p) waveform, resulting in less density.

Compensation for the configuration of the generator is most commonly accomplished by considering only the phasing and number of pulses. Conversion factors have been developed for these compensations (Table 23–1).

Example: If 80 kVp and 20 mAs produce a satisfactory image on a 1ϕ2p unit, what mAs should be used with the same patient and examination on a 3ϕ12p unit?

Answer:
mAs × conversion factor
20 mAs × 0.5 = 10 mAs

Focal Spot Size Larger focal spots utilize a greater incident electron stream than small focal spots. Most manufacturers carefully compensate for this effect by adjusting the actual mA at the filament for dual-focus tubes. The actual mA received by the filament when set at 100 mA for a large focal spot is less than the actual mA received when set at 100 mA for a small focal spot. There should be no difference between large and small focal spots when the unit has been calibrated properly. However, this effect may differ by the 30 percent necessary to alter image density in an improperly calibrated unit.

Large focal spots tend to bloom more at higher milliamperages and may occasionally reach a point where they alter image density. Blooming occurs with large milliamperages because the incident electron beam is not as easily focused by the focusing cup. It is rare for blooming to cause a visible density difference.

Because properly calibrated units will not exhibit image density changes when focal spots are changed, differences of this type should be reported as a quality control procedure. If den-

TABLE 23–1		
CONVERSION FACTORS		
EFFECT OF GENERATOR PHASE ON IMAGE DENSITY		
When Converting Generator Phase		**To Maintain Image Density, Multiply mAs**
From:	**To:**	**by a Conversion Factor of:**
1ϕ2p	3ϕ6p	0.6
1ϕ2p	3ϕ12p	0.5
3ϕ6p	1ϕ2p	1.6
3ϕ6p	3ϕ12p	0.8
3ϕ12p	1ϕ2p	2.0
3ϕ12p	3ϕ6p	1.2

Derived from Dupont Bit System.

sity differences are perceived due to focal spot blooming, replacement of the tube may be indicated.

Anode Heel Effect The anode heel effect alters the intensity of radiation, and therefore the image density, between the anode and cathode ends of the x-ray tube. Depending on the angle of the anode, this effect can cause a density variation of up to 45 percent between the anode and cathode ends of the image. Image density is always greater at the cathode end. The anode heel effect is more pronounced when the collimator is open wide than when it is closed because a greater portion of the peripheral beam, and therefore a greater portion of the intensity difference, reaches the image receptor when the collimator is wide open. The anode heel effect is also more significant when using extremely small angle anodes (12° or less).

When the anode heel effect becomes apparent, it can be minimized or converted to an advantage. It is minimized by collimating the beam and eliminating as much of the intensity difference at the periphery as possible. If a given film size is required (i.e., 14″×17″) collimation may be achieved by using a greater SID.

The anode heel effect may be converted to an advantage in examinations of objects with greater subject density at one end than at another. The advantage is utilized by placing the portion of the object with the greatest subject density toward the cathode end of the tube. This utilizes the greater intensity for the greater subject density and leaves the lesser intensity of the anode end of the tube for the lesser subject density. The anode heel effect can often be used to advantage in a number of examinations (Table 23–2).

Distance (SID and OID) Source-to-image receptor distance (SID), also known as focus-to-film distance (FFD), **alters the intensity of the beam reaching the image receptor, according to the inverse square law. The inverse square law affects density in inverse proportion to the square of the distance.** This is represented by the formula:

$$\frac{I_1}{I_2} = \frac{D_2^2}{D_1^2}$$

where: I_1 = old intensity

I_2 = new intensity

D_1^2 = old distance squared

D_2^2 = new distance squared

TABLE 23–2		
PROJECTIONS THAT MAY USE THE ANODE HEEL EFFECT TO ADVANTAGE		
Projection	**Body Part to Be Placed Toward**	
	Cathode End of Tube	**Anode End of Tube**
Femur (AP/lateral)	hip	knee
Lower leg (AP/lateral)	knee	hip
Humerus (AP/lateral)	shoulder	elbow
Forearm (AP/lateral)	elbow	wrist
Thoracic spine (AP)	abdomen	neck
Thoracic spine (lateral)	neck	abdomen
Lumbar spine (AP/lateral)	pelvis	abdomen

The law states that the intensity varies inversely with the square of the distance.

The inverse square law formula expresses the change in intensity when the distance changes. For example, as distance increases, radiation intensity and radiographic density decrease. However, the most common situation in radiography is a need to maintain an acceptable density while changing the distance. To maintain density, mAs (or an influencer) must be changed to compensate for the density change. The **density maintenance formula** is used for this purpose. This formula is based on the inverse square law but is reversed to a direct square law because mAs must increase when distance increases, and vice versa, in order to maintain density.

$$\frac{mAs_1}{mAs_2} = \frac{D_1^2}{D_2^2}$$

where: mAs_1 = original mAs mAs_2 = new mAs

D_1^2 = old distance squared

D_2^2 = new distance squared

Example: If a satisfactory density is obtained with 20 mAs at 72″, what mAs will be required to maintain the same density at 40″?

Answer:

$$\frac{mAs_1}{mAs_2} = \frac{D_1^2}{D_2^2}$$

$$\frac{mAs_1}{20\ mAs} = \frac{40″^2}{72″^2}$$

$$\frac{mAs_1}{20\ mAs} = \frac{1{,}600″}{5{,}184″}$$

$$mAs_1 = \frac{20\ mAs \times 1{,}600″}{5{,}184″}$$

$$mAs_1 = \frac{32{,}000″}{5{,}184″}$$

$$mAs_1 = 6.2\ mAs$$

It is more useful when algebraically changed to solve for the new mAs, which is the most common factor that must be calculated in clinical practice:

$$mAs_2 = \frac{mAs_1 \times D_2^2}{D_1^2}$$

Example: If a satisfactory PA chest radiograph is made at 72″ with 4 mAs, what mAs will be required at 56″?

Answer:

$$mAs_2 = \frac{mAs_1 \times D_2^2}{D_1^2}$$

$$mAs_2 = \frac{4\ mAs \times 56″^2}{72″^2}$$

$$mAs_2 = \frac{4\ mAs \times 3{,}136″}{5{,}184″}$$

$$mAs_2 = \frac{12{,}544″}{5{,}184″}$$

$$mAs_2 = 2.5\ mAs$$

The density maintenance formula is only accurate within a moderate acceptance range. The nonlinearity of some components in the imaging system (such as developer activity, intensifying screen phosphor emission and film silver halide response) makes it impossible to exactly quantify the relationship between radiation beam intensity and image density.

Table 23–3 illustrates the mAs change factors for the most common distances employed in radiography. The vast majority of diagnostic radiography today is done at 40″ to 72″. In addition 56″, which is halfway between 40″ and 72″, is useful in mobile radiography when circumstances do not permit either of the two preferred distances. A useful rule of thumb for doubling and halving distances can be derived from this table by considering the 30 percent range necessary to produce a visible density difference in the image:

Use only the distances 40″, 56″ and 72″. When increasing distance, double the

mAs for each change. When decreasing distance, halve the mAs for each change. For example, halve the mAs when changing from 72″ to 56″ and halve it again when changing from 56″ to 40″.

Distance doubling and halving will bring density within roughly 50 percent of the original

---

TABLE 23–3

mAs CHANGE FACTORS FOR APPROXIMATE DENSITY MAINTENANCE WHEN DISTANCE CHANGES

To calculate the new mAs, multiply the old mAs by the factor in the box corresponding to the distance change.

Old Distance	New Distance				
	36″	40″	48″	56″	72″
	90 cm	100 cm	120 cm	140 cm	180 cm
36″ (90 cm)	—	1.23	1.77	2.42	4.00
40″ (100 cm)	0.81	—	1.44	1.96	3.24
48″ (120 cm)	0.59	0.69	—	1.36	2.25
56″ (140 cm)	0.41	0.51	0.73	—	1.65
72″ (180 cm)	0.25	0.31	0.44	0.60	—

Example: If a satisfactory density is produced with 10 mAs at 40″, what mAs should be used to maintain the same density at 72″?

Answer: The mAs change factor for an old distance of 40″ and a new distance of 72″ is 3.24. 10 mAs × 3.24 = 32.4 mAs

---

density and are usually within image acceptance limits. This is only a rough rule of thumb for clinical practice. The exact conversion factors will produce much better mAs estimates.

Object-to-image receptor distance (OID), also known as object-to-film distance (OFD), has an effect on image density. The air-gap technique uses an increased OID to prevent scatter radiation from reaching the image receptor. This scatter radiation would normally contribute to the image density and its loss can cause a visible decrease in density when radiographing large patients. In most instances, OID variations are insufficient to cause visible density changes.

Filtration Filtration and its ability to alter beam intensity affect image density. All types of filtration—inherent, added and total—alter image density. Density decreases when filtration is increased.

X-ray units are calibrated with inherent, added and total filtration in place. When added filtration is changed, which is rare, a half-value layer calculation should be made to permit adjustment of mAs or other factors to maintain image density. When compensating filtration is used, image density must be established for both filtered and unfiltered regions. As with any other density problem, this is a matter of measurement of part size and clinical experience.

Beam Restriction Restricting the beam, collimating, or reducing the primary beam field size reduces the total number of photons available. This reduces the amount of scatter radiation and therefore reduces the overall density of the image.

The anatomical part size has a great influence on the beam restriction's effect on density. For example, a 20 cm abdomen technique that produces a satisfactory image with 14″ × 17″ collimation requires approximately twice the mAs to maintain the same density when collimation is reduced to 8″ × 10″, and about four times the original mAs at 4″ × 4″ collimation (Figure 23–5).

Anatomical Part Because the patient is the prime attenuator of the beam, the anatomical part being examined has a great deal of influence on the density on the film. The amount of attenuation is dependent on the thickness and type of the tissue being radiographed. The tissue type is affected by the average atomic number and the density (quantity of matter per unit volume) of the tissue. The use of contrast media will alter the average atomic number of the tissue and can affect density. Pathology can alter tissue thickness and/or type.

There is an inverse relationship between tissue thickness/type and radiographic density. In other words, as tissue thickness, average atomic number of the tissue, and/or tissue density increases, radiographic density decreases. **This is not a linear relationship** because of the multitude of variations in tissue composition. Depending on the type of contrast media or the type of pathology, an inverse or a direct relationship may exist.

Adjustments for changes in the anatomical part depend on the radiographer's ability to assess the tissue thickness and tissue type

85 **kVp**   1.0 **mAs**   40″SID
12:1 **grid**   400 **RS**   29.8 **mR**

85 **kVp**   1.0 **mAs**   40″ SID
12:1 **grid**   400 **RS**   31.6 **mR**

A

B

Figure 23–5A & B.   The effect of beam restriction on density. Although both radiographs were produced at the same technical factors, B exhibits less density.

while also considering the pathology and the use of contrast media. This ability is achieved only through clinical experience. Technique charts are designed to compensate for most changes in tissue thickness and type. Radiolucent contrast media (such as air) will increase radiographic density, while radiopaque contrast media (such as barium and iodine) will decrease radiographic density. Pathology can have either an additive or a destructive effect. Additive conditions decrease density while destructive conditions increase density.

A special problem related to part thickness occurs whenever severe tube angles (more than 15°) are used. The geometry of a severe tube angle causes a significant difference in tissue thickness between the edges of the image (Figure 23–6). Measurement of body parts for angles must occur at the central ray to average these differences. However, in some instances more than a 30 percent density difference may occur between the central ray and both ends of the image (more than a 60 percent difference between the ends of the image). Careful consideration of technical factors and use of the anode heel effect, when possible, may prevent some of these problems.

Casting materials present during orthopedic radiography affect the thickness of the anatomical part. Casting materials differ somewhat in composition but they attenuate the beam in a manner very similar to normal tissue attenuation. Adjustments for cast materials should be made for the increased thickness of the body part exactly as if an uncasted part of the same size were being radiographed. No adjustment should be made for the casting material itself.

Grids Grids absorb scatter which would otherwise add density to the film. The more efficient the grid, the less the density. Grids with high ratios, low frequency and dense interspace material; moving grids and improperly used grids (incorrect focal distance, etc.) all reduce density.

Compensation for varying grid ratios is generally accomplished by increasing mAs. The amount of mAs needed can be calculated using the grid conversion factors (see Table 16–2). Changes between grids, which is the most common clinical problem, are accomplished by using the following formula:

$$\frac{mAs_1}{mAs_2} = \frac{GCF_1}{GCF_2}$$

where: mAs_1 = original mAs

mAs_2 = new mAs

GCF_1 = original grid conversion factor

GCF_2 = new grid conversion factor

Because the primary purpose of a grid is the improvement of contrast, compensating for density changes by varying the kVp is not recommended because it may change the contrast in the opposite direction, thus negating the reason for using the grid in the first place.

Film/Screen Combination Both film and intensifying screens alter density according to their conversion efficiency. When the intensifying screen phosphors convert x-ray photons to the light photons that will expose the silver halides in the film, they attenuate the intensity of the light that has become the imaging beam. When the silver halide crystals in the film emulsion form latent image centers, they establish the physical foundation for the black metallic silver that is the definition of density. Relative speed (RS) numbers are the most useful parameters of intensifying screen combinations.

Relative speed (RS) numbers have been developed by manufacturers to permit easy

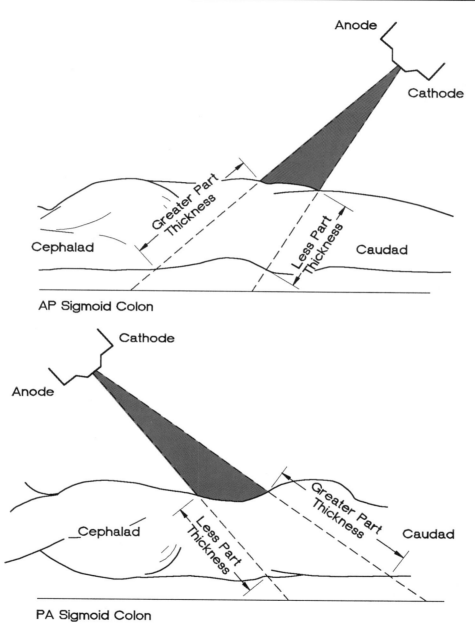

Figure 23–6.   The effect of severe tube angle on density. Note the changes in part thickness from the superior to inferior edges of the primary beam field.

adjustment of technical factors when changing film/screen combinations. Density and mAs are inversely proportional to relative speed. The relative speed conversion formula is:

$$\frac{mAs_1}{mAs_2} = \frac{RS_2}{RS_1}$$

where: mAs_1 = old mAs
mAs_2 = new mAs
RS_1 = old relative speed
RS_2 = new relative speed

Of course, the relative speed conversion formula may also be algebraically expressed as:

$$mAs_2 = \frac{RS_1 \times mAs_1}{RS_2}$$

Example: What is the proper mAs for use with an 80 RS system when technical factors of 55 kVp and 4 mAs produce an acceptable image with a 200 RS system?

Answer:

$$\frac{mAs_1}{mAs_2} = \frac{RS_2}{RS_1}$$

$$\frac{5}{mAs_2} = \frac{80}{200}$$

$$mAs_2 \times 80 = 5 \text{ mAs} \times 200$$

$$mAs_2 \times 80 = 1,000 \text{ mAs}$$

$$mAs_2 = \frac{10,000 \text{ mAs}}{80}$$

$$mAs_2 = 12.5 \text{ mAs}$$

Film Processing The condition of the film processing solutions can dramatically alter image density. Establishment of density, contrast and base plus fog parameters for the film processing system is part of the quality control program. Ascertaining that film processing density, contrast and base plus fog values are within parameters can remove film processing as a density factor.

Density will increase when the developer solution temperature increases, immersion time increases or replenishment rates increase. Density will decrease when the above factors decrease, as well as when contamination decreases solution strength.

SUMMARY

Density is one of the two photographic properties that comprise visibility of detail. Visibility of detail refers to the fact that the radiographic image is visible to the human eye only because sufficient density (and contrast) exists to permit the structural details to be perceived. The density of the radiographic image is the degree of overall blackening from the black metallic silver deposited in the emulsion.

The radiographic density on the film image is roughly doubled when mAs is doubled. When mAs is reduced by half, the resulting film image is about twice as light as the original. The effects of mAs and the other influencing factors in image density are not exact because of the multiple variables that are part of the imaging system.

A wide variety of factors affect radiographic density. These factors are classified as either controlling or influencing factors. The controlling factor is mAs and it should be used as the principle method for adjusting for insufficient or excessive radiographic density. The influencing factors include kilovoltage, focal spot size, anode heel effect, distance, filtration, beam restriction, anatomical part, grids, film/screen combination and film processing.

When the controlling or any of the influencing factors are altered, some change in density will occur. However, with some of the factors, the effect is often negligible. The following list illustrates the effect on density when the various factors are changed.

+ = increased density
− = decreased density
∅ = negligible effect

Controlling Factor

+ Increasing milliamperage-seconds
− Decreasing milliamperage-seconds

Influencing Factors

+ Increasing kilovoltage
− Decreasing kilovoltage
+ Increasing number of pulses in the generator waveform
− Decreasing number of pulses in the generator waveform
∅ Focal spot size
∅ Anode heel effect
− Increasing distance
+ Decreasing distance
− Increasing filtration
+ Decreasing filtration
− Increasing beam restriction/collimation
+ Decreasing beam restriction/collimation
− Increasing anatomical part thickness or tissue type
+ Decreasing anatomical part thickness or tissue type
+ Using radiolucent contrast media
− Using radiopaque contrast media
− Additive pathological conditions
+ Destructive pathological conditions
− Increasing grid ratio
+ Decreasing grid ratio
+ Increasing film/screen combination relative speed
− Decreasing film/screen combination relative speed
+ Increasing film processing developer time, temperature and/or replenishment rate
− Decreasing film processing developer time, temperature and/or replenishment rate

REVIEW QUESTIONS

1. Define radiographic density.
2. What is the controlling factor of radiographic density and how does it affect it?
3. How are density adjustments made for changes in kilovoltage?
4. How do the inverse square law and the density maintenance formulas differ from one another?
5. How do variations in the anatomical part affect density?
6. What are the relationships to density of grid ratio, frequency, interspace material and grid use?
7. What is the relationship to density of relative speed for film/screen combinations?
8. How does film processing affect density?

REFERENCES AND RECOMMENDED READING

Bauer, Richard G. High kilovoltage chest radiography with an air gap. *Radiologic Technology* 42, 10–14, 1970.

Bierman, A., and W. Hondius Boldingh. The relation between tension and exposure times in radiography. *Acta Radiologica* 35, 22–26, 1951.

Cahoon, John B. *Formulating X-Ray Techniques.* 8th ed. Durham, NC: Duke University Press, 1974.

Cahoon, John B. Radiographic technique: Its origin, concept, practical application and evaluation of radiation dosage. *The X-Ray Technician* 32, 354–364, 1961.

Carlton, Rick, and Arlene McKenna. Repeating radiographs: Setting imaging standards. *Postgraduate Advances in Radiologic Technology.* Berryville, VA: Forum Medicum, Inc., 1989.

Carroll, Quinn. *Fuchs's Principles of Radiographic Exposure, Processing and Quality Control*. 3rd ed. Springfield, IL: Charles C. Thomas Publisher, 1985.

Distance-technique relationship of angulated projections. *Radiologic Technology* 52:3, 301, 1980.

Donohue, Daniel P. *An Analysis of Radiographic Quality: Lab Manual and Workbook*. 2nd ed. Rockville, MD: Aspen Publishers, Inc., 1984.

Eastman Kodak Company, Health Sciences Markets Division. *The Fundamentals of Radiography*. 12th ed. Rochester, NY: Kodak Publication M1–18.

Eastman, T. R. Measurement: The key to exposure with manual techniques. *Radiologic Technology* 45, 75–78, 1973.

Files, Glenn W. *Medical Radiographic Technique*. Springfield, IL: Charles C. Thomas Publisher, 1952.

Files, Glenn W. Maximum tissue differentiation. *The X-Ray Technician* 7, 17–24+, 1935.

Fuchs, Arthur W. *Principles of Radiographic Exposure and Processing*. 1st ed. Springfield, IL: Charles C. Thomas Publisher, 1958.

Fuchs, Arthur W. *Principles of Radiographic Exposure and Processing*. 2nd ed. Springfield, IL: Charles C. Thomas Publisher, 1958.

Fuchs, Arthur W. The rationale of radiographic exposure. *The X-Ray Technician* 22, 62–68, 76, 1950.

Fuchs, Arthur W. Control of radiographic density. *The X-Ray Technician* 20, 271–273, 291, 1949.

Fuchs, Arthur W. Relationship of tissue thickness to kilovoltage. *The X-Ray Technician* 19, 287–293, 1948.

Fuchs, Arthur W. The anode 'heel' effect in radiography. *Radiologic Technology* 18:4, 158, 1947.

Fuchs, Arthur W. Balance in the radiographic image. *The X-Ray Technician* 12:3, 81–84, 118, 1940.

Gratale, Pete, Gilbert W. Turner, and Charles B. Burns. Using the same exposure factors for wet and dry casts. *Radiologic Technology* 57:4, 325–328, 1986.

Hiss, Stephen S. *Understanding Radiography*. Springfield, IL: Charles C. Thomas Publisher, 1978.

Jerman, Ed. C. *Modern X-Ray Technic*. St. Paul, MN: Bruce Publishing Co., 1928.

Lauer, O. Gary, John B. Mayes, and Rosemary P. Thurston. *Evaluating Radiographic Quality: The Variables and Their Effects*. Mankato, MN: The Burnell Company Publishers, Inc., 1990.

Mattsson, Ove. Practical photographic problems in radiography. *Acta Radiologica* Supplementum 120, 1–206, 1955.

Morgan, James A. *The Art and Science of Medical Radiography*. 5th ed. St. Louis, MO: Catholic Hospital Association, 1977.

Schwarz, Gerhart S. *Unit-Step Radiography*. Springfield, IL: Charles C. Thomas Publisher, 1961.

Seeman, Herman E. *Physical and Photographic Principles of Medical Radiography*. New York: Wiley & Sons, Inc., 1968.

Williams, William A. Radiographic effect formula: Its practical application. *The X-Ray Technician* 28, 1–6, 67, 1956.

Wilsey, R. B. The intensity of scattered x-rays in radiography. *American Journal of Roentgenology* 8, 328–338, 1921.

Winkler, Norlin T. A practical water phantom. *Radiologic Technology* 35:2, 65–70, 1963.

24 CONTRAST

The conclusion drawn from these experiments was that there was no mystery—that, other things being equal, contrast was determined solely by the voltage used. . . .

W. D. Coolidge, "Experiences with the Roentgen-ray tube."

OUTLINE

ASSESSING CONTRAST
RADIOGRAPHIC CONTRAST
EVALUATING CONTRAST
FACTORS AFFECTING CONTRAST

OBJECTIVES

Upon completion of this chapter, the student should be able to:

1. Identify contrast as a prime component of the photographic properties controlling visibility of detail of radiographic image quality.
2. Explain the various terms used to describe contrast.
3. Define radiographic contrast and the factors that affect it.
4. Describe the factors that affect image receptor (film) contrast.
5. Describe the factors that affect subject contrast.
6. Describe the effect of fog on image contrast.
7. Describe the effects of contrast changes on image appearance.
8. Determine the technical factor changes necessary to achieve optimal contrast.
9. Assess radiographic contrast on various radiographic images.
10. Recommend appropriate adjustments to improve contrast under various conditions.
11. Explain why kilovoltage peak is the controlling factor of contrast.
12. Explain how each influencing factor affects image contrast.

ASSESSING CONTRAST

Contrast is one of the two photographic properties that comprise visibility of detail. Visibility of detail refers to the fact that the radiographic image is visible to the human eye only because sufficient contrast (and density) exists to permit the structural details to be perceived. **Radiographic contrast is the difference between adjacent densities.** It can be mathematically evaluated as the percentage or ratio of the differences between densities. These differences can range from clear white through various shades of gray to black.

Because contrast consists of various densities, a thorough knowledge of the factors that control density is a prerequisite to understanding it. Although contrast must be considered an independent factor, the fact that it is composed of densities makes it very difficult to separate it from the evaluation of overall density. Any change in overall density will affect contrast. This makes contrast the most difficult of the prime technical factors to evaluate and adjust.

Describing Contrast

When the differences between adjacent densities that comprise contrast are great, the image is described as high contrast. The result is fewer discernible shades of gray. Conversely, when the differences are minimal, the image is described as low contrast. This produces more discernible shades of gray. Figure 24–1A has the fewest shades of gray and therefore has the highest contrast.

In Figure 24–1B–F, there are progressively more discernible shades of gray. Figure 24–1F has the lowest contrast image. This is analogous to a gray scarf on a gray coat, which has low contrast, versus a black scarf on a white coat, which has high contrast. Table 24–1 summarizes the relationships between the various terms used to describe contrast.

TABLE 24–1	
RELATIONSHIP BETWEEN TERMS USED TO DESCRIBE CONTRAST	
High Contrast	*Low Contrast*
Few shades of gray	Many shades of gray
Increased contrast	Decreased contrast
Low kVp	High kVp
Short scale contrast	Long scale contrast

As the differences between adjacent densities increase, there are fewer shades of discernible gray and the contrast is increased. Increasing contrast produces a high contrast image. As the differences between adjacent densities decrease, there are more shades of discernible gray and the contrast is decreased. Decreasing contrast produces a low contrast image.

The term "good contrast" is often applied to high contrast, but this is a misnomer and should be avoided because high contrast is not necessarily the most desirable. In fact, in most instances low contrast provides more information. Low contrast provides more differences in density even though the difference between densities is less. As long as the differences remain within the visible range of densities, low contrast provides more diagnostic information. Figures 24–2A and B are good examples of how high contrast fails to provide all the information that is obtained from a low contrast image. Although high contrast images may be perceived as more pleasing to the untrained eye, radiographers and radiologists realize that, although the lower contrast image is not as dramatic in its presentation, it often demonstrates more information. Without contrast there would be no image because all densities would appear identical. More information is visible simply because more densities are

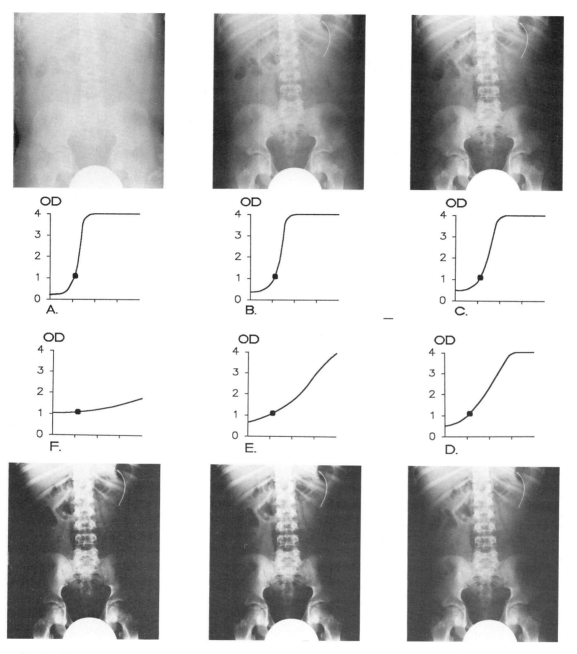

Figure 24–1. Pure contrast changes in a digital abdomen image produced with a fixed density point. These computerized images vary only in contrast as shown in the accompanying D log E curves. From A—F the contrast curve becomes steeper and shorter but the density point does not move up or down. C is considered optimal contrast for a diagnostic image. (Computed radiography images courtesy of Bruce Long, Indiana University Medical Center, Indianapolis.)

A   B

Figure 24–2. High and low contrast. (A) Chest radiograph produced using 80 kVp. (B) Chest radiograph of same patient using 110 kVp.

present, thus forming more possibilities for contrast differences.

Scale of contrast is the number of useful visible densities or shades of gray. Short scale contrast refers to an image that demonstrates considerable or maximal differences between densities and has a minimal total number of densities. Conversely, long scale contrast refers to an image that demonstrates slight or minimal differences between densities but has a maximal total number of densities (Figure 24–3). **Short scale contrast is also called high contrast, or increased contrast, while long scale contrast is called low contrast, or decreased contrast**.

The advent of computerized digital processing has made it useful to sometimes describe contrast as **physical** and **visible**. Physical contrast is the total range of density values recorded by the image receptor. It is the maximum contrast possible and is the most accurate representation of the varying intensities present in the x-ray beam after it has passed

through the subject. Visible contrast is the total range of density values that can be perceived by the human eye in a single image. It is a portion of the physical contrast and comprises the information from which diagnosis is made. Computers allow radiographers access to the entire range of densities available. Radiographers manipulate the physical contrast available into the visible range to produce the diagnostic image.

Manipulating Contrast

The image receptor records many densities that cannot be seen by the human eye. Depending on the desired contrast, the recorded densities are compressed or expanded to form a range of visible densities. This can be accomplished by changes in the film's D log E curve, adjustments in kVp, or by the use of a computer. Compression or expansion of the range of densities separates the physical contrast that is actually recorded by the image receptor from

| 40 kVp | 50 kVp | 60 kVp | 70 kVp | 80 kVp | 90 kVp | 100 kVp | 110 kVp | 120 kVp |

Figure 24–3.   Variations in scale of contrast. The number of shades of gray, the scale or range of contrast, increases as kVp increases.

the visible contrast that can be perceived by the viewer on a single image.

RADIOGRAPHIC CONTRAST

Radiographic contrast is the total amount of contrast acquired from both the anatomical part and the film. These are described as **subject and image receptor** (film) contrast, respectively.

Image Receptor (Film) Contrast

Image receptor (film) contrast is the range of densities that the image receptor is capable of recording. Mathematically, this is expressed as the slope of the D log E curve. Film contrast depends on four factors: the use of **intensifying screens, film density, the D log E curve, and processing**.

Intensifying Screens Intensifying screens create an inherently higher contrast image. Although the exact reason is unknown, contrast is always lower for a film exposed to x-rays only than it is for the same film exposed to light from intensifying screens. It is most likely related to the way in which the film responds to the x-ray photons. The D log E curve changes dramatically when a film designed for exposure by light is exposed directly to x-rays.

Film Density Film contrast also changes with changes in film density. This is especially true in the toe and shoulder regions of the curve. If the kVp remains constant, mAs and distance will determine the actual value of exposure, thereby determining the location of the exposure on the log relative exposure axis of the curve. If a film is exposed correctly, the film densities will fall within the visible range of the D log E curve. If the exposure places the developed densities on the toe (an underexposed film) or shoulder (an overexposed film), the slope is not as steep, resulting in a decrease in contrast (Figure 24–4).

D log E Curve The primary determinant of the shape of the D log E curve is the physical composition of the film emulsion. As the slope of the curve becomes steeper, contrast is increased. For example, in Figure 24–5, film A possesses higher contrast than film B. Because

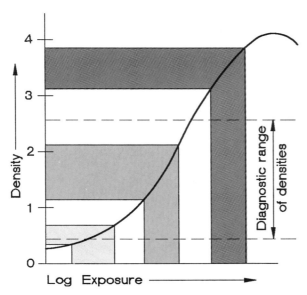

Figure 24–4. The effect of film density on contrast. When kVp remains constant, mAs and distance determine the location of the exposure on the log relative exposure axis. (A) When the film is correctly exposed the densities fall within the visible range. (B) An underexposed film occurs when the exposure places the developed densities into the toe. (C) An overexposed film occurs when the exposure places the developed densities into the shoulder. The decrease in contrast of under and overexposed films occurs because the slope is not as steep in the toe and shoulder.

of the steeper slope of the curve, the visible density range is compressed into a narrower exposure range. Film A is a high contrast, narrow latitude film. Film B is a low contrast, wide latitude film because the visible density range is expanded across a wider exposure range.

Processing Increasing film developer time, temperature, or replenishment rate will increase the chemical fog on the film. These changes produce a decrease in the slope of the curve (Figure 24–6). When any processing fac-

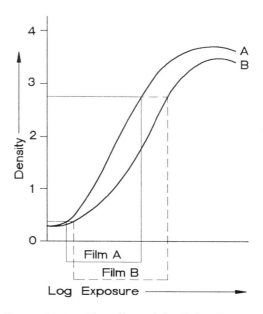

Figure 24–5. The effect of the D log E curve on contrast. As the slope of the curve becomes steeper, contrast is increased. Film A possesses higher contrast than film B, which compresses the visible density range into a narrower exposure range.

tor causes a change in base fog, contrast is affected. Developer temperature and immersion time, replenishment, and developer contamination are the primary processing factors that cause objectionable fog levels. Increased developer temperature, time, and replenishment rates cause increased fog and decreased contrast. Developer contamination by fixer causes increased fog and decreased contrast because the chemical ability of the developer reducing agents is seriously impaired by the pH change in the solution.

Subject Contrast

Subject contrast is the range of differences in the intensity of the x-ray beam after it has

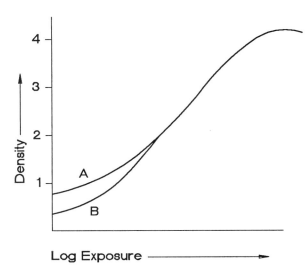

Figure 24–6. The effect of processing fog on contrast. Increased fog raises the toe of curve and decreases its slope, thus decreasing contrast.

been attenuated by the subject. It is dependent on kilovoltage and the amount and type of irradiated material.

Kilovoltage Kilovoltage peak (kVp) is the primary controller of subject contrast. As kVp increases, a wider range of photon energies is produced (Figure 8–6). The wider the range of photon energies, the greater the ability of the photons to penetrate the body tissues. This leads to a wider range of densities on the film, which results in an overall lower contrast.

As long as the kVp is adequate to penetrate the part being examined, low kVp will produce high subject contrast. When the kVp is too low, most of the photons do not reach the film because they are absorbed in the patient. Low kVp produces higher subject contrast because most of these low energy photons are absorbed by thicker parts while more penetrate the thin part. With high kVp, subject

contrast is decreased because more uniform penetration occurs between thick and thin parts.

The effect of kVp on subject contrast can be detailed by examining the D log E curve. Figure 24–7 shows the range of transmitted photon intensities forming the exposure to the film for both high and low kVp techniques for the same film type. High kVp produces a compressed range of relative exposures, which the slope of the D log E curve reflects within the visible density range. Low kVp produces an expanded range of relative exposures, which the slope of the D log E curve is unable to re-

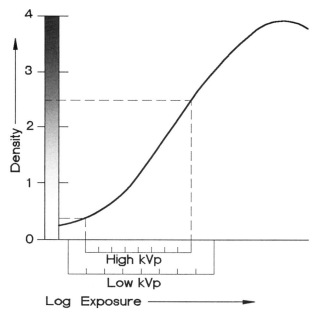

Figure 24–7. The effect of kVp on subject contrast. The range of transmitted photon intensities for high kVp produces a compressed range of relative exposures, which are reflected within the visible density range by the slope of the curve. The expanded range of exposures produced by low kVp is too wide for the curve to reflect within the visible density range. This causes some of the lowest and highest photon intensities not to be visible when low kVp is used.

flect within the visible density range. This causes some of the lowest and highest exposures to fall outside the visible density range. Increasing kVp causes density differences that were previously undetectable to become visible, resulting in an increase in the diagnostic information provided by the image.

This concept is demonstrated nicely by comparing chest radiographs to radiographs of the ribs. In chest radiography high kVps result in a wide range of radiographic densities that fall within the visible range. Both the air-filled lungs and the bony structures are demonstrated within the visible range. No structures appear under or overexposed. In rib radiography low kVps are used to enhance the differences between the air-filled lungs and the overlying bony structures. The air-filled lungs demonstrate increased radiographic density, while the bony structures demonstrate decreased radiographic density compared to the chest film.

In addition to kVp, radiation fog has a significant effect on contrast. It is the result of x-ray interactions with matter, primarily Compton scatter. As kVp increases the percentage of Compton interactions increases. As a result of this increase in the amount of scatter reaching the film, contrast is decreased. Scatter raises the base plus fog (the toe) and decreases the slope of the curve (Figure 24–6). These changes cause the lightest densities to be "fogged over" so they can no longer be distinguished from one another (Figure 24–8). The resulting image no longer includes a clear or pure "white" region, and therefore has less contrast.

Fog can be caused by factors other than scatter radiation. These include subjecting film to heat, low level ionizing radiation, or chemical fumes. Developer temperature, replenishment, and developer contamination may also cause objectionable fog levels. The effect of fog on contrast must be considered during clinical

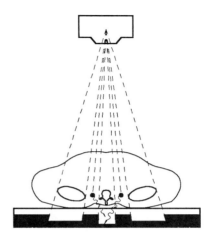

Figure 24–8. The effect of scatter radiation on contrast. Scatter radiation producing image density (and incorrect information) in a region of high subject density (under the vertebral column). The scatter interferes with the ability of the bone to cast a light shadow on the film.

radiography because it sets the acceptance limits for contrast regulation. The radiographer should remember that any factor that results in an increase in fog will decrease contrast.

Amount of Irradiated Material The amount of irradiated material depends on the thickness of the body part and the field size. Both these factors influence the number of x-rays transmitted to the image receptor. As body part thickness increases, x-ray absorption increases. Conversely, as body part thickness decreases so does absorption. This difference in absorption between various thicknesses influences subject contrast. When the difference between adjacent thicknesses of various body parts is great, subject contrast is increased. When little difference exists in the thickness of adjacent body parts, subject contrast is decreased.

When the overall thickness of a body part increases, or when field size increases, the amount of scatter created will increase. This results in a decrease in subject contrast. A decrease in overall body part thickness or field size results in increased subject contrast.

Type of Irradiated Material The type of irradiated material is influenced by the atomic number of the material and its density. Both these factors influence subject contrast.

Materials with a higher atomic number, such as lead and iodine, absorb a greater percentage of the x-ray beam than low atomic number materials, such as hydrogen, carbon, and calcium. This results from the presence of a greater number of electrons, which enables more interactions to occur. When the difference between the average atomic number of adjacent tissues is great, subject contrast is increased. When little difference exists between them, subject contrast is decreased. For example, bone has a higher average atomic number than soft tissue. Therefore, subject contrast between bone and soft tissue is greater than the contrast between adjacent soft tissue structures. Contrast media increase subject contrast by introducing greater differences in atomic number variations than those that exist naturally.

Tissue density describes how tightly the atoms of a given substance are packed together. When the difference between the densities of adjacent tissues is great, subject contrast is increased. When little difference exists between them, subject contrast is decreased. For example, bone tissue is a denser substance than lung tissue. Therefore subject contrast between bone and lung tissue is greater.

EVALUATING CONTRAST

The major consideration in evaluating visible contrast is **verification that a proper range of densities are visible throughout the ana-**tomical area of interest on the radiograph. Proper density alone is not enough. The anatomical structures of interest are visible only when sufficient contrast between the densities exists. Of course, these densities must be well within the range of human visibility (OD 0.25–2.50).

Unlike the evaluation of density, contrast assessment requires more than just sufficient density within the visibility range. Adequate contrast must demonstrate enough distinctly different densities within the range to satisfy diagnostic quality requirements for the particular examination. Much of this ability is the result of clinical experience. It is obvious that proper contrast is not the same for all tissues. Knowledge of anatomy and physiology, both normal and abnormal, as well as pathology and technical factors, is critical for proper contrast evaluation. Only when these skills are combined with an experienced and trained professional eye, can proper contrast evaluation occur.

Because there is more information recorded on a radiograph than is seen, the diagnostic importance of contrast is a matter of how many densities are included in the visible contrast range. To some extent, it can be said that low contrast images have more information. However, the critical point is that the various densities must be discernible.

The human eye is limited in its ability to discern light and dark. This essentially establishes an OD value for the lightest and darkest visible shades of gray. When additional shades of gray are added to the visible range of contrast, they must fit between these two densities. Each additional shade of gray reduces the magnitude of the density difference, or the contrast, between the lightest and darkest grays. Eventually a point is reached where additional shades of gray do not have enough density difference to be visible (Figure 24–1F). Of course, this occurs at different points, depending on individual visual abilities. A 30 percent density difference has been used as the minimum change to cause a visible difference because this magnitude is discernible by nearly everyone. However, some professionals may be able to discern as little contrast as a 15 percent density difference, which means they are capable of seeing twice as many shades of gray as someone who can discern only a 30 percent change.

Discerning contrast can be extremely difficult for even the experienced radiographer when the image exhibits poor density. **Contrast evaluation can be made only when sufficient density exists to permit the range of contrast to be seen**. The eye tends to consider nearby densities and contrast when evaluating image quality. It is so difficult for the eye to ignore nearby factors that a contrast mask is often helpful (Figure 24–9). A contrast mask is a simple tool to help focus on the contrast in a selected area. When a contrast mask is used with an image, adjacent information is eliminated. This makes the evaluation much easier as the contrast problem becomes evident as well as easier to evaluate (Figure 24–10). Because of the difficulty in ignoring nearby density problems (either too light or dark) even the experienced radiographer will find a contrast mask useful in making some evaluations.

Selecting The Appropriate kVp

There are no established rules concerning how much contrast is desirable in all situations. Experience and knowledge enable the radiographer to determine when a change in

Figure 24–9. A contrast mask.

contrast will increase the diagnostic quality of an image. Many radiologists find it desirable to have uniform contrast throughout a single examination to permit comparisons between projections. Low contrast can be achieved to some degree by utilizing a fixed kilovoltage technique system. Other radiologists prefer a higher contrast. This can be achieved to some degree by utilizing a variable kilovoltage technique system.

The radiographs in Figures 24–1 and 24–11 illustrate the effect of contrast on image quality. Notice in Figure 24–11 that the contrast varies as the kVp varies. Also notice that the contrast varies for the same kVp with different body part thickness (different subject densities). The exposure factors for these images used different mAs values to compensate for the differences in scatter radiation as the kVp was changed.

The radiographs in Figure 10–2 illustrate the effect of kVp on image density. To perceive a contrast change, density should be maintained at a uniform level. The 15 percent rule is an acceptable method of achieving uniform density when changing contrast. **A visible change in contrast will not be perceived until kVp is changed by 4–12 percent, depending on the kVp range** (Table 24–2). There is no reason to repeat an exposure for contrast reasons unless at least a 4–5 percent change is made,

TABLE 24–2		
CHANGES NECESSARY TO PRODUCE VISIBLE CONTRAST DIFFERENCES		
Level	*Change necessary to Produce Visible Change*	*Change to Equal Percent Change*
30–50 kVp	4–5 percent	1–3 kVp
50–90 kVp	8–9 percent	4–8 kVp
90–130 kVp	10–12 percent	9–16 kVp

A   B

Figure 24–10.   Using a contrast mask. (A) A radiograph of a chest that appears too light, making contrast evaluation difficult. (B) The same radiograph with the contrast mask applied to the right upper lobe of the lung, making contrast evaluation easier.

although higher kVps require even greater changes. The effects of mAs and the influencing factors on image contrast are not exact because of the wide variety of variables that are part of the imaging system. Many of the variables affect the contrast of the image as a side effect of other changes.

Both the quantity and quality of the x-ray beam will vary with changes in kilovoltage. There are too many variables to be quantified into a reliable formula. Because the 15 percent rule is used so much when maintaining image density, it is convenient to use it as the minimum practical change within the diagnostic range. Remember that the 15 percent rule is a misnomer as the actual changes necessary to maintain density vary from 15–25 percent (Figure 23–4).

When a radiograph is outside acceptance limits, it needs to be repeated. All acceptance limits permit some degree of variation, at least 8–15 percent change in contrast. **The rule for contrast changes is to make adjustments in increments of 15 or 8 percent**. If the radiograph does not require an 8 percent change in kVp and contrast, it seldom requires repeating. Exceptions to this rule are fine adjustments of 8 percent that are crucial to demonstrate small structures. Radiographers may adjust technique charts by an 8 percent margin, but will seldom subject the patient to a second exposure for such a minor change. As with density adjustments, contrast changes require bold action or no action at all.

In some instances it may be desirable to decrease kVp to increase contrast when mAs

60 kVp   38 mAs   40" SID
12:1 grid   400 RS   259 mR

A

60 kVp   102 mAs   40" SID
12:1 grid   400 RS   828 mR

D

80 kVp   7 mAs   40" SID
12:1 grid   400 RS   98.1 mR

B

80 kVp   18 mAs   40" SID
12:1 grid   400 RS   240 mR

E

100 kVp   3 mAs   40" SID
12:1 grid   400 RS   68.5 mR

C

100 kVp   7 mAs   40" SID
12:1 grid   400 RS   158 mR

F

Figure 24–11.   The effect of contrast on image quality. Skull radiographs produced at (A) 60 kVp; (B) 80 kVp; (C) 100 kVp. Abdomen radiographs produced at (D) 60 kVp; (E) 80 kVp; (F) 100 kVp. Compare these images, noting contrast changes due to anatomical part differences.

must be increased. A radiograph of a 30 cm abdomen produced at 90 kVp demonstrates a relatively low contrast (Figure 24–12B). When the same abdomen is radiographed at 70 kVp, a significantly higher contrast results (Figure 24–12A). The reduced kVp produced less scatter radiation, thus producing higher contrast. The natural tendency to increase kVp for thicker parts will not produce satisfactory radiographs if the effect of increased Compton scatter on contrast is not considered first.

Radiographic image contrast occurs due to the photoelectric effect's total absorption of photons in the subject. High contrast is directly related to the number of photoelectric effect interactions that occur in the subject. Because Compton interactions produce scatter, low contrast is directly related to the amount of Compton scatter that occurs in the subject. Image contrast can be controlled by adjusting kVp. The kVp controls the relationship between the number of photoelectric versus Compton interactions.

Contrast can be determined by matching the average incident photon energy with the average inner-shell binding energy of the predominant subject material, as shown in Figure 11–8. For example, when maximum contrast is desired for bone tissue, technical factors that increase the percentage of photoelectric interactions should be used. Photoelectric effect interactions increase as kVp decreases.

FACTORS AFFECTING CONTRAST

The controlling and influencing factors that affect contrast are shown in Figure 24–13. **The controlling factor that affects contrast has the most direct effect on the image**. When it is changed the image will change as a primary result. The influencing factors that control contrast have a **less direct effect** on the image or change other factors as well as contrast. When the influencing factors are changed the contrast is affected, but not as directly as with the controlling factor. With some of the factors this change is so small that it is essentially negligible.

Controlling Factor

Kilovoltage **Kilovoltage peak (kVp) is the controller of contrast**. As kVp increases contrast decreases. As kVp decreases contrast increases. In most instances the control of contrast rests with the radiographer by selecting an appropriate kVp setting from a technique chart developed for the particular x-ray unit in use. Other variables such as generator configuration (phase, falling load, or frequency) may also affect the final decision. A generator configuration that increases the effective kVp will result in a decrease in contrast. For example, for a given kVp a three-phase generator will produce a lower contrast than a single-phase unit.

Kilovoltage also controls the amount of scatter radiation produced. Increasing kVp increases the amount of radiation fog, thereby decreasing contrast.

The radiographer must adapt the suggested kVp setting for the individual procedure. Experience and study of various body habitus, pathologies, positioning, and equipment quickly provides the radiographer with clinical knowledge that can be used for these adjustments.

Influencing Factors

Milliampere-Seconds(mAs) Milliampere-seconds alters film density of the image and therefore affects contrast. When the change is sufficient to move density differences out of the range of human vision, either too dark or too light, the contrast is decreased (Figure 24–4).

Focal Spot Size The possibility of the focal spot size altering contrast enough to be visible is extremely unlikely. Focal spot sizes have

70 **kVp** 60 **mAs** 40″ **SID**
12:1 **grid** 400 **RS** 840 **mR**
phantom immersed in 20 cm water

A

90 **kVp** 60 **mAs** 40″ **SID**
12:1 **grid** 400 **RS** 387 **mR**
phantom immersed in 20 cm water

B

70 **kVp** 60 **mAs** 40″ **SID**
12:1 **grid** 400 **RS** 8,240 **mR**
phantom immersed in 30 cm water

C

90 **kVp** 60 **mAs** 40″ **SID**
12:1 **grid** 400 **RS** 3,010 **mR**
phantom immersed in 30 cm water

D

Figure 24–12. Increased contrast on 20 and 30 cm abdomens. (A) 20 cm abdomen at 70 kVp; (B) 20 cm abdomen at 90 kVp; (C) 30 cm abdomen at 70 kVp; (D) 30 cm abdomen at 90 kVp. All images were exposed with the same AEC and have the same overall density values. (Note the differences in mAs and mR dose.)

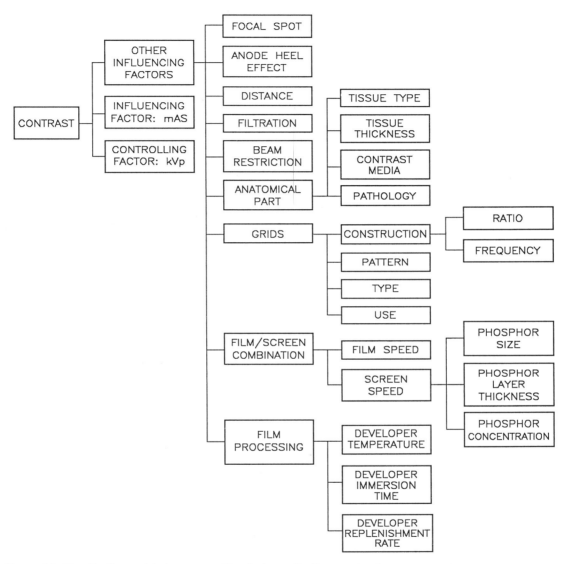

Figure 24–13.   Radiographic image quality: factors affecting contrast.

such a small effect on image density that it is unlikely that their effect on contrast could be detected.

Anode Heel Effect The anode heel effect alters the intensity of radiation, and therefore affects film density which can affect contrast. The intensity of radiation is greater at the cathode end of the tube. This difference would become visible only with open collimation and a small anode target angle (less than 12°). The anode heel has very little effect on contrast.

Distance Source-to-image receptor distance (SID) alters the intensity of the beam reaching the image receptor according to the inverse square law. This affects film density and therefore contrast. Greater distance decreases image density while less distance increases it. As distance alters density it can change the contrast exactly as does mAs.

Object-to-image receptor distance (OID) also has an effect on film density and contrast. An air-gap technique increases object-to-film distance and this permits scatter radiation to avoid the image receptor. This scatter radiation would normally contribute radiation fog to the image density. Removing scatter from the image will increase contrast.

Filtration Filtration increases the effect of kVp by changing the average photon energy of the beam. All types of filtration—inherent, added, and total—alter film density and contrast. Filtration affects contrast by changing the average photon energy and decreasing beam intensity. The increase in the average photon energy causes more Compton scatter production and this decreases contrast. The decreased intensity decreases density, which decreases contrast. This change is negligible, however, because most of these low energy photons do not exit the patient to contribute to film density. The predominant effect of filtration is caused by changes in average photon energy, therefore increased filtration decreases contrast. When filtration increases, kVp should be decreased slightly to maintain the same contrast.

Beam Restriction Restricting the beam, collimating, or reducing the primary beam field size reduces the total number of photons available. This reduces the amount of scatter radiation and therefore increases contrast.

Anatomical Part Because the patient is the prime attenuator of the beam, both the amount and type of tissue being examined greatly influence the density and contrast of the film. As the anatomical part size increases, the amount of scatter created by the part also increases, resulting in a decrease in contrast. As average atomic number and tissue density increase, the amount of scatter increases, which also results in a decrease in contrast.

As with density adjustments, compensation for anatomical part changes depends on an ability to assess tissue type, thickness, pathology, etc. This ability is achieved only through clinical experience.

Grids The primary function of a grid is contrast improvement (Figure 24–14). Grids improve contrast by removing scatter before it reaches the image. The contrast improvement factor (K) is the best measure of how well a grid accomplishes this function. The contrast improvement factor is dependent on the amount of scatter produced, which is controlled by the kVp and the amount and type of irradiated tissue. As the amount of scatter radiation increases, the lower the contrast and the lower the contrast improvement factor. The contrast improvement factor K is measured by using the average gradient (or gamma) of the straight line portion of the D log E curve:

$$K = \frac{\text{average gradient with the grid}}{\text{average gradient without the grid}}$$

If K = 1, then no improvement in contrast has occurred. Most grids have contrast improvement factors between 1.5 and 3.5 so their contrast is 1.5–3.5 times better than an identical non-grid film. The higher the K factor, the greater the contrast improvement.

Higher ratio grids remove more scatter and therefore have a greater contast improvement factor. This results in a higher contrast image.

Film/Screen Combinations The primary determinant of the shape of the D log E curve is the physical composition of the film emulsion. As the slope of the curve becomes steeper,

80 kVp	3.2 mAs	40″ SID
No grid	400 RS	45.2 mR

80 kVp	17 mAs	40″ SID
12:1 grid	400 RS	226 mR

A   B

Figure 24–14.   The effect of a grid on contrast. (A) 80 kVp without a grid; (B) 80 kVp with a grid. Both images were exposed with the same AEC and have the same overall density values. (Note the differences in mAs and mR dose.)

contrast is increased. Intensifying screens create an inherently higher contrast image. Contrast is always lower for a film exposed to x-rays only than it is for the same film exposed to light from intensifying screens.

Processing Increasing film developer time, temperature, or replenishment rate will increase the chemical fog on the film. These changes produce a decrease in the slope of the curve, which results in a decrease in contrast.

SUMMARY

Contrast is one of the two photographic properties that comprise visibility of detail. Visibility of detail refers to the fact that the ra-

diographic image is visible to the human eye only because sufficient contrast (and density) exists to permit structural details to be perceived. Radiographic contrast is the difference between adjacent densities. It can be mathematically evaluated as the percentage or ratio of the differences between densities. These differences can range from clear white through various shades of gray to black.

When the differences between adjacent densities that comprise contrast are great, the image is described as high contrast. The result is fewer discernible shades of gray. Conversely, when the differences are minimal the image is described as low contrast.

Short scale contrast is also called high contrast, or increased contrast, while long scale contrast is called low contrast, or decreased contrast. Physical contrast is the total range of density values recorded by the image receptor whereas visible contrast is the total range of density values that can be perceived by the human eye in a single image.

Radiographic contrast is the total amount of contrast acquired from both the anatomical part and the film. These are described as image receptor (film) contrast and subject contrast respectively. Image receptor (film) contrast is the range of densities that the image receptor is capable of recording. Film contrast depends on four factors: the use of intensifying screens, film density, the D log E curve, and processing. Subject contrast is the range of differences in the intensity of the x-ray beam after it has been attenuated by the subject. It is dependent on kilovoltage and the amount and type of irradiated material.

The major consideration in evaluating visible contrast is verification that a proper range of densities are visible throughout the anatomical area of interest on the radiograph. Proper density alone is not enough. The anatomical structures of interest can be visualized only when sufficient contrast between the densities exists. To perceive a contrast change, density should be maintained at a uniform level. The 15 percent rule is an acceptable method of achieving this.

A wide variety of factors affect radiographic contrast. These factors are classified as either controlling or influencing factors. The controlling factor is kVp and it should be used as the principle method for altering the contrast. The influencing factors include milliamperage-seconds, focal spot size, anode heel effect, distance, filtration, beam restriction, anatomical part, grids, film/screen combination, and film processing.

When the controlling factor or any of the influencing factors is altered, some change in contrast will occur, however with some of the factors the effect is often neglible. The following list illustrates the effect on contrast when the various factors are changed. For the purpose of this review, assume that compensation has been made for the changes in the radiographic density. Remember that if no compensation is made for the changes in density, and the resulting image is too light or too dark, contrast will always decrease.

+ = increases contrast
− = decreases contrast
∅ = negligible effect

Controlling Factor

− Increasing kilovoltage
+ Decreasing kilovoltage
− Increasing number of pulses in the generator waveform
+ Decreasing number of pulses in the generator waveform

Influencing Factors

∅ Increasing milliamperage-seconds*
∅ Decreasing milliamperage-seconds*
∅ Focal-spot size changes
∅ Anode heel effect
∅ Increasing SID
∅ Decreasing SID
+ Increasing OID
− Decreasing OID
− Increasing filtration
+ Decreasing filtration
+ Increasing beam restriction/collimation
− Decreasing beam restriction/collimation
− Increasing amount of irradiated tissue
+ Decreasing amount of irradiated tissue
− Increasing atomic number or density of tissue
+ Decreasing atomic number of density of tissue
+ Using contrast media
− Additive pathological conditions
+ Destructive pathological conditions

+ Increasing grid ratio
− Decreasing grid ratio
∅ Increasing film/screen combination relative speed
∅ Decreasing film/screen combination relative speed
+ Use of intensifying screens
− Increasing film processing developer time and temperature
+ Decreasing film processing developer time and temperature

*For example, changing mAs while maintaining density by SID changes.

REVIEW QUESTIONS

1. Define radiographic contrast.

2. How do high contrast images differ from low contrast images?

3. What is the difference between physical and visible contrast?

4. What factors affect image receptor (film) contrast and subject contrast?

5. How does film density affect image receptor contrast?

6. What is the controlling factor of subject contrast and how does it affect it?

7. How do variations in the anatomical part affect contrast?

8. What is the effect of a grid on contrast?

9. How does film processing affect contrast?

REFERENCES/SUGGESTED READINGS

Bierman, A. and Boldingh, W. Hondius. The relation between tension and exposure times in radiography. *Acta Radiologica*, 35, 22–26, 1951.

Cahoon, John B. *Formulating X-Ray Techniques.* 8th ed. Durham, NC: Duke University Press, 1974.

Cahoon, John B. Radiographic technique: Its origin, concept, practical application and evaluation of radiation dosage. *The X-Ray Technician*, 32, 354–364, 1961.

Carroll, Quinn. *Fuch's Principles of Radiographic Exposure, Processing and Quality Control.* 3rd ed. Springfield, IL: Charles C. Thomas Publishers, 1985.

Chow, Mai F. The effect of a film's sensitivity to its speed, contrast, and latitude. *The Canadian Journal of Medical Radiation Technology,* 19:4, 147, 1988.

Donohue, Daniel P. *An Analysis of Radiographic Quality: Lab Manual and Workbook.* 2nd ed. Rockville, MD: Aspen Publishers, Inc., 1984.

Eastman Kodak Company, Health Sciences Markets Division, *The Fundamentals of Radiography,* 12th ed. Rochester, NY: Kodak Publication M1–18.

Files, Glenn W. *Medical Radiographic Technique,* Springfield, IL: Charles C. Thomas Publishers, 1952.

Files, Glenn W. Maximum tissue differentiation. *The X-Ray Technician.* 7,17–24+, 1935.

Fuchs, Arthur W. *Principles of Radiographic Exposure and Processing.* 1st ed. Springfield, IL: Charles C. Thomas Publishers, 1955.

Fuchs, Arthur W. Relationship of tissue thickness to kilovoltage. *The X-Ray Technician,* 19, 287–293, 1948.

Fuchs, Arthur W. Balance and the radiographic image. *The X-Ray Technician,* 12:3, 81–84+, 1940.

Hiss, Stephen S., *Understanding Radiography,* Springfield, IL: Charles C. Thomas Publishers, 1978.

Jenkins, David, *Radiographic Photography and Imaging Processes,* Lancaster, England: MTP Press Ltd., 1980.

Jerman, Ed. C., *Modern X-Ray Technic,* St. Paul: Bruce Publishing Co., 1928.

Kodera, Yoshie; Robert A. Schmidt; Heang-Ping Chan and Kunio Doi. Backscatter from metal surfaces in diagnostic radiology, *Radiology,* Jan., 231, 1984.

Koenig, George F. Kilovoltage as a qualitative factor, *The X-Ray Technician* 29, 1–4, 13, 1957.

Lauer, O. Gary, John B. Mayes and Rosemary P. Thurston. *Evaluating Radiographic Quality: The Variables and Their Effects,* Mankato, MN: The Burnell Company Publishers, Inc., 1990.

Mattsson, Ove, Practical photographic problems in radiography. *Acta Radiologica* Supplementum 120 1–206, 1955.

Morgan, James A. *The Art and Science of Medical Radiography.* 5th ed. St. Louis, MO: Catholic Hospital Association, 1977.

Morgan, Russell H. An analysis of the physical factors controlling the diagnostic quality of roentgen images: Part III. Contrast and the intensity distribution function of a Roentgen image. *American Journal of Roentgenology and Radiation Therapy,* 55:1, 67–89, 1946.

Morgan, Russell H. An analysis of the physical factors controlling the diagnostic quality of roentgen images: Part IV. Contrast and the film contrast factor. *American Journal of Roentgenology and Radiation Therapy,* 55:5, 627–633, 1946.

Schwarz, Gerhart S. Kilovoltage conversion in radiography. *The X-Ray Technician.* 31:373–379, 436, 1960.

Schwarz, Gerhart S. Kilovoltage and radiographic effect. *Radiology,* 73:749–760, 1959.

Seeman, H. E. and H. R. Splettstosser. The effect of kilovoltage and grid ratio on subject contrast in radiography. *Radiology,* 64:572–580, 1955.

Seeman, Herman E. *Physical and Photographic Principles of Medical Radiography.* New York: Wiley & Sons, Inc., 1968.

Trout, E. Dale, D. E. Graves, and D. B. Slauson. High kilovoltage radiography. *Radiology,* 52:669–683, 1949.

Williams, William A. Radiographic effect formula: Its practical application. *The X-Ray Technician.* 28:1–6, 67, 1956.

25 RECORDED DETAIL

One look is worth a thousand listens.

Merrill C. Sosman, "A Radiologist's Opinion of the Stethoscope."

OUTLINE

ASSESSING RECORDED DETAIL
EFFECTS ON IMAGE APPEARANCE
FACTORS AFFECTING RECORDED DETAIL

OBJECTIVES

Upon completion of this chapter, the student should be able to:

1. Define recorded detail, including synonymous terms and derived units.
2. Explain the effect of various distances on recorded detail.
3. Describe the factors that affect penumbra size.
4. Describe the effect of film/screen combinations on the resolution of recorded detail.
5. Discuss the relationship of the three intensifying screen factors to recorded detail.
6. Describe appropriate techniques to prevent patient motion.
7. Synthesize various geometrical factors into a clinical protocol for improving resolution.
8. Recommend techniques for reducing motion, including immobilization devices.

ASSESSING RECORDED DETAIL

Recorded detail is one of the two geometric properties of radiographic image quality. Unlike the photographic properties of density and contrast, which control the visibility of detail, the geometric properties control detail itself. **Recorded detail is the degree of geometric sharpness or accuracy of the struc**tural lines actually recorded in the radiographic image. Good detail exists even when it cannot be seen due to poor visibility of detail or, in other words, when the density and/or contrast are poor. Recorded detail is one of the easiest of the prime technical factors to evaluate and adjust.

Recorded detail is also referred to as **definition, sharpness, resolution, or simply as**

detail. When the term detail is used by itself it usually refers to the recorded detail of the radiographic image. Detail is easily quantified and even has a derived unit. The term resolution is applied to quantified discussions of recorded detail. The **unit of resolution is** the line pairs per millimeter (lp/mm) or cycles per mm. A radiographic resolution tool is composed of pairs of lines a set distance from one another (Figure 25–1). The point at which the viewer can discern the closest pair of lines from each other represents the lp/mm reading. Most human visual acuity is limited to the range of 5 lp/mm. At this level each line is 0.1 mm wide, so a structure of this size could be discerned.

Figure 25–1. A resolution tool. The tool is read by discerning the point at which the finest lines are still visible as separated from one another. This point is then compared to the scale to determine the lp/mm reading. (Courtesy of Nuclear Associates, Inc., 100 Voice Road, Carle Place, NY 11514.)

Unfortunately, most radiographic imaging systems do not provide this level of resolution.

All radiographic images have less recorded detail than the object itself. In other words, the radiographic image exhibits some, but never all, of the detail of the anatomical part. The art of radiography involves controlling the degree of **unsharpness** so that it does not interfere with image diagnosis.

The effect of poor resolution on the image is seen as a lack of sharp definition of fine detail. This is caused by unacceptable levels of penumbra as compared to the umbral shadows that are expected from the part. Evaluation of resolution is best accomplished when an image has high contrast and a diagnostic quality density.

Recorded detail is usually evaluated during quality control testing by imaging a resolution test tool. In a clinical situation, small structures are the easiest to examine to evaluate recorded detail. The trabeculae of bone is an excellent guidepost to image resolution. Much of the ability to assess when the resolution is too poor to be of diagnostic quality is a matter of clinical experience (Figure 25–2).

EFFECTS ON IMAGE APPEARANCE

Resolution affects the image appearance by demonstrating fine detail structures, often very close to the size limits of the naked eye. When fine detail is lacking, the image will often appear blurred and gray.

Motion unsharpness is often not perceived by the beginning student, partially because students must learn to critically examine each image in a methodical manner. Another reason is that a thorough knowledge of how various anatomical structures should appear radiographically is necessary in order to recognize when motion causes them to appear unacceptable (Figure 25–3). The assessment of

A

B

Figure 25–2A & B.   Assessing resolution. (A) A pediatric wrist exhibiting good resolution. (B) An adult knee exhibiting fair resolution in the tibia and poor resolution in the femur.

motion is a matter of obtaining sufficient clinical experience. Progress in professional competence has been achieved when the beginning radiographer easily discerns motion unsharpness.

FACTORS AFFECTING RECORDED DETAIL

The factors that control recorded detail are shown in Figure 25–4. Close consideration of these factors will reveal that recorded detail is improved only through factors that increase the patient exposure dose. This makes consideration of how much resolution is necessary for a particular study a patient radiation protection issue. Resolution problems should be approached in this order:

1. Eliminate **motion**;
2. Reduce **OID (OFD)**;
3. Reduce **focal spot size**;
4. Reduce **intensifying screen phosphor size**; and
5. Increase **SID (FFD)**.

Geometry

The geometry of the beam is the most important factor in establishing the level of resolution desired for recorded detail. Because the x-ray beam emanates from a small point (the focal spot), the further the photons move from their source, the further they diverge. In Figure 25–5 note how much more tissue is imaged and exposed at the level of the spine than at the level of the collimator light beam. This is the basis of the inverse square law and it applies to the geometry of the beam as well.

Distance The distances between the source or focal spot (S), object or part (0) and image receptor (I) are critical in establishing sufficient recorded detail. These distances are referred

Figure 25–3. Motion unsharpness. The diaphragm, heart and bowel are all unsharp due to motion of this pediatric patient.

to, as shown in Figure 25–6, so that SOD + OID = SID. **Resolution is improved when OID decreases** and degraded whenever it increases. This is why the affected side or part of interest is always positioned as close to the film as possible.

Resolution is improved when SID increases and degraded when it decreases. Increasing SID improves the recorded detail of the image enough that numerous leaders in radiography are currently advocating a routine 48″ (120 cm) distance in place of the current 40″ (100 cm) distance.

When it is necessary to make adjustments in order to improve detail, OID should be eval-

uated first. **The minimum OID should be used to improve detail.** The details of the positioning and the equipment in use should be carefully considered. In many instances a change in positioning will accomplish a remarkable improvement in detail. In fact, most positioning routines were established with OID as a critical factor. For example, the PA chest projection is preferred because it places the heart closer to the film than does the AP projection. The left lateral stomach, AP kidney and AP lumbar projections were all developed for the same reason.

The OID can also be minimized by considering the distance between the surface supporting the part and the film cassette. Differences between the **tabletop-to-Bucky tray distance can have a considerable influence on OID.** Of course, the minimal OID is obtained with non-Bucky procedures that place the part directly on the cassette, as is routine in extremity radiography. However, once the need for a grid supersedes the resolution that is lost by using a Bucky tray, careful consideration can still result in significant differences in detail. For example, whereas a head unit will often permit an OID of 1–2 cm, a floating top table may permit an OID of only 10 cm. The differences in image quality are significant (Figure 25–7).

Once the OID has been minimized, **resolution is improved when SID increases** and degraded when it decreases. Again, positioning routines were established to take advantage of this relationship. For example, the lateral cervical is usually performed at 72″ (180 cm) instead of 40″ (100 cm) because the OID cannot be reduced due to the distance between the neck and shoulder. Increased SID is the only method that can produce a lateral image comparable to the AP and oblique projections, which have a much smaller OID.

Focal Spot Size Focal spot size is controlled by the line focus principle (see Figure

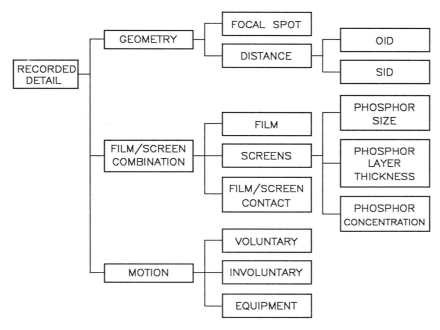

Figure 25–4.   Radiographic image quality: factors affecting recorded detail.

7–13). A multitude of tube designs have been used over the years to minimize the effective focal spot while maximizing the actual focal spot to absorb the heat.

The umbra is the distinctly sharp area of a shadow. **The penumbra is the imperfect, unsharp shadow surrounding the umbra**. It is also referred to as the edge gradient. The focal spot size is a major controller of image resolution because it controls penumbra. The fact that the source of the x-ray photons is not a point source, although it is sometimes convenient to think of it as such, is what causes penumbra. Figures 25–8A and B illustrate the umbra and penumbra caused by the focal spot size and configuration. As the focal spot decreases in size, penumbra also decreases, thus increasing resolution. Focal spots are usually not capable of imaging structures smaller than the focal spots themselves.

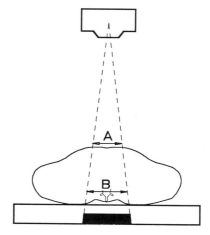

Figure 25–5.   Divergence of the x-ray beam. More tissue is imaged and exposed at the level of the spine (point B) than at the level of the collimator light beam (point A).

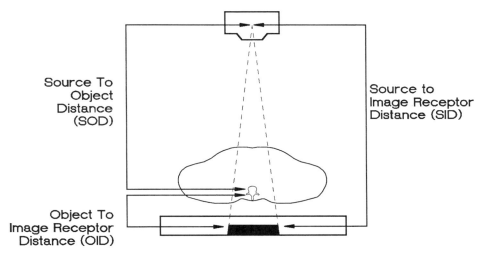

Figure 25–6.   Critical distances in radiography.

80 **kVp**	10 **mAs**	40″ **SID**
8:1 **grid**	400 **RS**	57.3 **mR**

80 **kVp**	10 **mAs**	40″ **SID**
8:1 **grid**	400 **RS**	57.3 **mR**

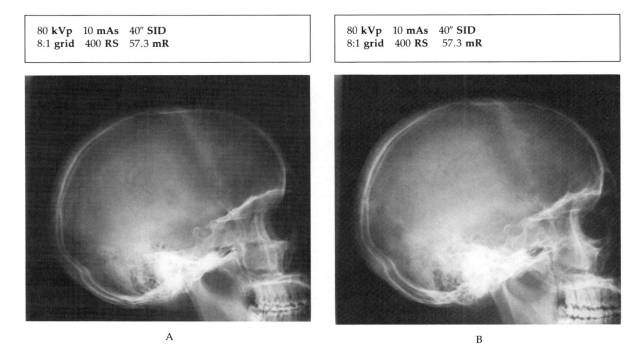

A   B

Figure 25–7A & B.   (A) 7 cm OID (FFD);   (B) 14 cm OID (FFD).

Figure 25–8A–F.   Umbra and penumbra. The umbral area receives essentially no photons. The penumbral area receives more photons at the outer edges with progressively fewer photons toward the umbral area, thus creating an imperfect, unsharp shadow around the umbra. (A&B) The effect of focal-spot size on resolution. The geometry of the beam reduces penumbra and increases resolution as focal-spot size decreases. (C&D) The effect of object-to-image receptor distance (OID) on resolution. As the OID decreases, penumbra is reduced and resolution increases. (E&F) The effect of source-to-image receptor distance (SID) on resolution. As SID increases, penumbra is reduced and resolution increases.

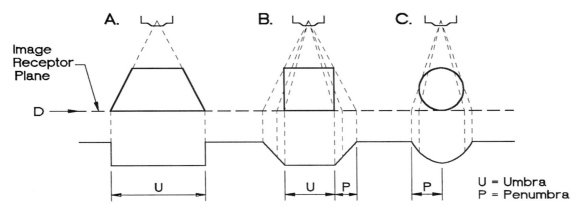

Figure 25–9A/C. Attenuation unsharpness. The D line represents the amount of density that would occur in the image receptor under each object. (A) A trapezoidal object shaped congruently to the divergence of the beam. (B) A square object produces density shadings that form the penumbra. (C) A round object produces a penumbra that is incorporated into the continuously varying density of the shape itself.

Figures 25–8C and D illustrate that as OID decreases, penumbra also decreases. Figures 25–8E and F illustrate that as SID increases, penumbra decreases. When penumbra decreases, resolution is increased.

Penumbra is increased by another phenomenon known as attenuation or absorption unsharpness. Because of the divergence of the incident x-ray beam, only an object that is trapezoidal would have a perfectly sharp edge (Figure 25–9A). A trapezoidal object would have a relatively equal object thickness that would attenuate the beam, causing an equal proportion of the beam to reach the image. A square object would project an edge with a gradually increasing attenuation (Figure 25–9B). Circular objects, which predominate in the human body, have an attenuation that varies throughout the entire object, reaching a maximum at a single point (Figure 25–9C). Consequently, the attenuation of the object itself causes a continuously varying projected density, which, when added to the penumbra, causes structures in the human body to have gradual instead of sharp edges.

Film/Screen Combinations

Film/screen combinations are most commonly classified by speed. Within a single phosphor type (for example, calcium tungstate or rare earth), there is an inverse relationship between film/screen combination speed and resolution. In other words, a slow film/screen combination will demonstrate better resolution than a fast one. This is such a definite relationship that many slow film/screen combinations are labeled as detail combinations.

Once the geometrical considerations of recorded detail have been maximized, the most common source of better resolution is the film/screen combination. Most institutions utilize at least two different film/screen combinations in recognition of the better detail required by extremity examinations. This policy permits higher speed film/screens to be used to reduce patient exposure dose for other examinations that do not require such high resolution.

Film Although various types of film have a wide variety of resolving capabilities, in radiography the intensifying screen always has

TABLE 25–1

EFFECTS OF INTENSIFYING SCREEN FACTORS ON RESOLUTION

Phosphor Change	Effect on Image Resolution	Effect on Patient Exposure Dose	Effect on Density
Crystal size			
increases	decreases	decreases	increases
decreases	increases	increases	decreases
Layer thickness			
increases	decreases	decreases	increases
decreases	increases	increases	decreases
Conversion efficiency			
increases	no change	decreases	increases
decreases	no change	increases	decreases

poorer resolution than the film. Radiographic film usually has resolving capabilities in the range of 100 lp/mm, far beyond the ability of any screen or human eye. As long as the film is sensitive to the light emitted by the screens, film speed and resolution are not important issues in radiographic imaging.

Although obsolete due to excessive patient exposure dose, nonscreen or direct exposure film possesses the highest resolution possible. Direct exposure film often required 20–100 times the mAs of a film/screen exposure.

Adjustment of film speed is seldom considered for resolution purposes. However, when a decision is made to use a higher resolution intensifying screen, its slower speed may be somewhat compensated for by using a higher speed film to help reduce patient exposure dose.

Intensifying Screens The resolving power of an intensifying screen depends on three factors: **phosphor size, phosphor layer thickness and phosphor conversion efficiency**. The relationship of these factors to recorded detail, patient exposure dose and density are shown in

Table 25–1. Note that to gain resolution, patient exposure dose must be increased. This creates a classical confrontation in radiography that pits recorded detail against patient exposure dose. The decision is often left to the radiographer, who must consider all elements of both sides of the issue. Detail speed screens can resolve about 15 lp/mm, par speed screens about 10 lp/mm, and high speed screens about 7 lp/mm. These differences in recorded detail are easily visualized (see Figure 21–3). In addition, because of their higher conversion efficiency, rare-earth phosphors have significantly better resolving abilities than similar speed calcium tungstate screens.

Quantum mottle is a phenomenon that may dramatically affect recorded detail when high speed intensifying screens are used with extremely low mAs. Modern intensifying screen technology is so advanced that it is now possible to obtain screens that are so sensitive that sufficient radiographic density can be achieved at extremely low mAs. If the total number of incident photons reaching the intensifying screen are insufficient to activate enough phosphors to emit light to cover the entire surface of the film, quantum mottle results (see Figure 20–6). When using diagnostic radiographic intensifying screens, quantum mottle is corrected **only** by increasing mAs.

When resolution is unsatisfactory and the geometric solutions have been exhausted, a higher resolution film/screen combination should be used. It is important to remember that this decision includes a significant increase in patient exposure dose. Conversely, if resolution is more than satisfactory for the examination, a lower resolution film/screen combination should be considered to reduce patient exposure dose.

Film/Screen Contact The radiographic film and intensifying screens are sandwiched together in the cassette by pressure pads that keep them in immediate direct contact with one another. When the film/screen contact is broken, even over a small area of the cassette, the image detail is not as sharp because of increased penumbra (see Figure 20–5).

The only adjustment for poor film/screen contact is repairing or discarding the cassette. The procedures for testing cassettes for film/screen contact are part of a quality control program.

Motion

Motion affects recorded detail because it fails to permit enough time for a well defined image to form. Instead, the image is spread over a distance and appears as a blurred series of densities in which no fine detail can be perceived.

Voluntary Motion Voluntary motion is that which is under the direct control of the patient. For the most part, this comprises the voluntary nervous system in cognizant adults (children and uncognizant adults may be excepted in some cases). For **all** patients, including children and uncognizant adults, **communication**, especially in a manner that establishes a professional and competent atmosphere, is the best method of controlling voluntary motion. There are a few examinations, such as most headwork, where immobilization greatly decreases the potential need for a repeated exposure.

For most examinations, when the radiographer effectively communicates positioning instructions, the patient is able to cooperate in reducing motion. Instructions must be given in a kindly and concerned manner. They must be in an understandable language, which includes avoiding medical terminology when appropriate, using proper pronunciation of foreign language instructions, is at a proper volume and is properly enunciated. Even infants and uncognizant adults will respond to a kindly tone of voice and gentle handling. Never assume that your patient is unable to understand your instructions. Many young children can be amazingly cooperative when they wish to be and uncognizant adults will often remember fragments of conversations when they regain full cognizance.

Involuntary Motion Involuntary motion is not under the conscious control of the patient. For the most part, involuntary motion is controlled by the involuntary nervous system and is physiological in nature. Heartbeat and parastalsis are the most common examples.

Equipment Motion Although often overlooked, motion of equipment can also be an occasional problem. If the movement of the reciprocating grid mechanism is not dampened, it can cause vibration of the cassette in the Bucky tray. If the x-ray tube suspension system is not balanced and isolated from other moving devices, especially overhead suspended units, it can vibrate or drift. This type of motion is extremely difficult to detect. It is usually suspected only when a variety of patients examined with the same x-ray unit appear to have motion problems.

Communication The best method of reducing motion is patient communication. It is assumed that appropriate aids to positioning, such as foam pads, angle sponges and sandbags, are already in use. The radiographer should consider the instructions that are given to be sure that they are clear, concise and understandable.

Exposure Time Reduction When the patient is cooperating, the best method is a reduction in exposure time with a corresponding increase in mA to maintain sufficient mAs and density. Involuntary motion can be reduced only by a reduction in exposure time. Other methods of decreasing exposure time while maintaining density include using higher speed film and screens, decreasing SID and increasing kVp. Increasing kVp is not a preferred method because of the accompanying contrast change. Table 25–2 summarizes the pros and cons of each method.

Immobilization When communication and exposure time reduction are not sufficient to reduce motion, partial immobilization must be considered. Immobilization devices, such as foam pads, angle sponges and sandbags, should be considered routine positioning aids. Patient motion can be expected when these aids are not provided. If students find it un-comfortable or difficult to hold radiographic positions during laboratory positioning practice, imagine how an ill patient who is in pain (most likely lying on the most acute area) must feel. The use of positioning aids is part of professionalism. Even when they are in short supply, the radiographer should try to locate the proper aids for the patient.

For some examinations, especially headwork, immobilization greatly reduces the potential need for repeated exposures and should be used routinely. A wide range of immobilization devices and techniques have been developed over the years; some are available commercially while others are homemade.

Experienced radiographers often say that tape is the radiographer's best friend. Tape should certainly be carried at all times by radiographers and used freely when warranted. A strip of tape across the forehead (folded sticky side out across skin surfaces) has avoided many repeated cranial exposures.

Some devices, especially in pediatrics, are designed to immobilize the entire body. Pediatric boards, mummy wrapping techniques, Pig-O-Stats™ and compression bands are common examples. Individual parts can usually be immobilized with combinations of tape, sandbags, long-handled paddles, compression bands and sheet wrapping. As a **last** resort, human immobilizers may be used to hold the patient in position. Male relatives are

TABLE 25–2

EFFECTS OF VARIOUS METHODS FOR REDUCING EXPOSURE TIME TO AVOID MOTION

Method	Density	Contrast	Resolution	Distortion
mA increase	maintains	maintains	maintains	maintains
kVp increase	maintains	decreases	maintains	maintains
Film/screen speed increase	maintains	maintains	decreases	maintains
SID decrease	maintains	maintains	maintains	increases

the first choice, female relatives second, then nonradiology hospital personnel and nonprofessional radiology personnel. Radiographers are the last choice. Under no circumstances should anyone be expected to routinely hold patients.

SUMMARY

Recorded detail is one of the two geometric properties of radiographic image quality. Unlike the photographic properties of density and contrast, which control the visibility of detail, the geometric properties control detail itself. Recorded detail is the degree of geometric sharpness or accuracy of the structural lines actually recorded in the radiographic image. Good detail exists even when it cannot be seen due to poor visibility of detail or, in other words, when the density and/or contrast are poor.

Recorded detail is also referred to as definition, sharpness, resolution, or simply as detail. When the term detail is used by itself, it usually refers to the recorded detail of the radiographic image. Detail is easily quantified and even has a derived unit. The term resolution is applied to quantified discussions of recorded detail. The unit of resolution is line pairs per millimeter (lp/mm) or cycles per mm.

The factors that affect recorded detail are geometry, including SID, OID and focal spot size; film/screen combinations, including film, intensifying screens and film/screen contact; and motion.

When the factors that affect recorded detail are altered, some change in the recorded detail will occur. No effect will occur unless one of these factors is altered. The following list illustrates the effect on recorded detail when the various factors are changed.

+ = increased recorded detail (resolution)
− = decreased recorded detail (resolution)

Geometry

+ Increasing SID
− Decreasing SID
− Increasing OID
+ Decreasing OID
− Increasing patient thickness
+ Decreasing patient thickness
− Increasing focal-spot size
+ Decreasing focal-spot size

Film/Screen Combination

− Increasing film/screen speed
+ Decreasing film/screen speed
+ Good film/screen contact
− Poor film/screen contact

Motion

− Increasing motion
+ Decreasing motion

REVIEW QUESTIONS

1. What is recorded detail?

2. How is resolution measured?

3. How do the SID and the OID affect recorded detail?

4. What is the relationship between focal spot size and recorded detail?

5. What is the difference between umbra and penumbra?

6. What three factors affect the resolving power of intensifying screens?

7. What is the difference between voluntary and involuntary motion?

8. What are the methods which can be used to reduce the possibility of motion?

REFERENCES AND RECOMMENDED READING

American Registry of Radiological Technologists. Use of 'penumbra' studied. *Radiologic Technology* 58:1, 74, 1987.

Cahoon, John B. *Formulating X-Ray Techniques.* 8th ed. Durham, NC: Duke University Press, 1974.

Cahoon, John B. Radiographic technique: Its origin, concept, practical application and evaluation of radiation dose. *The X-Ray Technician* 32, 354–364, 1961.

Calandrino, Goodelineas, and Allen. Parental participation in pediatric radiographic procedures: Help or hindrance? *Radiologic Technology* 58:3, 319–321, 1988.

Carroll, Quinn. *Fuchs's Principles of Radiographic Exposure, Processing and Quality Control.* 3rd ed. Springfield, IL: Charles C. Thomas Publisher, 1985.

Cullinan, Angeline M. *Producing Quality Radiographs.* Philadelphia, PA: Lippincott, 1987.

Donohue, Daniel P. *An Analysis of Radiographic Quality.* 2nd ed. Rockville, MD: Aspen Publishers, 1984.

Eastman Kodak Company, Health Sciences Markets Division. *The Fundamentals of Radiography.* 12th ed. Rochester, NY: Eastman Kodak Company, Publication M1–18, 1980.

Engel, Terry L. Effect of kilovoltage and milliamperage on focal spot size. *Radiologic Technology* 50:5, 559–561, 1979.

Files, Glenn W. *Medical Radiographic Technique.* Springfield, IL: Charles C. Thomas Publisher, 1952.

Files, Glenn W. Maximum tissue differentiation. *The X-Ray Technician* 7, 17–24+, 1935.

Fodor, Joseph III, and Jack C. Malott. *The Art and Science of Medical Radiography.* 6th ed. St. Louis, MO: The Catholic Health Association of the United States, 1987.

Fuchs, Arthur W. *Principles of Radiographic Exposure and Processing.* 2nd ed. Springfield, IL: Charles C. Thomas Publisher, 1958.

Fuchs, Arthur W. The rationale of radiographic exposure. *The X-Ray Technician* 22, 62–68, 76, 1950.

Fuchs, Arthur W. Balance and the radiographic image. *The X-Ray Technician* 12:3, 81–84+, 1940.

Geometrical Fallacies. *Radiologic Technology* 54:4, 297, 1983.

Hage, Stephen J. Modulation transfer function and film-screen combinations. *Applied Radiology* May/June, 1974.

Haus, Arthur G. Effects of geometric and screen-film unsharpness in conventional and 350 kVp chest radiography. *Radiology* Oct., 197, 1980.

Hiss, Stephen S. *Understanding Radiography.* Springfield, IL: Charles C. Thomas Publisher, 1978.

Jerman, Ed. C. *Modern X-Ray Technic.* St. Paul, MN: Bruce Publishing Co., 1928.

Lauer, O. Gary, John B. Mayes, and Rosemary P. Thurston. *Evaluating Radiographic Quality: The Variables and Their Effects.* Mankato, MN: The Burnell Company Publishers, Inc., 1990.

Morgan, Russell H. An analysis of the physical factors controlling the diagnostic quality of roentgen images: Part I. Introduction. *American Journal of Roentgenology and Radiation Therapy* 54:2, 128–135, 1945.

Morgan, Russell H. An analysis of the physical factors controlling the diagnostic quality of roentgen images: Part II. Maximum resolving power and resolution coefficient. *American Journal of Roentgenology and Radiation Therapy* 54:4, 395–402, 1945.

Morgan, Russel H. An analysis of the physical factors controlling the diagnostic quality of roentgen images: Part V. Unsharpness. *American Journal of Roentgenology and Radiation Therapy* 62:6, 870–880, 1949.

Seemann, Herman E. *Physical and Photographic Principles of Medical Radiography.* New York: Wiley & Sons, Inc., 1968.

Stears, John G., Joel E. Gray, and Eugene D. Frank. Radiologic exchange (resolution by focal spot size). *Radiologic Technology* 60:5, 429–430, 1989.

Stockley, Sybil M. *A Manual of Radiographic Equipment.* Edinburgh: Churchill Livingstone, 1986.

Sweeney, Richard J. Some factors affecting image clarity and detail perception in the radiograph. *Radiologic Technology* 46:6, 443, 1975.

THE CASE OF THE COLON IN THE SPIDER'S WEB

This radiograph of a barium-filled colon has strange vertical lines that seem to enclose the lower GI tract in a web. What is the cause of the lines?

Answers to the case studies can be found in Appendix E.

CHAPTER

26 DISTORTION

Hans Castorp peered through the lighted window, peered into Joachim Ziemssen's empty skeleton. The breast-bone and spine fell together in a single dark column. The frontal structure of the ribs was cut across by the paler structure of the back. Above, the collar-bones branched off on both sides, and the framework of the shoulder, with the joint and beginning of Joachim's arm, showed sharp and bare through the soft envelope of flesh. The thoracic cavity was light, but blood-vessels were to be seen, some dark spots, a blackish shadow.

Thomas Mann, *Der Zauberberg* (*The Magic Mountain*).

OUTLINE

ASSESSING DISTORTION
FACTORS AFFECTING SIZE DISTORTION
FACTORS AFFECTING SHAPE DISTORTION
EFFECT ON IMAGE APPEARANCE

OBJECTIVES

Upon completion of this chapter, the student should be able to:

1. Define size and shape distortion.
2. Explain the effects of SID and OID on image distortion.
3. Discuss various methods of minimizing distortion through variation of SID and OID.
4. Explain why elongation and foreshortening are relational definitions.
5. Describe the routine relationships between central ray, anatomical part and image receptor.
6. Explain the proper terms used to describe angulation direction and degree.
7. Differentiate distorted images from routine projections.
8. Calculate the magnification factor when given SID and SOD.
9. Calculate the actual size of an object when given the projected size, SID and OID.
10. Describe adjustments of SID and OID that will minimize magnification.
11. Describe adjustments of central ray, anatomical part and image receptor that will minimize shape distortion.

ASSESSING DISTORTION

Distortion is the second of the two geometric properties affecting radiographic image quality. Unlike the photographic properties of density and contrast, which control the visibility of detail, the geometric properties control detail itself. **Distortion is a misrepresentation of the size or shape of the structures being examined**. It creates a misrepresentation of the size and/or shape of the anatomical part being imaged. This misrepresentation can be classified as either size or shape distortion. Distortion, like detail, exists even when it cannot be seen due to poor visibility or, in other words, when the density and/or contrast are poor. The evaluation and adjustment of distortion require a thorough familiarity with normal radiographic anatomy. Unless the normal size and shape of a structure are known, comparison of the size and shape cannot be accomplished. Distortion can be difficult to determine even when normal sizes and shapes are known. Because the objective of radiography is to provide accurate images of structures, methods of minimizing distortion are important to diagnosis.

The factors that control distortion are shown in Figure 26–1. Careful examination of these factors will reveal that distortion is directly related to positioning. Only careful attention to the distances, direction and angulation between the anatomical part, central ray and image receptor can minimize distortion.

FACTORS AFFECTING SIZE DISTORTION

Size distortion can be only magnification in radiography. Radiographic minification is impossible, due to the divergent property of x-ray photons. Since it is not possible to reflect or refract x-ray photons by ordinary methods, they can only diverge from their point source. Thus, only magnification is possible and all size distortion is controlled by the radiographic distances, SID (FFD) and OID (OFD). In all instances, **reduced magnification size distortion increases the resolution of recorded detail**. Therefore, the objective in most radiography is to minimize magnification as much as possible. Magnification radiography is an exception to

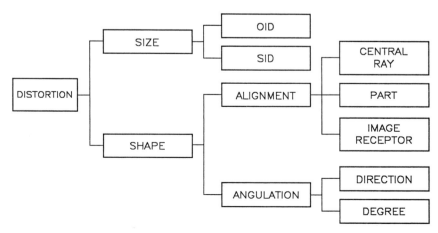

Figure 26–1. Radiographic image quality: factors affecting distortion.

this rule. In this instance, the principles of magnification geometry are used to increase the size of structures that are too small to be easily visualized. Special conditions must be created to achieve diagnostically acceptable magnification images.

Magnification size distortion is controlled by positioning the body part and tube to maximize SID while minimizing OID. This can be accomplished by various procedures and by positioning. For example, an upright oblique cervical vertebra projection can be performed at 72″ (180 cm) while a supine projection is performed at 40″ (100 cm). An AP chest may place the heart 6″ (15 cm) from the film while a PA projection would place it 2″ (5 cm) away.

Source-to-Image Receptor Distance

The SID has a major effect on magnification (Figure 26–2). **The greater the SID, the smaller the magnification**, because as SID increases the percentage of the total distance that makes up OID decreases. The OID is the critical distance for magnification and resolution.

Although 40″ (100 cm) has developed as the current routine SID, this was not always so. The popular SID has been increasing since the advent of radiography and will probably continue to do so. The first x-ray techniques book in the U.S. is generally recognized to be the 1918 *Extract from the United States Army X-Ray Manual,* in which 20″ (50 cm) is discussed as a reasonable SID. When Ed Jerman developed the first positioning and technique book, *Modern X-Ray Technic,* in 1928, he recommended distances varying from 25″ (63 cm) to 36″ (90 cm). Of course, in those days shorter distances were necessary because the x-ray tubes were not capable of handling the load required to provide sufficient density with the film and screens of the time. As generator technology advanced, the SID increased.

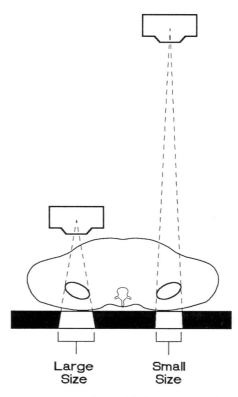

Figure 26–2. The effect of SID on image size magnification. Magnification size distortion is minimized by increasing SID.

Glenn Files' 1945 book, *Medical Radiographic Technic,* established the 40″ (100 cm) SID. For over 40 years this has remained the standard distance, but now there are institutions that use 48″ (120 cm) as a routine distance and the movement appears to be growing. Although a change demands new grids as well as careful consideration of x-ray unit design so that tube-to-tabletop distances can be achieved, and low table design so that radiographers can reach the tube, the increased resolution is worth the expense and trouble.

For many, many years chest radiography has routinely been performed at 72″ (180 cm) because the erect positioning arrangement permits a horizontal beam to be used and the increased SID effectively minimizes the magnification of the heart shadow. Any examination that permits a horizontal beam to be used can easily be established at an SID greater than 40″ (100 cm), and in many places the lateral cervical vertebral examination is performed at 72″ (180 cm) as well.

The source-to-object distance (SOD) is seldom discussed because it is included in descriptions of SID and OID, which are more critical. The SID is the distance that must be established by the radiographer when positioning.

The SID must be maximized to decrease magnification. Examinations of body parts with large inherent OID, such as the lateral cervical vertebra and the chest, use large SID

whenever possible. In addition, the historical trend to increase the routine SID should be continued.

Object-to-Image Receptor Distance

The OID is also a critical distance in both magnification and resolution. Figure 26–3 illustrates two major facets of OID. First, when objects within a structure are at different levels (Figure 26–3A and B) they will be projected onto the image as different sizes. This is similar to the manner in which the eye processes information for depth perception; smaller objects are perceived as more distant and larger objects as closer.

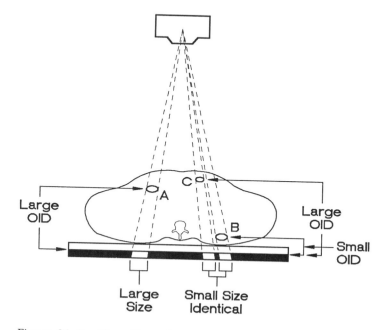

Figure 26–3. The effect of OID on image size magnification. Objects A and B are identical in size but their images as projected on the receptor are of significantly different sizes. Object C is significantly smaller than B, yet the image sizes are identical because of C's greater OID.

The radiographer should develop a stereoscopic perception of the radiographic image, which is difficult because radiographic perceptions are in reverse of the normal information the eye is accustomed to processing. This is because objects that are further from the image receptor will be magnified. For example, in a chest radiograph the ribs are seen as wider as they become more posterior. This effect should make them appear closer, which is the opposite of the truth for the PA projection. Nevertheless, the perception of three-dimensionality can be developed and then used to determine object-to-image receptor distance visually. When describing objects, it is important to remember that the size and distance relationship in a radiographically projected image is the opposite of that perceived visually.

A more important size relationship that is controlled by OID is shown in Figure 26–3 between objects B and C, where object C appears identical in size to object B. This is an illusion because object C is much smaller but is magni-

fied more because of its location in the part. This illustrates that a thorough knowledge of normal radiographic anatomy is a prerequisite to making judgements about size relationships. This is also one of the reasons radiographic examinations must include two projections, as close to 90° from one another as possible. When AP and lateral projections cannot be performed because of superimposing structures, as in an examination of the kidneys, it is important to include two oblique projections at 90° to one another. The two 90° opposing images can be used to verify the positional relationship of structures. This is also a shape distortion issue.

The OID is also important in dosimetry because it establishes the source-to-entrance skin distance that is the benchmark maximum dose to the patient. Because OID varies with the part size and position of the patient, it accounts for the increased exposure dose that is part of many examinations. For example, there is a significant difference in the OID between an AP and a lateral projection (Figure 26–4).

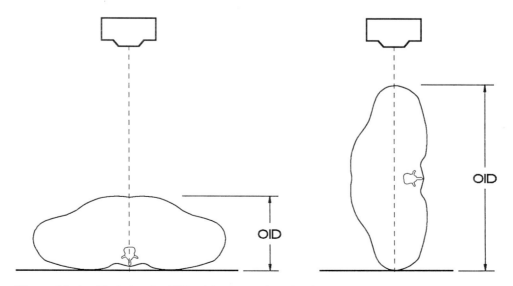

Figure 26–4.   Variation in OID with size and projection.

Obviously the entrance skin dose would be greater with the lateral, even if the same exposure factors were used. Consequently, larger patients receive a greater dose simply because their entrance skin surface is closer to the source. The increased mAs that is often used to provide sufficient density then increases the exposure dose even more.

The OID must be minimized to decrease magnification. Examinations of body parts with large inherent OID, such as the kidneys and chest, use positioning techniques to achieve as small an OID as possible.

Calculating Size Distortion

Size distortion is present in any radiographic image and can be measured very accurately by using simple geometry. **Magnification, or size distortion, can be assessed by calculation of the magnification factor.** The magnification factor is the degree of magnification and is calculated by:

$$M = \frac{SID}{SOD}$$

where M = magnification factor

Example: If the SID is 40″ (100 cm) and the SOD is 30″ (75 cm), what is the magnification factor?

Answer:

$$M = \frac{SID}{SOD}$$

$$M = \frac{40''}{30''} \quad or \quad M = \frac{100 \text{ cm}}{75 \text{ cm}}$$

$$M = 1.33$$

The magnification will be 33 percent or the image will be 133 percent of the object size.

Example: If the SID is 40″ and the OID is 2″, what is the magnification factor?

Answer:
Since the SOD is not supplied, it must be found by using the formula:

$$SID = SOD + OID$$
$$40'' = SOD + 2''$$
$$SOD = 40'' - 2''$$
$$SOD = 38''$$

then

$$M = \frac{SID}{SOD}$$

$$M = \frac{40''}{38''}$$

$$M = 1.05$$

The magnification factor permits calculation of the actual size of an object that is projected as an image by using the formula:

$$S = IM$$
where   S = actual size
I = image size
M = magnification factor

Example: If a projected image measures 5″ and the magnification factor is 1.02, what is the size of the actual object?

Answer:

$$S = IM$$
$$S = 5'' \times 1.02$$
$$S = 5.1''$$

Example: If object B in Figure 26–3 is 2″ in diameter on the image and is measured to be 3″ from the film (by using a lateral projection), what is its actual size if the SID is 40″?

Answer:
Since the SOD is not supplied, it must be found by using the formula:

$$SID = SOD + OID$$
$$40'' = SOD + 3''$$
$$SOD = 40'' - 3''$$
$$SOD = 37''$$

then

$$M = \frac{SID}{SOD}$$

$$M = \frac{40''}{37''}$$

$$M = 1.08$$

then

$$S = IM$$

$$S = 2'' \times 1.08$$

$$S = 2.16''$$

This magnification formula assumes that the focal spot is a point source. Because it is not, when the object size approaches the effective focal spot size or smaller, special problems develop from penumbral overlap (Figure 26–5). Therefore, **objects smaller than the effective focal spot cannot be demonstrated** and the

magnification formula must be modified to consider the width of the focal spot.

FACTORS AFFECTING SHAPE DISTORTION

Shape distortion is the misrepresentation by unequal magnification of the actual shape of the structure being examined (Figure 26–6). Shape distortion displaces the projected image of an object from its actual position and can be described as either elongation or foreshortening. **Elongation** projects the object so it appears to be longer than it really is while **foreshortening** projects it so it appears shorter than it really is. Elongation occurs when the tube or the image receptor is improperly aligned. Foreshortening occurs only when the

Figure 26–5. Objects smaller than the focal spot itself cannot be imaged due to penumbral overlap. The entire image is composed of overlapping penumbra with no umbra to define the edges.

Figure 26–6. Shape distortion due to unequal magnification. Note how the alignment of the part appears different depending on the degree of distortion. (Adapted with permission from Cullinan, Angeline M, *Producing Quality Radiographs*, copyright 1987 J. B. Lippincott, Philadelphia, PA.)

part is improperly aligned. Changes in the tube angle cause elongation, never foreshortening.

Shape distortion often results because structures lie normally at different levels within the body. Shape distortion also occurs because of the divergence of the x-ray beam. The projected length varies, depending on the angle between the object and the diverging beam (Figure 26–7).

Adjustment of shape distortion requires careful consideration of the beam-part-film geometry involved in the projection. This information must be combined with a knowledge of the normal projection of the structures to determine exactly how improvements can be achieved.

Alignment

Shape distortion can be caused or avoided by careful alignment of the central ray

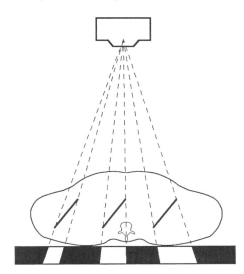

Figure 26–7. Shape distortion due to the angle between the object and the diverging beam. Although all three objects are at the same angle to the image receptor, the projected length varies according to the angle between the object and the diverging beam.

with the anatomical part and the image receptor. Proper positioning is achieved when the central ray is at right angles to the anatomical part and to the image receptor. This means the part and the image receptor must be parallel. When the position of the body part or object within the body does not permit this alignment, creative positioning must be utilized. The half-axial 30° angulation of the cranium to demonstrate the occipital bone, the 25° cephalad angulation of the pelvis to demonstrate the sigmoid colon, and the 10° caudad angulation of the coccyx, are all examples of routine procedures that were developed to minimize distortion.

Alignment adjustments involve bringing the tube central ray, the part and the film back into their correct relationship—part and film parallel to one another with the central ray perpendicular to both. Incorrect centering may occur from off-centering the tube (misalignment of the central ray), incorrectly positioning the part or off-centering the film (Figure 26–8). Off-centering of the film causes a small amount of shape distortion, although it will usually require a repeated exposure because nearby structures of interest are not imaged.

Central Ray The central ray is the theoretical photon that exits from the exact center of the focal spot. Ideally the central ray is intended to be projected **perpendicular to both the anatomical part and the image receptor**. Whenever the central ray is not perpendicular, some degree of shape distortion will result. This occurs in every image because only the central ray is truly perpendicular. Any structure that is not positioned at the central ray will be distorted because of the divergence of the beam—**the farther from the central ray, the greater the distortion**. This applies as distance from the central ray increases transversely as well as longitudinally. For example, an AP pelvis will have more distortion of an object

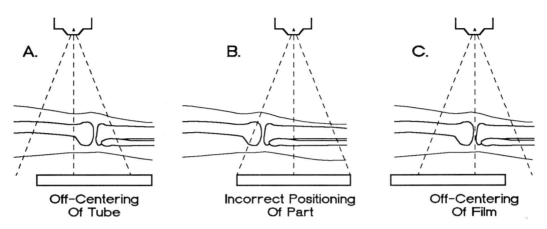

Figure 26–8.   Incorrect centering.

near the right greater trochanter than an object near the symphysis pubis. This is why it is so important to position according to standardized central ray locations.

Long bone length studies are an example of a procedure developed to ensure accurate central ray centering. The procedure shown in Figure 26–9 uses a radiopaque ruler, positioned from above the hip joint to below the ankle joint, as a measurement control. Spot films of the critical joints— hip, knee and ankle—are then made with the central ray perpendicular to the joint space to ensure accurate measurement.

Centering away from the specified central ray entrance point is equivalent to angling the tube away from perpendicular because the entire perspective of the anatomical part is distorted. Some projections take advantage of this type of distortion. For example, a PA lumbar projection uses the divergence of the beam to open the lordotically curved intervertebral joints (Figure 26–10).

The central ray is normally positioned perpendicular to the anatomical part and to the image receptor. When the part is superimposed over other structures, central angulation can be a useful tool to provide a projection that would otherwise be impossible to differentiate

from overlying structures. The use of the semi-axial AP projection of the skull to project the occipital region free of facial bone superimposition is an example. Failure to maintain the correct relationship between the part and the image receptor will produce a projected image that may not be comparable to norms and is therefore useless in the diagnostic process.

Anatomical Part The long axis of the anatomical part, or object, is intended to be positioned perpendicular to the central ray and parallel to the image receptor. When these positions are incorrect, distortion may occur. Elongation occurs when there is poor alignment of the tube and/or image receptor. Foreshortening occurs only when there is poor alignment of the part (Figure 26–11). Figure 26–11A shows the intended relationships of central ray, part and film. In Figure 26–11B the entire object is foreshortened because of the improper part-to-image receptor relationship. In addition to the entire object being foreshortened, one end is more magnified due to increased OID, which indicates that size distortion is also occurring.

In Figure 26–11C the entire object is again foreshortened with one end being more magnified due to increased OID. However, because of the differences in the actual size of the two ends, the increased size distortion of-

Figure 26–9. A long bone leg length study. Exact central ray location is critical to assuring an accurate measurement of the bone lengths. (A) Inaccurate leg lengths due to beam divergence at the joints from a single exposure. (B) Accurate leg lengths with three spot exposures, each perpendicular to a joint.

A. PA Projection

B. AP Projection

Figure 26–10.   Divergence of the beam used to advantage. The lordotic curvature of the lumbar spine and the divergence of the beam can be used to open the intervertebral joints in a PA projection.

the smaller end makes both ends appear the same size.

Note especially the vast differences in the projected images of these anatomical part relationships. Figure 26–11A projects an accurate image. Figure 26–11B projects distortion of both size and shape so the entire object is foreshortened and the large end appears larger than it really is. Figure 26–11C also projects distortion of both size and shape but has distorted the relationship so both ends appear the same size.

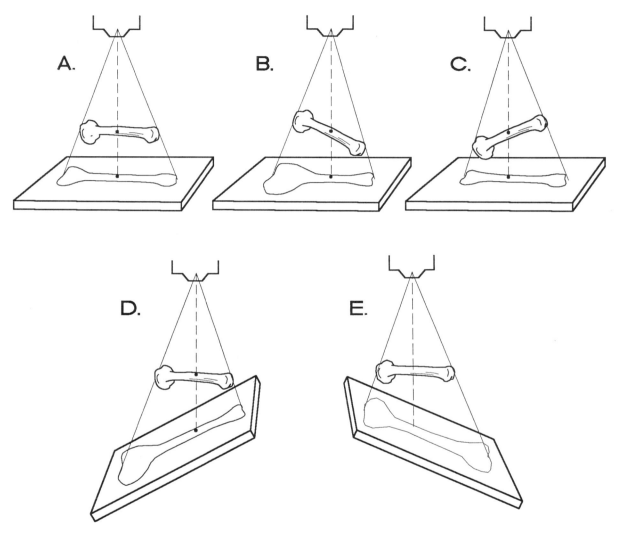

Figure 26–11. Foreshortening and magnification due to anatomical part and image receptor alignment. (A) Normal relationship between part and image receptor. (B-C) Foreshortening and magnification due to changes in anatomical part alignment. (D-E) Foreshortening and magnification due to changes in image receptor alignment.

The anatomical part is normally positioned with its long axis perpendicular to the central ray and parallel to the image receptor. As with the central ray, some routine projections are designed to vary from this standard to avoid superimposition. Failure to maintain the specified relationships between the central ray and the image receptor can result in an image that is not comparable to norms and therefore of limited value in the diagnostic process.

Image Receptor The image receptor, usually a radiographic film cassette, is intended to be positioned perpendicular to the central ray and parallel to the anatomical part. As long as the film plane is parallel to the object, the only result of off-centering of the image receptor is the clipping of a portion of the area of interest. Although this will usually result in a repeated exposure, there is no distortion of image size or shape.

However, when the film plane is not parallel to the object, or if the central ray is not centered to the part, serious shape distortion results exactly as if the object were not parallel. Figures 26–11D and E illustrate for the image receptor the same examples shown for the object in Figures 26–11B and C above.

The image receptor, or film plane, is normally positioned perpendicular to the central ray and parallel to the anatomical part. Even in routine projections designed to vary from this standard, the specified relationships must be maintained to obtain a useful diagnostic image.

Angulation

Angulation refers to the direction and degree the tube is moved from its normal position perpendicular to the image receptor. Numerous radiographic projections utilize angulation to avoid superimposition of parts. The semi-axial AP projection of the cranium, tangential os calcis and axial clavicle are all examples.

The angulation of the tube is designed to cause a controlled or expected amount of shape distortion to avoid superimposition. As long as the specified angulation is applied, the image is comparable to norms and is of diagnostic quality. Angulation of the tube also changes the SID, which, unless compensated for by a new SID, will produce unusual magnification.

Direction The most common direction of tube angle is longitudinal. Longitudinal angulations are usually termed **cephalad** when the tube is angled toward the head of the patient, and **caudad** when it is angled toward the patient's feet. Some radiographic tubes can also be angled transversely (sometimes referred to as "roll"). Transverse angulations are usually identified as right and left (in reference to the patient).

The direction of the tube angle is specified according to patient position and must be maintained as specified. When the patient position is reversed, the direction of tube angle must also be reversed to maintain the relationship. For example, 25° cephalad for an AP projection is identical to 25° caudad for a PA projection.

Degree Degree is simply a method of describing the exact amount of angulation **and is usually stated as the angle between the central ray and the film plane from the standard reference point of perpendicularity**. Because the

TABLE 26–1		
SID COMPENSATIONS FOR COMMON TUBE ANGULATIONS		
Tube Angulation	Overhead Scale	True FFD
5°	39.8″	40″
10°	39.4″	40″
15°	38.6″	40″
20°	37.6″	40″
25°	36.2″	40″
30°	34.6″	40″
35°	32.8″	40″

Table 2 from Robert J. English, *Radiologic Technology* 52:3, 304, 1980 by permission of the American Society of Radiologic Technologists.

standard reference point is 90° from the patient's head, radiographic angles must be added or subtracted from that point. For example, 5° cephalad is 5° from perpendicular as is 5° caudad. It is important to maintain the correct degree of angle specified for a given procedure. Tube angulations also change SID, which will produce changes in magnification. Table 26–1 provides conversions for common tube angulations.

Evaluating Shape Distortion

Shape distortion is a more subjective evaluation than size. It is much more difficult to assess because there is no effect that can be calculated, as in the magnification factor for size distortion. Instead, the entire assessment relies on the radiographer's knowledge of nor-

mal anatomy and the normal projected images for each position.

EFFECT ON IMAGE APPEARANCE

Size

Size distortion is simply a matter of magnification (Figure 26–12). All magnification involves a degree of loss of resolution, even when special systems are designed to minimize the loss.

Shape

Shape distortion involves both elongation and foreshortening and is a serious alteration in the projected image (Figure 26–13). There are

A

B

Figure 26–12.   Magnification size distortion. (A) Minimal heart size magnification in a PA chest. (B) An AP projection of the same patient demonstrating greater heart size magnification. (Courtesy of Tracy Thegze, R.T.(R), Community Hospital, Munster, IN.)

60 kVp	15 mAs	72″ SID	
No grid	100 RS	11.9 mR	

60 kVp	15 mAs	72″ SID	
No grid	100 RS	11.9 mR	

A

B

Figure 26–13. Shape distortion. (A) This radiograph was taken with the central ray perpendicular and centered to the center of the film. (B) This radiograph was taken with the central ray perpendicular but off center to the left (away from the pelvis). The effect on distortion is not significant; however, changes in the image appearance are evident, particularly when studying the pelvis which was furthest from the central ray. (C) This radiograph was taken with a central ray angle of 25° and centered to the center of the film. Notice the significant distortion created by angling the central ray.

60 kVp	15 mAs	72″ SID	
No grid	100 RS	11.9 mR	

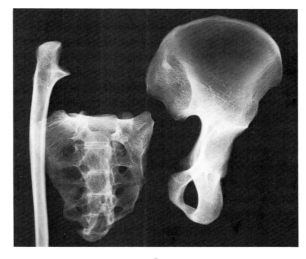

C

situations where shape distortion can be used to advantage, as in a tangential os calcis.

SUMMARY

Distortion is the second of the two geometric properties affecting radiographic image quality. Unlike the photographic properties of density and contrast, which control the visibility of detail, the geometric properties control detail itself. Distortion is the difference between the structures being examined and the recorded image. It creates a misrepresentation of the size and/or shape of the anatomical part being imaged. This misrepresentation can be classified as either size or shape distortion. Distortion, like detail, exists even when it cannot be seen due to poor visibility or, in other words, when the density and/or contrast are poor. The evaluation and adjustment of distortion require a thorough familiarity with normal radiographic anatomy. Unless the normal size and shape of a structure are known, comparisons of size and shape cannot be accomplished.

When the factors that affect size and shape distortion are altered, some change in distortion will occur. No change will occur unless one of these factors is altered. The following list illustrates the effect on distortion when the various factors are changed.

$\underline{+}$ = increased distortion
$\underline{-}$ = decreased distortion

Size Distortion

$\underline{-}$ Increasing SID
$\underline{+}$ Decreasing SID
$\underline{+}$ Increasing OID
$\underline{-}$ Decreasing OID
$\underline{+}$ Increasing patient thickness
$\underline{-}$ Decreasing patient thickness

Shape Distortion

$\underline{+}$ Improper central ray alignment
$\underline{+}$ Improper anatomical part alignment
$\underline{+}$ Improper image receptor alignment
$\underline{+}$ Improper direction of central ray angle
$\underline{+}$ Improper degree of central ray angle

REVIEW QUESTIONS

1. What is distortion?

2. What is the difference between size and shape distortion?

3. How do the SID and the OID affect size distortion?

4. What is the magnification factor formula?

5. What is the difference between elongation and foreshortening?

6. How does the alignment of the anatomical part affect shape distortion?

7. How do the direction and degree of angulation affect size distortion?

8. How can shape distortion be used to advantage?

REFERENCES AND RECOMMENDED READING

Cahoon, John B. *Formulating X-Ray Techniques.* 8th ed. Durham, NC: Duke University Press, 1974.

Cahoon, John B. Radiographic technique: Its origin, concept, practical application and evaluation of radiation dosage. *The X-Ray Technician* 32, 354–364, 1961.

Carroll, Quinn. *Fuchs's Principles of Radiographic Exposure, Processing and Quality Control.* 3rd ed. Springfield, IL: Charles C. Thomas Publisher, 1985.

Cullinan, Angeline M. *Producing Quality Radiographs*. Philadelphia, PA: Lippincott, 1987.

Distortion in imaging. *Radiography Today* 55:628, 31, 1989.

Donohue, Daniel P. *An Analysis of Radiographic Quality*. 2nd ed. Rockville, MD: Aspen Publishers, 1984.

Eastman Kodak Company, Health Sciences Markets Division. *The Fundamentals of Radiography*. 12th ed. Rochester, NY: Kodak Publication M1–18.

English, Robert J. Distance-technique relationship of angulated projections. *Radiologic Technology* 52:3, 301–304, 1980.

Files, Glenn W. *Medical Radiographic Technique*. Springfield, IL: Charles C. Thomas Publishers, 1952.

Hiss, Stephen S. *Understanding Radiography*. Springfield, IL: Charles C. Thomas Publisher, 1978.

Jenkins, David. *Radiographic Photography and Imaging Processes*. Lancaster, England: MTP Press Ltd., 1980.

Jerman, Ed. C. *Modern X-Ray Technic*. St. Paul, MN: Bruce Publishing Co., 1928.

Lauer, O. Gary, John B. Mayes, and Rosemary P. Thurston. *Evaluating Radiographic Quality: The Variables and Their Effects*. Mankato, MN: The Burnell Company Publishers, Inc., 1990.

Morgan, James A. *The Art and Science of Medical Radiography*. 5th ed. St. Louis, MO: Catholic Hospital Association, 1977.

Morgan, Russell H. An analysis of the physical factors controlling the diagnostic quality of roentgen images: Part II. Maximum resolving power and resolution coefficient. *American Journal of Roentgenology and Radiation Therapy* 54:4, 395–402, 1945.

Morgan, Russell H. An analysis of the physical factors controlling the diagnostic quality of roentgen images: Part V. Unsharpness. *American Journal of Roentgenology and Radiation Therapy* 62:6, 870–880, 1949.

Seeman, Herman E. *Physical and Photographic Principles of Medical Radiography*. New York: Wiley & Sons, Inc., 1968.

Stockley, Sybil M. *A Manual of Radiographic Equipment*. Edinburgh: Churchill Livingstone, 1986.

Tarrant, Ralph McConnell. Maintaining desired anode-film distance and alignment after angling the x-ray tube. *Radiologic Technology* 23:5, 349, 1952.

27 THE ART OF FILM CRITIQUE

If all the factors involved in the making of a . . . radiograph are known, it then becomes a simple matter, by means of . . . (a) method of analysis, to decide what may be done to improve the quality of that radiograph.

Ed. C. Jerman, The Father of Radiologic Technology.

OUTLINE

IMPLEMENTING IMAGING STANDARDS
IDENTIFYING AN IMAGING PROBLEM
AN EFFECTIVE FILM CRITIQUE METHOD
APPLYING THE FILM CRITIQUE METHOD

OBJECTIVES

Upon completion of this chapter, the student should be able to:

1. Discuss the elements of a diagnostic image as they relate to the art of film critique.
2. Identify the steps of the decision making process.
3. Describe an effective film critique method.
4. Use an effective film critique method.
5. Explain the differences between technical factor problems, procedural factor problems and equipment malfunctions.

IMPLEMENTING IMAGING STANDARDS

Radiographers are required to make decisions every day about the quality of their radiographic images. Critiquing an image is a very complex process which requires a thorough knowledge of all aspects of radiography. Deciding if an image is acceptable or unacceptable should be approached in a logical, organized manner. Film critique is an analytical process that involves many of the steps of diagnostic decision making.

The Diagnostic Image

The art of film critique revolves around the concept of deciding exactly where in the diagnostic quality spectrum a particular radiographic image lies. A practical technical definition of a diagnostic quality image has never been established because the artistic elements involved to produce the required medical information vary so much from one situation to another. The exponential number of variables involved make radiography as much an art as a science.

The production of a diagnostic image involves an overwhelming number of variables, including such elements as patient anatomy, pathological conditions, radiographic positioning, patient preparation, radiation protection, x-ray equipment, prime technical factor selections, collimation, film/screen combinations, film processing, density and contrast perceptions, detail and distortion. In other words, nearly all of the elements of anatomy, positioning, physics and principles of exposure are involved. **The art of film critique is the application of scientific knowledge to an analysis of the image.**

The Analytical Process

It is important to remember that not even radiologists are trained in the finer points of creating and analyzing the quality of a radiographic image. The radiographer is the expert and has the responsibility of proceeding with image analysis. Only with an acceptable image can a radiologist make an accurate diagnosis. It is the radiographer's professional responsibility to create the best possible image given each individual circumstance.

To determine whether an image is of diagnostic quality, the steps of an analytical decision making process must be followed.

The process begins with a review of the entire image. This is essential to avoid premature narrowing. During the review the radiographer watches for anything that is different from a diagnostic quality image. When differences are noticed, a pattern is sought, especially when there is more than one cue. Cues and patterns focus attention on a suspicious area, thus narrowing the search. Cues and patterns are then used to seek hypotheses. An effort is made to formulate a hypothesis that will explain all the cues. Cues that do not fit the hypothesis are held in reserve. The hypothesis is then tested by guided information seeking, with general questioning to produce more cue information. The last step is an evaluation of the final hypothesis. The hypothesis attempts to resolve the greatest number of cues and patterns.

There are myriad factors that can affect the quality of a radiographic image and these factors can act upon each other to create an astronomical number of possible imaging problems. A film critique system uses the diagnostic problem solving process to help resolve this situation.

IDENTIFYING AN IMAGING PROBLEM

The identification of an imaging problem requires the use of a full range of radiographic expertise. The radiographer must first recall that the purpose of the radiographic image is to provide information about the medical condition of the patient. The information needed may vary greatly, depending on the suspected medical problem and the anatomical region to be examined. For example, alignment of a nail during a hip-pinning operation requires a type of information different from that needed for detection of a small blood vessel constriction during cerebral angiography.

The meaning of the expression "diagnostic quality image" is quite different in these two cases. The hip pinning requires two images at right angles to one another as fast as possible with a major consideration being patient dose. The cerebral angiograph requires maximum visibility of detail and resolution from a high speed exposure with less consideration of patient dose. Any definition of a diagnostic quality image must consider the clinical situation while providing a good balance between visibility of detail (density and contrast) and the geometry of the image (recorded detail or distortion).

The primary problem encountered by radiographers in successfully critiquing images is the tendency to glance at radiographs instead of critically evaluating them for image quality. The professional approaches each image as a window in the diagnostic process.

In her introductory text for radiologists, *Fundamentals of Radiology*, Dr. Lucy Frank Squire emphasizes to aspiring radiologists that, "While the single-glance approach has its value, it is full of danger to the patient, because the presence of a very obvious abnormality tends to suppress psychologically your search for more subtle changes." She suggests that students utilize a systematic approach to evaluating radiographs, primarily by looking at various structures in a deliberate order, concentrating on each structure while excluding the superimposed shadows of other structures. Radiographers should adopt an identical process by looking at each technical and procedural factor in a systematic fashion before jumping to any "glancing" conclusions.

AN EFFECTIVE FILM CRITIQUE METHOD

An effective film critique method is a three-step process involving:

1. **the classification of the image,**
2. **the determination of the cause of the problem and**
3. **the recommendation of corrective action** (Figure 27–1).

This approach is designed to provide the radiographer with an organized and systematic protocol for critiquing a radiograph. When consistently used, the system will be found to be a thorough and dependable method for establishing and maintaining professional skills at the very highest level of competence. The form in Figure 27–2 illustrates the application of this film critique method.

Classification of the Image

The first step in classifying the image is to evaluate it to determine if it is within the diagnostic acceptance limits. If the image is within the acceptance limits it should be critically examined to determine if it is of **optimal** diagnostic quality. If it is satisfactory in every respect, the pride of professional competence is the radiographer's reward. If the image is within acceptance limits but not of optimal diagnostic quality, the radiographer should continue the critique to refine his or her technical skills. Although the radiograph may be submitted for diagnosis, a continued critique provides an opportunity to improve the quality of care for future patients.

If the film is outside the acceptance limits, a continued critique is mandatory prior to attempting to repeat the exposure. Failure to continue the critique is ethically unacceptable for a radiographer because it subjects the patient to additional radiation exposure without ascertaining how to produce an acceptable image.

Determination of the Cause of the Problem

The actual diagnostic problem solving begins with determination of the cause of the unacceptable or suboptimal image. In most instances there is more than one cause and this can complicate the problem solving process immensely. Searching for cues or patterns is primarily a matter of clinical experience. It is best to slowly narrow the search process by first trying to classify the problem into one of three major categories:

Figure 27-1. An effective film critique method.

FILM CRITIQUE FORM

I. CLASSIFY THE RADIOGRAPHIC IMAGE AS:

☐   WITHIN ACCEPTANCE LIMITS

      ☐ Optimal diagnostic information (critique is complete)
(all checkmarks below this line require completion of section II and III)
      ☐ Suboptimal diagnostic Information

☐   OUTSIDE ACCEPTANCE LIMITS

I I. DETERMINE THE CAUSE OF THE PROBLEM AS:

☐ **A: Technical Factors**

    ☐ Photographic problem with visibility of detail
        ☐ Density
        ☐ mAs _____
        ☐ Influencing factor (specify) _____
        ☐ Contrast
        ☐ kVp _____
        ☐ Influencing factor (specify) _____
    ☐ Geometric problem with detail
        ☐ Recorded Detail
        ☐ Geometry (specify) _____
        ☐ Film/Screen combination (specify) _____
        ☐ Motion _____
        ☐ Distortion
        ☐ Size (Magnification) (specify) _____
        ☐ Shape (Part/Film/Tube Alignment) (specify) _____

☐ **B. Procedural Factors**

    ☐ Patient Positioning
        ☐ Tube Alignment _____
        ☐ Part Alignment _____
        ☐ Film Alignment _____
    ☐ Patient Preparation (specify) _____

☐ **C. Equipment Malfunction**

    ☐ Processing Equipment (specify) _____
    ☐ Radiographic/Fluoroscopic Equipment (specify) _____

I I I. RECOMMEND CORRECTIVE ACTION For each cause specified above:

_____
_____
_____
_____

Figure 27–2.   Form used for film critique.

1. **a technical factor problem,**
2. **a procedural factor problem or**
3. **an equipment malfunction problem**.

All of these categories are then further subdivided in an effort to determine the exact cause of the problem.

Technical Factor Problems

Technical factor problems can be arranged into two categories: **a photographic problem with visibility of detail or a geometric problem with detail**. (Of course, some images will have problems with both visibility of detail and detail.) The photographic problems concern maintaining sufficient density and contrast to make the detail of the image visible. Even with good detail present, anatomical structures cannot be visualized unless appropriate density and contrast are also present. An image that appears totally black may still possess good detail; it is simply beyond the ability of the human eye to discern it. Geometric problems directly concern the production of detail (also called definition, sharpness and resolution). (See Unit III, Radiographic Image Quality Chart, p. 352.)

Photographic problems with visibility of detail are further classified as **density** or **contrast** problems. Density problems may be the result of the mAs selection and/or a variety of other influencing factors, including the film/screen combination, the selected kVp level, distance, grid selection, beam restriction, a pathology problem, etc. Contrast problems are the result of the kVp selection and/or a variety of influencing factors, including field size, patient thickness, grid selection, etc.

Geometric problems with detail are further classified as **recorded detail** or **distortion** problems. Recorded detail problems are the result of the geometry of the beam (focal spot size, focal film distance or object film distance), the film/screen combination, and/or patient motion. Distortion is further classified as size distortion (magnification) or shape distortion.

Size distortion problems are the result of SID or OID. Shape distortion problems are the result of improper tube, part and/or film alignment.

Procedural Factor Problems

A procedural factor problem can be classified as one that involves **patient positioning** or **patient preparation** for the x-ray examination. Proper patient positioning results when the part, the film and the tube (central ray) are correctly aligned with one another. The result is an image which demonstrates the anatomical structures of interest from the proper perspective. Of course, a thorough knowledge of the anatomy being visualized for a given radiographic procedure is essential to determine if the positioning is accurate. When studying an image for accuracy in positioning, three alignment factors should be reviewed separately:

1. the tube alignment,
2. the part alignment and
3. the film alignment.

The second procedural factor problem involves preparation of the patient for the examination. Proper patient preparation includes removing radiopaque objects from the area of interest (i.e., jewelry, safety pins, etc.), proper bowel cleansing for a gastrointestinal study, recording a thorough history, communicating clear instructions to the patient, etc.

Equipment Malfunction

The last major category in the classification of the causes of an imaging problem is equipment malfunction. While the technical and procedural factors may have been correctly determined, a problem can still result when the equipment being used for the examination does not function properly. Problems normally occur with the processing equipment or with the radiographic/fluoroscopic equipment. These problems can be kept to a minimum through an effective quality control program.

Recommendation of Corrective Action

Each identified cause requires an appropriate corrective action that will resolve the problem. Corrective action adjustments are based on knowledge and clinical experience. Clinical experience is gained through careful attention to problems and successes. Remember that clinical knowledge is gained by critiquing acceptable but suboptimal images, analyzing repeated images and recording successful results.

It is recommended that radiographers purchase or make a personal technique system booklet that can be easily carried while performing clinical examinations. This booklet should record appropriate technical factors, including the specific tube used (by room number or location), kVp, mAs, distance, grid, the relative speed of the film/screen combination,

anatomical projection, part thickness and any other variable factors (adjustable filtration, focal spot size, etc.). By using a personal technique system booklet, the radiographer has a quick reference for establishing the technical and procedural factors for a specific examination. Additionally, this guide can be useful for determining accurate adjustments in order to correct a problem.

APPLYING THE FILM CRITIQUE METHOD

Figure 27–3 illustrates how to use the film critique method that has been outlined. The radiograph in Figure 27–3A is classified as an image which is outside the acceptance limits of image quality. To determine the cause of this problem, the entire image should be studied for technical and procedural accuracy as

Figure 27–3A & B.   (A) Original radiograph. (B) Repeated radiograph.

well as for potential equipment malfunction problems.

From this review, it is determined that the image exhibits a technical factor problem and a procedural problem, but no apparent equipment problem. Further searching narrows the technical factor problem to a photographic problem of visibility of detail and the procedural problem to patient positioning. This narrowing is based on observations that the image is too dark and that not all of the anatomical structures of interest are demonstrated on the film. These two cues narrow the search by eliminating geometric problems of detail, patient preparation and equipment malfunction as probable causes. Once suspected problem areas are defined, the cues and patterns should be used to form a hypothesis about the probable cause of the problem.

The photographic problem of visibility of detail can be further narrowed to a density problem. The possible causes of excessive density are then reviewed to determine the most likely cause. Although too much mAs is the most common cause, a number of secondary factors, such as the film/screen combination, the grid selection and the kVp level, need to be considered and checked to test the hypothesis. This is a necessary part of evaluating the hypothesis.

Next, the procedural problem should be reviewed to determine the most likely cause. The problem is first narrowed to a patient positioning problem and then to an alignment problem.

The possible causes of alignment problems should then be reviewed to determine the most likely cause. Careful review of the image reveals that the central ray was not correctly aligned to the center of the film. Because of this improper central ray alignment, some of the anatomical structures of interest (the lower lungs and costophrenic angles) are not visualized.

The final step is recommending corrective action. In the example, the corrective action involves changes in technical factor selection and patient positioning. The mAs is reduced by one-half the original amount to correct the density problem and the central ray is properly aligned to the midline of the film. Figure 27–3B illustrates the result after these adjustments were made.

A thorough understanding of the concepts involved in producing an acceptable diagnostic quality image is important. Because of the large number of variables in the imaging process, acceptable images will not always result from the initial exposure. Even the best of radiographers will be required to repeat radiographs because of the vast number of variables. By applying a systematic film critique method, radiographers are practicing one of the most complex skills of the profession. This analytical and effective film critique method will help to ensure the best possible patient care by minimizing the need to repeat an exposure.

SUMMARY

Critiquing an image is a very complex process which requires a thorough knowledge of all aspects of radiography. Deciding if an image is acceptable or unacceptable should be approached in a logical, organized manner. Film critiquing is an analytical process that involves many of the steps involved in diagnostic decision making.

To determine whether an image is of diagnostic quality, the steps of an analytical decision making process must be followed.

The process begins with a review of the entire image to avoid premature narrowing. When differences are noticed, a pattern is sought, especially when there is more than one cue. Cues and patterns focus attention on a suspicious area, thus narrowing the search.

Cues and patterns are then used to seek hypotheses. An effort is made to formulate a hypothesis that will explain all the cues. The hypothesis is then tested by guided information seeking, with general questioning to produce more cue information. The last step is an evaluation of the final hypothesis. The hypothesis attempts to resolve the greatest number of cues and patterns.

An effective film critique method is a three-step process involving: 1) the classification of the image, 2) the determination of the cause of the problem and 3) the recommendation of corrective action.

In the first step, the image is classified to determine if it is within the diagnostic acceptance limits. If the image is within acceptance limits but not of optimal diagnostic quality, the radiographer should continue the critique to refine his or her technical skills. If the film is outside the acceptance limits, a continued critique is mandatory prior to attempting to repeat the exposure.

The actual diagnostic problem solving begins with determination of the cause of the unacceptable or suboptimal image. Searching for cues or patterns is primarily a matter of clinical experience. It is best to slowly narrow the search process by first trying to classify the problem into one of three major categories: 1) a technical factor problem, 2) a procedural factor problem or 3) an equipment malfunction problem.

Each identified cause requires an appropriate corrective action that will resolve the problem. Corrective action adjustments are based on knowledge and clinical experience. Clinical experience is gained through careful attention to problems and successes.

Even the best of radiographers will be required to repeat radiographs. Using an effective film critique method will help to assure the best possible patient care by minimizing the need to repeat an exposure.

REVIEW QUESTIONS

1. What is the purpose of film critique?

2. During the analytical process of critiquing a radiograph, how are cues and patterns used?

3. What are the three steps in an effective film critique method?

4. What are the three classifications of imaging problems?

5. What are the two categories of technical factor problems?

6. A necklace is seen on a chest radiograph. What type of imaging problem would this be?

7. A film is jammed in the processor and destroyed. What type of imaging problem would this be?

8. How does a radiographer determine the appropriate corrective action for an imaging problem?

REFERENCES AND RECOMMENDED READING

Carlton, Richard. Quality assurance in radiology. *Introduction to Radiologic Technology.* 2nd ed., Chapter 15, 149–166. Editors: Gurley, LaVerne T., and William J. Callaway. St. Louis, MO: Multi-Media Publishing, Inc.

Carnevali, Doris L., Pamela H. Mitchell, Nancy F. Woods, and Christine A. Tanner. *Diagnostic Reasoning in Nursing.* Philadelphia, PA: J. B. Lippincott Co., 1984.

Goldman, Lee W. Effects of film processing variability on patient dose and image quality. *Second Image Receptor Conference: Radiographic Film Processing: Proceedings of a Conference Held in Washington, D.C., March 31-April 2, 1977.*

Rockville, MD.: U.S. Department of Health, Education, and Welfare, Public Health Service, Food and Drug Administration, Bureau of Radiological Health, HEW Publication FDA 77–8036, 55–63, 1977.

Hiss, Stephen. *Understanding Radiography.* Springfield, IL: Charles C. Thomas Publisher, 1978.

Jerman, Ed. C. An analysis of the end-result: The radiograph. *Radiology* 6, 59–62, 1926.

Lauer, O. Gary. A method for radiographic film evaluation. *Principles and Practices of the College Based Radiography Program: Educational and Administrative Considerations.* Editor: Lauer, O. Gary. St. Louis, MO: W. H. Green, Inc., 1984.

Prior, John A., Jack S. Silberstein, and John M. Stang. *Physical Diagnosis: The History and Examination of the Patient.* St. Louis, MO: Mosby, 1981.

Squire, Lucy Frank, and Robert A. Novelline. *Fundamentals of Radiology.* 4th ed. Cambridge, MA: Harvard University Press, 1988.

THE CASE OF THE LINE IN THE STOMACH

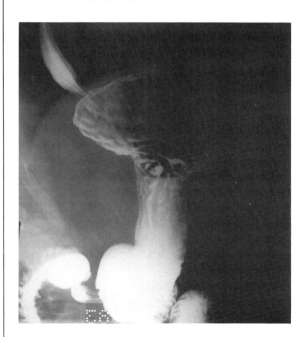

Although barium has been used to coat this stomach for the air contrast study, an odd line appears at its midpoint. What is causing the line?

Answers to the case studies can be found in Appendix E.

28 QUALITY CONTROL

. . . a quality assurance program maximizes the likelihood that the images will consistently provide adequate diagnostic information for the least possible radiation exposure and cost to the patient.

William R. Hendee and Raymond P. Rossi, *Quality Assurance for Radiographic X-Ray Units and Associated Equipment.*

OUTLINE

QUALITY ASSURANCE AND QUALITY CONTROL
PURCHASING EQUIPMENT
MONITORING EQUIPMENT PERFORMANCE
ANCILLARY EQUIPMENT
REPEAT FILM STUDIES
TROUBLESHOOTING

OBJECTIVES

Upon completion of this chapter, the student should be able to:

1. Define quality assurance and control and discuss their relationship to excellence in radiography.
2. Describe the process of identifying imaging requirements, developing equipment specifications, selecting equipment, installing and testing equipment, and training the technical staff.
3. Describe the objectives and responsibilities of monitoring equipment performance.
4. Discuss primary automatic film processor quality control monitoring and maintenance procedures.
5. Discuss primary quality control tests for external radiation beam monitoring of diagnostic radiographic systems, fluoroscopic systems, tomographic systems and automatic exposure controls.
6. List primary quality control tests for miscellaneous ancillary equipment, including cassettes and view boxes.

7. Explain the rationale behind the data collection process and the basic analysis of a radiographic repeat-rate study.
8. Describe a basic troubleshooting procedure.

QUALITY ASSURANCE AND QUALITY CONTROL

Quality Assurance

Quality assurance consists of activities that provide adequate confidence that a radiology service will render consistently high quality images and services. It is an evolutionary process that assesses everything that affects patient care. It may be medically, technically or managerially oriented. Quality assurance includes evaluating activities such as interpretation of examinations, maintenance of equipment, performance of procedures, filing systems, staff development, scheduling of examinations and supply lines.

The quality assurance process operates by identifying problems or potential problem areas, monitoring the problem and then resolving it. Monitoring problems involves several steps, including establishing criteria, performing monitoring, and collecting, analyzing and evaluating data. It is these steps of the monitoring process that are of greatest concern to the quality assurance radiographer.

Quality Control

Quality control is the aspect of quality assurance that monitors technical equipment to maintain quality standards. The concept of quality control is rooted in the need to stabilize the various equipment components of the radiographic imaging chain. From incoming line current through x-ray production to the processing of the radiograph, erratic equipment performance causes repeat radiographs and unnecessary patient exposure to radiation. The term quality control is sometimes used to describe the evaluation of individual radiographs according to acceptance limits standards. It is probably better to think of this image evaluation process as film critiquing or quality checking rather than quality control, although the quality control process is certainly a critical part of the critique evaluation.

Technical expertise will not ensure success in radiography unless the equipment is reliable. Because radiographic equipment changes as it ages, there are often great differences between the results obtained on one unit and those obtained on another. The same unit cannot be counted on to produce exactly the same beam for the radiographer to control and analyze unless it is properly checked on a regular basis. The system of checks to accomplish a measure of consistency in beam output is the quality control.

Ensuring the quality of the radiographic image is a prime responsibility of the radiologic technologist. Every patient expects to receive the highest possible quality, or excellence, of service, from a medical facility. No one wants to be exposed to ionizing radiation by a radiographer incapable of producing excellent images.

It is important that quality control be seen as a method of controlling the radiographic image from start to finish. To do this requires a series of procedures (Figure 28–1). Unfortunately, most quality control begins with the last step instead of the first. An effective program cannot be achieved simply by monitoring equipment performance, although this is unquestionably the most involved step. The thought process preceding equipment purchase is critical.

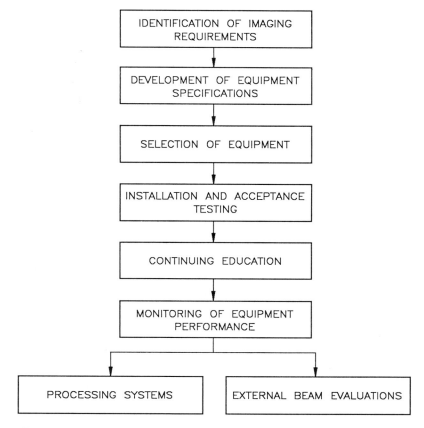

Figure 28–1.   A total quality control system. (Adapted from William R. Hendee and Raymond P. Rossi, *Quality Assurance for Radiographic X-Ray Units and Associated Equipment.* Rockville, MD: U.S. DHEW, PHS, FDA, Bureau of Radiological Health, HEW Publication FDA 79–8094, 1979.)

PURCHASING EQUIPMENT

Identification of Imaging Requirements

It is not always apparent exactly what type of equipment is needed when new purchases are being considered. Historically, this decision was made by the chief radiologist or administrative technologist. Rarely are the actual operators of the equipment, the radiogra-phers, consulted. The result has been that nearly every x-ray department owns a radio-logical monstrosity that is avoided by radiographers and radiologists alike. These units are often inconvenient, overly sophisticated, or unable to produce quality images. Careful identification of imaging requirements can prevent these problems.

It is not necessary to be an expert in imaging physics and technology in order to be capable of contributing to the process of identifying the imaging requirements. Each member of the radiological team can contribute his or her expertise. The person who will make the final decision should interview the radiologists, administrators, supervisors and staff technologists who will use the equipment. In many instances the needs of the radiologist will determine the basic parameters for the purchase. Administrators must often impose financial and space restraints, although they can also create new funds and space when necessary. Supervisors are often able to provide important information on patient flow and staffing needs. After the radiologists, the radiographers are the most important persons to have input because their experiences with equipment provide a wealth of information.

Development of Equipment Specifications

Generic equipment specifications should be developed from the interview information. It is important that the person formulating the specifications have the technical background to state exactly what is needed to meet the imaging requirements. An imaging physicist should be involved at this point. The best specifications include detailed statements of what the equipment should be capable of. For example, "Maintain mA linearity within ±10 percent to produce equal film density when mAs is maintained but mA is varied." This must include a change from highest to lowest setting. When the specifications are complete they are sent to vendors for bidding.

Selection of Equipment

The actual selection of equipment becomes simple if the investigation into the first two steps has been thorough. When the bids arrive they can be compared for meeting specifications, cost and service. The actual decision

is then academic. A pitfall in the process was identified by Bowers, et al.

> It was . . . very important . . . that the radiologists in the institution not show a preference to a particular vendor, thus weakening the bargaining position of . . . the department administrator.

In many institutions this pitfall should be expanded to include interference by administrative officers unfamiliar with imaging equipment.

Installation and Acceptance Testing of Equipment

Installation and acceptance testing of equipment is the responsibility of the vendor and/or manufacturer. The quality control technologist must verify that the equipment specifications have been met. Normally this includes supervising the testing procedures and results. It is suggested that the exact methods for acceptance testing be included in the original specifications. The data from these tests will form the standard for all future quality control monitoring.

Continuing Education

It is normally the responsibility of the vendor to familiarize the users of the equipment with its proper operation. With simple equipment, such as ancillary devices, the equipment manual may be sufficient for use in inservice training. More complex equipment should be demonstrated and explained by the vendor **to at least two persons** as part of the purchase contract. Continuing education **must** be an ongoing procedure. It is advisable to include both the quality control and in-service education coordinators in the initial training demonstrations. A good in-service program will include an orientation procedure as well as periodic updates on all complex equipment.

MONITORING EQUIPMENT PERFORMANCE

The final procedure of a total program is commonly considered to be the whole of quality control. Monitoring equipment performance includes routine checks of all radiographic equipment. Although they are interdependent, monitoring can be divided into two parts: (1) **film processing systems** and (2) **external beam evaluation**. Objectives for a performance monitoring system are to:

1. monitor the quality of the film processing systems,
2. measure the quality of the external radiation beams and
3. specify faults within these systems to allow corrective measures to be taken.

Evidence shows that a properly working quality control system will reduce equipment down-time and the number of repeated exposures. This will also reduce patient exposure dose, patient waiting time, and supply costs, as well as increase confidence in diagnostic consultation and boost departmental morale.

Responsibility

Professional service personnel or medical physicists are not required to perform routine quality control procedures. Many procedures must be done daily, and to use these experts would be too costly. Radiographers, who are more available and knowledgeable about potential problems, should do the equipment monitoring. An initial cost outlay for testing equipment is required. To maintain a program, staff technologists must be given time to perform the procedures and to evaluate them.

Processor Monitoring

Processor monitoring is designed to permit an automatic film processor to fluctuate within set limits. These tests may be performed by anyone who has been oriented to the use of the equipment involved. Only a radiographer or processor maintenance person should perform the corrective actions.

Action must be taken to correct problems whenever the limits are exceeded. A quality control program that is not backed up by a commitment to shut down processors that are outside limits is of little value. Manufacturers' suggestions should be followed for the start-up and for the regular maintenance of the processor.

There are also several monitoring tests that should be done on a daily basis. These include a darkroom fog test, also known as a safelight test, and processor sensitometry to monitor speed, contrast and base fog of film.

External Beam Evaluation

The second part of performance monitoring involves the evaluation of the external primary radiation beam. These tests must be performed by a radiographer who has a knowledge of the physical operation of the equipment and all related accessories. Corrective action should be taken only by an authorized service person.

Some monitoring equipment can be made very inexpensively; other equipment must be purchased. A dosimeter is an essential piece of equipment and reasonable quality control cannot be performed without one. Computerized dosimeters are available that permit readouts and printouts of many quality control parameters from a single exposure. Figure 28–2 illustrates common quality control equipment. A room log should be kept to record test results, maintenance, and repairs performed on each x-ray tube and other system in each room.

Diagnostic Radiographic Systems The tests that should be performed on diagnostic radiographic systems should be done on a **semi-annual** schedule. The tests for x-ray tubes should include:

Figure 28–2.   Radiographic quality control equipment. Clockwise from upper left: wire mesh film/screen contact tool, collimator accuracy tool, pinhole focal spot camera, digital dosimeter with laptop microcomputer, synchronous spinning top and penetrometer tool, and kVp test cassette with star pattern focal spot tool. In center: noninvasive beam evaluator (NERO™ computerized unit with ionization chamber box) and resolution pattern focal spot test tool.

Focal spot size estimation. An estimate of focal spot size is important so that it is kept within acceptable limits to ensure proper image detail. There are three types of focal spot test tools: line pair resolution tools, star test patterns, and pinhole cameras. Both line pair resolution tools and star test patterns function by imaging a resolution pattern on a film. The image can then be analyzed to estimate the focal spot size. A pinhole camera permits measurement of the focal spot by creating an image of the effective focal spot on a film (Figure 28–3).

The National Electrical Manufacturers Association (NEMA) specifies that focal spots of 0.3 mm and smaller may be measured with a star test pattern. Focal spots larger than 0.3 mm should be measured with a pinhole

A   B   C

2.0 mm   1.0 mm   1.0 mm

Figure 28–3.   Focal spot images produced on dental x-ray film with a pinhole camera. (Courtesy of J. E. Gray and M. Trefler, Pinhole cameras: Artifacts, modifications, and recording of pinhole images on screen film systems. *Radiologic Technology* 52:3, 277–282, 1980 by permission of the American Society of Radiologic Technologists from *Quality Control in Diagnostic Imaging*, Aspen Publishers, Inc., Rockville, MD 1983 by permission of the Mayo Foundation.)

camera. In clinical quality control assurance testing a pinhole camera is avoided because it is difficult to use accurately and requires massive tube loading. A star test pattern will satisfactorily monitor focal spot size growth in most instances. When the focal spot grows to an unacceptable size, the x-ray tube must be replaced. NEMA specifies that focal spots smaller than 0.8 mm may be 50 percent larger than the stated nominal size. Focal spots between 0.8 mm and 1.5 mm may be 40 percent larger than nominal and focal spots larger than 1.5 mm may be 30 percent larger than nominal. For example, a 0.5 mm focal spot may actually be 0.75 mm and still be considered acceptable.

Half-value layer. The amount of total filtration in the primary beam is important for both radiation protection and image quality. Radiation protection is assured by eliminating low-energy photons that are incapable of reaching the image receptor. Image quality is ensured by making appropriate contrast adjustments. Half-value layers are measured by using dosimetry equipment to detect the quality of aluminum filtration that will reduce the beam intensity to half the original value. Computerized quality control dosimeters provide a digital readout of the half-value layer. Half-value layer recommendations or requirements vary depending on the kVp. If insufficient filtration is present, the tube housing must be modified to supply additional aluminum filtration.

Collimator, central ray, and Bucky tray accuracy. The congruence of the projected centering light field and the central ray with the actual collimated primary x-ray beam and Bucky tray is of critical importance for radiation protection. Radiation protection is ensured by avoiding repeated radiographs due to overcollimation errors and by avoiding irradiation of tissue unless it will be imaged (U.S. federal law prohibits such practice through automatic positive beam limitation (PBL) requirements). A collimator test tool is simply a lead marker for each corner of the light beam plus crosshairs or a lead marker, placed several centimeters above the cassette surface, for the central ray. A 2 percent SID error is allowed between the primary-beam image and the light field size (this is a U.S. federal standard). The centering mark should be within 1 percent of the light field central ray. The PBL mechanism should not permit the primary beam to be larger than the cassette in the Bucky tray unless the overide lock is activated. When these margins of error are exceeded, the collimator light or PBL mechanism must be adjusted.

Distance and centering indicators' accuracy. Many older x-ray units have inaccurate distance indicators located on tube support stands or overhead readouts. In addition, both distance and centering locks, stops and detents may not be accurate. Assurance that distance and centering are accurate avoids the need for repeated exposures due to the inverse square law, misalignment of the central ray and primary beam collimation. Distance indicators should be checked with a tape measure (point zero should be measured from the focal spot, which is approximately 1 cm from the bottom of the tube housing end cap). Centering indicators can be checked by visual inspection of the collimator light beam (assuming a collimator and central ray accuracy test has been done). Distance indicators should be ±10 percent and centering indicators should be ±2 percent. If the indicators are not within these limits they should be adjusted.

Angulator or protractor accuracy. X-ray tables, Bucky units and tubes with angulators or protractors must provide accurate readings for positioning baselines. They can be evaluated by using a large protractor for angle measurements and a level to verify that locks, stops and detents are set to establish horizontal and perpendicular surfaces. Angles should be ±1 percent, with adjustments made when necessary.

The tests for x-ray generators should include:

Kilovoltage accuracy. Kilovoltage settings tend to drift over time, primarily as a result of tube aging. Their accuracy is essential in maintaining image quality. The scale of contrast and density cannot be predicted unless the kVp is accurate. Verification and calibration of the kVp ensure that technique exposure charts will produce diagnostic quality images. Computerized dosimeters provide digital readouts or printouts of average and single-pulse kVp. A kVp test cassette (sometimes called a modified Adran-Crookes or Wisconsin test cassette) may also be used, but it is less accurate, more time-consuming and difficult to use. If the settings drift beyond the ±5 kVp of the labeled setting, the generator must be recalibrated.

Timer accuracy. Exposure time settings also tend to drift over time. Their accuracy is essential in maintaining image quality because

image density cannot be predicted unless the time is accurate. Verification and calibration of the timer ensure that technique exposure charts will produce diagnostic quality images. Computerized dosimeters provide digital readouts or printouts of the exposure time, or a spinning top may be used to measure 1φ generators and a motorized synchronous top may be used for 3φ units. The tops are less accurate, more time-consuming and difficult to use. Exposure time settings should be maintained within ±5 percent of the label. If the settings drift beyond this limit the timing circuit or mechanism must be recalibrated.

mR/mAs and milliamperage linearity. Milliamperage settings also tend to drift over time, primarily as a result of tube aging. Their accuracy is essential to maintaining image quality because density cannot be predicted unless the mA is accurate. Assurance is needed that technique exposure charts will accurately produce diagnostic quality images. Milliamperage cannot be measured by noninvasive quality control methods. Consequently, mA station accuracy must be inferred by comparing mR/mAs measurements after both time and kVp accuracy have been verified. Comparative measurements are made for the same mAs at different mA and time settings to evaluate the linearity of the mA stations. Computerized dosimeters provide digital readouts or printouts of mR/mAs. Milliamperage stations should be maintained within ±10 percent of each other but Gray, et al., in *Quality Control in Diagnostic Imaging*, recommend maintaining the entire generator within ±10 percent. If the settings drift beyond the established limit the generator must be recalibrated.

Exposure reproduceability. Generators must be capable of repeating exposures accurately. This is ensured by measuring the mR/mAs of several different exposures with the same technical factors. Computerized dosimeters provide digital readouts or printouts of mR/mAs. Reproduceability should be maintained within ±5 percent. If the readings are beyond this limit the entire series of tube and generator tests should be analyzed to attempt to isolate the problem.

Specialized radiographic systems, such as fluoroscopy, tomography and automatic exposure controls, require additional tests.

Fluoroscopic Systems
The tests for fluoroscopic systems should include:

Exposure reproduceability. Fluoroscopic spot film devices use AECs and they should be evaluated according to the AEC tests below.

Exposure rate. Fluoroscopic exposure rates are measured by a dosimeter exactly as diagnostic mR/mAs. The exposure rate should not exceed 5 R/min. If the rate exceeds this limit the automatic brightness control or other systems may require calibration or repair.

Field size accuracy and beam alignment. As with collimation accuracy in diagnostic radiography, fluoroscopic units should not be capable of irradiating tissue outside the image receptor area. In addition to the evaluation performed for a diagnostic unit, fluoroscopic units should display everything within 1 cm of the edges of the image intensifier tube, and the primary beam should be aligned to the center of the image intensifier. Correction of the tube collimation, image intensification system or video display system may be required (further testing by a service engineer is necessary).

Source-to-skin distance limits. Fluoroscopic units should not be capable of placing the tube target closer than 15″ (38 cm) (or 12″ [30 cm] for a mobile fluoroscopy unit) to the patient's skin surface (this is a U.S. federal requirement). Without making any exposure, the source-to-image receptor distance should be verified. If it is not within limits, the unit should not be used until a mechanical device is fitted to set a minimum source-to-skin distance.

Intensifier viewing system resolution. Because fluoroscopic resolution is much poorer than radiographic resolution, periodic assurance that it has not deteriorated is critical in maintaining confidence in diagnosis. A fluoroscopic mesh test tool or a resolution pattern test tool can be imaged to permit visualization of the maximum resolving ability of the system. If the resolution appears to be deteriorating, a service engineer should be consulted.

Intensifier viewing system contrast. Because fluoroscopic contrast is much higher than radiographic contrast, it is important to periodically determine approximately how low contrast a structure may be imaged. Special low contrast fluoroscopic test tools are available that consist of two plates of aluminum with holes of 1–7 mm drilled in one of the plates. When the plates are sandwiched together and imaged on a fluoroscopy system, low contrast evaluation can be made based on the smallest visible hole.

TV monitors and recorders. The vast majority of modern fluoroscopic systems use video systems for image display because of the reduction in patient exposure dose. Although a video signal generator is the test tool of choice, its expense and limited application in radiography usually prohibit its use for routine testing. A fluoroscopic mesh test tool or a resolution test tool and a piece of wire mesh are more commonly used. The resolution test tool can be imaged on the fluoroscopy unit to permit visual measurement of the system resolution. The wire mesh can be imaged to permit visualization of distortion (Figure 28–4). When degradation in resolution or distortion is observed, a service engineer should be consulted.

Automatic brightness control. Although there are a number of types of automatic brightness controls, the term is used here in a generic sense. These controls are designed to function like an AEC in that variations in subject density are automatically compensated for, resulting in a relatively uniform image density.

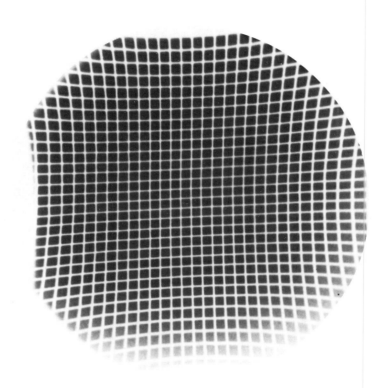

Figure 28–4. Normal distortion of a wire mesh test tool imaged with a conventional fluoroscopy system. (Reprinted from Joel E. Gray, Norlin T. Winkler, John Stears, and Eugene D. Frank, *Quality Control in Diagnostic Imaging*. Rockville, MD.: Aspen Publishers, Inc., 1983 by permission of Mayo Foundation.)

A computerized dosimeter can be used to measure exposure after the beam passes through a phantom. When the phantom thickness is decreased by half, the exposure dose should be similarly reduced. If there is a great discrepancy between phantom thickness and dose reduction, a service engineer should be consulted.

Tomographic Systems The tests for tomographic systems should include:

Uniformity and completeness of motion. Tomography relies on the motion of the tube dur-

ing exposure to produce a sectional image of the subject. Assurance of the uniformity and completeness of tube motion are basic tests. The test tool is simply a lead mask with a pinhole that is positioned several centimeters above the tomographic fulcrum. If the pinhole is centered to the film and then imaged with a full tomographic motion, images similar to Figure 28–5 may be obtained. Erratic tube motion is demonstrated by the uneven densities. If the motion were incomplete there would not be a full length of the tracing. If the motion is erratic or incomplete, the mechanisms involved

Figure 28–5. Tomographic uniformity and completeness of motion test with a pinhole trace image. Both exposures were erratic, as demonstrated by the uneven densities along the entire pinhole exposure. (Reprinted from Joel E. Gray, Norlin T. Winkler, John Stears, and Eugene D. Frank. *Quality Control in Diagnostic Imaging.* Rockville, MD: Aspen Publishers, Inc., 1983 by permission of Mayo Foundation.)

in the tomographic motion should be cleaned (rails, guidewheels, etc.) and the test repeated. If the problem continues, a service engineer should be consulted.

Section depth indicator accuracy. Tomographic units are designed to provide an image that is sharp (possessing good detail) only at the fulcrum level. Assurance that the fulcrum indicator is accurate is essential in diagnosing the location of structures within the subject. Commercial test tools are available or a penetrometer with lead numbered steps can be used. When a tomographic image is made of the test tool, the number that was at the level of the fulcrum should appear sharp. If it doesn't, the fulcrum indicator should be adjusted to the appropriate level. Additional testing may be required to ascertain the proper adjustment.

Section thickness accuracy. The sharp section of a tomograph should be of a known thickness, depending on the total arc of the tomographic motion (exact section thickness per arc is usually stated in the equipment manual). Commercial test tools are available or an angled wire mesh can be used. When the angled resolution mesh is imaged, the section thickness can be determined by measuring the region of sharpness on the image. If the section thickness is inaccurate, the pinhole trace should be consulted. If it appears unacceptable, a service engineer should be consulted.

Resolution. Tomographic resolution is determined by imaging a resolution test pattern at the fulcrum level. The resulting image can be visually inspected to determine the resolving capability of the system. When resolution deteriorates, standard diagnostic quality control measures should be consulted first, then a service engineer.

Automatic Exposure Controls The tests for automatic exposure controls should include:

Exposure reproduceability. The same reproduceability standards for diagnostic radiography systems are applied to AECs. Using the same procedure, with the addition of a subject phantom, densitometer readings of images produced with the AEC should be within OD ±0.1 in the same areas. Reproduceability cannot be achieved on an AEC with dosimeter mR/mAs readings. Radiographs must be produced and measured with a densitometer. If the readings are not within limits, the generator AEC circuits must be calibrated.

Ion chamber sensitivity. Most AECs utilize three ion chambers and permit activation of various combinations during exposures. It is important to ensure that each ion chamber is equally sensitive by comparing the reproduceability of each chamber individually. Exact chamber locations should be verified by producing an image of the ion chambers by using the AEC without a subject at extremely low kVp. After this step is completed, the test is done by using a lead brick to block all chambers but the one to be tested. The AEC reproduceability test is then performed for the unblocked chamber. If all chambers do not respond within ±10 percent, a service engineer should be consulted to recalibrate the generator AEC circuitry.

Density variation control accuracy. Nearly all AEC units provide controls to decrease and increase image density by changing the sensitivity of the ion chamber. These controls vary tremendously from one unit to another. Consultation of equipment manuals will provide the percentage of change each control is designed to produce. A computerized dosimeter can then be employed to obtain mR/mAs measurements to verify the intensity differences for each control. If the controls are not accurate, the generator AEC circuits must be calibrated.

Response capability. Each AEC has a minimum response capability (which varies with manufacturer and model). If the AEC cannot respond at the minimum time, there is no assurance that diagnostic quality images can be produced. Response capability is best evaluated by using a computerized dosimeter readout or printout to determine exposure time for AEC exposures made with a small lucite phantom. As the phantom thickness is reduced, the AEC should produce exposures within ±10 percent mR/mAs of one another until a time below the minimum exposure time is used. If the minimum response time is greater than specified, the AEC should not be used until the problem is corrected.

Back-up timer verification. Occasionally even the best radiographers will forget to activate the proper tube or AEC. When this occurs, patient radiation protection requires that AEC back-up timers be functioning to terminate exposures and protect both patient and tube. When a lead plate is placed over the AEC ionization chamber and an exposure is made, the back-up timer should terminate the exposure and a visual and an audible warning should occur. If the back-up timer or signals fail, the AEC should not be used until the problem is corrected.

ANCILLARY EQUIPMENT

Ancillary equipment must also be monitored on a regular basis. This includes cassette cleaning, film/screen contact tests and view box reproduceability.

Cassette Cleaning and Inspection

During normal use, radiographic intensifying screens are exposed to dust and other foreign particles as cassettes are opened during loading and unloading of film. Periodic cleaning of the screens with a specially formulated antistatic solution removes these artifacts and eliminates the potential for misdiagnosis. At the time they are cleaned, cassettes should also be inspected for wear at corners, edges and especially at hinges. When excessive wear is observed, the cassette should be tested to see if it is lightproof.

Film/Screen Contact

Cassette backs and fronts may warp due to improper storage or traumatic handling. This can lead to loss of contact between the film and the intensifying screen. When poor film-to-screen contact exists, the diverging light photons from the screen cause loss of detail and contrast. A wire mesh test tool should be imaged and the radiograph examined for areas of poor detail. Although rescreening cassettes will replace the pressure pads and sometimes resolve the problem, many institutions prefer to replace the entire cassette.

View Box Uniformity

View boxes, or illuminators, should emit a uniform intensity of light. One of the greatest sources of misunderstanding between radiographers and radiologists is the difference in light intensity of different view boxes because it directly affects the perceived radiographic density. When radiographs consistently exhibit different densities on different view boxes, they become difficult to evaluate. View boxes should be monitored with a light meter periodically to alleviate this problem. When inconsistencies are discovered, they should be brought to the attention of all professional staff.

Correction of the problem, when many view boxes are involved, can be expensive because most institutions have collected view boxes of different models and manfacturers over many years. The thickness and translucency of the plastic surface must be identical for all view boxes. Differences in the plastic are the most common cause of illumination problems. Old view boxes may require painting of their reflectors so the exact tone and reflecting ability of the paint matches newer models. Finally, the bulbs of all view boxes must not only be of the same manufacture and model but should be from the same production run. Attempts to solve view box problems should be carried out in the above order.

REPEAT FILM STUDIES

The careful analysis of repeated radiographs has proven a valuable aid in diagnosing the radiographic process. Repeated radiographs are also referred to as reject, retake, or double-dose studies. Even excellent repeat film studies need take little time or effort to pinpoint conditions that may be easily corrected. Significant reductions in patient exposure dose, radiographer time and effort and supply costs can be achieved with properly executed repeat film studies.

Obtaining Data

A repeat film study involves retaining all repeated radiographs, regardless of cause, for analysis. Any image outside the acceptance limits and scrap film should be included. Boxes labeled as to cause of repeat should be provided near each film processor and the room and tube used should be noted on each film before it is discarded. Typical causes of repeats are shown in Table 28–1.

The most important rule when analyzing repeated images is to not discipline radiographers based on the information obtained. The analysis must be used in a constructive manner to improve working conditions and to point out areas where further technical training may be helpful. Radiographers must be informed of the intent of the study and asked to cooperate in a positive manner to improve both patient care and working conditions. Most radiographers are aware of numerous items they believe contribute to repeat radiographs and welcome an opportunity to find justification for their change. Incompetent radiographers should be disciplined through normal administrative procedures based on actual performance, not as a finding of a repeat film study. Failure by management to follow this suggestion may result in inaccurate repeat-study data when films are not submitted for analysis.

Analysis of Data

The analysis of collected data begins with the classification and counting of images by cause of repeat, room, tube and radiographer. Data should also be separated according to

TABLE 28–1		
CAUSES OF REPEATED RADIOGRAPHS		
Light	34 percent	
Dark	21 percent	
Total exposure		55 percent
Positioning		30 percent
Motion		3 percent

time (weekly is most common). The compiled data should be examined for obvious problems. For example, a large number of images from a single room with an artifact in the same location might indicate a barium or iodine stain on a grid or table. Once obvious problems are addressed, the data should be examined for unequal distribution of repeats. Tables 28–2 and 28–3 illustrate how distributions can be diagnosed.

The **total repeat rate** is a valuable figure to monitor over long periods of time. It is calculated as a percentage of the total number of images produced during the period of the study. The total image figure can be extracted from institutional data in some cases or can be estimated by multiplying the number of examinations by the average number of images

TABLE 28–3

RETAKE PERCENTAGE BY TECHNOLOGIST

TECHNOLOGIST #

REASON	1	2	3	4	5
Dark	35	31	32	30	43
Light	32	31	31	34	30
Positioning	20	18	18	(30)	17
Centering	13	12	11	12	11
Motion	5	(11)	4	4	4
Error	(10)	4	5	3	3
Other	5	7	6	6	7
Total:	120	112	107	119	115

Needs to be more careful?

Has difficulty with some exams?

Using long exposure times?

Retake percentage by radiographer. (Adapted from: Lee W. Goldman and Scott Beech, *Analysis of Retakes: Understanding, Managing and Using an Analysis of Retakes Program for Quality Assurance.* Rockville, MD: U.S. DHEW, PHS, FDA, Bureau of Radiological Health, HEW Publication FDA 79–8097, 1979.)

TABLE 28–2

RETAKE PERCENTAGE BY ROOM

ROOM #

REASON	1	2	3	4	5
Dark	29	37	36	33	33
Light	(45)	31	32	32	37
Positioning	20	18	18	19	17
Centering	10	11	(20)	9	9
Motion	6	7	6	5	5
Other	8	6	7	7	6
Total:	118	110	119	105	107

Technique exposure chart error?

Collimator misaligned?

Retake percentage by room. (Adapted from Lee W. Goldman and Scott Beech, *Analysis of Retakes: Understanding, Managing and Using an Analysis of Retakes Program for Quality Assurance.* Rockville, MD: U.S. DHEW, PHS, FDA, Bureau of Radiological Health, HEW Publication FDA 79–8097, 1979.)

produced per examination. For example, a chest unit that produced 600 examinations in a week could be calculated to have produced 1,200 images (PA + lateral × 600). Repeat rates may suffer from a start-up effect where data may not be reliable for the first three weeks due to unfamiliarity with the requirements of the study or various psychological phenomena from stress to hypermotivation. U.S. data indicate that national radiographer repeat rates should be between 3 and 10 percent, with the average at 7 percent. Data also appear to indicate that when the rate drops below 3 percent there is a problem in data collection or an extremely wide acceptance limit in effect. It is important to realize that repeat rates are not only affected by film processing equipment, x-ray equipment, patient condition and radiographer competence, but also by the acceptance limits of the radiologists. In some instances a high repeat rate may indicate extremely high quality standards in the institution while the same rate may also indicate poor quality radiographers. Caution in interpretation is essential, and all aspects of the analysis should be carefully studied before conclusions are drawn.

TROUBLESHOOTING

Troubleshooting (locating problems when equipment malfunctions) is a diagnostic process. The same reasoning process that a physician uses to diagnose a disease can be applied to radiographic equipment. Beginning with the symptoms, the radiographer can work step-by-step through a problem solving procedure to eliminate possible problems until the source of trouble is isolated.

Although radiographers are not qualified to perform invasive procedures on electronic equipment, they can often pinpoint the general source of the problem. For example, an increase in image density could be caused by nearly all equipment in the radiographic imaging chain. However, a problem solving approach may discover that all radiographs have increased density, not just the radiographs from a single unit. This would focus attention on the film processor. If the developer temperature is checked and found to be within normal limits, the radiographer might then check the replenishment tank only to discover that it is empty. To solve the problem, the radiographer might fill the tank, remove air locks from the replenishment lines and restock the developer tank solution. A complete troubleshooting guide is provided in Appendix B.

SUMMARY

Quality assurance consists of activities that provide adequate confidence that a radiology service will render consistently high quality images and services. Quality assurance includes evaluating activities such as interpretation of examinations, maintenance of equipment, performance of procedures, filing systems, staff development, scheduling of examinations and supply lines. The quality assurance process operates by identifying problems or potential problem areas, monitoring the problem and then resolving it.

Quality control is the aspect of quality assurance that monitors technical equipment to maintain quality standards. The concept of quality control is rooted in the need to stabilize the various equipment components of the radiographic imaging chain. From incoming line current through x-ray production to the processing of the radiograph, erratic equipment performance causes repeat radiographs and unnecessary patient exposure to radiation.

Equipment purchasing decisions should involve each member of the radiological team. Specific imaging requirements should be identified and equipment specifications should be developed. Once the equipment is selected it is then installed and tested.

Monitoring equipment performance is an integral part of quality assurance. It involves the film processing systems as well as the external radiation beams. Ancillary equipment should also be checked.

Monitoring the quality of the film processing systems includes routine processor sensitometry and darkroom safelight testing. External beam evaluations involve monitoring the diagnostic radiographic systems, fluoroscopic systems, tomographic systems and automated exposure controls. A wide variety of tests on each of the systems are performed to assure equipment accuracy. Ancillary equipment, such as cassettes and view boxes, are also monitored.

A careful analysis of repeat radiographs is also a valuable aid in diagnosing the radiographic process. Significant reductions in patient exposure dose, radiographer time and effort and supply costs can be achieved with properly executed repeat-film studies.

REVIEW QUESTIONS

1. Why are quality assurance and control so important?

2. What factors should be considered when making equipment purchasing decisions?

3. How should film processing systems be monitored?

4. How often should tests be performed on diagnostic radiographic systems?

5. What tests should be performed routinely on the x-ray generator?

6. What tests should be performed routinely on automatic exposure controls?

7. Why are repeat film studies a valuable part of quality assurance?

REFERENCES AND RECOMMENDED READING

American Association of Physicists in Medicine. *Diagnostic Radiology Committee Task Force on Quality Assurance Protocol: Basic Quality Control in Diagnostic Radiology.* AAPM Report No. 4. Chicago, IL: AAPM, 1978.

American College of Radiology. *Quality Assurance in Diagnostic Radiology and Nuclear Medicine—The Obvious Decision.* Rockville, MD: U.S. Department of Health, Education, and Welfare, Public Health Service, Food and Drug Administration, Bureau of Radiological Health, HEW Publication FDA 81–8141, 1981.

Ardran, G. M., H. E. Crooks, and V. James. Testing x-ray cassettes for film-intensifying screen contact. *Radiography* 35:414, 143, 1969.

Barber, Triphy C., and Mike Thomas. *Radiologic Quality Control Manual.* Reston, VA: Reston Publishing Co., 1983.

Basart, Judith A. Developer pH: Its significance in quality control. *Radiographic Technology* 45:6, 413, 1974.

Berry, Gary C., Dale E. Starchman, and Willard J. Howland. Objective equipment selection and performance evaluation. *Radiology Management* 2:5, 14, 1980.

Bowers, J., P. Lin, and L. Rogers. Impact of equipment specifications on purchases. *Workshop in Purchase Specifications and Performance Evaluation of Radiologic Imaging Equipment Proceedings.* Chicago, IL: Midwest Chapter American Association of Physicists in Medicine, Northwestern University Medical School and Northwestern Memorial Hospital, May 12–13, 1978.

Brookstein, Joseph J., and Walter Steck. Effective focal spot size. *Radiology* 98, 31–33, 1971.

Burkhart, Roger L. *A Basic Quality Assurance Program for Small Diagnostic Radiology Facilities.* Rockville, MD: U.S. Department of Health and Human Services, Public Health Service, Food and Drug Administration, National Center for Devices and Radiological Health, HHS Publication FDA 83–8218, 1983.

Carlton, Rick. Establishing a total quality assurance program in diagnostic radiology. *Radiologic Technology* 52, 23–38.

Carroll, Quinn B. *Fuchs's Principles of Radiographic Exposure, Processing and Quality Control.* 3rd ed. Springfield, IL: Charles C. Thomas Publisher, 1985.

DeWerd, Larry A., and Frank Ranallo. kVp cassette measurements. *Radiologic Technology* 61:2, 145–146, 1989.

Dodd, Barry C. Repeat analysis in radiology: A method of quality control. *The Canadian Journal of Medical Radiation Technology* 14:2, 37, 1983.

Duffey, Ruth M. Quality assurance/department audits—new buzzwords in health care. *The Canadian Journal of Medical Radiation Technology* 15:4, 134, 1984.

Engel, Terry L. Effect of kilovoltage and milliamperage on focal spot size. *Radiologic Technology* 50:5, 559, 1979.

Everson, Jeffrey D., and Joel E. Gray. Focal-spot measurement: Comparison of slit, pinhole, and star resolution pattern techniques. *Radiology* 165:1, 261–264, 1987.

Fairbanks, R., and C. Doust. Methods for studying the focal spot size and resolution of diagnostic x-ray tubes. *Radiography* 45:533, 89, 1979.

Finney, William. Introduction to radiographic quality assurance. Chapter 41. Ballinger, Philip W. *Merrill's Atlas of Radiographic Positions and Radiologic Procedures.* 6th ed. 325–341. St. Louis, MO: C. V. Mosby Co., 1986.

Goldman, Lee W., and Scott Beech. *Analysis of Retakes: Understanding Managing and Using an Analysis of Retakes Program for Quality Assurance.* Rockville, MD: U.S. Department of Health, Education, and Welfare, Public Health Service, Food and Drug Administration, Bureau of Radiological Health, HEW Publication FDA 79–8097, 1979.

Gray, Joel E., Norlin T. Winkler, John Stears, and Eugene D. Frank. *Quality Control in Diagnostic Imaging.* Baltimore, MD: University Park Press, 1983.

Gray, Joel E., and Martin Trefler. Pinhole cameras: Artifacts, modifications, and recording of pinhole images on screen film systems. *Radiologic Technology* 52:3, 277, 1980.

Hendee, William R., and Raymond P. Rossi. *Quality Assurance for Radiographic X-Ray Units and Associated Equipment.* Rockville, MD: U.S. Department of Health, Education, and Welfare, Public Health Service, Food and Drug Administration, Bureau of Radiological Health, HEW Publication FDA 79–8094, 1979.

Hendee, William R., and Raymond P. Rossi. *Quality Assurance for Conventional Tomographic X-Ray Units.* Rockville, MD: U.S. Department of Health, Education, and Welfare, Public Health Service, Food and Drug Administration, Bureau of Radiological Health, HEW Publication FDA 80–8096, 1980.

Joint Commission on Accreditation of Healthcare Organizations. *Accreditation Manual for Hospitals.* 11–15. Chicago, IL: Joint Commission on Accreditation of Healthcare Organizations, Diagnostic Radiology Services, 1990.

Lam, Rebecca W., and Stan C. Price. The influence of film-screen color sensitivity and type of measurement device on kVp measurements. *Radiologic Technology* 60:4, 319–321, 1989.

Lam, Rebecca W., and Stan C. Price. In response—more on kVp measurements. *Radiologic Technology* 61:2, 146, 1989.

McLemore, J. M. *Quality Assurance in Diagnostic Radiology.* Chicago, IL: Yearbook Medical Publishers, 1981.

McKinney, William E. J. *Radiographic Processing and Quality Control.* Philadelphia, PA: J. B. Lippincott Co., 1988.

Midwest Region American Hospital Radiology Administrators. Equipment Specifications and Performance Standards Education Committee. *Radiology Management* 2:5, 27, 1980.

McFadden, Brenda. Half value layer calibration. *The Canadian Journal of Medical Radiation Technology* 20:2, 67, 1989.

National Electrical Manufacturers Association. Measurements of dimensions and properties of focal spots of diagnostic x-ray tubes. NEMA Standards Publication No. XR–5–1984, 1985.

Nelson, R. E., G. T. Barnes, and D. M. Witten. Economic analysis of a comprehensive quality assurance program. *Radiologic Technology* 49, 129–134, 1977.

Paleen, Robert, Patricia A. Skundberg, and Howard Schwartz. How much is quality assurance costing your department? *Radiology Management* 11:1, 24, 1989.

Price, Richard. The continuous assessment of x-ray tubes and generators. *Radiography* 47:553, 2, 1981.

Quality assurance programs for diagnostic radiology facilities, final recommendation. *Federal Register* 44, 71728–71740, 1979.

Rogers, K. D., I. P. Matthews, and C. J. Roberts. Variation in repeat rates between 18 radiology departments. *The British Journal of Radiology* 60, 463–468, 1987.

Rouse, Susan, and Arnold R. Cowen. Quality assurance of fluorographic camera systems. *Radiology* 49:587, 251, 1983.

Stears, John G., Joel E. Gray, William E. Webbles, and Eugene D. Frank. Radiologic exchange (kVp measurements). *Radiologic Technology* 60:3, 233–236, 1989.

Stears, John G., Joel E. Gray, William E. Webbles, and Eugene D. Frank. X-ray waveform monitoring for radiographic quality control. *Radiologic Technology* 57:1, 9–15, 1985.

Sweeney, Richard J. *Radiographic Artifacts: Their Cause and Control*. Philadelphia, PA: J. B. Lippincott Co., 1983.

Watkinson, S., M. Shaw, B. M. Moores, and E. Eddleston. Quality assurance: A practical programme. *Radiography* 49:578, 27, 1983.

Wheeler, William N. Equipment specifications and performance standards for equipment pertaining to the nuclear medicine department. *Radiology Management* 2:5, 43, 1980.

World Health Organization. *Quality Assurance in Diagnostic Radiology*. Geneva: World Health Organization, 1982.

Zimmer, E. A. *Artifacts and Handling and Processing Faults on X-Ray Films*. New York: Grune & Stratton, 1960.

UNIT IV: COMPARING EXPOSURE SYSTEMS

Once a thorough background knowledge has been acquired, the radiographer must then analyze the clinical conditions and synthesize the information into a workable exposure system. The objective is to provide a method of producing consistent image quality. Consistency facilitates the diagnostic process by permitting more valid comparisons between examinations and confidence in the amount of information presented in the image. A balance must exist between image quality, patient situation and exposure dose.

This unit presents various exposure systems and assists in evaluating which system is most appropriate for a particular clinical situation. All radiographers must have a thorough understanding of how an exposure system functions if it is to be used successfully. The practice of radiography involves so many nonroutine situations, unusual conditions and unique patients that simply following guidelines established by someone else does not permit the skilled radiographer to provide the patient with the highest quality of care.

Because of the tremendous number of variables in the radiographic imaging chain, the most successful exposure systems maintain them all except a single variable for a given range of conditions.

This unit begins with a technical discussion on **developing exposure charts** as a guide to establishing functional systems for clinical practice. The next two chapters detail the development of **fixed kVp systems** and **variable kVp systems**—the most popular exposure systems. Chapter 32 discusses **other exposure systems** that are more complicated and is followed by Chapter 33 on **the art of phototiming**, the most widely used exposure system. A full chapter of **exposure conversion problems** provides methods for solving the types of complex problems that arise in practice. The unit concludes with a chapter on **minimizing patient exposure dose**, the most important contribution made by the radiographer in his choice of exposure system.

29 DEVELOPING EXPOSURE CHARTS

[The radiograph] is not an anatomical snapshot taken at random.

Arthur W. Fuchs, Preface to the first edition of *Principles of Radiographic Exposure and Processing.*

OUTLINE

SYSTEM SELECTION
ANATOMICALLY PROGRAMMED RADIOGRAPHY
ESTABLISHING A TECHNIQUE CHART

OBJECTIVES

Upon completion of this chapter, the student should be able to:

1. Compare various exposure systems.
2. Describe the advantages and disadvantages of fixed and variable kVp systems.
3. Discuss other exposure systems that have influenced radiographic technique.
4. Explain why measurement of part thickness is critical to the accurate use of technique charts.
5. Describe the function of the radiographer when using automatic exposure control systems.
6. Describe how programmed exposure control systems function.
7. State the steps necessary to establish a technique chart.
8. Explain a basic phantom testing procedure.
9. Describe the process of selecting an optimal image range.
10. Extrapolate a technique chart from a limited number of phantom test images.
11. Describe the clinical trial and fine tuning processes.

SYSTEM SELECTION

The foundations of the principles of radiographic exposure technique were laid in the 1920s by Ed. C. Jerman, known as the father of radiologic technology in the United States, and were developed into a scientific system in the 1940s by Arthur W. Fuchs.

Because radiographic exposure is such a complex process, technique systems function best when the large number of variables can be held constant while a single factor is permitted to vary. The goal of any radiographic exposure system is to provide a method of consistency in the quality of image production. Each type of exposure system functions in a different way to accomplish this goal, but all require the routine use of technique charts. Radiographers should consult a technique chart prior to making each exposure. Failure to follow this practice results in a higher personal repeat rate and excessive, unwarranted, patient exposure dose.

A radiography department can expect to produce consistent results only when accurate technique charts are provided for each x-ray unit. Monitoring and revising these charts is part of the quality control function. Institutions that develop and enforce policies requiring radiographers to utilize posted technique charts experience lower repeat rates. Radiographers are advised to follow posted technique charts and to bring inaccuracies to the attention of quality control personnel immediately to avoid continued poor-quality images and excessive patient exposure dose.

Comparing Exposure Systems

Each exposure system has its advantages and disadvantages and professionals quickly develop a rationale for their favorite system. The student must study each system in detail to learn its advantages and disadvantages before forming a personal professional judgment.

It is important to recognize that any exposure system is designed to provide consistency in image quality and requires that all users of equipment in a single institution adhere to the same technique charts. Although personal philosophy may differ from institutional procedures and policies, the professional must let personal preference become secondary to the primary goal of widespread consistency in image quality. The following information outlines the various exposure systems that are explained in detail in this unit.

Fixed Kilovoltage Systems

Fixed kVp systems were developed by Fuchs in 1943 during World War II. They have strong theoretical support in the literature and among many radiographers because they tend to decrease patient dose, provide more information on the image, increase the consistency of image density and contrast, lengthen exposure latitude, reduce x-ray tube wear, decrease time settings and therefore patient motion, and are easier to remember. However, these systems produce more scatter radiation, which tends to provide a lower contrast than a variable kilovoltage system. Low contrast is usually perceived as less pleasing to the eye and for this reason many institutions have not adopted the fixed kVp system.

Variable Kilovoltage Systems

Variable kVp systems were the first methodical approach to radiographic technique. They were proposed by Jerman in 1925 and predominated until x-ray generators became powerful enough to support fixed kVp techniques in the 1940s. They permit small incremental changes in exposure to compensate for variation in body part thickness. Most x-ray generators permit finer adjustment of kVp stations than of time or mA settings. Variable kVp systems produce higher contrast images, which enhance the visibility of fine detail and increase the perception of resolution. Institutions that have not adopted a variable kVp system cite the overwhelming advantages of fixed kVp to patient dose, image information, tube wear, etc.

Other Exposure Systems

Over the years since the work of Jerman and Fuchs there have been many attempts to refine exposure systems. During the 1950s and 1960s attempts were made to use mathematical formulas to quantify the relationship between the primary factors, especially kVp and mAs. A number of these formulas have been proven invalid. Only the systems based on $\log_{10}$ have survived, although there is some support for body habitus and proportional anatomy systems. However, several exposure systems have been developed that have either had a major effect on thinking about radiographic technique or have proven to be accurate in clinical situations.

Du Pont Bit System The Du Pont Bit System is so called because it was developed, by computer analysis, by Robert Trinkle of E. I. Du Pont de Nemours and Company, Inc. Du Pont published the system in the 1970s and has supported it through numerous editions. The Bit System is a log-based system that utilizes points to quantify a vast number of radiographic variables, such as film density and contrast, distance, anatomical thickness, kVp, mAs, pathology, grids, development time, etc. The concept was simply that each projection required an established number of bits. Any balanced combination of variables that equaled the required bits would produce a diagnostic-quality image. The Bit System even permits calculation of approximate skin dose.

XVS System The X-Ray Value Scale (XVS) system was designed by Gerhart Schwarz in 1960. It was patterned after the photographic Exposure Value Scale (EVS) system, but with the addition of research into the effect of part thickness on kVp's effect on image density. The system was the first used to quantify the primary radiographic variables. It permitted variance of exposure factors, much as with the Bit System. The basis of the system was a caliper that measured part thickness in XVS numbers. Any total of XVS numbers that equaled the caliper measurement could be obtained from special markings on the x-ray machine's distance, mA, time and kVp indicators. The lack of standardization of all but a single factor resulted in too many variables for consistent diagnostic confidence. In addition, when manufacturers began to build units with XVS numbers replacing technical controls, radiographers experienced difficulty in adapting to specific clinical situations.

Siemens Point System The Siemens Point System was designed as a parallel system to the XVS system. It predated the Bit System, and although it was not as sophisticated, it permitted the radiographer to control the exposure variables much better than with the XVS system.

Supertech™ Calculator In 1973 a log-based, slide rule technique calculator was developed by Brice Kratzer, patented, trademarked, and marketed as the Supertech™ Calculator by Supertech, Inc. Circular and slide rule calculators had been presented in the radiographic literature by C. W. Reed in 1939 and 1949 and William A. Williams had developed a circular calculator technique system in 1960. Several of these calculators were distributed by commercial film companies, but only the Supertech™ Calculator has survived to the present and is updated continually. The most recent version includes an acrylic penetrometer with a calibration master film for elementary quality control testing of machine output. After a short testing procedure, each machine can be assigned a correction factor that takes into account such variations as kVp, mA, time, part thickness, patient age, projection, distance, grid, pathology, etc. In addition, the slide rule style calculator provides positioning instructions, principles of exposure and anatomy review and even serves as an angulator and basic quality control tool. The Supertech™ Calculator remains a viable technique system, especially in low volume clinics, physician's offices and in ancillary radiographic service situations, such as chiropractics and podiatry.

Proportional Anatomy Systems A body habitus system for chest radiography was proposed by Terry Eastman in 1969. Proportional anatomy systems were presented by Quinn Carroll in 1985 and by Eugene Frank and Norlin T. Winkler in 1987. These systems classify body parts and habitus into groups of similar subject density and contrast. The body habitus system determined technical factors for the chest from patient height and weight. The proportional anatomy systems use ratios or conversion factors to extrapolate a technique chart for the entire body from a control exposure.

Measurement of Part Thickness

Nearly all variables in exposure systems are changed according to the thickness of the anatomical part being radiographed and no exposure system can be expected to function accurately unless the radiographer measures part thickness. Part thicknesses for various regions in the average adult were detailed by Arthur Fuchs (Table 29–1).

Failure to measure consistently will cause unnecessary repeated exposures, resulting in excessive patient exposure dose. The device used to measure a part thickness is a **caliper**. Improper use of a caliper will result in improper technical factors and a repeated exposure. Caliper measurements are made either by central ray entrance and exit or by thickest

TABLE 29–1

AVERAGE ADULT PART THICKNESS BY REGION

Region		Average Thickness Adult—CMS			Percent Frequency
		AP	PA	Lat	
Thumb, Fingers		1.5–4			99
Hand		3–5			99
				7–10	93
Wrist		3–6			99
				5–8	98
Forearm		6–8			94
				7–9	92
Elbow		6–8			96
				7–9	87
Arm		7–10			95
				7–10	94
Shoulder		12–16			79
Clavicle			13–17		82
Foot		6–8			92
				7–9	91
Ankle		8–10			86
				6–9	96
Leg		10–12			85
				9–11	89
Knee		10–13			92
				9–12	92
Thigh		14–17			77
				13–16	76
Hip		17–21			76
Cervical Vertebrae	C1–3	12–14			77
	C4–7	11–14			98
	C1–7			10–13	90
Thoracic Vertebrae		20–24			76
				28–32	81
Lumbar Vertebrae		18–22			69
				27–32	77
Pelvis		19–23			78

(continued)

TABLE 29–1 (*continued*).				
Region	Average Thickness Adult—CMS			Per-cent Fre-quency
	AP	PA	Lat	
Skull		18–21		96
			14–17	88
Frontal		18–21		97
Sinuses Max.		18–22		88
			13–17	96
Mandible			10–12	82
Chest		20–25		82
			27–32	84

Reprinted with permission of the American Society of Radiologic Technologists from Arthur W. Fuchs's Relationship of tissue thickness to kilovoltage. *The X-ray Technician* [now *Radiologic Technology*] 19:6, 287–293, 1948.

Figure 29–1. Proper caliper measurement of part thickness by using the central ray entrance-to-exit method.

part. It is critical that all radiographers using a particular technique chart measure by the same method and in exactly the same manner.

Central ray measurements should be made from the point of central ray entrance to exit. For example, in Figure 29–1, the chest should be measured at point B, not point A or C. Thickest part measurements should be made at the thickest part of the area of interest. If another special measurement point or method has been established, it must be followed by all users of the chart.

Phototiming (AEC) Systems

When automatic exposure control (AEC) systems are used, the selection of exposure time factors, and thereby mAs selection, are eliminated. The radiographer must still exercise professional judgment to determine all other factors, including mA (which can be used to influence the time), kVp, distance, etc. Part of the art of phototiming is learning when to use AECs and when to avoid them.

ANATOMICALLY PROGRAMMED RADIOGRAPHY

The most exciting developments are currently in computerized exposure control systems. These systems are simply computerized technique charts utilizing existing exposure systems but storing the data in a memory bank that is an inherent part of the x-ray control console. Many of these units have anatomically based programming (Figure 29–2). For example, when the radiographer pushes a button to indicate a lumbar spine, a screen may provide a choice of projections. When the lateral projection is indicated, a suggested series of technical factors may be set on the x-ray console. If the exposure is begun, the computerized factors will be used. However, if the radiographer determines that nonroutine conditions exist, the technical factors can be modified prior to exposure. The computerized control can be programmed to display any desired exposure system and then be fine tuned to meet existing needs. If the programmed console or consoles

Figure 29–2. A programmed, computerized exposure control console. (Courtesy of GE Medical Systems.)

are monitored and maintained to display accurate techniques, they can be consulted for techniques for an entire department. Only an mAs correction factor would be needed for each room to make the chart accurate.

ESTABLISHING A TECHNIQUE CHART

The process of establishing a technique chart begins with collecting exposure data. The first step is to make a single exposure that produces an optimal diagnostic quality radiograph. This original image must be at the optimal center of the acceptance limits curve. Although any projection can be used as a starting point in collecting data, it is preferred that the first data be from a subject part size and kVp in the middle of the diagnostic range. Ideal part sizes are 10–25 cm and ideal kilovoltage is in the 60–80 range.

Figure 29–3 illustrates the steps in setting up a radiographic technique chart for any exposure system.

Initial Phantom Images

Initially, a series of test exposures is made to determine the optimal quality image.

ESTABLISHING A TECHNIQUE CHART

Figure 29–3. A systematic approach to establishing a technique chart.

This is accomplished by using an appropriate phantom to produce radiographs at a variety of technical factor combinations both above and below the average level. It is essential that the density remain the same at a control point to avoid misperception of the contrast range. It is preferred that the images be produced using an AEC to control the density. If an AEC is not available, or cannot be used due to other circumstances, a density reference control point must be established and measured with a densitometer. For example, the exact center of the body of L4 could be measured on each film. It would be necessary to adjust milliampere-second values until all images exhibited control point densities within OD 0.3 of one another.

Select Optimal Phantom Image

Once the series of phantom test images has been produced, it must be shown to all radiologists, who will be asked to diagnose the images, and to the supervisory radiographers, who will be responsible for image quality control checking. These professionals should not be asked to select the best image but to select those images they believe to be outside acceptance limits, because when any group of professionals is asked to select the best image there will be differences of opinion, leaving no concensus as to the best image. Conversely, elimination of those images that are not acceptable will often result in a series of images that are acceptable to all, although "perfect" to only a few.

Extrapolate Technique Chart

Next, a series of preliminary clinical trials should be performed by preparing a technique chart that adjusts current technical factors to those that are newly established as optimal. This is normally done by using the 15 percent rule and other guides for part thickness adjustments for particular exposure systems. Particular attention should be given to projections that have a narrow range of part thicknesses or few choices of technical factors. For example, the variations in a wrist or PA chest chart both require careful calculation, the wrist because the normal thickness range encompasses only about 3 cm and the PA chest because the extremely high kVp with a normal thickness range of only about 5 cm amplifies minute changes in mAs.

Phantom Testing

The new chart is then tested with a phantom to verify its effectiveness. Minimum phantom testing should include a median, small and large part thickness. At this point the chart is completed for all part thicknesses for each projection.

Clinical Trials

Finally, a limited series of clinical trial examinations should be performed using the new chart. Each examination should be recorded and all repeated images should be saved for analysis. The series of clinical examinations should then be shown to each person who participated in the determination of the original standards. If the new image quality is accepted, a new exposure technique chart should be designed and implemented. If the new image quality experiences limited acceptance, adjustments should be made to satisfy deficiencies and all of the phantom testing and clinical trial steps should be repeated. Under no circumstance should clinical trials be performed until phantom testing and the other preliminary steps have been properly completed. Whenever new equipment is added to the imaging chain, especially a new x-ray tube, intensifying screens, type of processing chemistry, or film, the phantom testing and/or clinical trial steps should be repeated until confidence in the chart is re-established.

Clinical Fine Tuning

Clinical fine tuning requires that the technical factors for each exposure be recorded, regardless of whether the image is within acceptance limits. Each image is then used to fine tune the chart. Excellent quality images permit technical factors for the part thicknesses to be verified, while all other images permit adjustments of the technical factors for their respective part sizes.

Ongoing Fine Tuning

It is important that a system of ongoing fine tuning be established as a quality control monitoring method. The quality control radiographer should be consulted whenever a technique chart produces an unacceptable image and the cause is not evident. A series of unexplained rejected images may signify a change in one of the system's components that can be determined by quality control testing. The problem can often be fixed by a service engineer, although aging processes (such as filament wear, focal spot deterioration and tube gas) may require adjustments of the technique chart.

SUMMARY

The goal of any radiographic exposure system is to provide a method of consistency in the quality of image production. Each type of exposure system functions in a different way to accomplish this goal, but all require the routine use of technique charts. Radiographers should consult a technique chart prior to making each exposure. Failure to follow this practice results in a higher personal repeat rate and excessive, unwarranted patient exposure dose.

A radiography department can expect to produce consistent results only when accurate technique charts are provided for each x-ray unit. Monitoring and revising these charts is part of the quality control program. Institutions that develop and enforce policies requiring radiographers to utilize posted technique charts experience lower repeat rates.

Each exposure system has its advantages and disadvantages and professionals quickly develop a rationale for their favorite system. It is important to recognize that any exposure system is designed to provide consistency in image quality and this requires that all users of equipment in a single institution adhere to the same technique charts. The two most popular exposure systems are the fixed kVp system and the variable kVp system. Other exposure systems include the Du Pont Bit System, the XVS System, the Siemens Point System, the Supertech™ Calculator, and various proportional anatomy systems.

A systematic process for establishing a technique chart involves producing initial phantom images, selecting the optimal phantom image, extrapolating a technique chart for a given exposure system, performing phantom testing using the extrapolated technique chart data, performing clinical trials, clinical fine tuning and, finally, establishing a system of ongoing fine tuning.

REVIEW QUESTIONS

1. What is the principle goal of a radiographic exposure system?

2. Why is it important for radiographers to utilize technique charts?

3. What are some of the advantages of the fixed kVp system?

4. What are some of the advantages of the variable kVp system?

5. What are the two methods used for taking caliper measurements?

6. What are the steps involved in establishing a technique chart?

7. What should be done when a technique chart produces an unacceptable image and the cause is not evident?

REFERENCES AND RECOMMENDED READING

Cahoon, John B., Jr. Radiographic technique—its origin, concept, practical application and evaluation of radiation dose. *Radiologic Technology* 32:4, 354, 1961.

Carroll, Quinn. *Fuchs's Principles of Radiographic Exposure, Processing and Quality Control.* 3rd ed. Springfield, IL: Charles C. Thomas Publisher, 1985.

Compton, Stephen. Bit conversion of technical factors in vascular procedures. *Radiologic Technology* 58:5, 413, 1987.

Eastman, Terry R. A history of radiographic technique. *Applied Radiology* July/August, 97–100, 1978.

Eastman, Terry R. Technique charts: The key to radiographic quality. *Radiologic Technology* 46:5, 365, 1975.

Fuchs, Arthur W. Radiography of entire body employing one film and a single exposure. *Radiography and Clinical Photography* 10, 9–14, 1934.

Hiss, Stephen S. Technique management. *Radiologic Technology* 46:5, 369, 1975.

Jerman, E. C. Potter-Bucky diaphragm technic. *Radiology* 6, 336–338, 1926.

Jerman, E. C. Extremity technic. *Radiology* 6, 252–254, 1926.

McFadden, Brenda. Principles of radiographic exposure: A new approach. *The Canadian Journal of Radiography, Radiotherapy, and Nuclear Medicine* 16:2, 45–54, 1985.

Williams, William A. Standardization of x-ray technique. *Radiologic Technology* 32:2, 137, 1960.

THE CASE OF THE MISSING LOWER PELVIS

For some unexplained reason, this patient's lower hips and pelvis disappeared. Why?

Answers to the case studies can be found in Appendix E.

30 FIXED KILOVOLTAGE SYSTEMS

The future trend is toward the use of optimum and higher kilovoltage values and a more widespread knowledge regarding the photographic function of each exposure factor.

John B. Cahoon, Jr., from the 15th Jerman Memorial Lecture at the 1961 Annual Meeting of the American Society of X-Ray Technicians.

OUTLINE

PRINCIPLES OF FIXED KILOVOLTAGE EXPOSURE SYSTEMS
ESTABLISHING A FIXED KILOVOLTAGE PEAK
TECHNIQUE CHART

OBJECTIVES

Upon completion of this chapter, the student should be able to:

1. Describe the principles of fixed kVp technique theory.
2. Discuss the primary advantages and disadvantages of fixed kVp technique systems.
3. Define optimal kilovoltage.
4. Explain how to establish fixed kVp for various subject parts.
5. Describe the steps in establishing a fixed kVp technique chart.
6. Synthesize a fixed kVp technique chart from control radiographs.

PRINCIPLES OF FIXED KILOVOLTAGE EXPOSURE SYSTEMS

Because radiographic exposure is such a complex process, technique systems function best when the large number of variables can be held constant while a single factor is permitted to vary. **In a fixed kilovoltage system, the kVp is held constant for a given range of subject** densities and contrasts while the mAs is varied to achieve an appropriate image density. The kVp has a profound effect on many radiographic factors, such as contrast, type of interaction, production of scatter radiation and average photon energy. In addition, it varies depending on generator phase, filtration, machine calibration, intensifying screen phosphor conversion efficiency, subject inner shell binding energy range, etc. Consequently, a technique chart that makes kVp a constant eliminates the effects of these variables on the exposure system. The basis of a fixed kilovoltage exposure system therefore becomes the concept of the optimal kilovoltage peak.

In keeping with the goal of any radiographic exposure system to provide consistency in the quality of image production, a fixed kilovoltage system provides a relatively uniform contrast and an easily remembered series of kilovoltages to which mAs values can be added to produce images within established acceptance limits. The uniform contrast contributes to radiologists' confidence in the information in the image as they do not have to contend with a variable gray scale.

Advantages and Disadvantages

There are a number of advantages to the fixed kilovoltage technique systems. These systems tend to decrease patient dose, as the kilovoltage is always at the maximum possible level, and this permits decreased mAs in compensation. The decreased mAs contributes to decreased patient exposure dose. In addition, the consistency in kVp levels results in uniform radiographic contrast, permitting the radiologist to compare radiographs of a given projection or patient, and provides more confidence in the diagnostic process. The higher average kVps that the optimal kVp concept produces lengthen exposure latitude. It also decreases mAs, thereby decreasing the average mA, which lowers x-ray tube heating and extends tube life, and/or decreasing time, which reduces the possibility of patient motion.

There are also disadvantages to a fixed kilovoltage technique system. These systems tend to provide a lower overall contrast than do variable kilovoltage systems and this is usually perceived by radiologists as less pleasing to the eye. Without question, the lower contrast produces much more scattered radiation

and films that are less artistically beautiful. Additionally, small incremental changes in exposure for variations in body part thickness may not be possible with systems that fix kVp and vary mAs, due to less variety in mA stations and exposure times as compared to the kVp settings.

Optimal Kilovoltage Peak

The optimal kVp is the maximum kVp level that will produce images with appropriate contrast that are consistently within acceptance limits. This kVp level must ensure sufficient penetration of the subject as well as provide acceptable radiographic contrast. Insufficient penetration of the area of interest, especially in contrast media studies, limits the diagnostic region to the edges of the contrast media. Sufficient penetration permits visualization through the contrast media and increases the diagnostic information available.

The use of the maximum kVp as optimal causes a corresponding decrease in the mAs required to produce acceptable image density. The mAs reduction contributes to both reduced mA and time. Reduced mA decreases x-ray tube heating and prolongs filament and anode life. Reduced time minimizes the possibility of patient motion. **The optimal kVp produces lower contrast and the minimum patient exposure dose.** The fixed kVp system takes advantage of the only situation in radiography where image quality can be increased (low contrast and therefore more diagnostic shades of gray) and patient exposure dose decreased (less mAs and therefore less mR/mAs).

Establishing Optimal Kilovoltage Peak

A number of optimal kVps are established for a fixed kVp system; each is specific for a range of subject densities and contrasts. In other words, the so-called "fixed kVp" is fixed only for a specific range of part thicknesses for a particular procedure. For example, where 80 kVp may be selected as the optimal kVp for noncontrast media abdominal examinations, 50 kVp may be determined to be the maximum for contrast that is acceptable for imaging the trabeculae of the smaller extremities. The optimal kVp should not be changed unless the conditions under which it was set have changed, or the acceptance limits are changed.

ESTABLISHING A FIXED KILOVOLTAGE PEAK TECHNIQUE CHART

The specific steps to setting up a fixed kVp technique chart follow the basic outline provided in Chapter 29.

Initial Phantom Images

Setting up a fixed kVp system requires that a series of test exposures be obtained to determine the optimal kVp. This is accomplished by using an abdomen or pelvis phantom to produce radiographs at a variety of kVps above and below the average level. It is essential that the density remain the same at a control point to avoid misperception of the contrast range (Figure 30–1). It is preferred that the images be exposed using an AEC, although a density reference control point can be used.

Select Optimal Phantom Image

Once the series of phantom test images has been produced, the optimal phantom image must be selected. The objective of optimal kVp is to determine the **highest** kVp and **lowest** contrast that is within acceptance limits, not the best image. The optimal kVp is the highest of the acceptable images. Remember that this process is one of elimination, not of selection. In other words, radiologists and

quality control radiographers should be asked to eliminate unacceptable images, not to choose the single best quality image.

Careful consideration must be given to the variety of subject densities and contrasts in the human body before establishing the optimal kVps for other procedures. Table 30–1 illustrates common optimal kVp ranges for the major body regions, but individual requirements often vary. For example, a slow film/screen combination that was chosen to achieve higher resolution for extremity radiography will often provide higher contrast than a faster combination. A higher kVp can be used than with a lower resolution system while still achieving high contrast. The higher kVp, although not compensating for the slower system's increased mAs and patient dose, does reduce the total exposure to a degree.

Extrapolate Technique Chart

Once the optimal kVp has been determined, an extrapolated technique chart should be obtained by adjusting current technical factors to the newly established optimal kVp. This is normally done by using the 15 percent rule to modify existing technical factors until the desired kVp has been achieved.

Milliampere-seconds is designed to be the primary variable for a fixed kVp exposure system. The mAs values for the technique chart must be set at minimum increments of 30 percent because values less than 30 percent are not visibly significant. Because there is no linearity of the film/screen combination and other variables, no accurate formula can be given for extrapolating mAs values. However, most systems have been found to operate in the range of doubling or halving the mAs for every 5 cm of subject thickness. For example, if 80 mAs produces a diagnostic quality image of a 20 cm part, a 15 cm part will require about 40 mAs, while a 25 cm part will require about 160 mAs. This is often applied to variable kVp technique

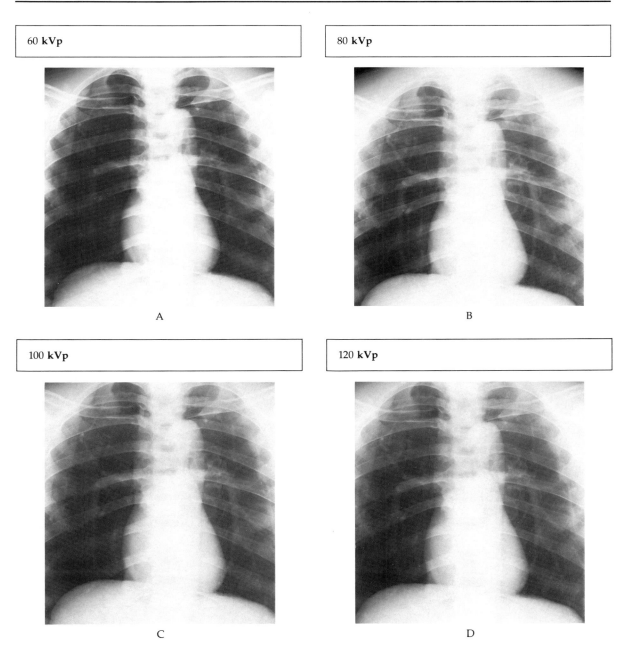

Figure 30–1A–D. A series of chest radiographs produced at 60, 80, 100 and 120 kVp to determine the optimal kVp. While 60 kVp may be selected as optimal for ribs, 120 kVp may be determined to be optimal for the chest.

TABLE 30–1	

COMMON OPTIMAL kVp RANGES FOR THE MAJOR BODY REGIONS

Region	Optimal kVp Range
Small extremities	50–60
Iodine-based contrast media studies	68
Large extremities	70
Skull	80
Abdomen and ribs	80
AP vertebral column	80
Lateral vertebral column	90
Chest	120
Barium-based contrast media studies	120

charts as a "2 kVp/cm rule," which is fairly consistent with the 15 percent rule and ensures sufficient penetration.

Phantom Testing

Phantom testing is recommended prior to performing patient examinations. As a minimum, phantom testing should be done for a median, small and large part size. Because of the nonlinearity of the exposure systems and the inadequacy of the 15 percent rule, phantom testing should always be employed when the part size is less than 10 cm or the kVp is outside the median diagnostic range of 60–80.

Phantom testing also serves as a fine tuning mechanism for the extrapolated chart prior to clinical use. Once several mAs values have been set, extrapolation of the mAs for subject thickness can be done accurately. For example, if 68 kVp is set as the optimal fixed kVp for iodine-based contrast media abdominal work, a technique chart might be established from a base diagnostic quality 20 cm phantom image

at 50 mAs (Table 30–2). Step 1 illustrates a blank chart with the phantom technique. Using the 15 percent rule, several additional mAs values can be extrapolated for phantom testing, as shown in Step 2. Upon phantom testing, the extrapolated mAs values may require fine tuning, as shown in Step 3. Once phantom fine tuning is accomplished, the extrapolation of the final mAs values can be completed, as shown in Step 4. At this point the chart has been proven within acceptance limits by phantom testing and is ready for clinical trials.

Clinical Trials

Limited clinical trials are permissible with the new chart. All images should be recorded, with repeated images saved for analysis. When clinical trials are proceeding without excess repeated exposures, the new technique chart can move into the clinical fine tuning stage.

Clinical Fine Tuning

The clinical fine tuning process will adjust and finally validate the entire chart. At this point the new technique chart can be adopted. However, ongoing fine tuning then begins as a permanent process.

Ongoing Fine Tuning

Ongoing fine tuning is the process that maintains the accuracy of the entire exposure system and gives radiographers and radiologists confidence in the exposure and diagnostic processes.

SUMMARY

Technique systems function best when the large number of variables can be held constant while a single factor is permitted to vary. In a fixed kilovoltage system the kVp is held constant for a given range of subject densities

TABLE 30–2	FIXED kVp TECHNIQUE CHART				
Blank Chart with Phantom Technique			Extrapolation of Additional mAs Values	Fine Tuning of Extrapolated mAs Values	Extrapolation of Final mAs Values
		Step 1	Step 2	Step 3	Step 4
cm	kVp	mAs			
16	68				10
17	68				20
18	68				30
19	68				40
20	68	50	50	50	50
21	68				60
22	68				70
23	68				80
24	68				90
25	68		100	100	100
26	68				115
27	68				130
28	68				145
29	68				160
30	68		200	180	180
31	68				215
32	68				250
33	68				285
34	68				320
35	68		400	360	360

and contrasts, while the mAs is varied to achieve an appropriate image density.

Fixed kilovoltage technique systems tend to decrease patient dose because the kilovoltage is always at the maximum possible level. In addition, the consistency in kVp levels results in a uniform radiographic contrast and a lengthened exposure latitude. There are also disadvantages to a fixed kilovoltage technique system. These systems tend to provide a lower overall contrast than do variable kilovoltage systems and this is usually perceived by radiologists as less pleasing to the eye. Additionally, small incremental changes in exposure for variations in body part thickness may not be possible with systems that fix kVp and vary mAs, due to less variety in mA stations and exposure times as compared to the kVp settings.

The optimal kVp is the maximum kVp level that will produce images with appropriate contrast that are consistently within acceptance limits. This kVp level must ensure sufficient penetration of the subject as well as provide acceptable radiographic contrast. A number of optimal kVps are established for a fixed kVp system and are specific for a range of subject densities and contrasts. In other words, the so-called "fixed kVp" is fixed only for a specific range of part thicknesses for a particular procedure.

Establishing a fixed kVp technique chart involves producing phantom images, selecting the optimal phantom image, extrapolating a technique chart, and performing phantom testing, clinical trials, clinical fine tuning and ongoing fine tuning.

REVIEW QUESTIONS

1. What is the principle of a fixed kVp exposure system?

2. What are the basic advantages of a fixed kVp exposure system?

3. What are the basic disadvantages of a fixed kVp exposure system?

4. Define optimal kVp.

5. How is the optimal kVp established?

6. What should be the minimal mAs increments used for variations in part thickness when using a fixed kVp exposure system?

REFERENCES AND RECOMMENDED READING

Cahoon, John B. *Formulating X-Ray Techniques.* 8th ed. Durham, NC: Duke University Press, 1974.

Cahoon, John B. Radiographic technique: Its origin, concept, practical application and evaluation of radiation dose. *The X-Ray Technician* 32, 352–364, 1961.

Carlstein, Charles J. Radiography of compressed air workers using optimum kilovoltage. *Radiologic Technology* 43:1, 10–14, 1971.

Carroll, Quinn. *Fuchs's Principles of Radiographic Exposure, Processing and Quality Control.* 3rd ed. Springfield, IL: Charles C. Thomas Publisher, 1985.

Clark, K. C. An introduction to high-voltage technique. *Radiography*, 19, 21–33, 1953.

Du Pont, E.I. de Nemours & Co. Medical Products Department, Customer Technology Center. *Bit System of Technique Conversion.* Wilmington, DE.

Eastman, Terry R. *Radiographic Fundamentals and Technique Guide.* St. Louis, MO: C. V. Mosby Co., 1979.

Eastman, Terry R. A history of radiographic technique. *Applied Radiology* July-August, 97–99, 1978.

Eastman, T. R. Technique charts: The key to radiographic quality. *Radiologic Technology* 46, 365–368, 1975.

Eastman, T. R. Measurement: The key to exposure with manual techniques. *Radiologic Technology* 45, 75–78, 1973.

Eastman, T. R. Chest technique through body habitus. *Radiologic Technology* 41, 80–84, 1969.

Files, Glenn W. *Medical Radiographic Technique.* Springfield, IL: Charles C. Thomas Publisher, 1955.

Fuchs, Arthur W. *Principles of Radiographic Exposure and Processing.* 2nd ed. Springfield, IL: Charles C. Thomas Publisher, 1958.

Fuchs, Arthur W. Control of radiographic density. *The X-Ray Technician* 20, 271–273, 291, 1949.

Fuchs, Arthur W. Relationship of tissue thickness to kilovoltage. *The X-Ray Technician* 19, 287–293, 1948.

Fuchs, Arthur W. Military photoroentgen technique employing optimum kilovolt (peak) principles. *The American Journal of Roentgenology* 53, 587–596, 1945.

Fuchs, Arthur W. The optimum kilovoltage technique in military roentgenography. *American Journal of Roentgenology* 50, 358–365, 1943.

Fuchs, Arthur W. Higher kilovoltage technic with high-definition screens. *Radiography and Clinical Photography* 14:3, 2–8, 1938.

General Electric Company Medical Systems Department. *How to Prepare an X-Ray Technic Chart*. Milwaukee, WI: Publication 4301A.

Gratale, Pete, Gilbert W. Turner, and Charles B. Burns. Using the same exposure factors for wet and dry casts. *Radiologic Technology* 57:4, 325–328.

Hiss, Stephen S. *Understanding Radiography*. Springfield, IL: Charles C. Thomas Publisher, 1978.

Hiss, Stephen S. Technique management. *Radiologic Technology* 46:5, 369–375, 1975.

Jerman, Ed. C. *Modern X-Ray Technic*. St. Paul, MN: Bruce Publishing Co., 1928.

Jerman, Ed. C. Potter-Bucky diaphragm technic. *Radiology* 6, 336–338, 1926.

Jerman, Ed. C. X-ray technic: From the old to the new. *Radiology* 5:6, 1925.

Koenig, George F. Potential. *Radiologic Technology* 37:4, 184–198, 1966.

Koenig, George F. Kilovoltage as a qualitative factor. *The X-Ray Technician* 29:4, 13, 1957.

Lyon, Neil J. Optimum kilovoltage techniques. *The X-Ray Technician* 33, 398–401, 1962.

McDaniel, Clarence Thomas. Tissue absorption theory applied to formulation of radiographic technique resulting in time as the variable factor. *Radiologic Technology* 37:2, 51–55, 1965.

Mahoney, George J. A slide rule for kVp-mAs adjustments facilitating the use of high kilovoltage. *The X-Ray Technician* 31, 35–38, 1959.

Merrill, Harley F. High kilovoltage radiography. *Radiologic Technology* 32:3, 259, 1960.

Morgan, James A. *The Art and Science of Medical Radiography*. 5th ed. St. Louis, MO: Catholic Hospital Association, 1977.

Sante, L. R. *Manual of Roentgenological Technique*. 9th ed. Ann Arbor, MI: Edwards Brothers, Inc., 1942.

Schwarz, Gerhart S. *Unit-Step Radiography*. Springfield, IL: Charles C. Thomas Publisher, 1961.

Schwarz, Gerhart S. Kilovoltage conversion in radiography. *The X-Ray Technician* 31, 373–379, 436, 1960.

Schwarz, Gerhart S. Kilovoltage and radiographic effect. *Radiology*, 73, 749–760, 1959.

Schwarz, Gerhart S. A simple universal unit system of radiographic exposures suited to departmental, national, and international standardization. *Radiology* 71, 573–574, 1958.

Schwarz, Gerhart S. Extended range radiography. *Radiology* 69, 419–423, 1957.

Thompson, Thomas T. *Cahoon's Formulating X-Ray Techniques*. 9th ed. Durham, NC: Duke University Press, 1979.

Trout, E. Dale, D. E. Graves, and D. B. Slauson. High kilovoltage radiography. *Radiology* 52, 669–683, 1949.

Van der Plats, G. J. *Medical X-ray Techniques in Diagnostic Radiology*. 4th ed. The Hauge: Martinus Nijhoff, 1980.

31 VARIABLE KILOVOLTAGE SYSTEMS

Norlin T. Winkler

The [radiographer] who does his work by the "hunch method" can never successfully compete with one who having mastered the fundamentals is enabled to develop a proper procedure and put into the film any quality that may be desired.

Ed. C. Jerman, the Father of Radiography in the United States.

OUTLINE

PRINCIPLES OF A VARIABLE KILOVOLTAGE PEAK EXPOSURE SYSTEM
ESTABLISHING A VARIABLE KILOVOLTAGE PEAK EXPOSURE CHART

OBJECTIVES

Upon completion of this chapter, the student should be able to:

1. Describe a variable kilovoltage technique system.
2. Discuss the primary advantages and disadvantages of variable kVp technique systems.
3. State the 2 kVp rule.
4. Explain why more than a single kilovoltage scale is required.
5. Calculate new exposure factors from a single satisfactory exposure when mAs ratios are provided.
6. Synthesize a stepped variable kVp technique chart from control radiographs.

PRINCIPLES OF A VARIABLE KILOVOLTAGE PEAK EXPOSURE SYSTEM

A variable kilovoltage x-ray exposure technique system is one in which the kilovoltage to be used for a particular projection is varied depending on measured body part thickness. The thicker the body part, the higher the value of kilovoltage assigned. A milliampere-second value is specified for each body part to be

476

52 kVp 1200 mAs 42″ SID
16:1 grid 300 RS 1550 mR

A

Figure 31–1A. High contrast produced at low (52) kilovoltage.

115 kVp 10 mAs 42″ SID
16:1 grid 400 RS 106 mR

C

Figure 31–1C. Low contrast produced at high (115) kilovoltage.

70 kVp 160 mAs 42″ SID
16:1 grid 300 RS 580 mR

B

Figure 31–1B. Ideal contrast produced at appropriate (70) kilovoltage.

examined. Its value depends on image receptor speed and other parameters.

In use, the radiographer sets the mAs specified for the part and measured part thickness. The value of kVp corresponding to that thickness is found on the chart. For example, in Table 31–1, a 12 cm-thick part will require 54 kVp (i.e., an average shoulder).

Advantages and Disadvantages

Technique systems that use variable kilovoltage offer the advantage of permitting small incremental changes in exposure to compensate for variation in body part thickness. These changes in exposure may not be possible with systems that fix kilovoltage and vary milliampere-seconds because of an insufficient number of settings on the exposure timers of many x-ray generators.

A potential disadvantage of the variable kilovoltage technique arises when one consid-

TABLE 31–1					
2 kVp PER cm TABLE					
cm	10	11	12	13	14
kVp	50	52	54	56	58

ers the complexity of the effect of changing kilovoltage on the way the subject is imaged on the radiograph. Increasing kilovoltage reduces radiographic contrast. Reducing contrast may be helpful if the initial kilovoltage is too low to provide adequate penetration of the part (Figure 31–1A). A reduction in contrast that occurs when kilovoltage is too high can reduce the radiologist's ability to see fine detail in the image (Figure 31–1C). A useful variable kilovoltage system must use values of kilovoltage that provide adequate penetration of the part and result in a level of contrast that is acceptable to the radiologist (Figure 31–1B).

The radiation exposure to the patient is strongly dependent upon the kilovoltage used for the view. In general, the higher the kilovoltage, the lower the patient dose. When kilovoltage is at an appropriate level for the body part examined, patient dose considerations need not enter into the decision of whether to establish an exposure system using fixed or variable kVp.

Historical Development

In the early days of radiography it was common practice to use a change of 2 kVp for every one centimeter of tissue thickness. A kilovoltage progression could be readily computed by taking two times the centimeter measurement. To this value a constant, such as 30 kVp, was added to achieve a kVp value high enough to penetrate the part.

$$(2 \text{ kVp} \times \text{part cm}) + 30 \text{ kVp} = \text{new kVp}$$

Example: What is the proper kilovoltage for a 20 cm part thickness?

Answer:

$$(2 \text{ kVp} \times \text{part cm}) + 30 \text{ kVp} = \text{new kVp}$$
$$(2 \text{ kVp} \times 20 \text{ cm}) + 30 \text{ kVp} = \text{new kVp}$$
$$(40 \text{ kVp/cm}) + 30 \text{ kVp} = 70 \text{ kVp}$$

It was found that multiple kilovoltage scales were needed because the values selected from the progression could be too low to provide adequate penetration of body parts, such as the shoulder or cervical spine, which contain dense bone with little soft tissue (Table 31–2A). Higher kilovoltage scales were created by increasing the base kilovoltage added. For example, if kilovoltage were computed using 40 kVp instead of 30 kVp, the formula would be:

$$(2 \text{ kVp} \times \text{part cm}) + 40 \text{ kVp} = \text{new kVp}$$

Example: What is the proper kilovoltage for the same 20 cm part thickness, using the new formula?

Answer:

$$(2 \text{ kVp} \times \text{part cm}) + 40 \text{ kVp} = \text{new kVp}$$
$$(2 \text{ kVp} \times 20 \text{ cm}) + 40 \text{ kVp} = \text{new kVp}$$
$$(40 \text{ kVp/cm}) + 40 \text{ kVp} = 80 \text{ kVp}$$

All values would be correspondingly higher with the new formula. For example, the values of shoulder and cervical spine views measuring 12 cm would be 64 kVp instead of the 54 kVp previously obtained. By increasing or decreasing the value of kVp added as a constant, it is possible to create an array of kilovoltage scales. The scales shown in Tables 31–2A–C were computed using 30, 40 and 50 kVp as the constant:

$$(2 \text{ kVp} \times \text{part cm}) + 30 \text{ kVp} = \text{new kVp}$$
$$(2 \text{ kVp} \times \text{part cm}) + 40 \text{ kVp} = \text{new kVp}$$
$$(2 \text{ kVp} \times \text{part cm}) + 50 \text{ kVp} = \text{new kVp}$$

Note that the kilovoltage values for a 20 cm-thick body part are shown as 70 kVp, 80 kVp and 90 kVp, depending on the scale selected.

TABLE 31–2A		TABLE 31–2B	
KILOVOLTAGE SCALES		**KILOVOLTAGE SCALES**	
2 kVp/cm + 30		2 kVp/cm + 40	
cm	kVp	cm	kVp
2	34	2	44
3	36	3	46
4	38	4	48
5	40	5	50
6	42	6	52
7	44	7	54
8	46	8	56
9	48	9	58
10	50	10	60
11	52	11	62
12	54	12	64
13	56	13	66
14	58	14	68
15	60	15	70
16	62	16	72
17	64	17	74
18	66	18	76
19	68	19	78
20	70	20	80
21	72	21	82
22	74	22	84
23	76	23	86
24	78	24	88
25	80	25	90
26	82	26	92
27	84	27	94
28	86	28	96
29	88	29	98
30	90	30	100
31	92	31	102
32	94	32	104
33	96	33	106
34	98	34	108
35	100	35	110
36	102	36	112

TABLE 31–2C	

KILOVOLTAGE SCALES
2 kVp/cm + 50

cm	kVp
2	54
3	56
4	58
5	60
6	62
7	64
8	66
9	68
10	70
11	72
12	74
13	76
14	78
15	80
16	82
17	84
18	86
19	88
20	90
21	92
22	94
23	96
24	98
25	100
26	102
27	104
28	106
29	108
30	110
31	112
32	114
33	116
34	118
35	120
36	122

Changes of 10 kVp in the base number added were used in the belief that a change of ±10 kVp would compensate for doubling and halving mAs. In practice 30, 40 or 50 can be easily added to centimeters doubled by the radiographer mentally and the assigned value of kVp can thus be readily determined when charts are not available. Milliampere-second values were found by trial and error but, once determined, were listed for a particular body part and kilovoltage selected by measuring the part. A useful technique chart was thus created.

It was found in practice that 80 kVp for a 20 cm abdomen using equipment and image receptors of the time was nearly ideal. Fuchs suggested that kVp be fixed at 80 for the abdomen, with mAs varied to compensate for the size difference of patients. Fixed kilovoltage techniques, sometimes called optimum techniques, are described in Chapter 30. They are mentioned here to point out that similar results may be obtained regardless of the system employed in order to handle the variables of kVp, mA, and time.

Although the kilovoltage scales shown in Tables 31–2A, B, and C were useful in practical patient radiography, and in fact would still be useful, two assumptions used in their computation were found to be false. The notion that a ±10 kVp change will balance a change of double or half mAs has largely given way to the so-called 15 percent rule. This rule suggests decreasing kVp by 15 percent to reduce density by half and increasing kVp by 15 percent to double density. Although the 15 percent rule better reflects the exponentially nonlinear changes that occur when kilovoltage is altered, it is not totally accurate either. These relationships are among the most complex in radiography and remain difficult to quantify.

When the 15 percent rule is applied, it can be readily seen that a 7.5 kVp change is required at 50 kVp (15 percent × 50 kVp) to balance a 50 percent reduction in mAs, while at 100 kVp, a 15 kVp change (15 percent × 100 kVp) is required. This reflects the fact that at low kilovoltage a small change in kVp can have a large effect on film exposure, while at higher kilovoltage a larger change will be required to produce the same effect. A uniform change of 2 kVp per centimeter in tissue thickness will not function satisfactorily over a wide range of tissue thicknesses. At a fixed value of mAs and proper exposure of an average patient, radiographs of thicker patients will become increasingly underexposed as patient size increases.

Early users of variable kilovoltage techniques computed kVp scales using 2 kVp per centimeter plus a constant and ±10 kVp between the scales. They were able to use such charts successfully chiefly because the range of variation in adult body part thicknesses is small (see Table 29–1). Thus, kilovoltage values used for a particular body part are within a relatively narrow range. Since mAs values were found by trial and error using kilovoltage from the scales according to patient measurement, problems due to the use of ±10 kVp change between the scales were minimized, if not entirely eliminated. In addition, a patient whose body habitus varies from the norm is easily recognized by an experienced radiographer, and it was common practice then, as now, to increase or decrease the mAs according to the radiographer's professional judgment in compensation for body habitus and known pathological conditions.

The variable kilovoltage technique systems used today have evolved from the earlier systems. A modern version of a variable kilovoltage chart currently in use in the Mayo Clinic Department of Diagnostic Radiology is shown in Table 31–3. A precursor to this chart was originally established by Raymond Runge of Mayo Clinic about 1925. As was common practice, the first versions were constructed using kilovoltage corresponding to two times the centimeter measurement plus a constant. Runge recognized the deficiencies of this approach and made revisions in his later experiments by using a water phantom, which greatly improved the results. Modifications were made by Winkler to further refine the kilovoltage progressions and, most recently, by Stears and Frank with the introduction of rare-earth intensifying screens.

The Kilovoltage Scale

The kilovoltage versus measured centimeter thickness chart shown in Table 31–3 has the kilovoltage values arranged in seven columns plus one column corresponding to centimeter thickness of the part examined. For a given centimeter thickness there are up to seven kVp values that may be selected. For a 21 cm patient thickness these values are 52, 58, 63, 72, 80, 95 and 115 kVp. Note that the kilovoltage columns are labeled Scale 8, Scale 4, Scale 2, Scale 1, ½ Scale, ¼ Scale and ⅛ Scale. The kilovoltage change from one scale to the next at any given centimeter thickness is that amount that will be equal to reducing mAs by half or doubling it. For example, using kilovoltage values from Scale 1 as a base at the 21 cm level (72 kVp), a shift to ½ Scale (80 kVp) will permit reducing mAs by ½. A change from Scale 1 to ¼ Scale allows mAs to be reduced to ¼ the value for kVp Scale 1, while kVp from the ⅛ Scale would allow use of ⅛ the mAs. Use of the lower kVp values obtained from Scale 2, Scale 4 and Scale 8 would require the use of two times, four times or eight times the mAs used with the kVp from Scale 1.

Radiographs obtained are similarly exposed but, because of the extreme range of kilovoltage used (52–115), vary widely from too high to too low contrast (see Figures 31–1A-C). In practice, the column from which kilovoltage is selected is specified to produce a level of contrast preferred by radiologists. For a patient

TABLE 31–3

KILOVOLTAGE VS. MEASURED CENTIMETER THICKNESS CHART

SCALE 8	SCALE 4	SCALE 2	SCALE 1	CM	1/2 SCALE	1/4 SCALE	1/8 SCALE
		47	52	6	58	63	72
		48	53	7	59	64	73
		49	54	8	60	66	74
		50	55	9	61	68	76
	SCALE 4	51	56	10	62	70	78
	47	52	58	11	63	72	80
	48	53	59	12	64	73	82
	49	54	60	13	66	74	84
	50	55	61	14	68	76	87
SCALE 8	51	56	62	15	70	78	91
47	52	58	63	16	72	80	95
48	53	59	64	17	73	82	98
49	54	60	66	18	74	84	101
50	55	61	68	19	76	87	105
51	56	62	70	20	78	91	110
52	58	63	72	21	80	95	115
53	59	64	73	22	82	98	120
54	60	66	74	23	84	101	125
55	61	68	76	24	87	105	130
56	62	70	78	25	91	110	135
58	63	72	80	26	95	115	140
59	64	73	82	27	98	120	
60	66	74	84	28	101	125	
61	68	76	87	29	105		
62	70	78	91	30	110		
63	72	80	95	31	115		
64	73	82	98	32	120		
66	74	84	101	33	125		
68	76	87	105	34	130		
70	78	91	110	35	135		
72	80	95	115	36	140		
73	82	98	120	37			
74	84	101	125	38			
76	87	105	130	39			
78	91	110	135	40			
80	95	115	140	41			

EXTREMITY CASSETTE

CM	kVp
1	45
2	47
3	49
4	52
5	55
6	58
7	61
8	64
9	67
10	70

EXTREMITY — Non-Bucky	TIME	mA	kVp			TFD	CASSETTE
REGULAR CASSETTE						45″ (ALL)	
Ankle/Elbow	.016	200	1/4			48″	24 x 30 cm
Tibia-Fibula	.016	200	1/4			48″	14 x 17 in
Calcaneous	.016	200	1/2			48″	8 x 10 in
Wrist-Carpal Tunnel	.033	200	65 kVp			48″	8 x 10 in
Cast - Plaster	.033	200	1/4			48″	
Cast - Fiberglass	.016	200	1/4			48″	
EXTREMITY CASSETTE			SM	MED	LG		
Hand/Wrist PA/OBL	.025	200	58	60	62	48″	24 x 30 cm
Hand/Wrist LAT	.025	200	63	65	67	48″	8 x 10 in
Forearm	.025	200	Extremity Scale			48″	7 x 17 in
Toes	.025	200	58	60	62	48″	24 x 30 cm
Foot	.025	200	63	65	67	48″	24 x 30 cm
Lateral Calcaneous	.025	200	63	65	67	45″	8 x 10 in.

By permission of Mayo Foundation.

21 cm in thickness, the ½ Scale value, 80 kVp, is used if the generator is single phase. Lower kVp from Scale 1 (72 kVp) is chosen to maintain similar radiographic contrast if a three-phase generator is used. Arrangement of the kilovoltage columns such that the kVp changes by moving from any column to its neighbor permits halving or doubling mAs while allowing great flexibility in the use of the scales. This also permits selection of a kVp value to provide adequate penetration of any examined part, and thus produces optimum radiographic contrast.

The kilovoltage change necessary between the scales to balance doubling or halving mAs was initially derived from water phantom experiments. Kilovoltage progression (the increase in kilovoltage needed for each increase of one centimeter of tissue thickness) was obtained by using a doubling increase in kilovoltage for each 5 cm increase in part thickness. For example, in Table 31–3, the kVp value for a 21 cm measurement shown in ½ Scale (80 kVp) is listed in Scale 1 for a 26 cm measurement and the ½ Scale value for 26 cm (95 kVp) is listed in Scale 1 corresponding to 31 cm. All scales have been constructed using a double technique kVp value for each 5 centimeter change in thickness. Values for centimeters between the technique doubling points are chosen to provide a smooth progression but rounded off to the nearest whole kVp.

Determination of kilovoltage, though important, gives only one of the primary exposure factors. In a variable kVp technique system, kilovoltage selection is made by first measuring the examined part and then selecting a value from the kVp tables, as previously described. Values of distance, milliamperage and time must also be determined in any useful technique system.

Source-to-Image Receptor Distance

The inverse square relationship between SID (FFD) and radiation intensity at the film permits a small difference in SID to translate into a large difference in exposure of the radiograph. For this reason, the SID should be specified for each examination.

As a practical matter, and to avoid off focal distance grid cut-off of primary radiation, the focal distance of the x-ray table Bucky should be used. Because some table grids are difficult to examine without dismantling the x-ray table, it may be helpful to know that most equipment manufacturers provide 40″ focal distance grids for most x-ray tables. For this reason, a 40″ SID is often the best choice, unless the particular Bucky grid employed is known to have been manufactured for use at another focal range.

A useful SID selection for most routine radiography would be 40″ (100 cm) for flat Bucky work and extremities, with 72″ (180 cm) used for upright chest work. It is important that whatever SID is selected, the value be noted on the technique chart, and that all users of the chart recognize that an alteration in technique must be made if the specified SID is not used for a particular examination.

Milliampere-Seconds A useful technique system requires determination of the value of mAs that will provide proper exposure to the film when used in combination with the kilovoltage chosen. During phantom testing, milliamperage-seconds are increased or decreased in doubling or halving increments for sequential radiographs until proper exposure is achieved. The mAs value that has been determined is then recorded in terms of mAs or mA and time use on the technique chart. This method of determining mAs by trial and error was thoroughly described by Fuchs. Kratzer's Supertech™, Trinkle's Du Pont Bit System, the Siemens Point System, and Schwartz's XVS system are examples of other systems and devices that have been designed to assist in the process of x-ray technique development. Although the number of trial and error exposures that must be made can be dramatically reduced with the use of any of the systems mentioned above, the development of an effective x-ray technique system for an individual x-ray department can be successfully accomplished only by that department.

mAs Ratios

In the late 1980s Frank and Winkler presented a method of computing an x-ray exposure technique with the use of mAs ratios. The system of mAs ratios was devised by Winkler, who set up mathematical relationships from trial and error exposure determinations for various body parts that had been made by Runge. Reference to the kilovoltage scales in Table 31–3 is made to select values of kVp for use with mAs values for the examined part, which are computed using the mAs ratios after a base exposure is found. The advantage of the system lies in the radiographer's ability to compute mAs values for all body parts once the mAs value for only one body part has been found by trial and error. The need to examine large numbers of patients with multiple trials is eliminated. Minor changes in computed mAs values found for some views may be desirable following a period of use.

The resulting technique system of mAs ratios combined with kilovoltage varied with part thickness may be categorized as **variable kVp within an optimal range**. For example, the average thickness for an adult shoulder ranges from 12–16 cm. Kilovoltage for these extremes will be 64–72 kVp (from ½ Scale, shown in Table 31–3). Thus, the actual kilovoltage range typically used is narrow for any given body part. The best features of variable kVp techniques (small incremental changes) and fixed kVp techniques (optimal contrast) are obtained.

As previously described, the thickness of the examined part is measured where specified or along the path of the central ray. The value of the kVp corresponding to the thickness of the part is selected from the kVp chart. For example, for a shoulder measuring 14 cm, ½ Scale is specified with a three-phase generator and a value of 68 kVp is found, while the mAs is fixed.

The mAs ratios used in technique computation are shown in Table 31–4. Computed mAs values are used with kilovoltage corresponding to part thickness from the chart in Table 31–3. In this system, the AP projection of the lumbar spine is assigned a value of 1.0. Existing exposure techniques, which had been established by Runge using trial and error exposure for each body part, were used in computing the ratios by the following formula:

$$\frac{\text{mAs for body part}}{\text{mAs for AP lumbar}} = \text{mAs ratio for body part}$$

ESTABLISHING A VARIABLE KILOVOLTAGE PEAK EXPOSURE CHART

Initial Phantom Images

When a new technique chart is computed using the mAs ratios, mAs for the AP lumbar spine is first found by patient examination. In the process, the patient's thickness is measured, kVp is selected from the kilovoltage chart found in Table 31–3 and the required mAs is estimated based on previous experience. Only those patients referred for a lumbar spine examination should be involved in the process.

Select Optimal Phantom Image

If the resulting radiograph is too light or dark, a repeat radiograph with an appropriate mAs adjustment is made. This process is continued on subsequent patients until ideal diagnostic quality radiographs are obtained. The

TABLE 31–4 — mAs RATIOS FOR BODY PARTS

Examination	mAs Ratios	kVp 3–Phase	kVp 1–Phase
Skull AP & LAT Adult	.45	½ scale	¼ scale
Cervical AP	.60	½	¼
Lateral (Cross Table)	.15	½	¼
OBL (Tabletop)	.20	½	¼
Swimmers	.75	1	½
Odontoid (30″)	.25	½	¼
Pillar	1.00	¼	⅛
Thoracic AP (Filter)	1.50	1	½
(without Filter)	.75	1	½
Thoracic LAT (Filter)	3.04	2	1
(without Filter)	.50	2	1
Thoracic Lower LAT (No Filter)	.60	2	1
Lumbar AP and Abdomen (19–23 cm)	1.00	1	½
Lumbar OBL (19–23 cm)	1.50	1	½
Lumbar LAT	1.50	1	½
Lumbar LOC LAT	1.50	1	½
Lumbar Graft LAT (L5–S1)	3.04	2	1
Lumbar Flexion/Extension	3.04	2	1
Pelvis & Hip/OBL	1.50	1	½
Hips LAT	1.50	1	½
Sacrum AP	1.50	1	½
Coccyx AP	1.50	1	½
Sacrum, Coccyx LAT	3.00	2	1
S-I Joints	1.50	1	½
Shoulder AP	.30	½	¼
Y or Neer View	.30	½	¼
Transthoracic Lateral	.13	½	¼
Axillary (Grid)	.30	½	¼
Scapula AP & LAT OBL	.39	½	¼
Clavicle	.30	½	¼
Humerus	.30	½	¼
Femur	.60	½	¼
LAT & OBL for Vessels	.40	½	¼
Knee	.19	¼	⅛
Intercondylar Notch	.075	½	¼
Patella (Merchants)	.075	¼	⅛
Chest, AP Supine, All	.025	½	¼
Bucky Chest	.17	½	¼
Chest, Lateral Supine (Bucky)	.25	1	½
Chest, Lateral Decubitus (Grid)	.13	½	¼
Lateral Sternum	1.50	1	½
Ribs Above Diaphragm	.25	1	½
Ribs Below Diaphragm (19—23 cm)	1.00	1	½

TABLE 31–4 (continued)	EXTREMITIES[1]		
Examination	**mAs Ratios**	**kVp 3–Phase**	**kVp 1–Phase**
Regular cassette: Non-Bucky			
Ankle/Elbow	.075	½ scale	¼ scale
Tibia-Fibula	.075	½	¼
Calcaneus	.075	¼	⅛
Wrist-Carpal Tunnel	.075	65 kVp	73 kVp (no caliper)
Cast-Plaster	.15	½	¼
Cast-Fiberglass	.10	½	¼
Extremity cassette: Non-Bucky			
Hand/Wrist-PA/OBL	.25	58 60 62	
Hand/Wrist-LAT	.25	63 65 67	
Forearm	.25	EXT Scale (use caliper)	
Toes	.25	58 60 62	
Foot	.25	63 65 67	

—mAs ratios are based on: Lumbar AP, 21 cm technique and a film density of 1.4 (± 0.10) from the standard phantom.[2] Always use this *base technique* for the calculations.
—All values are for bucky/grid unless specified.
—All values are for adult techniques.
—All values are for 48″ unless specified.
—The following examinations each have three exposure time and kVp values. The mAs ratio is for the *middle measurement* (19–23 cm): Lumbar AP and Abdomen; Lumbar Oblique; Ribs below diaphragm.
[1] May vary depending upon tabletop attenuation and speed of system.
[2] Gray, Winkler, Stears, Frank. *Quality Control in Diagnostic Radiology*. Aspen Publishers Incorporated, Rockville, 1983. © 1988 Mayo Clinic Foundation, Rochester, MN. (By permission of Mayo Foundation.)

kVp should not be altered from the value shown for part thickness in Table 31–3.

The use of a patient equivalent phantom can reduce or eliminate the need for patient exposures. The American National Standards Institute (ANSI) patient equivalent phantom (PEP) is recommended for this purpose. Technical factors required to produce a film density of OD 1.4 with the PEP are suited for use on a 21 cm AP lumbar spine patient. Use the kVp for a 21 cm patient from the chart and find the mAs required by trial exposures.

Extrapolate Technique Chart

Once the mAs value that produces an optimal diagnostic quality image for the AP lumbar spine has been established, a complete technique chart is computed from that value as follows:

1. Values are substituted in the mAs ratio formula. For example, if 66 mAs was found to be a good value for the AP lumbar, it becomes the constant for all further calculations.

2. The mAs ratio for the body part is found in Table 31–4 and the formula is used to calculate the new mAs for the body part.

Example: The shoulder has an mAs ratio of 0.30. What is the appropriate mAs value that should be used for a system that produces a satisfactory AP lumbar at 66 mAs?

Answer:

$$\frac{\text{mAs for body part}}{\text{mAs for AP lumbar}} = \text{mAs ratio for body part}$$

$$\frac{\text{mAs for body part}}{66 \text{ mAs}} = 0.30$$

$$\text{mAs for body part} = 66 \text{ mAs} \times 0.30$$

$$\text{mAs for body part} = 19.8 \approx 20 \text{ mAs}$$

The kilovoltage is selected from ½ Scale (Table 31–3), which yields 64 kVp for a shoulder measuring 12 centimeters. Technical factors for the shoulder are 20 mAs, 64 kVp. An appropriate mA and time selection for 20 mAs might be 200 mA at 0.10 second.

Computed techniques should be entered in a technique chart that is prominently posted in the x-ray control booth for ready reference by the radiographers (Table 31–5).

It is usually most advantageous to list values of mA and time rather than mAs unless only mAs is shown on the control. This approach frees the radiographer from being required to calculate appropriate mA and time values and reduces the likelihood of errors that could cause repeats. Additionally, the use of a single mA setting eliminates the potential for exposure problems caused by variations in x-ray output that may exist between the mA stations available on a generator, and calculations of technical factors are simplified.

Example:

Assume that 66 mAs was found to be appropriate for the AP lumbar spine and the 200 mA station at 0.33 seconds was used. If the 200 mA station is chosen as a constant, only the exposure time for the AP lumbar needs to be used with the mAs ratio to compute the exposure time for other body parts. What exposure time should be used for a pelvis, when the pelvis ratio is 1.5?

Answer:

$$\frac{\text{mAs for body part}}{\text{mAs for AP lumbar}} = \text{mAs ratio for body part}$$

When the mA station is a constant, only the exposure time needs to be calculated:

$$\frac{\text{sec for body part}}{0.33 \text{ sec}} = 1.5$$

$$\text{sec for body part} = 0.33 \text{ sec} \times 1.5$$

$$\text{sec for body part} = 0.495 \approx 0.5 \text{ sec}$$

In this example, the technique for the pelvis is found to be 0.5 second at 200 mA, with the kVp measured from kVp Scale 1. Time values for other body parts are computed in the same way and entered in the technique chart. When an exact match between the time value computed cannot be made because of the limited number of time selections available on the x-ray control, the next greater time value should be used.

mA Station Selection The speed of image receptors currently used, in combination with thermal load capacities of x-ray tubes usually supplied with x-ray equipment, will generally allow the use of the small focal spot at 100 mA single phase and 200 mA three phase for nearly all common procedures. However, reference must be made to the single exposure rating chart for the tube to assure that exposures computed are indeed within the capacity of the small focal spot. For example, the 1ϕ tube rating chart that was previously shown in Figure 7–23 would permit a maximum of 0.2 second at 200 mA and 80 kVp. Thus the exposure computed for the pelvis in the preceding example (0.5 sec, 200 mA and kVp as measured) would not be allowed with a single-phase generator and this x-ray tube on the small focal spot. Use of the large focal spot would be necessary. However, for a 150 mA small focal spot, a maximum exposure of 4 sec at 80 kVp is per-

TABLE 31–5

VARIABLE KILOVOLTAGE TECHNIQUE CHART

EXAMINATION	TIME	mA	kVp	mAs	TFD	CASSETTE
SKULL						45″(ALL)
SKULL, AP, LAT Adult	.20	200	1/4	40	48″	24 x 30 cm
CERVICAL SPINE						
Cervical AP 10° ↑	.15	200	1/4	30	48″	8 x 10 in
Lateral (Cross Table) (NON-GRID)	.05	200	1/4	10.2	48″	24 x 30 cm
OBL (Table Top)	.066	200	1/4	13.2	48″	24 x 30 cm
Swimmer's	.40	200	1/2	80	48″	24 x 30 cm
Odontoid	.20	200	1/4	40	30″	8 x 10 in
Piller 30° ↓	.30	200	1/8	60	48″	24 x 30 cm
THORACIC SPINE						
Thoracic AP (Filter)	.40	200	1/2	80	48″	35 x 43 cm
Thoracic LAT (Filter)	.60	↓	1	120	48″	35 x 43 cm
THIN 100 mA AVERAGE 150 mA PORTLY 200 mA						
Thoracic Lower LAT (No Filter)	.30	200	1	60	48″	24 x 30 cm
LUMBAR SPINE/ABDOMEN						
Lumbar AP 5° ↑ and Abdomen						
– 18 cm	.15	200	1/4	30	48″	35 x 43 cm
19 - 23 cm	.30	200	1/2	60	48″	35 x 43 cm
24 cm -	.60	200	1	120	48″	35 x 43 cm
Lumbar OBL 42° 5° ↑						
– 18 cm	.10	200	1/8	20	48″	24 x 30 cm
19 - 23 cm	.20	200	1/4	40	48″	24 x 30 cm
24 cm -	.50	200	1/2	100	48″	24 x 30 cm
Lumbar LAT Meas L-2	.40	200	1/2	80	48″	30 x 35 cm
Lumbar Loc LAT Meas L-5	.40	200	1/2	80	48″	8 x 10 in
Lumbar Graft LAT	.40	200	1/2	80	48″	24 x 30 cm
Lumbar Flexion & Extension	.40	200	1/2	80	48″	30 x 35 cm

Technique charts of the type used at the Mayo Clinic, Rochester, Minnesota. Computed for a single-phase generator using mAs ratios in Table 31–4. By permission of Mayo Foundation, Rochester, MN.

TABLE 31–5 *(continued)*

EXAMINATION	TIME	mA	kVp	mAs	TFD	CASSETTE
PELVIC REGION						
Pelvis & Hips AP / OBL 5° ↓	.40	200	1/2	80	48"	35 x 43 cm
Hips LAT	.80	200	1/2	160	48"	24 x 30 cm
Sacrum AP 5° ↑	.40	200	1/2	80	48"	24 x 30 cm
Coccyx AP 10° ↓	.40	200	1/2	80	48"	24 x 30 cm
Sacrum, Coccyx LAT	.80	200	1	160	48"	24 x 30 cm
S-I Joints (R & LPO 20°)	.40	200	1/2	80	48"	24 x 30 cm
SHOULDER						
Shoulder AP	.10	200	1/4	20	48"	24 x 30 cm
Neer View	.10	200	1/4	20	48"	24 x 30 cm
Transthoracic Lateral	.10	200	1/2	20	48"	35 x 43 cm
Axillary (Grid)	.10	200	1/4	20	48"	24 x 30 cm
Scapula AP & LAT OBL	.10	200	1/4	20	48"	24 x 30 cm
Clavical	.10	200	1/4	20	48"	24 x 30 cm
Humerus	.10	200	1/4	20	48"	35 x 43 cm
Westpoint View (non-grid)	.033	200	1/4	6.6		
FEMUR, KNEE						
Femur	.10	200	1/4	20	48"	35 x 43 cm
LAT & OBL for Vessels	.10	200	1/4	20	48"	35 x 43 cm
Knee	.05	200	1/8	10	48"	24 x 30 cm
Intercondylar Notch	.025	200	1/4	5	48"	Non-Bucky
Patella (Merchants)	.033	200	1/8	6.6	48"	Non-Bucky
Ingrowth Knee	.066	200	1/8	13.2	45"	35 x 43 cm
CHEST						
AP Supine, All (non-grid)	.10	200	1/4	20	48"	Non-Bucky
Bucky Chest	.05	200	1/4	10	45"	
Lateral Supine (Bucky)	.066	200	1/2	13.2	48"	35 x 43 cm
Lateral Decubitus (Grid)	.05	200	1/4	10	48"	35 x 43 cm
Lateral Sternum	.40	200	1/2	80	48"	30 x 35 cm
RAO AP-Sternum	.20	200	1	40	45"	24 x 30 cm
RIBS						
Ribs Above Diaphragm	.10	↓	1/2	varies	48"	24 x 30 cm

THIN   AVERAGE   PORTLY
150 mA   200 mA   300 mA

EXAMINATION	TIME	mA	kVp	mAs	TFD	CASSETTE
Ribs Below Diaphragm						
- 18 cm	.15	200	1/4	30	48"	24 x 30 cm
19 - 23 cm	.30	200	1/2	60	48"	24 x 30 cm
24 cm -	.60	200	1	120	48"	24 x 30 cm

mitted. Thus the 150 mA station could be used at the small focal spot. It is important to check the tube's single exposure rating chart and to be certain that the correct chart for the focal spot size, generator type, and rotor speed is used as the tube's ratings are strongly dependent on these factors.

Measurement of Part Thickness

Effective use of a variable kVp technique chart requires precise measurement of part thickness. This is accomplished with a measuring caliper. As a rule, measurement of part thickness along the path of the central x-ray beam is used. For accuracy in measurement, the measuring caliper should be angled if the x-ray beam is angled. However, if the technique chart was constructed by someone using different measuring standards, the same rules used for the chart must be followed by everyone who uses it.

There are two exceptions to this general rule of measuring along the path of the central x-ray beam when the mAs ratio system in Table 31–4 is used. These are the AP projection of the lumbar spine and/or abdomen and the lateral lumbar spine. The AP lumbar or abdomen should be measured just below the tip of the sternum. The lateral lumbar spine should be measured at L2.

Special Considerations

The range of part thickness found in patients is relatively narrow for most body parts, such as the skull, knee or shoulder (see Table 29–1). For this reason, the use of a single kVp progression can be specified for these examinations without the kVp becoming so low on the thinner patients as to result in underpenetration and such high contrast or so high on the thicker patients as to produce radiographs with insufficient contrast. However, in abdominal examinations patient thickness in the AP dimension varies over an extremely wide range. Though most patients

will fall into the range of 19–23 cm, patients who measure as little as 17 cm or as much as 34 cm will frequently be found. Although the kilovoltage range used with a 1ϕ generator for most patients (19–23 cm) will be relatively narrow, 76 to 84 kVp (Table 31–3, ½ Scale), extended use of the same variable kVp scale for the 17 cm thick patient would show 73 kVp and for the 34 cm patient 130 kVp. Body part penetration and the resultant radiographic contrast are strongly influenced by kVp level. Should these values be used, it will quickly be noted that 73 kVp is too low and 130 kVp too high for the best results. To avoid this problem in practice, the mAs should be reduced to half and the kVp value increased for the small patients. The mAs should be doubled and the kVp value decreased for the larger patients, resulting in the following modification to the AP lumbar technique chart:

Part thickness	Chart scale to be used with 1ϕ generator	Chart scale to be used with 3ϕ generator
18 cm and below	¼ Scale	½ Scale
19–23 cm	½ Scale	Scale 1
24 cm and above	Scale 1	Scale 2

In practice, this maintains kVp within the range of 76–84 kVp for a 1ϕ unit, and image contrast problems attendant with the use of too low or too high kVp are avoided.

Phantom Testing

Phantom testing is recommended prior to performing patient examinations. As a minimum, phantom testing should be done for a median, small and large part size as a fine tuning mechanism for the extrapolated chart prior to clinical use.

Clinical Trials

Limited clinical trials are permissible with the new chart. All images should be recorded, with repeated images saved for analysis. When clinical trials are proceeding without excess repeated exposures, the new technique chart can move into the clinical fine tuning stage.

Clinical Fine Tuning

The clinical fine tuning process will adjust and finally validate the entire chart. At this point the new technique chart can be adopted. However, ongoing fine tuning then begins as a permanent process.

Ongoing Fine Tuning

Ongoing fine tuning is the process that maintains the accuracy of the entire exposure system and gives radiographers and radiologists confidence in the exposure and diagnostic processes.

SUMMARY

A variable kilovoltage x-ray exposure technique system is one in which the kilovoltage to be used for a particular projection is varied depending on measured body part thickness. A milliampere-second value is specified for each body part to be examined.

Technique systems that use variable kilovoltage offer the advantage of permitting small incremental changes in exposure to compensate for variation in body part thickness. A potential disadvantage of the variable kilovoltage technique arises when one considers that the effect of changing kilovoltage on the way the subject is imaged on the radiograph is complex. Increasing kilovoltage reduces radiographic contrast. Reducing contrast may be helpful if the initial kilovoltage is too low to provide adequate penetration of the part. A reduction in contrast that occurs when kilovolt-

age is too high can reduce the radiologist's ability to see fine detail in the image. A useful variable kilovoltage system must use values of kilovoltage that provide adequate penetration of the part and result in a level of contrast that is acceptable to the radiologist.

Initially, variable kVp systems were established using a 2 kVp change for each centimeter of tissue thickness. A constant was added to this value, such as 30, 40 or 50 kVp, to get the kVp level up to a value that would provide adequate penetration. Application of the 15 percent rule shows that a uniform increase of 2 kVp for each centimeter change will not work satisfactorily over a wide range of tissue thicknesses.

Based on a number of years of field testing, a variable kVp system was established which reflects the need to adjust the kVp level based on the examination being performed. Seven scales were developed with the kVp change from one scale to the next at any given centimeter of thickness being the amount that will balance cutting the mAs in half or doubling it. Once the selected kVp scale is determined, the mAs values are computed using mAs ratios after a base exposure is found. The AP lumbar projection is used for the base exposure. This eliminates the need for multiple trial and error exposures.

The effective use of a variable kVp system requires precise measurement with the use of calipers.

REVIEW QUESTIONS

1. Which exposure factor(s) become constant(s) in a variable kilovoltage technique system?

2. What are the primary advantages and disadvantages of variable kVp technique systems?

3. What is the 2 kVp rule?

4. Why is more than a single kilovoltage scale required?

5. What is the formula that is used to calculate new exposure factors from a single satisfactory exposure when mAs ratios are provided?

REFERENCES AND RECOMMENDED READING

Cahoon, John B. *Formulating X-Ray Techniques.* 8th ed. Durham, NC: Duke University Press, 1974.

Cahoon, John B. Radiographic technique: Its origin, concept, practical application and evaluation of radiation dosage. *The X-Ray Technician* 32, 354–364, 1961.

Eastman, T. R. Technique charts: The key to radiographic quality. *Radiologic Technology* 46, 365–368, 1975.

Eastman, T. R. Measurement: The key to exposure with manual techniques. *Radiologic Technology* 45, 75–78, 1973.

Eastman, T. R. Chest technique through body habitus. *Radiologic Technology* 41, 80–84, 1969.

Files, Glenn W. *Medical Radiographic Technique.* Springfield, IL: Charles C. Thomas Publisher, 1952.

Frank, Eugene D., Winkler, Norlin T. Preparing an accurate x-ray exposure technique chart. Lecture, American Society of Radiologic Technologists 60th Annual Meeting. Albuquerque, NM. June 1988.

Fuchs, Arthur W. *Principles of Radiographic Exposure and Processing.* 2nd ed. Springfield, IL: Charles C. Thomas Publisher, 1958.

Fuchs, Arthur W. The rationale of radiographic exposure. *The X-Ray Technician* 22, 62–68, 76, 1950.

Fuchs, Arthur W. Control of radiographic density. *The X-Ray Technician* 20, 271–273, 291, 1949.

Fuchs, Arthur W. Relationship of tissue thickness to kilovoltage. *The X-Ray Technician* 19, 287–293, 1948.

Funke, T. Pegged kilovoltage technic. *Radiologic Technology* 37:4, 202–213, 1966.

General Electric Company Medical Systems Department. *How to Prepare an X-Ray Technic Chart.* Milwaukee, WI: Publication 4301A.

Gray, Joel E., Winkler, Norlin T., Stears, John G., Frank, Eugene D. *Quality Control in Diagnostic Imaging.* Aspen Systems Corp., 1983.

Hiss, Stephen S. *Understanding Radiography.* Springfield, IL: Charles C. Thomas Publisher, 1978.

Jenkins, David. *Radiographic Photography and Imaging Processes.* Lancaster, England: MTP Press Ltd., 1980.

Jerman, Ed. C. *Modern X-Ray Technic.* St. Paul, MN: Bruce Publishing Co., 1928.

Jerman, E. C. Extremity technic. *Radiology* 6, 252–254, 1926.

Koenig, George F. Kilovoltage as a qualitative factor. *The X-Ray Technician* 29, 1–4, 13, 1957.

McDaniel, Clarence. Tissue absorption theory applied to formulation of radiographic technique resulting in time as the variable factor. *Radiologic Technology* 37:2, 51, 1965.

Morgan, James A. *The Art and Science of Medical Radiography.* 5th ed. St. Louis, MO: Catholic Hospital Association, 1977.

Morgan, R. H. An analysis of the physical factors controlling the diagnostic quality of roentgen images. *American Journal of Roentgenography and Radium Therapy* 54, 128; 54, 395; 55, 67; 55, 627.

Runge, Raymond K. Technical Assistant, Department of Diagnostic Radiology, Mayo Clinic, Rochester, MN (personal communications).

Sante, L. R. *Manual of Roentgenological Technique.* 9th ed. Ann Arbor, MI: Edwards Brothers, Inc., 1942.

Schwarz, Gerhart S. Kilovoltage conversion in radiography. *The X-Ray Technician* 31, 373–379, 436, 1960.

United States War Department. *Technical Manual: Roentgenographic Technicians.* TM 8–240, July 3, 1941.

THE CASE OF THE ANIMAL WITH THE LARGE CALCIFIED TUMOR-LIKE MASS

What is the huge mass in the lower abdomen of this animal?

(Reprinted by permission of the International Society of Radiographers and Radiological Technicians from the K. C. Clark Archives, Middlesex Hospital, London, England)

Answers to the case studies can be found in Appendix E.

32 OTHER EXPOSURE SYSTEMS

Pride in one's profession is demanded . . . a vital feeling of belonging to a favored profession, which gives many rights but also requires many duties. All our ambitions should be directed toward a faithful fulfillment of duties toward others as well as toward ourselves. . . .

W. C. Röntgen, upon assuming the position of Rector of the University of Wurzburg.

OUTLINE

XVS UNIT STEP SYSTEM
DU PONT BIT SYSTEM
SIEMENS POINT SYSTEM
SUPERTECH™ CALCULATOR
PROPORTIONAL ANATOMY SYSTEMS

OBJECTIVES

Upon completion of this chapter, the student should be able to:

1. Describe the concept of a log-based point system for technique chart conversion and development.
2. Discuss the value of exposure systems other than fixed or variable kVp when developing technique charts.
3. Validate a fixed or variable kVp system by using another exposure system.
4. Explain the concept of proportional anatomy exposure systems, including extrapolation of a technique chart from control images via constants or ratios.

Although fixed and variable kVp exposure systems are the most popular systems in use, there are situations where other exposure systems are easier to use or more accurate. Each of the following exposure systems has advantages and disadvantages. Students can test their

knowledge of the principles of radiographic exposure and increase their understanding of the relationships between technical factors by careful study of each of these systems.

Each system was developed by a radiographer, except for the XVS unit step system, step system, which was developed by a radiologist. Except for the proportional anatomy systems, they are all based on logarithmic scales. Each was subjected to extensive study and experimentation and was designed to provide consistency in image quality while quantifying variables into a useful format. These systems have either had a major effect on thinking about radiographic technique or have proven to be accurate in clinical situations and are still in use.

XVS UNIT STEP SYSTEM

Considerable attention was given to the quantification of radiographic exposure factors during the 1950s. Many authors, notably Reed (in 1939) and Williams (in 1956, 1958 and 1960) attempted to prove a radiographic effect (RE) formula as a corollary to the photographic effect (PE) formula that had gained acceptance for measuring photographic image density. The problems these researchers encountered stemmed from their failure to recognize the full effect of subject density and contrast, primarily through part thickness, on the production of scatter radiation. In 1959, Gerhart Schwarz published a study of these effects and from this work continued his research to develop the X-Ray Value Scale (XVS) system, which was published as a book entitled *Unit-Step Radiography* in 1960.

The XVS system was patterned after the photographic Exposure Value Scale (EVS) system but with the addition of Schwarz's research into the effect of subject thickness on kVp's effect on image density. The system was not strictly log-based, although the basis of this type of system was present. The XVS system was the first to quantify the primary radiographic variables. It permitted variance of kVp, mA, time and filtration, as the Bit System would later, but did not address other variables.

The system functioned by using a caliper to measure subject part thickness in XVS num-

bers instead of centimeters. Any total of XVS numbers that equaled the caliper measurement could be obtained from special markings on the x-ray machine's mA, time and kVp indicators. Schwarz proposed mechanical systems that would automatically set the x-ray control after measuring patient thickness with photocells. One major manufacturer even built a control console that gave XVS numbers instead of radiographic exposure factors. In later years this concept was adopted in a revised form and marketed by another major manufacturer. Of course, radiographers are crippled by these types of systems because they effectively blindfold the operator by requiring him or her to guess at technical factors. One of the greatest triumphs of the professionalism of radiographers occurred when this type of equipment labeling was rejected by purchasers because it limited the skills of the operators.

An interesting note in Schwarz's book is that he had to impose rigid requirements on radiographers during the original clinical trials of the XVS system because it became an easy game to discover which XVS numbers were hiding which exposure factors on the control consoles. The radiographers then proceeded to improve image quality by ignoring the XVS units when necessary. Schwarz conceded that the radiographer must retain the right to exercise his or her professional judgment by deviating from average values.

Although Schwarz proposed several modifications of the system, the lack of standardization of all but a single factor, plus the ignorance of the many other variables, resulted in the eventual demise of the system. However, the theory of the interrelationships between the variables is a basic concept in understanding radiographic exposure factors and remains worthy of study.

Equipment with variations of unit step labeling is available for use in regions of the world where it is not possible to adequately train x-ray operators. For a time, the benefit of providing basic radiographic services far outweighs the risk of inadequate training. The Basic Radiological System (BRS), which operates on this principle, is supported by the International Society of Radiographers and Radiological Technicians (ISRRT) and the World Health Organization (WHO).

DU PONT BIT SYSTEM

The Du Pont Bit System was developed by Robert J. Trinkle of E.I. Du Pont de Nemours and Company, Inc., in 1957. The system is similar to the Polaroid light value exposure (LVS) system, the XVS unit step system of Schwarz described above, and the Siemens Point System described below. Trinkle used a computer to analyze vast quantities of exposure system data, and named the system after the computer processing bit to emphasize the use of computerized data. The Du Pont company publishes a pocket guide to the system and routinely revises it. The system uses log-base$_2$ points to quantify variables with the objective of maintaining image density within acceptance limits. Each point, or bit, either doubles or halves the density.

The Bit System is designed as a technique conversion system, although an experienced radiographer can make valid extrapolations using guide totals for the major subject density and contrast regions of the body. The 9th edition of the Bit System, with step-by-step instructions on its use, is provided in Appendix C.

The system is used as the basis for the computerized Du Pont technique charts that are available to customers. As with any other system, following the steps to establish a technique chart will produce a functional system. Each projection must be rated for an established number of bits. Any balanced combination of variables that equal the established bits

will produce a diagnostic quality image. The key is to maintain a balanced combination of variables. Conversion of a technique by more than a full bit (doubling or halving) is not recommended. The Bit System also permits calculation of approximate skin dose by applying distance, mAs and converted kVp bits to a dose table.

SIEMENS POINT SYSTEM

The Siemens Point System, developed in 1950 by the Siemens Corporation, was based on work by F. Claassen. Siemens publishes and revises the system, which is more commonly used in Europe than elsewhere. The system uses log-base$_{10}$ points to quantify variables, with the objective of maintaining image density within acceptance limits. The system requires three points to double or halve the density.

The Siemens Point System is designed to serve as a complete technique chart system. It must be calibrated by determining an initial exposure value point for each anatomical area. If the suggested initial exposure values do not produce an optimal image, correcting points must be established for all subsequent exposures. The chart provided by Siemens is usually modified by the correcting points to establish normal exposure value points. The normal exposure value points provide an accurate exposure system. Each anatomical area is listed on the chart as an average part thickness. Compensation for part size variations is one point per centimeter except for chest radiography, where the compensation is one point per 1.5 cm. The ancillary charts must be consulted to estimate appropriate technical factor changes when correction points must be added or subtracted. The system can be easily used for technique conversions in the same manner as the Du Pont Bit System. A current version of the system is provided in Appendix D.

SUPERTECH™ CALCULATOR

Brice Kratzer published an article in 1973 reporting on research experience with a log-based slide rule technique calculator. It was later developed, patented, trademarked and marketed as the Supertech™ Calculator by Supertech, Inc. Slide rule-style calculators, both circular and linear, had been developed by Reed in 1939 and 1949 and Williams had developed a circular calculator technique system in 1960. These calculators were limited to the relationship between 1–2 factors, for example the relationship between kVp and mAs. Two commercial film companies in the United States published and distributed the calculators for many years. The Supertech™ Calculator is the only one that has survived to the present and is revised regularly.

Supertech™ includes elements of quality control testing, positioning guidelines, principles of exposure and anatomy review, and can serve as an angulator. It is sold as a kit with an acrylic penetrometer and calibration master film for elementary quality control testing of machine output (Figure 32–1). After a short testing procedure, each machine can be assigned a correction factor that takes into account over a dozen different variables. Supertech™ remains

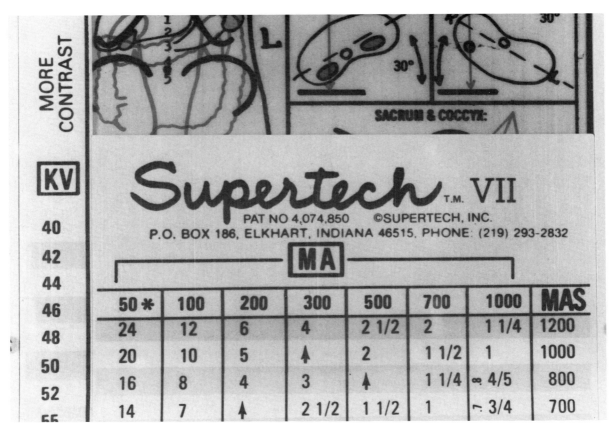

Figure 32–1.   The Supertech™ Calculator. (Courtesy of Supertech, Inc.)

a viable technique system and has found acceptance in low volume clinical sites, and in situations where radiography is an ancillary service, such as physicians' offices, chiropractics and podiatry.

PROPORTIONAL ANATOMY SYSTEMS

Proportional Anatomy Systems are based on the concept that the body can be classified into regions of similar subject densities and contrasts and that these similarities can be correlated to exposure factors.

Terry Eastman reported on a body habitus technique system for chest radiography in 1969. The system was based on observations that chest density and contrast were closely related to various body habitus factors, especially height and weight. Eastman collected data on adult averages and then codified an effective technique chart that correlated exposure factors with the patient's height and weight. Although limited to chest radiography, the system remains in use in some institutions where a high volume of essentially normal chest radiography is performed.

To date, two true Proportional Anatomy Systems have been presented, one by Quinn Carroll in 1985 and the other by Norlin T. Winkler and Eugene Frank in 1987. Carroll's system is presented in his revision of *Fuchs's Principles of Radiographic Exposure, Processing and Quality Control*. Winkler and Frank have presented their data at the annual meetings of the American Society of Radiologic Technologists. Their data are the cumulation of research begun by Raymond Runge and encompass experiences at the Mayo Clinic in Rochester, Minnesota, since 1925. Both of these systems classify body parts, habitus and projections into groups of similar subject density and contrast. Carroll uses conversion factors while Winkler and

Frank use mAs ratios to extrapolate a technique chart for the entire body from a control exposure. Winkler presents the Mayo Clinic system as the current state of the art for variable kVp systems (see Table 31–4).

SUMMARY

Although fixed and variable kVp systems are the most popular systems in use, there are situations where other systems are easier to use or more accurate. These other systems include the XVS Unit Step System, the Du Pont Bit System, the Siemens Point System, the Supertech™ Calculator and Proportional Anatomy Systems.

The XVS system was patterned after the photographic Exposure Value Scale (EVS) system but with the addition of Schwarz's research into the effect of subject thickness on kVp's effect on image density. The XVS system was the first to quantify the primary radiographic variables. The system functioned by using a caliper to measure subject part thickness in XVS numbers instead of centimeters. Any total of XVS numbers that equaled the caliper measurement could be obtained from special markings on the x-ray machine's mA, time and kVp indicators.

The Du Pont Bit System was developed using a computer to analyze vast quantities of exposure system data, and it was named after the computer processing bit to emphasize the use of computerized data. The system uses log-base$_2$ points to quantify variables with the objective of maintaining image density within acceptance limits. Each point, or bit, either doubles or halves the density. Each projection is rated for an established number of bits. Any balanced combination of variables that equal the established bits will produce a diagnostic quality image.

The Siemens Point System uses log-base$_{10}$ points to quantify variables with the objective of maintaining image density within acceptance limits. The system requires three points to double or halve the density. Each anatomical area is listed with an average part thickness. Compensation for part size variations is one point per centimeter except for chest radiography, where the compensation is one point per 1.5 cm.

The Supertech™ Calculator is a log-based slide rule technique system. After a short testing period, each machine can be assigned a correction factor that takes into account over a dozen different variables.

Proportional Anatomy Systems are based on the concept that the body can be classified into regions of similar subject densities and contrasts and that these similarities can be correlated to exposure factors. Two true Proportional Anatomy Systems (Carroll and Frank/Winkler) classify body parts, habitus and projections into groups of similar subject density and contrast. Carroll uses conversion factors while Winkler and Frank use mAs ratios to extrapolate a technique chart for the entire body from a control exposure.

REVIEW QUESTIONS

1. What do all of the various exposure systems have in common?

2. What four primary radiographic variables were quantified in the XVS System?

3. Why was the Du Pont Bit System so named?

4. What is the relationship between a bit and radiographic density?

5. What is the Supertech™ Calculator?

6. On what concept are Proportional Anatomy Systems based?

REFERENCES AND RECOMMENDED READING

Cahoon, John B. *Formulating X-Ray Techniques.* 8th ed. Durham, NC: Duke University Press, 1974.

Compton, Stephen C. Bit conversion of technical factors in vascular procedures. *Radiologic Technology* 58:5, 413–416, 1987.

Cullinan, Angeline M. *Producing Quality Radiographs.* Philadelphia, PA: Lippincott, 1987.

Du Pont Company Photosystems & Electronic Products Department. *Bit System of Technique Conversion.* 8th ed. Wilmington, DE.

Eastman, T. R. Chest technique through body habitus. *Radiologic Technology* 41, 80–84, 1969.

Funke, T. Pegged kilovoltage technic. *Radiologic Technology* 37, 202–213, 1966.

General Electric Company Medical Systems Department. *How to Prepare an X-Ray Technic Chart.* Milwaukee, WI: Publication 4301A.

Kratzer, Brice. A technique computer: Scientific approach to radiologic technology. *Radiologic Technology* 42, 142–150, 1973.

Palmer, P. E. S. The World Health Organization—basic radiological system. *Radiography* 51:597, 169–178, 1985.

Picot, Joselyne. A computerized system for calculating technique guides. Unpublished paper presented at the International Society of Radiographers and Radiological Technicians 6th World Congress, Rio de Janeiro, Brazil, October, 1977.

Schwarz, Gerhart S. *Unit-Step Radiography.* Springfield, IL: Charles C. Thomas Publisher, 1961.

Schwarz, Gerhart S. Kilovoltage conversion in radiography. *The X-Ray Technician* 31, 373–379, 436, 1960.

Schwarz, Gerhart S. Kilovoltage and radiographic effect. *Radiology* 73, 749–760, 1959.

Schwarz, Gerhart S. A simple universal unit system of radiographic exposures suited to departmental, national, and international standardization. *Radiology* 71, 573–574, 1958.

Schwarz, Gerhart S. Extended range radiography. *Radiology* 69, 419–423, 1957.

Stopford, James E. Log$_{10}$ technique charts. *Radiologic Technology* 51:3, 331–333, 1979.

Thompson, Thomas T. *Cahoon's Formulating X-Ray Techniques.* 9th ed. Durham, NC: Duke University Press, 1979.

Trinkle, Robert J. The bit system of technic conversion. Unpublished paper presented at American Society of Radiologic Technologists annual meeting, Boston, June 1966.

World Health Organization. *Manual of Radiographic Technique.* Geneva: World Health Organization Publications, 1985.

THE CASE OF THE LAST DINNER

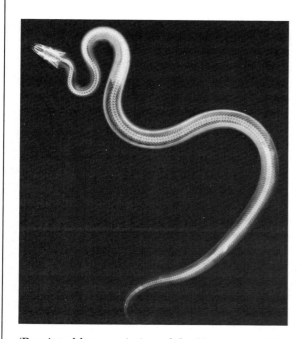

Of course this is a snake, but can you tell if its last dinner is still intact within the GI tract?

(Reprinted by permission of the International Society of Radiographers and Radiological Technicians from the K. C. Clark Archives, Middlesex Hospital, London, England)

Answers to the case studies can be found in Appendix E.

33 THE ART OF PHOTOTIMING

The art of phototiming is the art of positioning.

OUTLINE

IONIZATION CHAMBERS
POSITIONING SKILLS

OBJECTIVES

Upon completion of this chapter, the student should be able to:

1. Explain why the art of phototiming is the art of positioning.
2. Accurately identify configuration size, shape and position for various brands of ionization chambers.
3. Describe how to modify image density, contrast and time when using an automatic exposure control.
4. Describe various common subject density and subject contrast problems when phototiming.
5. Explain the effect of collimation on phototimed image quality.
6. Provide solutions to minimum response time and back-up time problems.
7. Explain how to modify the suggested technical factors on an anatomically programmed control unit.
8. Discuss the advisability of creative phototiming.

The operation of both phototiming and ionization chamber automatic exposure controls (AECs) were discussed in Chapter 6, X-Ray Equipment. It is important to remember that although phototiming is the common term used in clinical practice, the generic terms automatic exposure control (AEC) and automatic exposure device (AED) refer to both antique photo-timing devices and the ionization chambers currently in use. Although commonly referred to as phototiming, the term actually refers to the use of ionization chambers. In nearly all instances the principles are applicable to phototimers as well as ionization chambers.

AECs have been popular since their introduction by Russell H. Morgan in 1942. He designed the first phototimer for use with mass chest screening photofluorographic units. It was designed to react to the dominant area of the radiograph that is proportional to the general appearance of the entire image.

The ionization chamber is designed for a single purpose, best illustrated by the proper term for the device—**automatic exposure control**. The single function of an AEC is to eliminate the need for the radiographer to set an exposure time. The radiographer loses control over **time**, and as a result **mAs**, when using an AEC. All other factors, **especially mA and kVp**, must still be set manually.

Radiographers can fall into the habit of depending on AECs to produce diagnostic radiographs in situations for which they were never designed. When using an AEC it is critical that the **location** of the ionization chamber be determined and the precise **positioning** of tissue over that location be achieved. These factors can be remembered by thinking of the use of AECs as another of the radiographic **arts** based on professional expertise and a sound technical understanding.

IONIZATION CHAMBERS

The most critical element in using AECs is the exact position of the ionization chambers because positions differ for various brands and models of equipment (Figure 33–1). **Automatic exposure devices provide a diagnostic quality density only for structures positioned directly above the ionization chambers.** Therefore the most important fact to remember when using automatic exposure devices is that **the art of phototiming is the art of positioning**. Experienced radiographers become extremely adept, often to the point of being artistic, in carefully positioning exactly the right amount of tissue over the chambers.

Ionization chamber AECs are usually used in a three chamber configuration. The most common relationship of the three chambers is with the center chamber at the center of the image receptor with right and left chambers slightly higher. This configuration places the center chamber below the duodenum and transverse colon for most abdominal examinations, thus eliminating problems with gastric and bowel gas being placed over the chamber. This configuration also places the right and left chambers away from the mediastinum and completely within the lobes of the lungs during chest radiography. As long as the exact chamber locations are known, this configuration will not affect phototiming ability during other examinations.

Determining Configurations

Determining the location of the AEC chambers can be a difficult task. Some manufacturers provide plastic inserts for collimators that project an image of the chamber location, size and shape with the positioning light beam (Figure 33–2). These inserts are accurate for only the specified SID (usually printed in a corner of the insert.) When projection inserts are not provided, the radiographer must be capable of determining the location, size and shape. This can be accomplished by producing a radiograph without a body part as the subject, phototimed at very low kVp for maximum contrast (Figure 33–1).

Controlling Configurations

Phototiming console controls permit various combinations of the ionization chambers to be activated in order to control the exposure. Most units permit any single cell or all three cells to be activated. Some units permit other combinations to be utilized, for example, right and left chambers together or all three at once. In these situations, the signals from the cells are sent to a special operational amplifier which sums the voltages received from each

52 **kVp**   4 **mAs**   72″ **SID**
16:1 **grid**   200 **RS**   3.12 **mR**

A

40 **kVp**   5.1 **mAs**   40″ **SID**
10:1 **grid**   200 **RS**   9.66 **mR**

B

40 **kVp**   3.5 **mAs**   40″ **SID**
10:1 **grid**   200 **RS**   6.64 **mR**

C

D

Figure 33–1A–D.   Automatic exposure control ionization chamber configurations. (A) A radiograph of a General Electric configuration with square ionization chambers. The middle cell is centered to the image receptor while the outside cells are placed high. (B) A radiograph of a Philips configuration with both square and circular chambers. The middle cell is square and centered to the image receptor while the outside cells are round and high. (C) A radiograph of a CGR configuration with irregularly shaped cells. The middle cell is square and centered to the image receptor while the outside cells are irregular and high. (D) Actual square ionization chambers of a Siemens configuration. The middle cell is centered to the image receptor while the outside cells are high. Note the wire leads to each ionization chamber. (Photograph courtesy of Eugene Frank, Mayo Foundation.)

Figure 33–2.   Projection of AEC locations from collimator positioning light.

cell and divides by the number of cells that have been activated. When the appropriate voltage for a diagnostic quality density is reached, the exposure is terminated by the operational amplifier. When more than one cell is activated, the cell receiving the most radiation will contribute the greatest electrical signal and therefore have the most influence on image density. For example, if three cells are activated and an abdomen is positioned so that barium is over one cell and normal tissue over the other two cells, the resultant image will be slightly overexposed because the operational amplifier was dividing the incoming voltage by all three cells but only two cells were contributing to the signal. If the cell under the barium was the only one activated, the image would

be greatly overexposed, probably to the back-up time limit, because insufficient radiation was received to terminate the exposure. Cell selection is therefore determined by the radiographer based on knowledge of anatomy and positioning.

Density Controls

All AEC systems permit the adjustment of the amount of radiation necessary to send the exposure termination signal. These controls regulate the image density but often have different labels, depending on the manufacturer. Typical AEC density control labels are −3, −2, −1, 0, 1, 2, 3, or ¼, ½, N, 1¼, 1½. Most labels use the center control as the normal density (0 and N in the two examples) and permit both increases and decreases. Some units use a single density control while others use a major and a minor control. Major controls operate large density changes while minor controls operate fine adjustment.

The density controls should not be used to compensate for patient part thickness or kVp changes. The AEC system is designed to calculate this compensation automatically. Proper use of the density controls is accomplished when the configuration of the ionization chamber cells cannot be adapted to the necessary positioning, for example, when an image is produced that is slightly too dark for the lung fields and a decrease in density is desired even though the patient and ionization chambers are properly positioned.

Exposure Technique Charts

Automatic exposure controls require the use of exposure technique charts that specify the technical parameters to be used. The only difference from nonphototimed charts is that cell locations are given while time settings are eliminated, as the AEC fulfills that function automatically.

POSITIONING SKILLS

The AEC will produce a diagnostic density for whatever tissue is placed directly over the chamber. When the radiographer possesses good positioning skills, the vast majority of phototimed exposures will produce diagnostic quality results. Poor positioning skills result in an increased repeat rate when phototiming. There are numerous instances when variables in tissue density and contrast may complicate the precise location of the tissue of interest over the ionization chamber. Knowledge of when these instances are likely to occur and the experience to adequately compensate for them are important. When not enough of the structure of interest is positioned over the activated ionization chamber, the AEC cell will attempt to produce a diagnostic quality density for whatever is over it (Figures 33–3 and 33–4).

The skilled radiographer detects the majority of these conditions through careful observation of the patient and consideration of

Figure 33–4. Improper AEC cell selection. Although this PA chest is too dark, note that the region at the center of the film, where the AEC cell was activated, is of perfect density for the thoracic spine.

the patient's history. A proper clinical history can reduce the number of repeated radiographs and produce excellent images.

Subject Density and Contrast Problems

Phototiming problems with subject density and contrast occur whenever an unexpected density is present or when an expected density is lacking. For example, fluid in the lungs causes increased subject density and contrast, for which the AEC would remain on longer, making an aerated lung much too dark for diagnosis. A case of emphysema would produce the opposite result.

Collimation

Collimation of the primary beam is another important consideration when phototiming. Attempts to tightly collimate should be

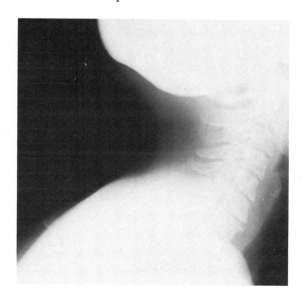

Figure 33–3. Improper positioning over AEC cell. Although this lateral cervical spine is too light, note that the region at the center of the film, where the AEC cell was activated, is of nearly perfect density.

avoided near ionization chamber locations. If the primary beam is collimated from an activated chamber, the chamber operates as if the tissue is extremely dense. The resulting long exposure will create a dark radiograph.

The use of wider collimation can also create problems because the full primary beam will produce scatter radiation that may undercut the patient (Figure 33–5). This undercutting scatter will cause the AEC to terminate the exposure while some areas of the image are still too light.

Timing Problems

Minimum response time and the proper use of a back-up time during phototiming are important considerations. The minimum re-sponse time is the length of time necessary for the AEC to respond to the ionization and send a signal to terminate the exposure. Modern AECs have a minimum response time in the region of 0.001 second. However, the use of extremely high speed intensifying screens for smaller part sizes can cause problems when AECs need less than 0.001 second to produce a diagnostic quality density. In these instances, mA should be decreased to permit longer AEC time.

The back-up time should be set at 150 percent of the anticipated manual exposure time, although U.S. public law requires that generators automatically terminate AEC exposures at 600 mAs or 60 kilowatt seconds (kWs) (kVp × mA × time) above 50 kVp, and 2,000 mAs below 50 kVp. When the back-up time is

Figure 33–5A & B. Undercutting scatter. (A) The uncollimated primary beam produces scatter that undercuts the patient and causes the AEC to prematurely terminate the exposure. (B) An image that is too dark in the upper right quadrant due to undercutting. (Reprinted from "Automatic Exposure Control: A Primer," *Radiologic Technology*, Vol. 59, No. 5, 1988, p. 425. Radiograph courtesy of Seymour Sterling.)

too short, it will terminate the exposure before the AEC signal, thus producing a light image. In these instances, the back-up time should be increased to a level where the AEC is terminating the exposure at the proper time.

Anatomically Programmed Radiography

Anatomically programmed radiography (APR) units combine a phototiming system with a technique chart that is computerized to correspond to anatomical procedures. The control console permits the choice of an anatomical region (for example, the chest) and the projection (for example, PA). This choice results in the computer entering the suggested average technique (for example, 120 kVp, 600 mA, with the right and left ionization chambers activated). The radiographer may override the suggested technique when patient condition, pathology or other factors make it desirable to do so.

Creative Positioning

The experienced radiographer often becomes extremely adept at positioning exactly the right amount of tissue over the chambers.

Experienced radiographers should remember that **a manual technique will always provide a precisely repeatable exposure** whereas a phototimed exposure leaves the radiographer guessing.

Care must be taken when AEC cells are not completely covered by tissue. The most common compensation in this circumstance is to deactivate the uncovered cell. However, if no cell is covered by normal tissue for the area of interest, deactivation is not the answer. In these instances, creative techniques must be used. For example, if a cell is covered by an appropriate percentage of tissue, it may react with an appropriate density. These techniques require much experience and should not be attempted by inexperienced radiographers.

SUMMARY

The ionization chamber is designed for a single purpose, best illustrated by the proper term for the device—automatic exposure control. The single function of an AEC is to eliminate the need for the radiographer to set an exposure time. The radiographer loses control over time, and as a result mAs, when using an AEC. All other factors, especially mA and kVp, must still be set manually.

When using an AEC, it is critical that the location of the ionization chamber be determined and that the precise positioning of tissue over that location be achieved. AEC locations differ for various brands and models of equipment. Automatic exposure devices provide a diagnostic quality density only for structures positioned directly above the ionization chambers. AECs are usually used in a three chamber configuration. The most common relationship of the three chambers is with the center chamber at the center of the image receptor with right and left chambers slightly higher.

Phototiming console controls permit various combinations of the ionization chambers to be activated in order to control the exposure. When more than one cell is used, the signals from the cells are sent to a special operational amplifier which sums the voltages received from each cell, divides by the number of cells that have been activated, and then terminates the exposure.

All AEC systems permit the adjustment of the amount of radiation necessary to send the exposure termination signal. These controls regulate the image density but often have different labels, depending on the manufacturer. Typical AEC density control labels are −3, −2, −1, 0, 1, 2, 3, or ¼, ½, N, 1¼, 1½. Some units use a single density control while others use a major and a minor control.

Problems can result with the use of AEC devices when variations occur in subject density or contrast. Collimation must also be used consistently to assure proper results. The AEC's minimum response time can also cause exposure problems when very fast film/screen combinations are used. Back-up times should be set at 150 percent of the expected manual technique time.

REVIEW QUESTIONS

1. What is the principle function of the automatic exposure control?

2. What are the typical number and configuration of the ionization chambers?

3. What is the purpose of an operational amplifier?

4. When should the density controls be used?

5. How can changes in subject density result in phototiming problems?

6. How can collimation affect phototimed image quality?

7. What is minimum response time?

REFERENCES AND RECOMMENDED READING

Bruce, Geoffrey. Automatic exposure control—a few notes. *Radiography* 42:503, 235, 1976.

Bushong, Stewart C. *Radiologic Science for Technologists.* 4th ed. St. Louis, MO: C. V. Mosby Co., 1988.

Carroll, Quinn B. *Fuchs's Principles of Radiographic Exposure, Processing and Quality Control.* 3rd ed. Springfield, IL: Charles C. Thomas Publisher, 1985.

Coulehan, John L., and Marian R. Block. *The Medical Interview: A Primer for Students of the Art.* Philadelphia, PA: F. A. Davis Co., 1987.

Croft, Melanie J. Filtration, the answer to the automatic exposure control response problem. *Radiologic Technology* 57:5, 447, 1986.

Cullinan, Angeline M. *Producing Quality Radiographs.* Philadelphia, PA: Lippincott, 1987.

Curry, Thomas S., James E. Dowdey, and Robert C. Murry, Jr. *Christensen's Physics of Diagnostic Radiology.* 4th ed. Philadelphia, PA: Lea & Febiger, 1990.

Eastman, Terry R. Automated exposures in contemporary radiography. *Radiologic Technology* 43:2, 80, 1971.

Fodor, Joseph III, and Jack C. Malott. *The Art and Science of Medical Radiography.* St. Louis, MO: The Catholic Health Association of the United States, 1987.

Hiss, Stephen S. *Understanding Radiography.* Springfield, IL: Charles C. Thomas Publisher, 1978.

Jenkins, David. *Radiographic Photography and Imaging Processes.* Lancaster, England: MTP Press Limited, 1980.

Karila, Kauko T. K. Manual or automatic exposure controller imaging in mammography. *Radiography Today* 54:618, 35, 1989.

Morgan, R. H. The automatic control of exposure in photofluorography. *Public Health Reports* 58, 1533–1541, 1943.

Morgan, R. H. A photoelectric timing mechanism for the automatic control of roentgenographic exposure. *American Journal of Roentgenography and Radium Therapy* 48, 220–228, 1942.

Seeram, Euclid. *X-Ray Imaging Equipment.* Springfield, IL: Charles C. Thomas Publisher, 1985.

Selman, Joseph. *The Fundamentals of X-Ray and Radium Physics.* 7th ed. Springfield, IL: Charles C. Thomas Publisher, 1985.

Sprawls, Perry. *Principles of Radiography for Technologists*. Rockville, MD: Aspen Publishers, Inc., 1990.

Stears, John G., Joel E. Gray, and Eugene D. Frank. Radiologic exchange (automatic exposure control function). *Radiologic Technology* 59:6, 521–522, 1988.

Sterling, Seymour. Automatic exposure control:

A primer. *Radiologic Technology* 59:5, 421–427, 1988.

Thompson, Thomas T. *A Practical Approach to Modern Imaging Equipment*. 2nd ed. Boston, MA: Little, Brown, and Co., 1985.

Thompson, Thomas T. *Cahoon's Formulating X-Ray Techniques*. 9th ed. Durham, NC: Duke University Press, 1979.

THE CASE OF THE VERY DENSE OBJECT

What could be causing the image of the very dense object on the right side of the fourth cervical vertebrae?

Answers to the case studies can be found in Appendix E.

34 EXPOSURE CONVERSION PROBLEMS

Never lose your courage.

Professor Wilhelm Röntgen.

OUTLINE

STANDARD CONVERSION RELATIONSHIPS AND TABLES
SOLVING COMPLEX EXPOSURE PROBLEMS

OBJECTIVES

Upon completion of this chapter, the student should be able to:

1. Discuss the limitations of standard conversion tables.
2. Explain the concept of direct and inverse relationships versus proportions.
3. Calculate appropriate new exposure factors for multiple changes in exposure factor variables.

STANDARD CONVERSION RELATIONSHIPS AND TABLES

A primary concern when using conversion tables is their tendency to oversimplify complex exposure problems. It is safer to think of radiographic exposure factors as relationships to one another rather than as direct conversions. The radiographer uses conversion tables as guidelines, with the realization that the great number of variables in any imaging system make all conversion factors variables, not constants. Conversion tables are designed to assist in producing an image within acceptance limits. Production of an image of optimal

diagnostic quality usually requires fine tuning. Conversion tables, like all other factors, require fine tuning before being integrated into an exposure system.

Most conversion tables are designed to provide a method of maintaining image density. It is important to understand the interrelationship between variables and their effects on the four image quality factors: density, contrast, recorded detail and distortion.

The effect of a particular variable is best described as either a direct relationship, in which an increase in the variable causes an increase in the effect, or an inverse relationship, in which an increase in the variable causes a decrease in the effect, and vice versa. The description of a relationship as direct or inverse does not necessarily indicate that the relationship is **proportionally** direct or inverse. In other words, a proportionally direct relationship would indicate that a linear relationship exists between the variable and the effect, whereas a direct relationship would simply indicate that as the variable changes, the effect changes in the same direction, not necessarily in a linear manner.

Table 34–1 is a master table indicating the relationship of most radiographic image variables on density, contrast, recorded detail and distortion. Conversion tables are provided for the factors that are commonly considered when converting from one exposure factor or system to another, especially regarding maintaining image density. (Tables 34–2 through 34–9).

SOLVING COMPLEX EXPOSURE PROBLEMS

The most difficult part of developing technique exposure factor skills is learning how to use the information in actual clinical situations. The difficulty lies in the fact that clinical problems usually present complex situations with more than one variable. Now that each variable has been explored in detail, it is necessary to learn how to solve complex exposure problems with many variables.

Methodology

A very simple method can be used to assess a complex exposure problem. Although the analytical decision making process can be used, it is simpler to work through the variables. If the same variables are considered for each problem, it is less likely that a factor will be missed.

Radiographic variables that should be considered when solving a clinical exposure problem can be classified into four major areas: equipment, tube, patient and image receptor. Each of these four areas has its variables, as shown in Table 34–1. The variables are easier to remember than it first appears. Equipment is composed of phase plus the four primary factors (kVp, mA, time and distance). The tube is focal spot, filtration and field size. The subject consists of part density and contrast. The image receptor includes grid and film/screen variables.

Mistakes in solving complex exposure problems are invariably caused by failure to consider one of these variables. Even when the solution to a problem appears self-evident, a moment taken to consider all the variables may reveal a hidden factor that would have been missed otherwise.

The following problems demonstrate this methodology.

Example: A satisfactory radiograph is produced as follows:
1φ2p, 80kVp, 40 mAs, 40″ SID, 8:1 grid, 250 RS. If a new radiograph is to be produced with the following changes—3φ6p, 12:1 grid, 400 RS—what changes should be made to maintain the original density?

Answer: The following variables must be considered:
Equipment: generator phase from 1φ2p to 3φ6p.
Image receptor: grid from 8:1 to 12:1.
Image receptor: film/screen combination from 250 RS to 400 RS.

Each variable must be converted for the new exposure:
Equipment: generator phase from 1φ2p to 3φ6p.

The conversion factor for 1φ2 to 3φ6 = mAs × 0.38.

40 mAs × 0.38 = 15.2 mAs.
Image receptor: grid from 8:1 to 12:1.

TABLE 34–1

EFFECTS OF RADIOGRAPHIC EXPOSURE VARIABLES
ON THE PRIMARY FACTORS

D = direct relationship (when the variable changes, the effect changes in the same direction).
I = inverse relationship (when the variable changes, the effect changes in the opposite direction).
NOTE: Many effects are not linearly proportional.
0 = no effect.

Effect On

Variable	Density	Contrast	Recorded Detail	Distortion
EQUIPMENT				
Generator Phase	D	I	0	0
Kilovoltage	D	I	0	0
Milliamperage-seconds	D	0	0	0
SID	I	0	D	I
OID	I	I	I	D
TUBE				
Focal Spot Size	0	0	I	D
Filtration	I	I	0	0
Beam Restriction	D	D	0	0
SUBJECT				
Part Thickness	I	I	I	D
Tissue Type	I	I	0	0
Additive Pathology	I	I	0	0
Destructive Pathology	D	D	0	0
IMAGE RECEPTOR				
Grid Ratio	I	D	0	0
Film/Screen Relative Speed	D	0	I	0
Film Processing				
Developer Time	D	I	0	0
Developer Temperature	D	I	0	0
Developer Replenishment	D	I	0	0

The conversion factor formula for grid changes is

$$\frac{mAs_1}{mAs_2} = \frac{GCF_1}{GCF_2}$$

The conversion factor for an 8:1 grid = 4

The conversion factor for a 12:1 grid = 5.5, so

$$\frac{15.2 \ mAs}{mAs_2} = \frac{4}{5.5}$$

$$mAs_2 \times 4 = 15.2 \ mAs \times 5.5$$

$$mAs_2 \times 4 = 83.6 \ mAs$$

$$\text{mAs}_2 = \frac{83.6 \text{ mAs}}{4}$$

$$\text{mAs}_2 = 20.9 \text{ mAs}$$

Image receptor: film/screen combination from 250 RS to 400 RS.

TABLE 34–2

CONVERSION FACTORS: EFFECT OF GENERATOR PHASE ON IMAGE DENSITY

When Converting Generator Phase		To Maintain Image Density, Multiply mAs by a Conversion Factor of:
From:	To:	
$1\phi2p$	$3\phi6p$	0.6
$1\phi2p$	$3\phi12p$	0.5
$3\phi6p$	$1\phi2p$	1.6
$3\phi6p$	$3\phi12p$	0.8
$3\phi12p$	$1\phi2p$	2.0
$3\phi12p$	$3\phi6p$	1.2

Adapted from the Du Pont Bit System, 9th edition, E. I. Du Pont de Nemours, Inc., Wilmington, DE.

TABLE 34–3

THE FIFTEEN PERCENT RULE

To maintain radiographic density when increasing kVp: increase kVp 15 percent and reduce mAs to half.

To maintain radiographic density when decreasing kVp: decrease kVp 15 percent and double mAs.

TABLE 34–4

THE mAs FORMULA

$$\text{mA} \times \text{seconds} = \text{mAs}$$

TABLE 34–5

THE DENSITY MAINTENANCE FORMULA

$$\frac{\text{mAs}_1}{\text{mAs}_2} = \frac{D_1^2}{D_2^2}$$

where	mAs_1	=	original mAs
	mAs_2	=	new mAs
	D_1	=	original distance
	D_2	=	new distance

The same formula can be expressed as:

$$\text{mAs}_2 = \frac{\text{mAs}_1 \times D_2^2}{D_1^2}$$

TABLE 34–6

RECOMMENDED COMPENSATION FOR SUBJECT PART THICKNESS

$$\text{mAs} = 2X \text{ or } 0.5X \text{ mAs per 5 cm} =$$
$$15\%\text{–}20\% \text{ mAs per cm}$$
$$\text{kVp} = 2 \text{ kVp per cm}$$

NOTE: Because scatter production varies with total part thickness, these figures are based on 60–80 kVp for a 20 cm part. The recommendations for changes are less accurate further from this average range.

TABLE 34–7

GRID RATIO CONVERSION FORMULA

$$\frac{\text{mAs}_1}{\text{mAs}_2} = \frac{\text{GCF}_1}{\text{GCF}_2}$$

TABLE 34-8

GRID RATIO CONVERSIONS

(Approximate values based on clinical tests of pelvis and skull.)

Grid Ratio	60 kVp	85 kVp	110 kVp
No grid	1	1	1
5:1	3	3	3
8:1	3.75	4	4.25
12:1	4.75	5.5	6.25
16:1	5.75	6.75	8

Adapted with permission from *Characteristics and Applications of X-Ray Grids*, Liebel-Flarsheim division of Sybron Corporation, Cincinnati, Ohio.

TABLE 34-9

RELATIVE SPEED FORMULA

$$\frac{mAs_1}{mAs_2} = \frac{RS_2}{RS_1}$$

The conversion formula for RS changes is

$$\frac{mAs_1}{mAs_2} = \frac{RS_2}{RS_1}$$

The RS change is from 250 RS to 400 RS, so

$$\frac{20.9 \text{ mAs}}{mAs_2} = \frac{400}{250}$$

$$mAs_2 \times 400 = 20.9 \text{ mAs} \times 250$$

$$mAs_2 \times 400 = 5{,}225 \text{ mAs}$$

$$mAs_2 = \frac{5{,}225 \text{ mAs}}{400}$$

$$mAs_2 = 13 \text{ mAs}$$

So the new exposure factor conditions require a change to 13 mAs to duplicate the density of the original exposure factors.

Example: A satisfactory radiograph is produced as follows:
3φ6p, 80 kVp, 20 mAs, 72" SID, 12:1 grid, 400 RS.
If a new radiograph is to be produced with the following changes—3φ12p, 68 kVp, 100 mA, 10:1 grid, 200 RS—what changes should be made to maintain the original density?

Answer: The following variables must be considered:
Equipment: generator phase from 3φ6p to 3φ12p.
Equipment: kVp from 80 to 68.
Equipment: mAs = time × 100 mA.
Image receptor: grid from 12:1 to 10:1.
Image receptor: film/screen combination from 400 RS to 200 RS.

Each variable must be converted for the new exposure:
Equipment: generator phase from 3φ6p to 3φ12p.
The conversion factor for 3φ6p to 3φ12p = mAs × 0.8.
20 mAs × 0.8 = 16 mAs
Equipment: kVp from 80 to 68.
The conversion when decreasing kVp by 15 percent is doubling the mAs.
80 kVp × 15% = 12 kVp
80 kVp − 12 kVp = 68 kVp
so, 16 mAs × 2 = 32 mAs
Image receptor: grid from 12:1 to 10:1.
The conversion factor formula for grid changes is

$$\frac{mAs_1}{mAs_2} = \frac{GCF_1}{GCF_2}$$

The conversion factor for an 8:1 grid = 3.75.
The conversion factor for a 12:1 grid = 4.75, so

$$\frac{8 \text{ mAs}}{mAs_2} = \frac{3.75}{4.75}$$

$$mAs_2 \times 3.75 = 32 \text{ mAs} \times 4.75$$
$$mAs_2 \times 3.75 = 152 \text{ mAs}$$
$$mAs_2 = \frac{152 \text{ mAs}}{3.75}$$
$$mAs_2 = 40.5 \text{ mAs}$$

Image receptor: film/screen combination from 250 RS to 400 RS.

The conversion formula for RS changes is

$$\frac{mAs_1}{mAs_2} = \frac{RS_2}{RS_1}$$

The RS change is from 250 RS to 400 RS, so

$$\frac{10.1 \text{ mAs}}{mAs_2} = \frac{400}{250}$$
$$mAs_2 \times 400 = 40.5 \text{ mAs} \times 250$$
$$mAs_2 \times 400 = 10{,}125 \text{ mAs}$$
$$mAs_2 = \frac{10{,}125 \text{ mAs}}{400}$$
$$mAs_2 = 25.3 \text{ mAs}$$

Equipment: mAs = time × 100 mA

$$\frac{25.3 \text{ mAs}}{100 \text{ mA}} = \text{time}$$
$$0.25 = \text{time}$$

So the new exposure factor conditions require a change to 25.3 mAs to duplicate the density of the original exposure factors. Using 100 mA, the exposure time would be set at 0.25 seconds.

SUMMARY

A primary concern when using conversion tables is their tendency to oversimplify complex exposure problems. It is safer to think of radiographic exposure factors as relationships to one another rather than as direct conversions. Conversion tables are designed to assist in producing an image within acceptance limits. Most conversion tables are designed to provide a method of maintaining image density. It is important to understand the interrelationships between variables and their effects on the four image quality factors: density, contrast, recorded detail and distortion.

The effect of a particular variable is best described as either a direct relationship, in which an increase in the variable causes an increase in the effect, or an inverse relationship, in which an increase in the variable causes a decrease in the effect, and vice versa. A proportionally direct relationship would indicate that a linear relationship exists between the variables.

The most difficult part of developing technique exposure factor skills is learning how to use the information in actual clinical situations. It is necessary to learn how to solve complex exposure problems with many variables. A very simple method can be used to assess a complex exposure problem. If the same variables are considered for each problem, it is less likely that a factor will be missed.

Radiographic variables that should be considered when solving a clinical exposure problem can be classified into four major areas: equipment, tube, patient and image receptor. Mistakes in solving complex exposure problems are invariably caused by failure to consider one of the variables. Even when the solution to a problem appears self-evident, a moment taken to consider all of the variables may reveal a hidden factor that would otherwise have been missed.

REVIEW QUESTIONS

1. What is the primary purpose of conversion tables?

2. When making exposure factor conversions, it is important to consider the effect on which of the image quality factors?

3. What is the meaning of a direct relationship?

4. What is the difference between a relationship and a proportion?

5. When solving complex exposure problems, the variables can be classified into what four major areas?

REFERENCES AND RECOMMENDED READING

Cahoon, John B. *Formulating X-Ray Techniques.* 8th ed. Durham, NC: Duke University Press, 1974.

Carroll, Quinn. *Fuchs's Principles of Radiographic Exposure, Processing and Quality Control.* 3rd ed. Springfield, IL: Charles C. Thomas Publisher, 1985.

Cullinan, Angeline M. *Producing Quality Radiographs.* Philadelphia, PA: Lippincott, 1987.

Du Pont Company Photosystems & Electronic Products Department. *Positioning and Exposure Guide for General Radiography.* Wilmington, DE: Publication R–53806–1.

Du Pont Company Photosystems & Electronic Products Department. *Bit System of Technique Conversion.* 8th ed. Wilmington, DE.

Eastman, Terry R. *Radiographic Fundamentals and Technique Guide.* St. Louis, MO: C. V. Mosby Co., 1979.

Eastman, T. R. *The Radiographic Technique Guide.* Wilmington, DE: Du Pont de Nemours, Inc. Photo Products Department Publication A–99101.

Frank, Eugene D., and Norlin T. Winkler. Preparing an accurate x-ray exposure technique chart. Rochester, MN: Mayo Foundation, postgraduate course from American Society of Radiologic Technologists annual meetings, 1987–1988.

General Electric Company Medical Systems Department. *How to Prepare an X-Ray Technic Chart.* Milwaukee, WI: Publication 4301A.

Hiss, Stephen S. *Understanding Radiography.* Springfield, IL: Charles C. Thomas Publisher, 1978.

Jenkins, David. *Radiographic Photography and Imaging Processes.* Lancaster, England: MTP Press Ltd., 1980.

Kratzer, Brice. A technique computer: Scientific approach to radiologic technology. *Radiologic Technology* 42, 142–150, 1973.

Thompson, Thomas T. *Cahoon's Formulating X-Ray Techniques.* 9th ed. Durham. NC: Duke University Press, 1979.

35 MINIMIZING PATIENT EXPOSURE DOSE

I became acquainted very early with the destructive effect of roentgen rays upon living tissue. In fact, it was only a few months after the announcement of Röntgen's discovery that I required medical care for a roentgen burn covering most of the back of one hand.

W. D. Coolidge, "Experiences with the Roentgen-ray tube."

OUTLINE

ESTIMATING APPROXIMATE ENTRANCE SKIN EXPOSURE DOSE
TYPICAL ENTRANCE SKIN EXPOSURE DOSES
REDUCING EXPOSURE DOSE WITH COMMUNICATION
REDUCING EXPOSURE DOSE WITH POSITIONING
REDUCING EXPOSURE DOSE WITH TECHNICAL FACTORS
DISCUSSING RADIATION RISK VERSUS BENEFIT WITH PATIENTS

OBJECTIVES

Upon completion of this chapter, the student should be able to:

1. Explain the relationship of entrance skin dose exposure to other measurement points.
2. Calculate mR/mAs from a calibration dose total.
3. Calculate total exposure when given subject part thickness, SID, kVp, mAs and an mR/mAs chart.
4. Describe typical entrance skin exposure doses for common radiographic procedures.
5. Discuss methods of reducing patient exposure dose through effective communication.
6. Describe various methods of reducing patient exposure dose through effective positioning.

7. Explain the interrelationship of the prime factors.
8. Evaluate various exposure factors for the most effective methods of reducing patient exposure dose under various clinical conditions.
9. Describe an effective method of minimizing patient exposure dose by emphasizing radiation risk factors.
10. Describe an effective method of maximizing patient diagnostic information by emphasizing radiation benefit factors.
11. Analyze various approaches to discussing radiation risk versus benefit with patients, physicians and radiologists.

A predominant concern of radiographers is how to reduce the radiation exposure dose to the patient. This concern is reflected in every decision made, especially when choosing technique exposure factors. The conscientious radiographer can reduce the patient exposure dose by at least 50 percent in most examinations by choosing appropriate exposure factors.

One of the most important characteristics of the professional is the ability to decide when it is appropriate to tip the radiation benefit versus risk issue in favor of the risk by reducing the patient exposure dose while compromising the diagnostic quality of the image, and when to tip the issue in favor of the benefit by increasing the patient exposure dose while maintaining the diagnostic quality of the image. There are circumstances that dictate when each choice should be made, and this chapter will attempt to lay the foundation necessary to make these decisions.

ESTIMATING APPROXIMATE ENTRANCE SKIN EXPOSURE DOSE

Figure 35–1 illustrates a typical radiographic examination with the exposure dose indicated at various points. It is obvious that the maximum exposure dose received by the patient is not at the area of interest but at the skin entrance to the body. This is known as the entrance skin dose and is calculated at the minimum SOD. Note that the minimum SOD is not equal to the SOD of the area of interest and that the entrance skin receives a greater exposure. Although radiobiologists and physicists often discuss organ doses and gonadal doses, the entrance skin dose is the most common expression to approximate patient exposure dose because it is safer to assume a maximum effect when attempting to minimize exposure to ionizing radiation.

Diagnostic Radiography mR/mAs Charts

Exposure to patients can be estimated by recording mR/mAs when the x-ray unit is calibrated. This is calculated by recording a dose reading for any average exposure and then dividing the dose reading in mR by the total mAs used. The expression mR/mAs represents the formula itself. The mR/mAs measurements are usually recorded for an SID of 40″ (100 cm). To estimate the entrance skin exposure dose, the inverse square law must be applied to determine the exposure for the source-to-entrance skin distance.

The mR/mAs readings vary according to the kVp used, with higher kVp producing greater mR/mAs. Consequently, mR/mAs readings should be recorded for each kVp range within the normal expectations of the unit. A typical mR/mAs chart is shown in Table 35–1.

Figure 35–1.   Exposure doses at various locations in the imaging process.

A quick estimate of entrance skin exposure can be made from this chart, as shown in the example below.

Example: What is the approximate entrance skin exposure for a 20 cm AP abdomen produced at 80 kVp and 20 mAs on the unit for the chart in Table 35–1?

Answer:
Table 35–1 indicates that 80 kVp=3.5 mR/mAs. The exposure required 20 mAs, so the exposure at 100 cm = 3.5 mR/mAs × 20 mAs and the exposure at 100 cm = 70.0 mR.

$$SID = SOD + OID$$
$$100\ cm = SOD + 20\ cm$$
$$SOD = 100\ cm - 20\ cm$$
$$SOD = 80\ cm$$

$$\frac{mR_1}{mR_2} = \frac{SOD^2}{SID^2}$$

$$\frac{70\ mR}{mR_2} = \frac{80\ cm^2}{100\ cm^2}$$

$$\frac{70\ mR}{mR_2} = \frac{6,400\ cm}{10,000\ cm}$$

$$mR_2 \times 6,400\ cm = 70\ mR \times 10,000\ cm$$

$$mR_2 = \frac{70\ mR \times 10,000\ cm}{6,400\ cm}$$

$$mR_2 = \frac{700,000}{6,400}$$

$$mR_2 = 109.4$$

Example: What is the total approximate entrance skin exposure for an intravenous pyelogram of a 24 cm abdomen if an AP preliminary scout; 5 min AP; 10 min AP, RPO and LPO; 15 min PA; and 30 min AP radiographs of the abdomen were produced at 70 kVp and 15 mAs on the unit for the chart in Table 35–1?

TABLE 35–1

A TYPICAL mR/mAs CHART

SID = 40″ (100 cm)

kVp	mR/mAs
50	0.9
60	1.7
70	2.5
80	3.5
90	4.5
100	5.6
110	6.9
120	7.9

Answer:

Table 35–1 indicates that 70 kVp=2.5 mR/mAs. Each exposure required 15 mAs, so the approximate entrance skin exposure = 2.5 mR/mAs × 15 mAs and the approximate entrance skin exposure = 37.5 mR per exposure; 37.5 per exposure × 7 exposures = 262.5 mR = 0.2625 R.

$$SID = SOD + OID$$
$$100 \text{ cm} = SOD + 24 \text{ cm}$$
$$SOD = 100 \text{ cm} - 24 \text{ cm}$$
$$SOD = 76 \text{ cm}$$

$$\frac{mR_1}{mR_2} = \frac{SOD^2}{SID^2}$$

$$\frac{262.5 \text{ mR}}{mR_2} = \frac{76 \text{ cm}^2}{100 \text{ cm}^2}$$

$$\frac{262.5 \text{ mR}}{mR_2} = \frac{5,776 \text{ cm}}{10,000 \text{ cm}}$$

$$mR_2 \times 5,776 \text{ cm} = 262.5 \text{ mR} \times 10,000 \text{ cm}$$

$$mR_2 = \frac{262.5 \text{ mR} \times 10,000 \text{ cm}}{5,776 \text{ cm}}$$

$$mR_2 = \frac{2,625,000}{5,776}$$

$$mR_2 = 454.5$$

Fluoroscopic mR/min Charts

Approximate entrance skin exposure for fluoroscopic equipment is measured in R/min. Estimation of approximate entrance skin exposure dose is calculated in the same manner.

Example: What is the approximate entrance skin exposure for a fluoroscopic examination of the abdomen performed for 5.5 minutes at 110 kVp at 1.7 R/min?

Answer:

The exposure required 5.5 min, so the approximate entrance skin exposure = 1.7 R/min × 5.5 min and the approximate entrance skin exposure = 9.35 R = 9,350 mR.

Example: What is the total approximate entrance skin exposure for a fluoroscopic examination of an 18 cm abdomen performed for 7 min and 45 sec at 110 kVp at 1.7 R/min and then followed by an AP, at 10 mAs, left lateral, at 25 mAs, and LPO projection, at 20 mAs, of the stomach at 120 kVp on the unit for the chart in Table 35–1?

Answer:

The exposure required 7.75 min, so the approximate entrance skin exposure = 1.7 R/min × 7.75 min and the approximate entrance skin exposure = 13.175 R = 13,175 mR. The total mAs for the three projections = 10 + 25 + 20 mAs = 55 mAs. Table 35–1 indicates that 120 kVp = 7.9 mR/mAs, so the approximate entrance skin exposure = 7.9 mR/mAs × 55 mAs and the approximate entrance skin exposure = 434.5 mR; 13,175 fluoro mR + 434.5 diagnostic mR = 13,609.5 mR = 13.61 R.

$$SID = SOD + OID$$
$$100 \text{ cm} = SOD + 18 \text{ cm}$$
$$SOD = 100 \text{ cm} - 18 \text{ cm}$$
$$SOD = 82 \text{ cm}$$

$$\frac{mR_1}{mR_2} = \frac{SOD^2}{SID^2}$$

$$\frac{13{,}609.5 \text{ mR}}{\text{mR}_2} = \frac{82 \text{ cm}^2}{100 \text{ cm}^2}$$

$$\frac{13{,}609.5 \text{ mR}}{\text{mR}_2} = \frac{6{,}724 \text{ cm}}{10{,}000 \text{ cm}}$$

$$\text{mR}_2 \times 6{,}724 \text{ cm} = 13{,}609.5 \text{ mR} \times 10{,}000 \text{ cm}$$

$$\text{mR}_2 = \frac{13{,}609.5 \text{ mR} \times 10{,}000 \text{ cm}}{6{,}724 \text{ cm}}$$

$$\text{mR}_2 = \frac{136{,}095{,}000}{6{,}724}$$

$$\text{mR}_2 = 20{,}240 = 20.24 \text{ R.}$$

TYPICAL ENTRANCE SKIN EXPOSURE DOSES

Numerous studies have been done regarding the exposure dose delivered to patients during diagnostic radiographic examinations. Diagnostic radiography is by far the greatest source of ionizing radiation exposure for the public. It is estimated that 15 percent of the radiation dose received by the general public is a result of diagnostic radiographic exami-

nations. Table 35–2 shows the average patient exposure guides for entrance skin exposure as published by the Conference of Radiation Control Program Directors. Within an acceptance range of ±20 percent, this guide is considered to be the standard for current practice in the United States.

Radiography of the lumbar spine, pelvis and hip contributes the greatest exposure doses. These examinations deserve special attention from radiographers because careful consideration of the need for the examination, positioning, patient instructions, technical factors and shielding can result in significant reduction in the total exposure dose to the patient.

REDUCING EXPOSURE DOSE WITH COMMUNICATION

Radiographers often overlook the importance of gaining the trust and confidence of the patient. This is accomplished by a professional approach that includes technical competence, empathy for the patient and effective communication and questioning skills. When the pa-

---

TABLE 35–2

MEDICAL ENTRANCE SKIN EXPOSURES (ESE) IN mR
(Measurements in air with no phantom)

Projection	Patient Thickness (in cm)	Grid	SID (in inches)	ESE in mR	
				200 speed	400 speed
Abdomen–AP	23	Yes	40	490	300
Lumbar Spine–AP	23	Yes	40	450	350
Full Spine–AP	23	Yes	72	260	145
Cervical Spine–AP	13	Yes	40	135	95
Skull–LAT	15	Yes	40	145	70
Chest–PA	23	No	72	15	5
		Yes	72	25	15

Reprinted with permission from *Average Patient Exposure Guides: 1988*, Conference of Radiation Control Program Directors, Inc., Frankfort, KY: CRCPD Publication 88–5, 1988.

tient has confidence in the radiographer there is a higher probability that detailed instructions will be followed, which helps to reduce motion and degradation of positioning.

REDUCING EXPOSURE DOSE WITH POSITIONING

An effective method of reducing patient exposure dose is through accurate and effective positioning. Avoidance of repeated exposures far outweighs all other methods of reducing patient exposure. However, once positioning skills have been developed to a degree of competence, several positioning details may further reduce the total exposure dose.

Radiographic Projection

Some organs are especially sensitive to the effects of radiation, for example, the female breast, the kidneys and the lens of the eye. Increased recorded detail and decreased distortion result when the area of interest is placed as close to the image receptor as possible. In most instances a significant reduction in the total exposure dose is achieved because this positioning also places the organ as far from the entrance exposure as possible. For example, a PA chest reduces the exposure to the breast, an AP abdomen reduces exposure to the kidneys, and a PA skull reduces exposure to the lens of the eye. Deviation from these projections should occur only when unusual circumstances dictate an alternate projection.

Immobilization

Proper immobilization is a necessary part of achieving satisfactory recorded detail and diminishing the need for repeat exposures. Elimination of motion and decreased tissue density through compression both contribute to a reduction of patient exposure dose.

REDUCING EXPOSURE DOSE WITH TECHNICAL FACTORS

The radiographer can significantly reduce the approximate entrance skin exposure dose to the patient by judicious selection of technique exposure factors. Studies have shown that over 50 percent of repeated exposures are the result of improper technical factor selection. Table 35–3 illustrates the effect each of the major technical factors has on patient exposure dose. In most instances when a technical factor is varied, other factors will be modified to maintain image density. Therefore, the important information is not the direct result of the technical factor change, but the result of compensation to maintain image density or other components of image quality.

Interrelationship of the Prime Factors

The radiation intensity from a diagnostic x-ray unit will vary in a direct relationship with mAs, directly with the square of kVp and inversely with the square of the distance. This total relationship is often expressed as:

$$\frac{(\text{mAs})\,(\text{kVp})^2}{d^2}$$

Although this formula includes only the four primary factors, it is useful to understand that they are interrelated and can all be used to influence the total exposure dose.

Kilovoltage Range

When kVp is increased without compensating for other factors, patient exposure is increased. Therefore, a decrease in kVp is desired when attempting to reduce patient exposure. However, when an increase in kVp is compensated for by a decrease in mAs to

TABLE 35–3

EFFECTS OF RADIOGRAPHIC EXPOSURE VARIABLES ON PATIENT EXPOSURE DOSE

| | | Effect of Patient Dose When: | |
| | Variable Is Increased without Compensation | Variable Is Increased but Image Density Is Maintained By Compensating | |
Variable		with kVp Only	with mAs Only
Kilovoltage	+	NA	−
Milliamperage	+	+	0
Time	+	+	0
Distance			
SID	−	−	0
SOD	−	−	0
OID	+	+	+
Focal spot size	0	NA	NA
Filtration	−	−	+
Field Size	+	varies	varies
Gonadal shielding	−	NA	NA
Subject part density	+	+	+
Grid Ratio	0	+	+
Intensifying screens	0	−	−
Film speed	0	−	−
Film processing			
Developer time	0	−	−
Developer temperature	0	−	−
Developer replenishment	0	−	−

maintain image density, a significant reduction in patient dose is achieved. **Selection of the highest possible kilovoltage is the best method of using exposure factors to reduce patient exposure dose**. With fixed kilovoltage systems, care must be taken to achieve an optimal kVp that is within acceptance limits. Because fixed kVp technique systems tend to utilize higher optimal kVp levels, they usually reduce patient exposure doses. A comparison of approximate dose levels with the two systems is illustrated in Table 35–4.

Remember that generator phase also has an effect on kilovoltage output. Although an increase in the number of pulses from the generator will increase the patient dose because of the increased average photon energy, in most instances there is no appreciable difference in the exposure dose when image density is compensated for through decreased mAs or kVp.

Milliamperage and Time

When mAs is decreased, patient exposure is also decreased. When an increase in mAs is

TABLE 35-4

COMPARISON OF APPROXIMATE EXPOSURE DOSE WITH FIXED AND VARIABLE kVp TECHNIQUE SYSTEMS

Variable— 56 kVp, 5 mAs = 12.8 mR
Fixed— 65 kVp, 2.5 mAs = 9.5 mR

Variable— 68 kVp, 40 mAs = 175.1 mR
Fixed— 80 kVp, 20 mAs = 135.4 mR

Variable— 102 kVp, 20 mAs = 222.0 mR
Fixed— 120 kVp, 10 mAs = 156.3 mR

These examples would produce equivalent image density.

compensated by a decrease in kVp, patient exposure will increase. An inverse relationship exists between mAs and kVp in maintaining image density. To decrease patient exposure, mAs should be maintained at the lowest possible level because there is a direct relationship between mAs and dose. Because variable kVp technique systems tend to utilize lower kVp levels with higher mAs, the result can be higher average patient exposure doses than with fixed kVp systems.

Distance

Distance cannot be discussed alone because SID, SOD and OID have differing relationships to patient exposure dose. When SID or SOD is increased, patient exposure decreases. When kVp is used to compensate for image density, the dose will decrease but the use of mAs for compensation will usually increase the total exposure. In most instances, when OID decreases, SOD increases and this will reduce patient exposure. This holds true regardless of whether kVp or mAs is used to compensate for the air-gap contrast and density changes.

Focal Spot Size

Focal spot size has no effect on patient exposure dose.

Filtration

An increase in filtration will reduce the exposure dose, even when kVp is compensated to maintain image density. However, when mAs is used to compensate for lost image density, the result is often an increase in the total exposure dose. This applies only to the small filtration increases used in diagnostic radiography, usually not more than 0.5 mm Al/eq. Any significant increase in filtration (1.0 mm Al/eq or more) would have an overall dose reduction effect.

Field Size

When the primary-beam field size decreases, the patient exposure dose also decreases. An increased field size will increase the total exposure dose even when mAs or kVp is adjusted to compensate for image density because a greater tissue area is irradiated. An increase in the primary technical factors is necessary to compensate for lost scatter radiation density when the field size is decreased. Although this appears to increase exposure dose, the elimination of a greater percentage of tissue from the beam is a greater protective method than the increased factors.

Modern x-ray tube collimators utilize two sets of shutters or leaves to eliminate most of the off-focus radiation. When an aperture diaphragm is used instead of a collimator, off-focus radiation can increase the peripheral exposure dose adjacent to the primary beam field.

Gonad Shielding

Gonad shielding is extremely effective in reducing exposure to the gonads. There are three major types of gonad shields: flat contact, shadow and shaped contact. Flat contact shields are positioned over the gonads at the skin surface. Shadow shields are positioned in the primary beam immediately below the collimator. Shaped contact shields are worn by the patient to surround the gonads.

Subject Part Density

A decrease in subject part density will decrease scatter production and reduce the patient exposure dose. When compensation for lost scatter is made by increasing mAs or kVp, a reduction in total exposure usually holds.

Grids

Because the grid is placed after the patient in the imaging sequence, a change in grid ratio has no effect on patient exposure dose. However, when the grid ratio is decreased, and image density is maintained by decreases in mAs or kVp, a significant dose reduction can be achieved. The use of a grid of unnecessarily high ratio causes routine increases in patient exposure dose and should be avoided.

Intensifying Screens

Because the intensifying screens are placed after the patient in the imaging sequence, a change in screens has no effect on patient exposure dose. However, whenever the screen speed is increased, a significant reduction in mAs or kVp can be achieved while maintaining image density. **The second most effective method of reducing patient exposure dose is to use the highest possible film/screen combination.**

Film

Because the film is placed after the patient in the imaging sequence, a change in film has no effect on patient exposure dose. Base plus fog is a factor that should not be related to patient exposure dose reductions. If base plus fog becomes too high, the detrimental effect on image quality will result in repeated exposures. However, a decrease in patient dose can be accomplished when a higher speed film is used and mAs or kVp is reduced to maintain image density. Because higher contrast films also exhibit greater speed, the same effect is achieved with a higher contrast film. Film latitude becomes wider as speed and contrast decrease. Consequently, a narrow latitude film is desirable when attempting to reduce patient exposure dose. This approach requires radiographers to be extremely accurate in selecting technical factors.

Film Processing

Because film processing occurs after the patient in the imaging sequence, a change in processing has no effect on patient exposure dose. However, the compensations that are required to overcome reductions in developer time, temperature or replenishment can result in unnecessarily high patient exposure doses. Developer time, temperature and replenishment cannot be effectively increased to reduce patient exposure dose. Film processing is a system that must be maintained at an optimal level to ensure satisfactory image quality. Failure to do so can result in increased exposure rates, but success in maintaining the system cannot be considered a direct cause of decreased exposure rates.

DISCUSSING RADIATION RISK VERSUS BENEFIT WITH PATIENTS

The radiographer is often in the position of discussing radiation risk versus benefit with patients. To the attending physician, and sometimes even to the radiologist, the radiographer must represent the patient's interest in reducing dose. At the same time the radiographer must represent, to the patient, the physician's interest in maximizing diagnostic information. These points of view generally oppose one another. One exception is the use of higher kVp to produce a lower contrast. In this example, patient dose is decreased and the diagnostic information is increased.

Minimizing Exposure Dose by Emphasizing Risk

The patient's interest in reducing the total exposure dose must be represented even when the patient does not express such an interest. Some patients even express an opposite interest, as often occurs with minor complaints, such as lung congestion or a sprained ankle, when the patient arrives in the physician's office, a clinic or an emergency room with a request for an x-ray examination. When patients assume this attitude, the physician may prescribe an x-ray examination as a placebo. Most medical ethicists consider the prescription of a procedure for the purpose of deceiving the patient, or a procedure known to be without specific efficacy, to be unethical. This includes unnecessary radiographic examinations, which are known to be potentially detrimental.

In such a situation, the radiographer should perceive an obligation to act in such a way as to eliminate the request for the examination or at least to reduce the number of exposures. Through demonstration of professional competence, the radiographer can obtain the stature necessary to permit consultation regarding modification or elimination of examination requests.

Part of gaining this type of respect is the ability to make well considered judgments on when to advocate reductions in patient exposure dose and when to advocate additional examinations. These judgments require all the radiographer's knowledge of anatomy, physics, radiation biology, positioning, pathology, im-

aging equipment and, especially, clinical experience. For example, a radiographer should advocate an additional projection of the abdomen when an erect radiograph for an abdominal obstruction series fails to demonstrate the top of both diaphragms. Conversely, the radiographer is acting professionally when advocating the elimination of separate wrist projections when both hand and wrist examinations have been requested but there is visible trauma only to the hand, the patient has no complaint of wrist pain, and the clinical history does not indicate a high probability of referred stress to the wrist joint.

For examinations that are of questionable need, the radiographer is within professional rights to inform the patient of his or her right to refuse an examination. **Under no circumstances should this be perceived by the radiographer as cause to inform the patient that an examination is not needed or to give a personal opinion regarding medical treatment or diagnosis**. The radiographer must have an introductory background in medical law in order to make judgments of this type. For example, minors, persons who have had their civil rights suspended (such as persons in the custody of law enforcement officers), mentally incompetent persons and some other categories of patients do not have the right to refuse examinations.

The selection of patients for x-ray examinations has been the focus of considerable study, particularly when the chest, lumbar spine and skull are involved. Patients can be divided into asymptomatic and symptomatic groups when determining which should be exposed to radiation. Asymptomatic patients should be examined only when there is significant cause, after considering the incidence and severity of the condition, the detection reliability of the examination, and the usefulness of the examination in treatment. The most common examples of asymptomatic patients are those undergoing screening procedures. Although mass chest and lumbar spine screening are now discouraged, mammography screening is encouraged for women of certain age groups. Symptomatic patients are more likely to require x-ray examination but should fit two major criteria: the examination must be capable of providing the desired information, and the information, even if negative, is expected to contribute to the management of the patient. The radiographer has a responsibility to contribute to these criteria whenever possible, primarily through history-taking. When circumstances that appear to routinely violate these principles are encountered, the radiographer should consider withdrawing from participation in the examinations.

Maximizing Diagnostic Information by Emphasizing Benefit

While advocating a reduction of patient exposure dose, the radiographer must simultaneously impress on the patient the physician's primary concern of maximizing diagnostic information. This includes establishing credibility with the patient by demonstrating competence in answering questions, taking a medical history, manipulating the x-ray equipment, exhibiting a professional demeanor and myriad other details. Established credibility permits the radiographer to convince the patient to follow breathing instructions, endure an additional uncomfortable projection or permit a repeated exposure.

The benefit of radiographic procedures has been an unquestionable aspect of medicine since Röntgen's discovery in 1895. Although this is generally accepted by the public, some patients have a heightened anxiety about exposure, and there are periodic increases in publicity that cause concern over medical radiation exposures. These issues must be addressed by the radiographer as the primary professional contact with the patient. **The radiographer has a responsibility to advocate medically necessary examinations and to assure the patient that the benefit outweighs the risk.**

The primary duty of the radiographer on this issue is to provide the patient with sufficient information to permit the patient to make an informed decision regarding the examination. This can be a very sensitive topic and must be approached in a thorough and professional manner. One of the best accepted methods of providing this information to the patient is through comparison of relative radiation risks. Table 35–5 illustrates comparative risks of chest x-ray examinations to other radiation risks that are common public knowledge. Another effective method of illustrating relative radiation risk is through a catalog of risks, such as the extract shown in Table 35–6.

When a patient requests information about the exact dose for a particular examination, the radiographer has an obligation to attempt to provide that information. However, it is important that the patient have a basic understanding that only an **approximate entrance skin dose** can be provided. The radiographer should inform the patient that the entrance skin dose is the maximum exposure dose and that the actual dose to the area of interest would be significantly less.

The Center for Devices and Radiological Health of the United States Food and Drug Administration has advocated the use of radiation record cards for patients. Proposals have been made for credit card style cards with magnetic record tapes for running totals of approximate entrance skin exposure dose. There are currently x-ray units available with print-out capability so this information can be given to patients upon request. As the public becomes more informed about the potential risks of

TABLE 35–5

GROSS COMPARISON OF RELATIVE RADIATION LEVELS*

	Scaled Relative Dose[†]
Natural background	50–100 chest examinations/year
Diagnostic radiology	0.1–500 chest examinations/study[‡]
Nuclear imaging	50–1,000 chest examinations/study[¶]
Start of acute radiation syndrome	30,000 chest examinations in *one* day
Lethal dose (LD50$_{30}$)	300,000 chest examinations in *one* day
Radiation therapy (small volumes of tissue)	100,000–1,000,000 chest examinations in a few weeks
Ultrasound	This scale does not apply
NMR	This scale does not apply

* Due to differential tissue distributions and sensitivities, such estimates are intended to be rough comparisons (50–100 chest examinations will have different biologic effects from that resulting from 100–200 mrads of natural background.

[†]1 PA chest examination = 5 millirad average tissue dose in thorax, which corresponds to a whole body equivalent dose of 2 millirads.

[‡]Dependent on examination types and techniques.

[¶]Does not properly account for doses received in those tissues in which the radionuclide concentrates.

(Reprinted with permission of Joseph P. Whalen and Stephen Balter, *Radiation Risks in Medical Imaging*, Chicago: Yearbook Medical Publishers, Inc., 1984.)

TABLE 35–6

ESTIMATED LOSS OF LIFE EXPECTANCY DUE TO VARIOUS CAUSES*

Lifestyle	Estimated Loss in Days
Being unmarried—male	3,500
Cigarette smoking—male	2,250
Being unmarried—female	1,600
Cigarette smoking—female	800
Dangerous job	300
Motor vehicle accidents	207
Alcohol (U.S. average)	130
Accidents at home	95
Average job	74
Radiation job	40
Accidents to pedestrians	37
Safest job	30
Natural radiation	8
Medical x-rays	6

Individual Action	Estimated Loss in Minutes
Buying a small car	7,000
Coast to coast drive	1,000
Coast to coast flight	100
Smoking a cigarette	10
Calorie-rich dessert	50
Non-diet soft drink	15
Diet soft drink	0.15
Crossing a street	0.4
Extra driving	0.4/mile
Not fastening seat belt	0.1/mile
1 mrem of radiation	1.5

* Adapted from Cohen and Lee. Reproduced from *Health Physics*. 36:707, 1979. Used by permission of the Health Physics Society.

Adapted with permission of Bernard L. Cohen and I-Sing Lee, "A catalog of risks," *Health Physics* 36, 707–722, 1979.

medical radiation exposure, additional developments in this arena can be expected.

The patient has the right to refuse radiographic examination. The radiographer is bound by professional duty to respect this right and to advocate it to physicians, including radiologists, if necessary. As long as the patient has the right to refuse treatment, proceeding with an examination under protest from the patient may place the radiographer at risk of malpractice action (usually as assault and battery).

SUMMARY

A predominant concern of radiographers is how to reduce the radiation exposure dose to the patient. This concern is reflected in every decision that is made, especially when choosing technique exposure factors. The conscientious radiographer can reduce the patient exposure dose by at least 50 percent in most examinations by choosing appropriate exposure factors.

The maximum exposure dose received by the patient is not at the area of interest but at the skin entrance to the body. This is known as the entrance skin dose and is calculated at the minimum SOD. Exposure to patients can be estimated by recording mR/mAs when the x-ray unit is calibrated. This is calculated by recording a dose reading for any average exposure and then dividing the dose reading in mR by the total mAs used. The expression mR/mAs represents the formula itself. The mR/mAs measurements are usually recorded for an SID of 40″ (100 cm). To estimate the entrance skin exposure dose, the inverse square law must be applied to determine the exposure for the source-to-entrance skin distance. For fluoroscopy, the estimated dose is calculated in mR/min instead of mR/mAs.

Radiographers can reduce exposure dose to the patient through their communication skills, their positioning skills, and through proper selection of technical exposure factors. Technical factors include the kilovoltage range, mA, exposure time, distance, filtration, field size, gonadal shielding, subject part density, grids, intensifying screens, film and film processing.

The radiographer is often in the position of discussing radiation risk versus benefit with patients. To the attending physician, and sometimes even to the radiologist, the radiographer must represent the patient's interest in reducing the dose. At the same time the radiographer must represent to the patient the physician's interest in maximizing diagnostic information.

REVIEW QUESTIONS

1. What is the relationship between entrance skin dose exposure and other measurement points?

2. What is the mR/mAs for a calibration exposure of 80 kVp at 40 mAs that produces a total dose of 86 mR?

3. What is the total exposure for a patient measuring 26 cm when the SID is 40″ for an exposure of 70 kVp and 35 mAs and the mR/mAs at 70 kVp is 2.6 at 40″?

4. How can patient exposure dose be reduced through effective communication?

5. How can patient exposure dose be reduced through effective positioning?

6. What changes should be made in kVp, mA, time and distance if each is the only factor changed to reduce patient dose?

7. What are the variables, other than the four prime factors, that can be used to reduce patient dose?

8. What risk factors could be mentioned to answer a patient's inquiry about exposure dose for an examination?

9. What diagnostic benefits could be mentioned to answer a patient's inquiry about the need for an examination?

10. Describe an approach to discussing radiation risk versus benefit with patients, physicians and radiologists.

REFERENCES AND RECOMMENDED READING

Anderson, P. E., P. E. Anderson, and P. Vander-Kooy. Dose reduction in radiography of the spine for scoliosis. *Acta Radiologica* 23, 251–253, 1982.

Appleton, Margaret B., and Stephen R. Carr. Radiation protection in a neonatal intensive care unit: A practical approach. *Radiography* 50:592, 137, 1984.

Baker, D. G. How significant are the risks from occupational exposure to ionizing radiation? *Applied Radiology* 18:9, 19, 1989.

Ball, J. L. Does high kV reduce the dose?. *Radiography* 64:523, 163, 1978.

Barnhard, Howard J. The bedside examination: A time for analysis and appropriate action. *Radiology* 129, 539–540, 1978.

Baxter, A. Choice of kilovoltage. *Radiography* 64:524, 196, 1978.

Beauchemin, Roch. Telescopic gonad protector: Analysis and experimentation of a telescopic gonad protector. *The Canadian Journal of Medical Radiation Technology* 15:1, 39, 1984.

Bednarek, D. R. A protocol for exposure limitation in radiography. *Radiologic Technology* 53, 229–234, 1981.

Belanich, Mark M., Philip Iorio, Ruthellen Jonason, and James Summers. A simple, cost-effective method for determination of entrance skin exposures for diagnostic radiology examinations. *Applied Radiology* 16, 39–41, 1987.

Brown, Reynold F., John W. Shaver, and David A. Lamel. *The Selection of Patients for X-Ray Examinations.* Rockville, MD: U.S. Department of Health, Education, and Welfare, Public Health Service, Food and Drug Administration, Bureau of Radiological Health, HEW Publication FDFA 80–8104, January 1980.

Burkhart, Roger L. *Patient Radiation Exposure in Diagnostic Radiology Examinations: An Overview.* Rockville, MD: U.S. Department of Health, Education, and Welfare, Public Health Service, Food and Drug Administration, Bureau of Radiological Health, HEW Publication FDFA 83–8217, August 1983.

Bushong, Stewart. Radiation Protection. Chapter 2 in *Merrill's Atlas of Radiographic Positions and Radiologic Procedures.* 6th ed. 15–30. Philip W. Ballinger. St. Louis, MO: C. V. Mosby Co., 1986.

Butler, Priscilla F., Burton J. Conway, Orhan H. Suleiman, George H. Koustenis, and Charles K. Showalter. Chest radiography: A survey of techniques and exposure levels currently used. *Radiology* 156, 533–536, 1985.

Butler, Priscilla F., Alvin W. Thomas, William E. Thompson, Mary Ann Wollerton, and Jay A. Rachlin. Simple methods to reduce patient exposure during scoliosis radiography. *Radiologic Technology* 57:5, 411–416, 1986.

Cade, W. J. S., and M. J. Haddaway. Measurement of absorbed skin dose in tomography. *Radiography* 49:577, 24, 1983.

Cahoon, John B., Jr. Radiographic technique — its origin, concept, practical application and evaluation of radiation dosage. *Radiologic Technology* 32:4, 354, 1961.

Caprio, Michael L. The pregnant x-ray tech— providing adequate radiation safety for the fetus. *Radiologic Technology* 52:2, 161, 1980.

Cohen, Bernard L., and I-Sing Lee. A catalog of risks. *Health Physics* 36, 707–722, 1979.

Collen, Morris F., and Philip M. McClean. *Utilization of Diagnostic X-Ray Examinations.* Rockville, MD: U.S. Department of Health, Education, and Welfare, Public Health Service, Food and Drug Administration, Bureau of Radiological Health, HEW Publication FDFA 83–8208, August 1983.

Conference of Radiation Control Program Directors, Inc. Committee on Quality Assurance in Diagnostic Radiology. *Average Patient Exposure Guides: 1988.* Frankfort, KY: Conference of Radiation Control Program Directors, Inc., 1988.

Coulehan, John L., and Marian R. Block. *The Medical Interview: A Primer for Students of the Art.* Philadelphia, PA: F. A. Davis, 1987.

Coulehan, John L. Personal communication, January 6, 1990.

Davies, Jackie, and J. G. B. Russell. Carbon fibre faced cassettes in neonatal radiography: Their use and cost effectiveness. *Radiography* 52:603, 113, 1986.

Downey, Edward F., and Priscilla Butler. Less radiation and better images: A new scoliosis radiography system. *Military Medicine* 149, 526–528, 1984.

Frank, Eugene D. Use of the posteroanterior projection: A method of reducing x-ray exposure to specific radiosensitive organs. *Radiologic Technology* 54, 343–347, 1983.

Frank, Eugene, John Stears, Joel Gray, Norlin T. Winkler, and Alan D. Hoffman. Use of the P. A. projection: A method of reducing x-ray exposure to specific radiosensitive organs. *The Canadian Journal of Medical Radiation Technology* 15:2, 63, 1984.

Gibbs, S. Julian. Approaches to radiation risk estimation. *The Physical Basis of Medical Imaging.* 329–342. Editors: Coulam, Craig M., John J. Erickson, F. David Rollo, and A. Everette James, Jr. New York: Appleton-Century-Crofts, 1981.

Godderidge, Cecilie. A radiology department's response to consumer concerns regarding the hazards of low-dose radiation. *Radiology Management* 4:3, 1, 1981.

Huda, Walter, and Karen Gordon. Radiation risks to medical radiation technologists during pregnancy. *The Canadian Journal of Medical Radiation Technology* 17:3, 121, 1986.

Hall, Eric J. *Radiobiology for the Radiologist.* 3rd ed. Philadelphia, PA: J. B. Lippincott, 1988.

Herman, Martin W. A comparative study of scattered radiation levels from 80 kVp and 240 kVp x-rays in the surgical ICU. *Radiology* 134, 552, 1980.

Hilger, Martin T. J. Radiation exposure to nursing personnel from portable radiographic procedures. *Radiology Management* 6:2, 16, 1983.

Hummel, Rudy H., Richard L. Wesenberg, and Gary M. Amundson. A computerized x-ray dose-monitoring system. *Radiology* 231, 1985.

Joseph, Lireka P., and Mary Ann Wollerton. *Extremity Radiography Following Trauma: An Overview.* Rockville, MD: U.S. Department of Health, Education, and Welfare, Public Health Service, Food and Drug Administration, Bureau of Radiological Health, HEW Publication FDFA 84–8232, August 1984.

Light, Mary C., Sabee Y. Molloi, Donald R. Yandouo, and Frank N. Ranallo. Scatter radiation exposure during knee arthrography. *Radiology,* 867, 1987.

Maillie, H. D., A. Segal, and J. Lemkin. Effect of patient size on doses received by patients in diagnostic radiology. *Health Physics* 42, 665–670, 1982.

Manny, Edward F., Harvey Rudolph, and Mary Ann Wollerton. *Pre-Employment Low Back X-Rays: An Overview.* Rockville, MD: U.S. Department of Health, Education, and Welfare,

Public Health Service, Food and Drug Administration, Bureau of Radiological Health, HEW Publication FDFA 81–8173, August 1981.

Manny, Edward F., and Roger L. Burkhart. *Measurement Techniques for Use with Technique/ Exposure Guides.* Rockville, MD: U.S. Department of Health, Education, and Welfare, Public Health Service, Food and Drug Administration, Bureau of Radiological Health, HEW Publication FDFA 85–8248, August 1985.

Mayes, Christopher D. Tomography—measurement of skin dose—were the results invalid?. *Radiography* 49:583, 173, 1983.

McClean, Philip M., and Lireka P. Joseph. *Plain Skull Film Radiography in the Management of Head Trauma: An Overview.* Rockville, MD: U.S. Department of Health, Education, and Welfare, Public Health Service, Food and Drug Administration, Bureau of Radiological Health, HEW Publication FDFA 81–8172, August 1981.

McCullough, E. C. Exposure requirements in diagnostic roentgenologic procedures. *Applied Radiology*, 95–101, 1976.

McGlone, W. E. Radiation protection of the reproductive organs during radiography of the hip joints. *Radiologic Technology* 41, 277–279, 1970.

McDormand, C., and T. Pel. Scoliosis radiography—let's reduce patient exposure. *The Canadian Journal of Medical Radiation Technology* 17:1, 37, 1986.

Miller. Biological effects of diagnostic irradiation. *Radiologic Technology* 48:1, 11–16, 1976.

Milner, S. C., and E. Naylor. An estimation of doses received by patients in a diagnostic x-ray department. *Radiography Today* 55:622, 16, 1989.

National Council on Radiation Protection and Measurements. *Exposure of the Population in the United States to Ionizing Radiation.* Report 93. Bethesda, MD: NCRP, 1987.

Novitch, Mark. Evaluation of radiation exposure in diagnostic radiology examinations. *Radiology Management* 5:4, 33, 1983.

Noz, Marilyn E., and Gerald Q. Maguire. *Radiation Protection in the Radiologic and Health Sciences.* 2nd ed. Philadelphia, PA: Lea & Febiger, 1985.

Overutilization of x-rays. *Radiologic Technology* 51:2, 241, 1979.

Pagel, John W. Radiation protection in diagnostic radiology. *The Physical Basis of Medical Imaging.* 303–328. Editors: Coulam, Craig M., John J. Erickson, F. David Rollo, and A. Everette James, Jr. New York; Appleton-Century-Crofts, 1981.

Phillips, Leon A. *A Study of the Effect of High Yield Criteria for Emergency Room Skull Radiography.* Rockville, MD: U.S. Department of Health, Education, and Welfare, Public Health Service, Food and Drug Administration, Bureau of Radiological Health, HEW Publication FDFA 78–8069, July 1978.

Radiation exposure from diagnostic radiology exams: General recommendations. *Radiology Management* 8:2, 49, 1986.

Radiation safety program for diagnostic radiology departments. *Radiologic Technology* 52:3, 321, 1980.

Ragozzino, Mark W. Average fetal depth in utero: Data for estimation of fetal absorbed radiation dose. *Radiology*, 513, 1986.

Robinson, T., J. A. Becker, and A. P. Olson. Clinical comparison of high-speed rare-earth screen and par-speed screen for diagnostic efficacy and radiation dosage. *Radiology* 145, 214–216, 1982.

Rosenstein, Marvin. *Handbook of Selected Tissue Doses for Projections Common in Diagnostic Radiology.* Rockville, MD: U.S. Department of

Health, Education, and Welfare, Public Health Service, Food and Drug Administration, Bureau of Radiological Health, HEW Publication FDFA 89–8031, December 1988.

Rossi, Raymond P., Burdell Harnisch, and William R. Hendee. Reduction of radiation exposure in radiography of the chest. *Radiology* 144, 909–914, 1982.

Shleien, B., T. T. Tucker, and D. W. Johnson. *The Mean Active Bone Marrow Dose to the Adult Population of the United States from Diagnostic Radiology.* Rockville, MD: U.S. Department of Health, Education, and Welfare, Public Health Service, Food and Drug Administration, Bureau of Radiological Health, HEW Publication FDFA 77–8013, January 1977.

Shrimpton, P. C. Monitoring the dose to patients undergoing common x-ray examinations. *Radiography Today* 54:619, 38, 1989.

Shrimpton, P. C. Monitoring the dose to patients undergoing common x-ray examinations. *Radiography Today* 54:619, 1988.

Skubic, Stanley E., and Panos P. Fatouros. Absorbed breast dose: Dependence on radiographic modality and technique and breast thickness. *Radiology,* 263, 1986.

Statkiewicz, Mary Alice, and E. Russell Ritenour. *Radiation Protection for Student Radiographers.* Denver, CO: Multi-Media Publishing, Inc., 1983.

Stears, John G., Joel E. Gray, and Eugene D. Frank. Radiologic exchange (dose reduction with 105 mm spot films). *Radiologic Technology* 60:6, 515–516, 1989.

Strategies for reducing health hazards from medical x-rays. *The Canadian Journal of Medical Radiation Technology* 13:4, 159, 1982.

Travis, Elizabeth LaTorre. *Primer of Medical Radiobiology.* 2nd ed. Chicago, IL: Yearbook Medical Publishers, 1989.

Trefler, Martin. Radiation exposure reduction using carbon fiber. *Radiology,* 751, 1982.

Trout, E. Dale, John P. Kelley, and George A. Cathey. The use of filters to control radiation exposure to the patient in diagnostic roentgenology. *The American Journal of Roentgenology 67,* 946–963, 1952.

Tyndall, Donald A., and Susan M. Bedsole. Exposure reduction and image quality for pantomographic radiography. *Radiologic Technology* 59:1, 51–53, 1987.

U.S. Department of Health, Education, and Welfare. *Gonad Shielding in Diagnostic Radiology.* Rockville, MD: U.S. Department of Health, Education and Welfare, Public Health Service, Food and Drug Administration, Bureau of Radiological Health, HEW Publication FDFA 75–8024, June 1975.

U.S. Department of Health, Education, and Welfare. *Specific Area Gonad Shielding: Recommendation for Use on Patients During Medical Diagnostic X-Ray Procedures.* Rockville, MD: U.S. Department of Health, Education, and Welfare, Public Health Service, Food and Drug Administration, Bureau of Radiological Health, HEW Publication FDFA 76–8054, August 1976.

U.S. Department of Health, Education, and Welfare. *The Selection of Patients for X-Ray Examinations: The Pelvimetry Examination.* Rockville, MD: U.S. Department of Health, Education, and Welfare, Public Health Service, Food and Drug Administration, Bureau of Radiological Health, HEW Publication FDFA 80–8128, July 1980.

U.S. Department of Health, Education, and Welfare. *Procedures to Minimize Diagnostic X-Ray Exposure of the Human Embryo and Fetus.* Rockville, MD: U.S. Department of Health, Education, and Welfare, Public Health Service, Food and Drug Administration, Bureau of Radiological Health, HEW Publication FDFA 81–8178, August 1981.

U.S. Department of Health, Education, and Welfare. *The Selection of Patients for X-Ray Examinations: Chest X-Ray Screening Examinations.* Rockville, MD: U.S. Department of Health, Education, and Welfare, Public Health Service, Food and Drug Administration, Bureau of Radiological Health, HEW Publication FDFA 83–8204, August 1983.

U.S. Department of Health, Education, and Welfare. *Nationwide Evaluation of X-Ray Trends (NEXT)—Eight Years of Data (1974–1981).* Rockville, MD: U.S. Department of Health, Education, and Welfare, Public Health Service, Food and Drug Administration, Bureau of Radiological Health, HEW Publication FDFA 84–8229, April 1984.

U.S. Department of Health, Education, and Welfare. *The Selection of Patients for X-Ray Examinations: Presurgical Chest X-Ray Screening Examinations.* Rockville, MD: U.S. Department of Health, Education, and Welfare, Public Health Service, Food and Drug Administration, Bureau of Radiological Health, HEW Publication FDFA 86–8261, April 1986.

U.S. Department of Health, Education, and Welfare. *The Selection of Patients for X-Ray Examinations: Skull X-Ray Examination for Trauma.* Rockville, MD: U.S. Department of Health, Education, and Welfare, Public Health Service, Food and Drug Administration, Bureau of Radiological Health, HEW Publication FDFA 86–8263, June 1986.

Watkins, Gary L. Public health risks from low dose medical radiation. *Radiologic Technology* 59:2, 160, 1988.

Weatherburn, G. C. Reducing radiation doses to the breast, thyroid and gonads during diagnostic radiography. *Radiography* 49, 151–156, 1983.

Wesenberg, Richard, and Gary M. Amundson. Fluoroscopy in children: Low-exposure technology. *Radiology* 153:1, 243–247, 1984. Wesenberg, Richard L., Joel D. Blumhagen, Raymond P. Rossi, Sashia W. Hilton, Joan M. Gilbert, and Deborah J. Nedeau. Low-dose radiography of children. *Radiologic Technology* 51:5, 641, 1980.

Whalen, Joseph P., and Stephen Balter. *Radiation Risks in Medical Imaging.* Chicago, IL: Yearbook Medical Publishers, Inc., 1984.

Winkler, Norlin T. Minimizing radiation exposure of patients and personnel. *Radiologic Technology* 41:3, 142–149, 1969.

Wochos, John F., and John R. Cameron. *Patient Exposure from Diagnostic X-Rays: An Analysis of 1972–1974 NEXT Data.* Rockville, MD: U.S. Department of Health, Education, and Welfare, Public Health Service, Food and Drug Administration, Bureau of Radiological Health, HEW Publication FDFA 77–8020, April 1977.

Yoshizumi, Terry T., Kenneth T. Drummond, Jill O. Freeman, and Martha Mullett. Radiation safety and protection of neonates in radiological exams. *Radiologic Technology* 58:5, 405, 1987.

Young, Anthony T. Surface shield: A device to reduce personnel radiation exposure. *Radiology*, 801, 1986.

UNIT V: SPECIAL IMAGING SYSTEMS

To complete a basic foundation in the principles of radiographic imaging, several special imaging systems deserve consideration. These include the use of specialized diagnostic equipment for **mobile radiography, fluoroscopy**—the oldest and most common dynamic radiographic modality—and conventional **tomography**. Several **specialized techniques** that use diagnostic radiography, including stereoradiography, magnification, duplication, subtraction and xeroradiography, should be employed when they can enhance the diagnostic image.

Many modern imaging modalities utilize computers to accomplish digital **image processing**. These include **computed tomography** and **magnetic resonance imaging**, which, although recognized as specialty areas within radiologic technology, continue to serve as extensions of the radiographer's knowledge.

The specialty areas of ultrasound, nuclear medicine and radiation therapy (oncology), although within the scope of departments of radiology, are not addressed in this text because they are recognized as separate established professional disciplines with their own accreditation and certification processes. Proper study of these professions generally requires a recognized educational program of one or more years encompassing the study of subjects beyond the realm of this text.

A thorough study of the five units of this text—**Creating the Beam, Creating the Image, Analyzing the Image, Comparing Exposure Systems** and **Special Imaging Systems**—provides the thorough physical basis required of the radiographer.

A basic knowledge of physics and imaging must be combined with a thorough understanding of anatomy, physiology, pathology and positioning to give the radiographer the scientific foundation essential to making him competent in his field. Only when this foundation is coupled with an elementary understanding of human interactions and some clinical experience does the truly professional radiographer emerge.

36 MOBILE RADIOGRAPHY

Come, come, and sit you down. You shall not budge!
You go not till I set you up a glass
Where you may see the inmost part of you.

Shakespeare, *Hamlet*, III, iv, 18.

OUTLINE

SPECIAL PATIENT CONSIDERATIONS
SPECIAL RADIATION PROTECTION CONSIDERATIONS
TYPES OF EQUIPMENT
SPECIAL TECHNICAL FACTOR SELECTION
CONSIDERATIONS

OBJECTIVES

Upon completion of this chapter, the student should be able to:

1. Determine factors that contribute to the difficulty of mobile radiography.
2. Explain appropriate communications methods for mobile examinations.
3. Describe items that must be considered when arranging a patient room for a mobile examination.
4. Recommend methods for accomplishing acceptable variations of standard radiographic projections, especially chest examinations for air-fluid levels.
5. Assess the radiation protection rules for mobile radiography.
6. Differentiate light duty portable x-ray units from full power mobile units.
7. Evaluate the advantages of capacitor discharge and battery powered mobile units.
8. Explain why technical factor selection is more difficult during mobile radiography.
9. Describe the effect of various generator waveforms on kVp.
10. Identify advantages of standardizing mobile SID to one of 40″ (100 cm), 56″ (140 cm) or 72″ (180 cm).

11. Determine appropriate grids for mobile examinations.
12. Appraise various film/screen combinations for mobile applications.

The mobile radiographic examination is often the ultimate test of the radiographer's competence and skill. Accomplishing an optimal quality image without stationary equipment on the most difficult patients is a prime achievement. An understanding of the special considerations involved in mobile examinations is important for the radiographer.

SPECIAL PATIENT CONSIDERATIONS

Mobile examinations are more difficult to accomplish because there are so many additional variables—variables that would be constants with a stationary unit—when manipulating and positioning both patient and equipment. In many instances the reason an examination is requested at the bedside is to avoid transporting the patient because of his physical condition. Special adaptations of routine projections, imaginative equipment manipulation and innovative technical factor considerations are often required.

In surgery or the emergency unit, the stress of performing in a high tension environment may be added to the patient problems. These situations often include limitations to aseptic conditions and the presence of additional critical equipment (e.g., ventilators, multiple intravenous solutions, cardiac lines, etc.).

Communication

Although good communication with the patient is not a special consideration during mobile examinations, it is advisable for the radiographer to park the mobile unit outside a patient's room before entering to establish the proper rapport. The patient's permission must be obtained before proceeding with the examination, an explanation of the procedure should be given, and some rearrangement of equipment and room furnishings must usually be accomplished before bringing the mobile unit into the room.

The unconscious or incognizant patient requires the same explanation that a cognizant patient would receive. In many instances conscious but incognizant patients will be more cooperative if they hear a kindly voice of explanation prior to being touched. In surgery, the attending physician or operating room nurse must be consulted before entering, and this procedure should be followed even in an emergency suite.

Manipulating Equipment

Extreme care must be taken when manipulating equipment in a high technology environment such as intensive care, surgery or the emergency unit. The importance of other equipment must be considered, especially when it must be moved to make room for the x-ray unit. Care must be exercised to ensure that power supplies, oxygen tubes, catheters, intravenous lines, etc., have enough slack to permit movement. Finally, the radiographer must take care not to bump the bed or other equipment when moving the mobile unit out of the way or when driving it into position. Although this seems to be an obvious consideration, it is easily overlooked when one's mind is on the examination. Wall suspended television units are especially hazardous to both the x-ray tube and the radiographer's head. Neither the radiographer nor the patient can afford to be in a hurry when preparing for a mobile examination. It is the radiographer's duty to return all items to their original locations prior to leaving the area.

Positioning and Pathology

Patients requiring examinations with mobile equipment are often unable to assume standardized positions. Clinical experience and a thorough knowledge of acceptable positioning variants are required for this problem. For example, the inability of the patient to sit on the side of a bed requires an AP projection of the chest instead of the preferred PA projection. A patient in orthopedic traction may not be able to straighten the knee. Thus, a distal knee joint, mid-shaft and proximal hip exposure will be required to avoid gross distortion and to satisfactorily demonstrate the entire femur from a single projection. However, routine positioning practices should still be carried out to the extent possible. For example, during chest radiography most cognizant patients are capable of moving the scapula from the lung fields by rolling their shoulders forward, as they would if the examination were performed on stationary equipment.

Even with difficult or uncooperative patients, chest radiography should be performed with the patient in a semi-erect position in the vast majority of instances. Patients who have been confined to a bed, especially when pathology is present, are prone to disease processes that cause collections of fluid. Even elevating the thorax to the level of a pillow (perhaps only 10° from supine) may provide an opportunity to demonstrate a fluid level. Ideally, air-fluid level demonstration is best accomplished with the patient in a completely erect position, utilizing a horizontal beam (Figure 36–1). Demonstration of air-fluid levels when a patient is unable to assume an erect position causes gross distortion of anatomical structures (Figure 36–2). This distortion may be great enough to render the image useless for normal chest diagnosis. **When it is determined that air-fluid demonstration is a priority, two projections may be required: one for air-fluid levels and the other for a normal projection of the chest.**

The radiographer must not assume that an apparently well patient is able to be transported to stationary equipment. For example, an ambulatory patient on whom a mobile chest examination is requested, may in fact be under observation for myocardial infarct and may be susceptible to the sudden onset of potentially serious symptoms.

The radiographer must also not assume that every mobile examination will result in a poorer image quality than examinations performed in the radiology department. The same myocardial infarct patient may be capable of providing a detailed history that makes delineation of the heart shadow the primary image quality goal, of assuming an erect position on the edge of a bed, and of holding a cassette to permit a 72″ (180 cm) PA projection essentially identical in quality to an image produced with a stationary unit.

Because the mobile examination is performed at the patient's bedside, there is an increased possibility of artifacts, such as personal items (e.g., dropped hair pins, jewelry, etc.), layers of coverings (e.g., insulated blankets, several sheets, etc.), and medical equipment (e.g., nasogastric tubes, intravenous lines, catheters, electrocardiographic leads, clamps, etc.). A careful and tactful examination of the area of interest should be performed prior to exposure to locate and remove as many of these artifacts as possible. It is usually possible to carry out this examination during positioning, which also presents an opportunity to check for a necklace, bra, brace, etc. Clamps holding various tubes and lines should be moved as far from the area of interest as possible. For example, intensive care unit chest radiography often requires movement of intra-

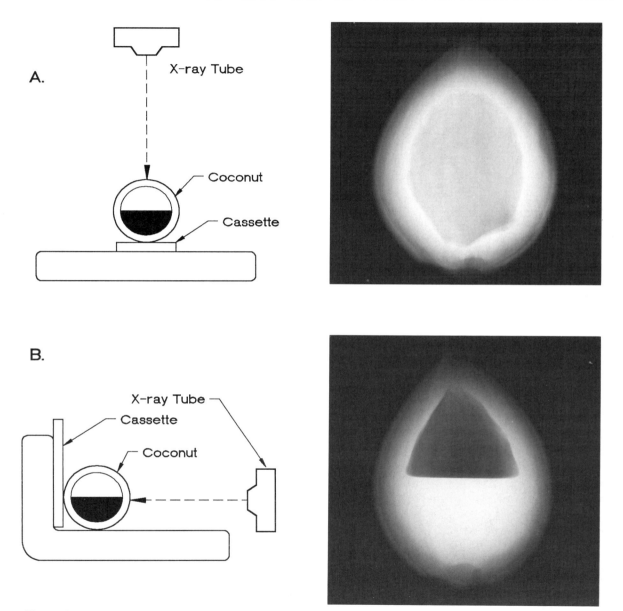

Figure 36–1A & B.   Demonstration of air-fluid levels. A coconut was used to demonstrate the effect of various positions and tube angles on air-fluid levels. (A) Recumbent AP projection with beam perpendicular to the air-fluid level. (B) Upright AP projection with beam parallel to the air-fluid level.

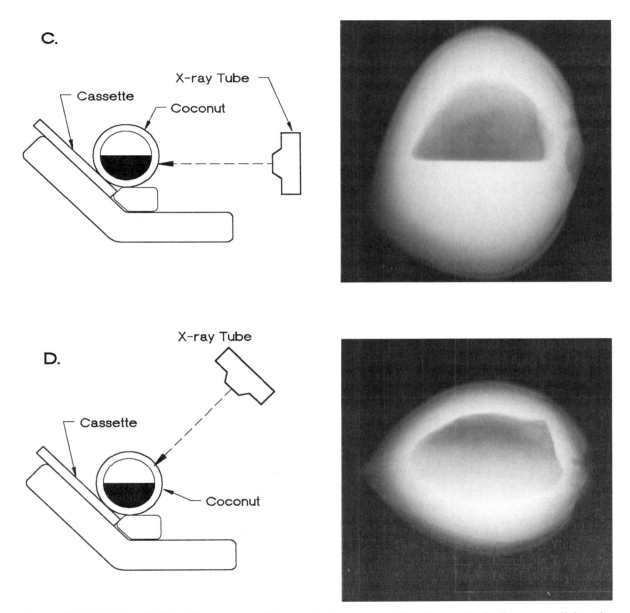

Figure 36–1C & D. (C) The film was at a 45° angle to the plane of the floor with the beam parallel to the air-fluid level and therefore parallel to the floor. (D) The film was at a 45° angle to the plane of the floor and therefore at a 45° angle to the air-fluid level, with the beam perpendicular to the film. Note that the central ray must be parallel to the floor in order to demonstrate distinct air-fluid levels.

Figure 36–2.   A chest radiograph demonstrating distortion due to improper source-to-image receptor alignment during a mobile examination. The central ray and film were not perpendicular to one another.

venous, respiratory and cardiac lines from over the lung fields. **A nursing staff member or physician should be consulted before moving any lines, especially venous and arterial**. It is desirable to limit coverings to a single smoothed layer of gown or sheet.

SPECIAL RADIATION PROTECTION CONSIDERATIONS

During a mobile examination the radiographer is bringing a radiation hazard into an

area not designed for radiation protection. Professional responsibility for ensuring radiation protection becomes a fundamental operating procedure during all mobile radiography. This is a prime opportunity for radiographers to educate the public, health professionals, physicians and other patients concerning proper radiation protection practices. A duty exists to protect the patient, health workers, the public and oneself. The rules shown in Table 36–1 should never be violated. The mobile unit should not be used as a portable shield. When standing behind a mobile unit, a lead apron is required to ensure sufficient protection. Radiographers should also move to a maximum distance from the mobile unit by extending the exposure control cord prior to making the exposure.

TYPES OF EQUIPMENT

X-ray units are available in a wide array of sizes and capabilities, many of which can be classified as mobile. Although often described as portable units (the truly portable unit can be hand carried), the proper description is mobile. The need for mobile x-ray equipment has been apparent from the earliest days of radiography; one unit was designed to fit in a suitcase. During World War I, the Picker Corporation developed a mobile unit that has remained popular for bedside radiography in hospitals. Today there are two major classifications of mobile equipment: portable light duty units and full power institutional units (Figure 36–3).

Power Supplies

Light duty mobile units and some full power units obtain power from wall outlets. Although some older units required 220 volts, modern units are usually designed to use 110 volts. The more advanced full power units use batteries for a power supply and are capable of greater voltages. Units that are not battery-equipped may be susceptible to line voltage

TABLE 36–1
RADIATION PROTECTION RULES FOR MOBILE RADIOGRAPHY

1. Recognize a duty to protect your patient, health professionals, physicians, the public and yourself.
2. Request the public, health professionals, physicians and other patients to leave the immediate area prior to exposure.
   (Always inform these persons that you will be finished in a moment, request them to remain nearby, and inform them promptly when you are finished.)
3. Announce in a loud voice your intent to make each exposure and permit sufficient time for others to leave.
4. Carry at least two lead aprons: one for yourself, the other for your patient. If you have an assistant, he too must have an apron.
5. Never place your hand or any other body part within the primary beam.
6. Provide gonadal protection for your patient.
7. Achieve maximum distance from the patient (not the tube) immediately prior to exposure, in accordance with rules requiring the use of a 6' cord on mobile units.
8. Label and handle each cassette carefully to avoid repeats.

fluctuations due to other resistances operating from the same circuit.

When using a mobile unit that is drawing power from a wall outlet, the voltage compensator must be accurately adjusted immediately prior to exposure. Battery units are usually equipped with circuitry to monitor battery strength, and normal maintenance procedures include periodic replacement of old batteries. However, battery cell failure is a potential cause of erratic exposures.

Figure 36–3. A typical full powered mobile radiographic unit. (Courtesy of GE Medical Systems.)

Generators

Specialized generators have been developed specifically for mobile equipment. Capacitor discharge units and battery powered units are the most common. Capacitor discharge units produce a constant potential output while battery operated units produce output that is essentially 3ϕ (Figure 36–4).

Power Drive

An additional advantage of a battery powered unit is that power is available to drive the unit itself. In large institutions, power driven units quickly become the radiographer's best friend. The drive switch on a mobile unit should be of the dead-man type so that its release immediately disengages the power drive. The size and weight of a battery powered mobile x-ray unit are considerable and extreme care must be observed when piloting it. Patients and staff could be seriously injured by careless driving. Radiographers must be cau-

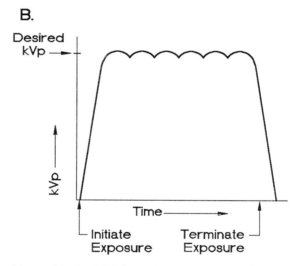

Figure 36–4. Mobile unit generator waveforms. (A) A capacitor discharge unit. (B) A battery powered unit.

tious in looking ahead, especially at corners and intersections, just as when driving a car.

AUTOMATIC EXPOSURE CONTROL

Automatic exposure control (AEC, AED or phototiming) is available for most mobile units in the form of a paddle ionization chamber, the Mobil-AID® Automatic Exposure Control (a registered trademark of Advanced Instrument Development, Inc.) (Figure 36–5). This unit functions exactly as an ionization chamber AEC in a stationary unit except that the chamber is contained within a paddle that can be positioned behind the cassette. The critical element in the use of the Mobil-AID® AEC is the accuracy of the positioning of the ionization chamber. All the elements of positioning used with stationary AECs must be applied to the positioning of the paddle and the positioning of the patient.

SPECIAL TECHNICAL FACTOR SELECTION CONSIDERATIONS

Establishing technical factors for mobile units almost always involves conversion of multiple variables (i.e., generator phase, filtration, grid, etc.) from stationary equipment technique systems. Because multiple conversions increase the risk of error, it is advis-

Figure 36–5. Mobil-AID® Automatic Exposure Control for mobile procedures. (Courtesy of Advanced Instrument Development, Inc.)

able to establish individual technique charts for each mobile unit. There are numerous special considerations when establishing these charts.

Kilovoltage

Most mobile units produce an x-ray beam with an average photon energy that is quite different from that of stationary equipment. Full power rotary 3φ units that are battery powered produce a waveform, as shown in Figure 36–4B. Because this waveform has essentially no ripple, it is actually more efficient and will produce a higher average photon emission than a 3φ, 12 pulse unit.

Capacitor discharge units have serious kilovoltage limitations. Careful examination of the waveform in Figure 36–4A illustrates the difference from pulse generators. With a capacitor discharge unit, voltage drops approximately 1 kV/mAs. Therefore voltage is about 0.5 kV/mAs less than initial kVp. The total voltage drop may be as much as 30 percent. (For example, an exposure at 80 kVp and 40 mAs would end at 56 kVp and average only 68 kV.) The mAs used with a capacitor unit should not exceed 30 percent of the kVp. For example, not more than 24 mAs should be used at 80 kVp.

Milliampere-Seconds

Low power units may not be capable of the high mAs required for grid radiography and may even require the use of kVp instead of mAs to obtain sufficient density for some examinations. When these problems are present, a motion problem will invariably develop because longer exposure times are used. For a relatively healthy and cooperative patient, a double or even triple exposure may be considered in order to overcome this problem. However, the radiographer must be **extremely** cautious not to overload the tube in this situation.

Distance

A primary cause of repeated mobile exposures is failure to measure distance. **Every mobile projection must have SID measured.** Radiographers who estimate SID must be within 15 percent to avoid producing a visible image density difference. A 72″ (180 cm) chest radiograph must be exposed between 61″ (153 cm) and 83″ (208 cm) to produce an optimal image from 72″ (180 cm) factors.

Figure 36–6 illustrates common problems encountered in mobile chest radiography. The size of the room and the location of the bed and ancillary equipment may not permit a mobile unit to be manipulated into a position from which a standard 40″ (100 cm) or 72″ (180 cm) projection can be obtained. Position A may be unobtainable because of tube height limitations. Position B is usually obtainable but does not optimize information because at an SID of 40″ (100 cm) it magnifies the heart and, when the patient cannot sit erect, does not provide the geometry to demonstrate air-fluid levels. Positions C and D may be obtainable

when air-fluid levels are required, but position C causes magnification.

The most reliable method of eliminating density fluctuations due to distance is to use only the two standardized distances, 40″ (100 cm) and 72″ (180 cm), with the addition of 56″ (140 cm) for mobile radiography. The 56″ (140 cm) distance should be employed only when 40″ (100 cm) is undesirable because of magnification, yet 72″ (180 cm) is not possible due to room and/or equipment limitations. As seen earlier in Table 23–3, mAs conversions are provided to maintain density at these distances according to the rule of doubling or halving mAs with each distance change (i.e., 40″ [100 cm] to 56″ [140 cm] to 72″ [180 cm]).

Grids

Proper alignment to a grid is difficult when the patient is supine but the grid is on a soft bedding surface, which easily permits the grid to tilt, unless the patient's weight is almost exactly distributed around the center of the grid. Proper alignment is even more diffi-

Figure 36–6.   Common distance problems during mobile chest radiography.

cult when the film is at an angle other than parallel or perpendicular.

Figure 36–7 illustrates the problems created by this common situation. The radiographer must attempt to align the central ray and the cassette perpendicular to one another. Although this is a relatively simple task when the relationships are as shown in Figure 36–7A, it becomes very difficult when the reference points are not parallel or perpendicular.

Most people can draw a simple angle, such as 45°, quite accurately, but accuracy becomes more difficult when the baseline is at an angle. Figure 36–8 demonstrates this difficulty. Angling off-center to a focused grid by as little as 5° can result in sufficient grid cut-off to visibly reduce image density.

Grids that permit wide exposure and centering latitude assist in these problems. **Low-ratio grids (5:1 and 6:1) are often preferred for mobile radiography**. Use of a linear instead of a focused grid also increases latitude.

Film/Screen Combinations

Because there are more variables with mobile radiography, it is appropriate to permit a wider latitude film and intensifying screen combination to be used. Wider latitude films usually exhibit slower speed, greater resolution and lower contrast. It is also appropriate to take the opposite position and utilize a high speed film/screen combination to reduce patient exposure dose and overcome the limitations of lower power equipment. However, when rotary 3ϕ battery powered units are available, their output capabilities remove equipment limitation rationales.

Other Factors

Other technical factors are not significantly different between mobile and stationary equipment, although the exact specifications for equipment will vary. For example, mobile equipment seldom requires fractional focal spots.

SUMMARY

Mobile examinations are more difficult because there are so many additional variables—variables that would be constants with

Figure 36–7. Alignment problems during mobile chest radiography. (A) A simple alignment problem correctly resolved. (B) A difficult alignment problem correctly resolved.

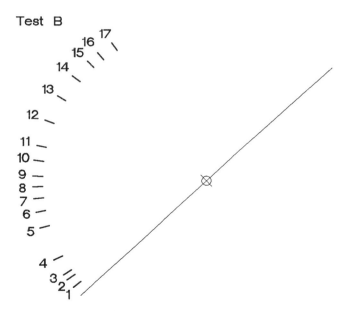

Figure 36–8.   Difficulty of angle estimation with an angled baseline. If a line is drawn from one of the numbers to the dot, which number would create a 90° angle? A 15° angle? A 37° angle? Record your answers for both tests A and B and then look on page 550 for the correct answers. Do not tilt your head or the book when completing test B.

a stationary unit—when manipulating and positioning both patient and equipment. In many instances the reason an examination is re-

quested at the bedside is to avoid transporting the patient because of his physical condition. Special adaptations of routine projections, imaginative equipment manipulation and innovative technical factor considerations are often required. Good communication with the patient is a necessary part of all radiographic procedures. The unconscious or incognizant patient requires the same explanation that a cognizant patient would receive.

Extreme care must be taken when manipulating equipment in a high technology environment such as intensive care, surgery or the emergency unit. Care must be exercised to ensure that power supplies, oxygen tubes, catheters, intravenous lines, etc., have enough slack to permit movement.

Patients requiring examinations with mobile equipment are often unable to assume standardized positions. Clinical experience and a thorough knowledge of acceptable positioning variants are required for this problem. Because the mobile examination is performed at the patient's bedside, there is an increased possibility of artifacts, such as personal items, layers of coverings and medical equipment.

During a mobile examination the radiographer is bringing a radiation hazard into an area not designed for radiation protection. A duty exists to protect the patient, health workers, the public and oneself.

X-ray units are available in a wide array of sizes and capabilities, many of which can be classified as mobile. There are two major classifications of mobile equipment: portable light duty units and full power institutional units. Light duty mobile units and some full power units obtain power from wall outlets. The more advanced full power units use batteries for a power supply and are capable of greater voltages. Specialized generators have been developed specifically for mobile equipment. Capacitor discharge units and battery-powered units are the most common. Capacitor discharge units produce a constant potential output while battery operated units produce output that is essentially 3φ.

Establishing technical factors for mobile units almost always involves conversion of multiple variables (i.e., generator phase, filtration, grid, etc.) from stationary equipment technique systems. Because multiple conversions increase the risk of error, it is advisable to establish individual technique charts for each mobile unit. A number of factors should be considered when establishing mobile technique charts, including kilovoltage, milliamperage, distance, grids and film/screen combinations.

REVIEW QUESTIONS

1. Why are mobile procedures often more difficult than those performed using stationary units?

2. What should the radiographer do before bringing mobile equipment into a patient's room?

3. What must be considered when manipulating mobile equipment in a high technology environment?

4. What must a radiographer do to adequately visualize air-fluid levels on a chest radiograph?

5. What are the two most common generators used for mobile equipment?

6. What type of generator waveform is produced with a full powered battery operated mobile unit?

7. Why is it important to measure distance (SID) for all mobile procedures?

8. What type of grids are preferred for mobile procedures?

REFERENCES AND RECOMMENDED READING

Barnhard, Howard J. The bedside examination: A time for analysis and appropriate action. *Radiology* 129, 539–540, 1978.

Cantwell, Kathleen G., Harry C. Press, Jr., Javan E. Anderson. Bedside radiographic examinations: Indications and contraindications. *Radiology* 129, 383–384, 1978.

Chesney, D. Noreen, and Muriel O. Chesney. *X-Ray Equipment for Student Radiographers*. 3rd ed. Oxford: Blackwell Scientific, 1984.

Cullinan, Angeline M. *Producing Quality Radiographs*. Philadelphia, PA: J. B. Lippincott, 1987.

Drafke, Michael W. *Trauma and Mobile Radiography*. Philadelphia, PA: F. A. Davis Company, 1990.

Ehrlich, Ruth Ann, and Ellen Doble McCloskey. *Patient Care in Radiography*. 3rd ed. St. Louis, MO: C. V. Mosby Co., 1989.

Eisenberg, Ronald L., John R. Akin, and Marcus W. Hedgcock. Optimal use of portable and stat examination. *The American Journal of Roentgenology* 134, 523–524, 1980.

Evans, S. A., Loyce Harris, C. P. Lawinski, and I. R. F. Hendra. Mobile x-ray generators: A review. *Radiography* 51:595, 89–107, 1985.

Osborn, Royce R. Improved portable radiographs of the trunk without the use of grids or Bucky. *Radiologic Technology* 32:2, 145, 1960.

Rossi, Raymond, Burdell D. Harnisch, and William R. Hendee. Evaluation of an automatic exposure control device for mobile radiography. *Radiology* Dec., 823, 1982.

Seeram, Euclid. *X-Ray Imaging Equipment*. Springfield, IL: Charles C. Thomas Publisher, 1985.

Trew, D. J. The 'cordless' mobile x-ray machine. *Radiography* 36:427, 159–164, July 1970.

Weaver, Kenneth E., Gregory J. Barone, and Thomas R. Fewell. Selection of technique factors for mobile capacitor energy storage x-ray equipment. *Radiology* 128, 223–228, 1978.

Answers to Figure 36–8

Test A	Test B
90° = 15	90° = 15
15° = 3	15° = 4
37° = 8	37° = 7

37 FLUOROSCOPY

. . . in February, 1896, fantastic, vague, and startling reports emanated from the foreign press regarding a wonderful device "invented" by Professor Salvioni of Perugia, Italy, called the cryptoscope, that permitted instantaneous visualization of human, living, and moving bones. . . . At about the same time Professor McGie of Princeton University also developed a . . . skiascope. Edison also constructed a similar device about which extensive publicity soon developed. He named it the fluoroscope.

Arthur W. Fuchs, "Edison and Roentgenology."

OUTLINE

HISTORICAL DEVELOPMENT
FLUOROSCOPIC USES
TYPES OF EQUIPMENT
FLUOROSCOPIC X-RAY TUBES
IMAGE INTENSIFICATION TUBES
FLUOROSCOPIC GENERATORS
IMAGE QUALITY
VIEWING SYSTEMS
RECORDING THE FLUOROSCOPIC IMAGE
MOBILE FLUOROSCOPIC EQUIPMENT
RADIATION PROTECTION DURING FLUOROSCOPY

OBJECTIVES

Upon completion of this chapter, the student should be able to:

1. Differentiate fluoroscopic examinations from static diagnostic radiographic examinations.
2. Describe a typical basic fluoroscopic image chain.
3. Explain the difference between the operation of a fluoroscopic and a diagnostic x-ray tube.

4. Describe the advantages of image intensified fluoroscopy over conventional screen fluoroscopy.
5. Explain the functions and operation of the image intensification tube input screen, photocathode, electrostatic focusing lenses and anode and output screen.
6. Explain the operation of multifield magnification image intensification tube.
7. Discuss the effects of minification and flux gain on total brightness gain.
8. Explain the basic function of a fluoroscopic automatic brightness control.
9. Discuss the factors that affect fluoroscopic image contrast, resolution, distortion and quantum mottle.
10. Explain the operation of an optical mirror viewer system, video camera CCD, video camera tube and video monitor.
11. Evaluate the three basic types of fluoroscopic viewing systems.
12. Explain the uses of dynamic and static fluoroscopic recording systems.
13. Evaluate various types of fluoroscopic recording systems for various clinical situations.
14. Explain the operation of a cineradiographic camera, a spot film recording system, 105 mm chip film and 70 mm roll film recording systems and magnetic and laser video disc recorders.
15. Discuss the resolving ability of various videotape recording equipment.
16. Relate problems with mobile radiographic equipment to mobile fluoroscopic equipment.
17. Discuss various methods of reducing exposure dose to the patient, the radiographer and the radiologist during a fluoroscopic examination.

HISTORICAL DEVELOPMENT

Fluoroscopy (fluoro) is a dynamic radiographic examination, compared to diagnostic radiography, which is static in character. Fluoroscopy involves active diagnosis during an examination. For this reason, fluoroscopy is primarily the domain of the radiologist. The radiographer's role becomes that of an assistant during the examination, although routine post-fluoroscopic radiography is the responsibility of the radiographer. **Radiographers should perform fluoroscopy only for static examinations** where diagnosis is not involved, such as spot filming the terminal ilium.

The invention of the fluoroscope is credited to Thomas A. Edison in 1896, the year after Röntgen's discovery of x-rays. However, technically speaking, Röntgen discovered x-rays fluoroscopically when he noticed their ability to demonstrate skeletal anatomy as he brought a lead disc into the beam and observed the dynamic movement of his own fingers projected onto a fluorescent screen. Fluoroscopic procedures have, therefore, been a part of diagnostic radiography since its inception.

A fluoroscopic imaging chain consists of a specialized x-ray tube with an image receptor, called the **fluoroscopic screen**, that can be viewed during an x-ray exposure. The first fluoroscopes were held by hand in front of the patient and x-ray tube and included a viewing hood to eliminate extraneous light. Later units attached the fluoro screen to the x-ray table. In both systems, the radiologist's face and eyes received the full primary beam. A great number of the pioneers in radiology became martyrs of the science because of the design of early fluoro units. Once the biological hazards of radiation became apparent, the design of the fluoroscope was changed to permit viewing by an arrangement of mirrors. This arrangement shielded the primary beam in a leaded enclosure while the mirrors transmitted the optical image to the viewer. **Image intensification tubes** were developed in 1948 and they resulted in video camera and monitor systems (see Figure 6–1) which began to replace mirror viewers. However, there is still a significant loss of detail with a video system, a fact that cannot be appreciated unless an opportunity to view a fluorescent screen through a mirror system arises.

FLUOROSCOPIC USES

Although the fluoroscopic image was preferred originally, the need to document findings, coupled with immense improvements in the resolution capabilities of diagnostic radiography, not to mention reductions in the exposure dose to the patient, caused fluoroscopy to become less popular. It is currently used only for studies that require observation of dynamic physiological functions, e.g., the flow of barium through the gastrointestinal tract, swallowing, the injection of a contrast medium into the heart, etc.

Fluoroscopic Positioning Previewing

Fluoroscopy is not intended to be used as a preview to positioning. Radiographers spend two years or more learning how to position the patient properly. There should be no reason for a radiographer to use fluoroscopy as a positioning guide. This procedure would cause unnecessary patient exposure to ionizing radiation. Radiographers should obtain a satisfactory image 95 percent of the time, and this

degree of expertise entails not just positioning but technical factors and equipment variations as well.

TYPES OF EQUIPMENT

The fluoroscopic x-ray tube and image receptor are mounted on a C-arm to maintain their alignment at all times (Figure 37–1). In the United States, federal regulations prohibit the use of a fluoroscopic x-ray tube when the entire primary beam is not resulting in an image. The C-arm permits the image receptor to be raised and lowered to vary the beam geometry for maximum resolution while the x-ray tube remains in position. It also permits scanning the length and width of the x-ray table. There are two types of C-arm arrangements, both described by the location of the x-ray tube. Under-table units have the x-ray tube under the table while over-table units suspend the tube over the patient.

The arm that supports the equipment suspended over the table is called the **carriage**. It typically includes an image intensification tube (on an under-table unit) or the x-ray tube (on an over-table unit), controls for power drive to the carriage, brightness (which regulates the tube mA), spot film selection, tube shutters, spot filming and/or cine camera, video input tube and other controls. Although it can be disengaged and pushed away from the table to gain access to the patient, exposure cannot commence until the carriage is returned to a full beam intercept position.

FLUOROSCOPIC X-RAY TUBES

Fluoroscopic x-ray tubes are very similar to diagnostic tubes except that they are designed to operate for longer periods of time at much lower mA. Where a typical diagnostic tube operates at 50–1,200 mA, **the fluoroscopic mA range is 0.5–5.0 mA.** The tube target must

Figure 37–1.   C-arm alignment of fluoroscopic x-ray tube and image receptor.

be fixed to prevent an SOD of less than 15″ (38 cm). The fluoroscopic tube is operated by a foot switch, which permits the fluoroscopist to have both hands free to operate the carriage and position and palpate the patient. Care must be taken to not accidentally activate the foot switch when the unit is in operating mode before or after examinations. Fluoroscopic tubes are equipped with electrically controlled shutters that permit maintenance of close collimation from the fluoro carriage during both fluoroscopy and spot filming.

IMAGE INTENSIFICATION TUBES

Early fluoroscopic screens were very dim. Dark adaptation, a procedure in which light levels are reduced for a period of at least 10–15 minutes to permit the rods of the eye to be-

come activated, was a time-consuming and irritating part of the radiologist's work routine. The exclusive use of the rod cells constituted a serious threat to diagnostic accuracy because visual acuity is controlled by the cones, which require daylight (photopic) levels of light in order to function. Photopic visual acuity is about 10 times greater than scotopic acuity. The brightness of the fluoro image was not raised to daylight levels until image intensification technology was developed in 1948.

An image intensification tube is designed to electronically amplify the brightness of an image. Modern image intensifiers are capable of increasing image brightness 500–8,000 times. Photopic visual acuity becomes active when the brightness is about 1,000 times that of a fluoroscopic screen. Their primary use is in fluoroscopy equipment, although variations of the design are used in other modalities.

A typical image intensifier is shown in Figure 37–2. The primary x-ray beam exits the patient and strikes the input screen of the image intensifier tube, which is a vacuum tube with a cathode and an anode. The fluorescent screen is built into the image intensifier as its input screen. **The fluorescent screen absorbs the x-ray photons and emits light photons,** which immediately encounter the photocathode (the cathode of the tube) that is in contact with the input screen to prevent divergence of the light beam. **The photocathode absorbs the light photons and emits electrons.** The electrons are then accelerated from the cathode toward the anode and the output screen by the potential difference that exists between the cathode and anode. At the same time the electron beam is focused onto the output screen, which is much smaller than the input screen. **Electrostatic lenses are used to accelerate and focus the electrons. The primary brightness gain occurs from the acceleration and focusing of the electron beam.** The acceleration of the electron beam increases its energy and its ability to emit light at the output screen. The focusing of the electron beam intensifies the image into a smaller area. **The output screen absorbs the electrons and emits light photons,** which are then available for viewing or further electronic processing by a video system. Note

Figure 37–2. An image intensification tube. The quantity of photons and electrons in the image changes at each stage of the intensification process, with the output significantly greater than the input.

the changes in the quantity of photons and electrons in the image at each stage of the intensification process.

The entire image intensification tube is encased in a lead lined housing that effectively absorbs the primary beam while permitting the intensified light photon image to be transmitted to the viewer. An ion pump device called a getter is used to remove ions produced during operation and to maintain the vacuum within the tube.

Input Screen and Photocathode

The input fluorescent screen consists of a 0.1–0.2 mm layer of sodium-activated cesium iodide (CsI) phosphors coated onto the concave surface of the image intensification tube. This surface may be made of glass, titanium, steel or aluminum and ranges from 6″ (15 cm) to 23″ (58 cm) in diameter, depending on the manufacturer and use. The screen is concave to maintain the same distance between each point on the input screen and its corresponding location on the output screen. Failure to maintain this distance would result in distortion of the image because points farther from the center would be more magnified. The CsI phosphors are packed together very tightly so they absorb about 66 percent of the incident beam, producing a good conversion efficiency, or quantum yield. The phosphors then emit light photons vertically, in proportion to the absorption, thus reducing the lateral spread of light photons that would reduce the image detail. As an example, a single 25 keV incident photon would typically produce over 1,500 light photons. This conversion efficiency permits the fluoro system to function with minimal activation of the phosphors.

An extremely thin protective coating is applied to the input screen to prevent a chemical interaction with the photocathode. The photocathode material is composed of photoemissive metals, usually cesium and antimony compounds, which are applied to the protective coating. The two materials appear to be a single coating when examined. The photoemissive materials absorb the light photons and emit electrons in a process called photoemission. The process is similar to thermionic emission except that the stimulation is light instead of heat.

Electrostatic Lenses

The electrostatic lenses are a series of positively charged electrodes located inside the glass envelope of the tube. Because the electrons are negative, the positive charge of the lenses accelerates and focuses the electron stream, which carries the fluoroscopic image. As with an optically focused image, the focal point reverses the image so the output screen image is reversed from the input screen image (right becomes left and superior becomes inferior). The concave input screen reduces distortion by maintaining the same distance between all points on the input screen and their corresponding locations on the output screen, regardless of the position of the focal point.

Magnification Tubes The greater the voltage supplied to the electrostatic lenses the greater the acceleration, and the closer the focal point moves toward the input screen. Image intensification tubes can be designed to magnify the image electronically by changing the voltage on the electrostatic lenses. They are often called multifield, dual-field, triple-field or quad-field intensifiers.

Increased voltage focuses the electrons at a point closer to the input screen and this causes the image to be magnified when it reaches the output screen (Figure 37–3). Magnification image intensifiers are capable of 1.5–4 × magnification, which is usually controlled at the fluoro carriage. Some tubes are capable of up to four different magnifications. Resolution can be increased from ≈4 lp/mm to

9" Mode

6" Mode

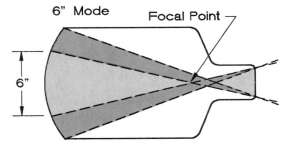

Figure 37–3. A magnification image intensification tube. Changes in the focal point produce the magnification.

≈6 lp/mm when the magnification mode is used. The tubes are described according to the diameter of the area of the input screen that will be imaged. For example, a 23/15 dual-focus tube has a 9″ (23 cm) input screen when operating normally and uses a 6″ (15 cm) area when magnifying. The magnification factor is calculated as:

$$\text{magnification} = \frac{\text{input screen diameter}}{\text{diameter of input screen used during magnification}}$$

Example: What is the magnification for an image viewed with an image intensification tube with an input screen diameter of 9″ (23 cm) that is using a 5″ (13 cm) diameter area during magnification?

Answer:

$$\text{magnification} = \frac{\text{input screen diameter}}{\text{diameter of input screen used during magnification}}$$

$$\text{magnification} = \frac{9''}{5''}$$

$$\text{magnification} = 1.8$$

The excess edges of the image are not transmitted by the output screen; therefore the primary beam field should be collimated to the viewing field when these tubes are operated in magnification mode. Minimal magnification is used for most studies because it reduces contrast problems due to minification and flux gain and permits viewing of the entire primary beam field.

Anode and Output Screen

The anode is positively charged and is normally supplied with about 25 kV. This charge causes a tremendous attraction of the negative electrons from the photocathode. The anode is positioned inside the glass envelope, immediately in front of the output screen. It has a hole in its center that permits the accelerated electrons to pass through the anode field and onto the output screen.

The output screen is also a glass fluorescent screen. It is a silver-activated zinc-cadmium sulfide phosphor (ZnS-CdS:Ag) that was also used as the input phosphor in early tubes. The electrons that strike the screen are converted into light photons that exit the tube. Because all phosphors emit light isotropically, an opaque filter is used under the output phosphor layer to prevent most of the light emitted in that direction from returning to the input screen, where it would degrade the image. Some newer intensifiers use a fiber optic disc in place of the glass output screen. Fiber optics eliminate the isotropic emission problem and are capable of transmitting the image some distance without loss of resolution.

Total Brightness Gain

Total brightness gain is a measurement of the increase in image intensity achieved by an image intensification tube. It is determined by two factors: minification gain and flux gain.

Minification Gain Minification gain occurs as a result of the same number of electrons that were produced at the large input screen being compressed into the area of the small output screen. Most image intensification tubes have input screens of 6″ (15 cm) or 9″ (23 cm), although 12″ (30 cm) and larger tubes have been available for special applications. The typical output screen has a diameter of 1″ (2.5 cm). The minification gain is calculated as the ratio between the area of the input and output screens.

$$\text{minification gain} = \frac{\text{input screen diameter}^2}{\text{output screen diameter}^2}$$

Example: What is the minification gain for an image intensification tube with an input screen diameter of 6″ (15 cm) and an output diameter of 1″ (2.5 cm)?

Answer:

$$\text{minification gain} = \frac{\text{input screen diameter}^2}{\text{output screen diameter}^2}$$

$$\text{minification gain} = \frac{6^2}{1^2}$$

$$\text{minification gain} = \frac{36}{1}$$

$$\text{minification gain} = 36$$

Minification gain is simply an increase in brightness or intensity, not an improvement in the quality or number of photons making up the image.

Flux Gain Flux gain is a measurement of the increase in light photons due to the conversion efficiency of the output screen. For example, if the output phosphor produces 50 light photons for each electron that strikes it, the flux gain would be 50. Flux gain does not take into account the conversion efficiency of the input screen. It deals only with the gain accomplished by the electron to light conversion at the output screen. Flux gain causes a decrease in image quality exactly as intensifying screens decrease resolution in diagnostic images as a result of the penumbral effect of individual phosphor crystals.

Total Brightness Gain Total brightness gain can be calculated by several methods. As a function of minification and flux gain, the formula is:

$$\text{brightness gain} = \text{minification gain} \times \text{flux gain}$$

Example: What is the total brightness gain for an image intensification tube with a minification gain of 36 and a flux gain of 60?

Answer:

$$\text{brightness gain} = \text{minification gain} \times \text{flux gain}$$

$$\text{brightness gain} = 36 \times 60$$

$$\text{brightness gain} = 2{,}160$$

However, the original formula was:

$$\text{brightness gain} = \frac{\text{intensity of output phosphor}}{\substack{\text{intensity of Patterson B–2} \\ \text{fluoroscopic screen}}}$$

A Patterson B–2 fluoro screen was chosen as the reference point because it was in common use at the time. This formula has lost acceptance because the Patterson B–2 screens vary from one batch to another and their deterioration is not linear. Although it appears that the term brightness gain will continue in use, its measure is a conversion factor that is the ratio of the intensity of the output phosphor to the input exposure rate.

$$\frac{\text{conversion}}{\text{factor}} = \frac{\text{intensity of output phosphor}}{\text{mR/sec}}$$

Output phosphor intensity is measured in candelas (cd), the unit of luminous intensity.

$$\text{conversion factor} = \frac{\text{cd/m}^2}{\text{mR/sec}}$$

Typical values for modern image intensifier systems are $80-250 \frac{\text{cd/m}^2}{\text{mR/sec}}$

This represents a gain of 8,000–25,000 times.

Brightness gain deteriorates as much as 10 percent per year because, just as with intensifying screen phosphors, the input and output screen phosphors age. Although difficult to measure, brightness gain can be evaluated by monitoring the radiation dose required to obtain a diagnostic image from a standard phantom, such as an abdomen or pelvis.

FLUOROSCOPIC GENERATORS

The generators used for static radiography are also used for fluoroscopy. Usually the operator's console includes a control that activates the fluoroscopic system and bypasses the static radiography system.

Brightness Control

A wide variety of systems with different names are used to automatically maintain satisfactory fluoroscopic image density and contrast. Automatic brightness control (ABC) is the most common term although automatic dose control (ADC) and automatic brightness stabilization (ABS) accomplish the same result. They maintain the brightness of the image by automatically adjusting the exposure factors as necessary according to subject density and contrast. Most ABC systems monitor the current flowing between the cathode and anode of the image intensification tube or the intensity of the output screen. In all systems, the primary beam is changed when current and intensity fall below established levels. Regulation of the primary beam can be accomplished by varying kVp, mA and pulse time. Most ABCs use combinations of these methods in a manner similar to a stepped variable kVp technique system. For example, kVp is gradually increased to the maximum acceptable contrast level, then mA is doubled while kVp is stepped down to the lowest acceptable contrast level and the procedure is started over again. All ABCs have a relatively slow response time, which is noticeable during routine fluoroscopic scanning because the image density adjustment lags a moment behind rapid changes in tissue density. Automatic gain control (AGC) is part of the video camera control system. It responds very quickly but does not change the x-ray exposure factors.

IMAGE QUALITY

Because the imaging chain of a fluoroscopic system is so complex, there are more factors that affect each of the quality elements of the image than in static radiography. In addition to contrast, resolution and distortion, quantum mottle must also be considered.

Contrast

Contrast is controlled by increasing the amplitude of the video signal, although it is affected by other factors. Image intensified fluoroscopic contrast is not only affected by scattered ionizing radiation but is also affected by penumbral light scatter in the input and output screens, and light scatter within the image intensification tube itself. Scattered ionizing radiation not only produces scatter photons arriving at the input phosphor but also produces some background fog from incident photons that are transmitted through the tube to the output screen or that backscatter from the output to the input screen. Light photons also scatter as they are reflected and refracted within the tube. Since light is emitted isotropically from the output phosphor, some of it will strike the input screen, causing a backscatter effect. All these effects combine to produce a background fog that raises the base density of the image. This affects image contrast exactly as film processing base plus fog affects film contrast. By raising the lowest density value, it decreases the total visible contrast. The overall effect is of reduced contrast. There is also a decrease in image contrast near the edges of the images.

Resolution

The primary limitation on most fluoroscopic resolution is the 525-line raster pattern of the video monitor. For nonvideo recording, such as spot filming or direct optical viewing, the ability to resolve recorded detail in a fluoroscopic system will vary depending on the geometrical factors, just as in static radiography. However, the geometrical factors are different, including minification gain, electrostatic focal point, input and output screen diameter and viewing system resolution (especially television system resolution), as well as OID and phosphor size and thickness. CsI image intensifiers are capable of ≈4 lp/mm. Optical mirror systems that permit indirect viewing of the fluoro screen are capable of ≈3 lp/mm. Magnification or multifield image intensifiers are capable of up to ≈6 lp/mm in the magnification mode.

Distortion

Size distortion is caused by the same factors that affect static radiographic magnification, primarily OID. Magnification image intensifiers that produce a magnified image by changing the electrostatic focal point within the tube do not significantly affect actual size distortion. Although a magnified image often appears to have more distortion, the distortion is also present in the minified image. It is simply easier to detect when enlarged.

Shape distortion is caused primarily by geometric problems in the shape of the image intensification tube. Although the input screen is concave, it does not completely eliminate edge distortion at the output screen. Electrons at the outer edges of the image tend to flare outward as they are electrostatically focused. Part of this problem is caused by the repulsion of electrons from one another due to their like charges. Figure 28–4 illustrates the edge distortion problem in image intensification tubes. This effect is called vignetting or pincushion distortion and may comprise 8–10 percent of the image area. Some of the vignetting effect is also caused by the effect of the divergence of the primary beam from the x-ray tube focal spot. Vignetting also causes image intensity to be greater at the center of the image and less at the edges. Consequently, distortion is minimized and contrast is improved at the center of the fluoro image.

Quantum Mottle

Quantum mottle is a blotchy or grainy appearance caused by insufficient radiation to create a uniform image. Since the quantity of photons is controlled by the mA and time settings, with static radiography any mA and time combination can be used to accumulate sufficient radiation to create a uniform image. With fluoroscopy, the time factor is controlled by the length of time the eye can integrate, or accumulate, light photons from the fluoro imaging chain. Because this period is 0.2 second, fluoroscopy must provide sufficient photons, through mA, to avoid mottle. Quantum mottle is also a large part of video noise and is a special problem during fluoroscopy because the units operate with the minimum number of photons possible to activate the fluoro screen. The factors that influence mottle are those that affect the total number of photons arriving at the retina of the eye. This includes radiation output, beam attenuation by the subject, the conversion efficiency of the input screen, minification gain, flux gain, total brightness gain, viewing system and the distance of the eye from the viewing system. Increasing the efficiency of any of these factors can assist in reducing quantum mottle, but the most common solution is to increase the fluoro tube mA.

VIEWING SYSTEMS

A number of viewing systems have been developed to deliver the image from the output screen to the viewer. These include optical mirror, video, cine and spot film systems. Some of these systems permit dynamic real-time viewing while others are for static images. The viewing time, resolution and processing time vary. Table 37–1 illustrates the characteristics of each system.

Optical Mirror Viewers

Optical mirror viewers are arrangements of mirrors and lenses to direct the output screen image to the viewer (Figure 37–4). The final mirror is adjustable to the height of the viewer's eye. However, a disadvantage is that the viewer must remain positioned exactly within a few degrees to view the reflected image. It is difficult to move in order to palpate a patient or do anything else without losing sight of the fluoroscopic image. In addition, only a single viewer can see the image, a disadvantage when several viewers could benefit from seeing it. The radiographer is at a distinct disadvantage with an optical mirror system because positioning landmarks cannot be located to assist in post-fluoroscopic positioning.

An optical viewing system does permit a beam splitter to be established by using a partially silvered mirror (e.g., 10 percent, 50 percent, etc.) to permit part of the light image to be transmitted instead of reflected. The transmitted light can then be directed to a cine or spot film camera. This permits simultaneous

TABLE 37–1

COMPARISON OF VARIOUS IMAGE INTENSIFICATION VIEWING SYSTEMS

System	Dynamic/Static	Real-time/Delayed	Resolution	Processing Time
Optical mirror	dynamic	real-time	highest	short
Video				
Real-time	dynamic	real-time	7th highest	short
Videotape	dynamic or static	delayed	lowest	short
Cine film				
16 mm	dynamic or static	delayed	6th highest	highest
35 mm	dynamic or static	delayed	5th highest	highest
Spot film				
Cassette	static	delayed	2nd highest	high
105 mm chip	static	delayed	3rd highest	high
70 mm roll	static	delayed	4th highest	high

Figure 37–4. An optical mirror viewing system.

viewing and recording of an image. However, the loss of light at the beam splitter requires additional intensity at the output screen, which can be achieved only by increasing the number of incoming x-ray photons and thereby increasing the exposure dose to the patient.

The most commonly used fluoroscopic viewing system is video. Closed circuit video is used with all transmission through cables to avoid broadcast interference. A system includes a video camera attached to the image intensification tube output phosphor and a display monitor for viewing. Fluoroscopic video cameras use a vidicon or Plumbicon™ tube or a charge-coupled device (CCD).

Video Camera Tubes

The vidicon and Plumbicon™ tubes are similar in operation, differing mainly in their target layers. A Plumbicon™ tube has a faster response time than a vidicon tube. The tube consists of a cathode with a control grid, a series of electromagnetic focusing and electrostatic deflecting coils, and an anode with face plate, signal plate and target (Figure 37–5).

Cathode The cathode consists of a heating assembly that forms an electron gun by thermionically emitting electrons that are shaped into a beam by a control grid. The electron beam is then accelerated toward the target but

Figure 37–5. A video camera tube.

is decelerated by the anode and a wire mesh in front of the target. This arrangement brings the electrons to a near standstill where they are straightened so the beam strikes the target perpendicularly. At the same time the focusing coils bring the electron beam to a point to maintain resolution. Pairs of deflecting coils serve to cause the electron beam to scan the target in a path known as a raster pattern (Figure 37–6). Commercial television uses a 525 horizontal line raster pattern, but high resolution video systems now offer 1,050 line systems. The speed of the electron gun movement is difficult to comprehend. The electron beam scans across the screen nearly 1,000,000 times per minute. However, to avoid flicker each scan is divided into two halves, with the first half scanning even-numbered lines and the second half scanning odd-numbered lines. This permits the 30 scans to be projected as 60 half frames per second and flickering is eliminated. (European systems operate at 25 scans for 50 half frames per second to match the 50 Hz current.) The raster pattern significantly reduces the resolution of the image and is the primary disadvantage of a video viewing system.

Anode The output phosphor of the image intensification tube is coupled with the face plate of the vidicon tube by fiber optics or optical lenses. This permits the light photons to be transmitted to the signal plate and target. The signal plate consists of a thin film of graphite charged with a positive voltage. It is thin enough to transmit light yet thick enough to conduct the electronic signal out of the tube. The target consists of a thin insulating mica coating in which globules of a light sensitive photoconductive material are suspended in a matrix.

Vidicon tubes use antimony trisulfide (Sb_2S_3) while Plumbicon™ tubes use lead oxide (PbO). The globules are approximately 0.001 inch in diameter and their size determines the resolving power of the tube. Each globule is capable of absorbing light photons and then releasing electrons equivalent to the intensity of the absorbed light. The loss of electrons creates a positive charge at the globule, which in turn causes the signal plate to become negatively charged. When the electron gun's beam scans the target, it discharges the globules. This sequential discharging of the globules releases the signal plate's charge as a pulsed signal.

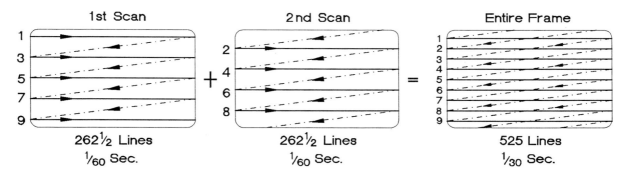

Figure 37–6. A video monitor raster scanning pattern. The electron beam scans the diagonal lines as active traces while the horizontal lines are inactive retraces to position for the next active trace. The electron beam scans 262½ alternate lines every ¹⁄₆₀ second and the second set of lines the next ¹⁄₆₀ second. Consequently, the entire 525-line raster pattern is scanned every ¹⁄₃₀ second. This is 30 times per second, which is 15,720 scan lines per second.

This sequential pulsing is the video signal, which can be translated back into an image via the electron gun of the viewing monitor.

The vidicon tube is connected to the output screen of the image intensification tube by either fiber optics or an optical lens system. Fiber optics are bundles of extremely small, light conducting cable. They are very durable but do not permit the image intensification tube output to be intercepted for spot filming. Spot filming requires an optical lens system similar to the old mirror optical viewing system. The use of beam splitting mirrors permits the image to be recorded by a spot filming device while being viewed. Other systems use a fully silvered mirror to interrupt viewing while deflecting the image for spot filming. Optical lens systems are considerably larger and are easily distinguished by the large size of the housing on top of the image intensification tube. They must be handled gently to avoid trauma to the lenses and mirrors.

Video Camera Charge-Coupled Devices (CCD)

A CCD is a semiconducting device capable of storing a charge from light photons striking a photosensitive surface. When light strikes the photoelectric cathode of the CCD, electrons are released proportionally to the intensity of the incident light. As with all semiconductors, the CCD has the ability to store the freed electrons in a series of P and N holes, thus storing the image in a latent form (see Chapter 5). The video signal is emitted in a raster scanning pattern by moving the stored charges along the P and N holes to the edge of the CCD, where they are discharged as pulses into a conductor. The primary advantage of CCDs is the extremely fast discharge time, which eliminates image lag. This is extremely useful in high speed imaging applications such as cardiac catheterization. Other advantages

are that CCDs are more sensitive than video tubes, they operate at much lower voltages, which prolongs their life, they have acceptable resolution and they are not as susceptible to damage from rough handling.

Video Monitor

A video monitor (or television tube) is a cathode ray tube (CRT) that consists of a vacuum tube with a fluorescent phosphor coated on the inside of the front screen and an electron gun with deflecting and focusing electromagnets (Figure 37–7). The electron gun is the cathode while the anode is plated onto the front screen. The monitor creates an image as the gun sprays the pulsed stream of electrons from the camera onto the screen phosphor. The gun follows the same raster pattern used by the camera. The phosphor crystals emit light when struck by electrons and transmit it as a visual image through the glass of the

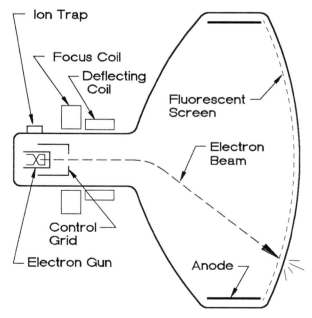

Figure 37–7. A video monitor [cathode ray tube (CRT)].

screen to the viewer. The video monitor is the most restrictive element in the fluoro imaging chain resolution. A 525 line monitor is capable of displaying between 1–2 lp/mm. Magnification of this image by the video camera or an optical system can increase resolution significantly. Video monitors often operate in the low kilovoltage range and can emit low energy x-rays.

The video monitor viewing conditions change with viewing distance, raster pattern and screen size. A 525 line pattern on a 9″ monitor has a minimum viewing distance of 37″ while 70″ is suggested for a 17″ monitor. High resolution patterns (1,050 lines) may be viewed closer; a 9″ monitor has a minimum viewing distance of 17″ while 36″ is suggested for a 17″ monitor. Contrast and brightness can be adjusted with controls on the monitor itself. However, these controls cannot compensate for contrast and brightness problems within the imaging chain. Conversely, the monitor should be checked prior to assuming a problem is in the imaging chain.

RECORDING THE FLUOROSCOPIC IMAGE

Dynamic Systems

Dynamic recording of fluoroscopic images has been limited to cine film and videotape, although laser videodisc would be possible if the recorders were not so expensive.

Cine Film Systems Cinematic or cine film imaging systems are sometimes referred to as cinefluorography. They consist of a cine (movie) camera positioned to intercept the image produced by the output screen of the image intensification tube. They require about 90 percent of the image intensity for proper exposure levels. Both 16 mm and 35 mm formats are currently in use. Although they dramatically increase resolution when compared to video

systems, they also require significantly greater patient exposure dose.

Cine cameras operate by recording a series of static images at high speed. When the images on processed film are projected at the same high speed, the eye becomes incapable of differentiating the separate images and perceives them as a single image in motion. Cine cameras must be synchronized to ensure that the pulses of radiation from the generator coincide with the opening of the shutter to expose the film. This is usually accomplished by operating the camera at either 30 or 60 frames (images) per second to coordinate with the 60 Hz rectified current operating the x-ray tube. Without synchronization, the output screen intensity would vary during the $\frac{1}{30}$ or $\frac{1}{60}$ second the shutter was open, resulting in some frames being underexposed. To assist in synchronization, the x-ray tube is grid biased or grid pulsed by placing a negatively charged wire across the cathode focusing cup. When the grid wire is turned off and on in pulses, it permits the cathode to pulse electrons to the x-ray tube anode, thus producing a pulse synchronized x-ray beam.

Cineradiographic film is usually viewed as both movie and stop-action film. It must be shown at 16 frames per second if smooth motion is to be perceived. Because the eye can perceive flicker at up to 50 frames per second, movie projectors operate at 24 frames per second and show each frame twice, thus pulsing the light 48 times per second and eliminating flicker.

The generator and fluoro x-ray tube in a cine system must be able to handle large heat loads. Although individual exposure factors for a single frame are minimal, when multiplied by the 30–60 frames per second required to produce cine, a significant heat load is produced. A 3ϕ, 12 pulse, 70–80 KW generator and a liquid cooled, 50–60 KW tube with a 0.6 mm focal spot are suggested.

Videotape Recording Both ½″ (VHS) and ¾″ (U-Matic) videotape recorders are used to record fluoroscopic images. The ¾″ format provided higher resolution until the advent of ½″ VHS-S high resolution recorders. The VHS-S system requires high resolution cameras, recorders, tape and monitors but offers a significant increase in resolution that is highly desirable in fluoroscopic systems. All systems utilize tape cassettes and operate the same as home video systems. Magnetic recording and playback heads produce and read a pattern of magnetic particles on the tape, producing a pulsed video signal. In most medical applications only the video track on the tape is used. The audio and synchronization tracks are left empty.

Static Spot Filming Systems

Spot film systems, although part of the fluoroscopic imaging chain, must be considered separately because they are limited to static images. They are necessary when a permanent record of the fluoroscopic examination is desired to document findings. They are therefore used with nearly every fluoro examination.

Spot filming permits a permanent static record to be made when information important to diagnosis (either positive or negative) is observed fluoroscopically. Spot filming remains extremely popular due to the ease with which it can be done, its low cost and the format (transilluminated hard copy films that are easily stored and viewed with other static images).

It is possible to use spot filming equipment to rapidly record a series of static images in a manner that functions as a dynamic record. Angiographic procedures that use serial static exposures can use spot filming when the image resolution is satisfactory.

Spot filming may be accomplished by several methods. Cassettes (radiographic film and intensifying screens in cassettes), 105 mm chip film and 70 mm roll film are the most common formats. Each has its merits.

Cassettes Cassette spot filming uses standard radiographic cassettes equipped with a pair of intensifying screens. Standard sizes are 9″ × 9″ (24 cm × 24 cm) although some units will accept 8″ × 10″ (18 cm × 24 cm) cassettes.

The cassette, stored in a lead lined compartment in the fluoroscopic carriage, can be moved into the primary beam field via controls located on the fluoro carriage. The x-ray tube current is simultaneously boosted to radiographic levels (100–1,200 mA). The carriage controls permit selection of the area of the cassette to be exposed, automatically collimate the tube and spot film mask shutters to the appropriate size, and position the cassette properly. Common selections are a full frame exposure, known as 1-on-1, two half frame exposures, 2-on-1 vertical and 2-on-1 horizontal, and four exposures, 4-on-1. The radiographer is usually responsible for replacing exposed cassettes when a radiologist is spot filming with them. In these circumstances the radiographer must observe the exposure selections to anticipate when a new cassette will be required. After the exposure is initiated an AEC terminates it and the cassette is automatically returned to the storage compartment. The process is slow because of the time required to move the cassette into place for exposure.

Cassette spot filming causes the highest exposure dose to the patient. Cassettes may require up to 300 μR per exposure at the entrance to the cassette. This may translate into a 30 mR entrance skin dose per exposure. It has been estimated that each spot film may be equal to more than a minute of fluoroscopic time. As with any radiographic examination, images should not be produced unless they will contribute significantly to the management of the patient. There is a definite tendency in the United States to overdocument negative findings because of malpractice litigation experiences.

105 mm Chip Film Chip spot filming uses 105 mm × 105 mm cut film. The process is relatively fast, up to 12 frames per second, as the only movement necessary prior to exposure is the beam splitting of the mirror.

70 mm Roll Film Roll spot filming uses a roll of film 70 mm wide. As with 105 mm chip film, the process is fast, up to 12 frames per second, as the only movement necessary prior to exposure is the beam splitting of the mirror.

Videodisc Recorders Videodisc recorders operate in a way similar to videotape recorders. The difference is that the videodisc unit records only a single image. In playback mode it displays the same image over and over 30 times per second. The process is extremely fast and playback can be instantaneous. Both magnetic and laser videodisc equipment are available. The magnetic format is less expensive and easier to operate but the laser format provides higher resolution. The magnetic format uses the arrangement of magnetized particles on the moving disc to cause a magnetic field to fluctuate and produce the video signal. The laser format uses a laser light to scan the disc surface, causing the light to be reflected to a photodiode to produce the video signal.

MOBILE FLUOROSCOPIC EQUIPMENT

Mobile C-arm fluoroscopic units are extremely popular for surgical procedures (Figure 37–8). When coupled to a videodisc unit, both static and dynamic imaging can be instantly available. The units operate exactly as do stationary fluoroscopic units, although controls may have different labeling. All the cautions and adaptations for mobile radiography are applicable to mobile fluoroscopy.

Figure 37–8. A mobile C-arm fluoroscopic unit. (Courtesy of GE Medical Systems.)

RADIATION PROTECTION DURING FLUOROSCOPY

The Patient

Fluoroscopic units operate with the minimum radiation output possible for the efficiency of the imaging system. There is no appreciable difference in the patient exposure dose between an optical mirror viewing system and a video system. The entrance skin dose for the patient is the surface closest to the source. With an under-table unit the entrance skin dose is measured from the surface next to the table top. With an over-table unit it is measured from the surface toward the fluoro carriage. The tabletop dose rate should not exceed 10 R/min and for most units should range from 1–3 R/min. The minimum source-to-skin distance is 12″ (30 cm) for mobile fluoroscopic equipment and 15″ (38 cm) for stationary equipment.

In the United States, federal law requires an audible five-minute timer. Although it can be reset as many times as necessary to complete a procedure, it is intended to serve as a reminder to the radiologist of how much total exposure time is being used. Fluoroscopy is interrupted when the five minutes have elapsed and the radiographer must reset the timer to continue the procedure.

Magnification image intensifiers cause increased patient exposure dose because the automatic brightness control (ABC) will increase the tube output to compensate for the loss of electrons within the image intensification tube during magnification. The x-ray tube should have the collimation shutters closed to the viewing image size when in the magnification mode. When magnifying, the output screen of the image intensification tube does not receive the entire image from the input screen so it is possible to irradiate tissue that cannot be viewed. Although these image intensifiers may have interlocks that automatically collimate when magnifying, attention to this detail decreases patient exposure dose.

Patient exposure dose for cinefluorography is significant. The minimum exposure dose required at the entrance to the image intensification tube is 20 μR per frame. This often translates into an entrance skin dose of 2,000 μR/frame (2 mR/frame). At 60 frames per second this results in 2 mR/frame $\times$ 60 frames/sec = 7,200 mR/min = 7.2 R/min.

Spot film recorders vary in exposure dose to the patient. Cassettes often require 30 mR per exposure while 105 mm or 70 mm film averages about 10 mR per exposure. Of course, these rates may vary with the sensitivity of the image intensification system and the exact mechanics of and film used in the recording system.

The Radiographer and Radiologist

A lead apron of at least 0.25 mm Pb/eq must be worn by all persons (other than the patient) who are present in the fluoroscopic room during exposure. An apron designed to cover the front and sides of the body is usually sufficient, although a wrap-around apron for both front and back should be considered if the radiographer is required to turn his/her back to the patient and x-ray tube during the procedure. Radiographers assisting during fluoroscopy must develop the ability to back and sidle around the room during exposures, always keeping the front of the body with its lead apron facing the patient and tube. If the hands must be placed within the primary beam, lead gloves of at least 0.25 mm Pb/eq must be worn.

The primary source of exposure to the radiographer and radiologist is the patient. It is worth noting that the highest energy scatter occurs at a 90° angle to the incident beam and that the patient on an x-ray table is usually at the same level (90° from a primary photon angle of incidence) as the gonads of the radiographer. It is also worth remembering that according to the inverse square law, a single step back from the patient will decrease the exposure dose exponentially (Figure 37–9). The slot immediately under the tabletop where the Bucky tray is positioned for diagnostic radiography is also at the gonadal level. Fluoroscopic units must have a lead shield to cover this slot. However, it must be brought into position by moving the Bucky tray to the head or foot of the table prior to beginning fluoro. Strips of lead rubber, forming a drape, are positioned between the fluoroscopist and patient to absorb the majority of the patient scatter. The radiographer has one advantage during fluoroscopy in that he/she may position himself/herself behind the radiologist. This not

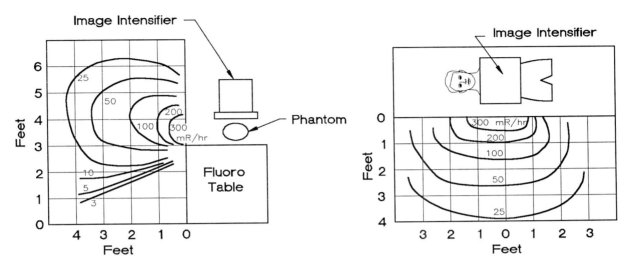

Figure 37–9. An isodose curve for a typical fluoroscopic unit. The shape of the curve illustrates areas of lesser dose during fluoroscopic procedures. (Adapted with permission from Wold, G. J., Scheele, R. V., and Agarwal, S. K. "Evaluation of Physician Exposure During Cardiac Catheterization," *Radiology*, Vol. 99, April 1971, p. 188–190.)

only adds an additional lead apron, but the entire body of the fluoroscopist is there to protect the radiographer.

Fluoroscopy units with cassette spot filming devices are available in front and rear loading models. The front loading models require the fluoroscopist to eject the cassette and lift the arm to permit the radiographer to remove the exposed cassette and insert an unexposed replacement. During this procedure it is difficult to operate the fluoroscopic unit, but if it is operated, the radiographer is protected from scatter by a lead drape, the fluoroscopist, and the fluoroscopist's lead apron as well as his/her own lead apron. Rear loading models require the radiographer to lift the exposed cassette from the rear of the carriage. This usually requires stepping onto a platform at the rear of the fluoroscopy table and places the radiographer within inches of the patient (the source of scatter radiation). Fluoroscopy units

should not be operated during replacement of spot film cassettes from rear loading units.

Others

The radiographer has a duty to require that anyone present in the fluoroscopy room during an examination wear a lead apron. All persons, regardless of rank or authority, should be informed of this requirement. Fluoroscopy should not be initiated until everyone complies.

SUMMARY

Fluoroscopy (fluoro) is a dynamic radiographic examination that involves active diagnosis during the examination. For this reason fluoroscopy is primarily the domain of the radiologist. The radiographer's role becomes that of an assistant during an examination.

Fluoroscopy is currently used for studies that require observation of dynamic physiological functions, e.g., the flow of barium through the gastrointestinal tract, swallowing, the injection of a contrast medium into the heart, etc.

The fluoroscopic imaging chain consists of a specialized x-ray tube with an image receptor, called the fluoroscopic screen, that can be viewed during an x-ray exposure. The fluoroscopic x-ray tube and image receptor are mounted on a C-arm to maintain their alignment at all times. Fluoroscopic x-ray tubes are very similar to diagnostic tubes except that they are designed to operate for longer periods of time at much lower mA. Where a typical diagnostic tube operates at 50–1,200 mA, the fluoroscopic mA range is 0.5–5.0 mA. An image intensification tube is designed to electronically amplify the brightness of an image. Modern image intensifiers are capable of increasing image brightness 500–8,000 times.

During fluoroscopy, the primary x-ray beam exits the patient and strikes the input screen of the image intensifier tube, which is a vacuum tube with a cathode and an anode. The fluorescent screen is built into the image intensifier as its input screen. The fluorescent screen absorbs the x-ray photons and emits light photons, which immediately encounter the photocathode (the cathode of the tube) that is in contact with the input screen to prevent divergence of the light beam. The photocathode absorbs the light photons and emits electrons. The electrons are then accelerated from the cathode toward the anode and the output screen by the potential difference that exists between the cathode and anode. At the same time, the electron beam is focused onto the output screen, which is much smaller than the input screen. Electrostatic lenses are used to accelerate and focus the electrons. The primary brightness gain occurs from the acceleration and focusing of the electron beam. Brightness gain is a measurement of the increase in image intensity and is determined by minification gain and flux gain. The acceleration of the electron beam increases its energy and its ability to emit light at the output screen. The focusing of the electron beam intensifies the image into a smaller area. The output screen absorbs the electrons and emits light photons, which are then available for viewing or further electronic processing by a video system. The primary factors that affect the quality of the fluoroscopic image include contrast, resolution, distortion, and quantum mottle.

A number of viewing systems have been developed to deliver the image from the output screen to the viewer. These include optical mirror, video, cine and spot film systems. Some of these systems permit dynamic real-time viewing while others are for static images. The viewing time, resolution and processing time vary. During fluoroscopy, it is possible to record either a dynamic or a static image. Dynamic imaging systems include cine film systems and videotape recording. Static spot filming systems include cassettes, 105 mm chip film, 70 mm roll film and videodisc recorders.

Fluoroscopic units operate with the minimum radiation output possible for the efficiency of the imaging system. The entrance skin dose for the patient is the surface closest to the source. The tabletop dose rate should not exceed 10 R/min and for most units should range from 1–3 R/min.

A lead apron of at least 0.25 mm Pb/eq must be worn by all persons (other than the patient) who are present in the fluoroscopic room during exposure. The primary source of exposure to the radiographer and radiologist is the patient, with the highest energy scatter occurring at a 90° angle to the incident beam. The radiographer has a duty to require that anyone present in the fluoroscopy room during an examination wear a lead apron.

REVIEW QUESTIONS

1. Why is fluoroscopy the domain of the radiologist?

2. What is the typical basic fluoroscopic imaging chain?

3. How does a fluoroscopic x-ray tube differ from a diagnostic x-ray tube?

4. Why is an image intensification system a significant advantage over the conventional screen fluoroscopy?

5. What is the basic function of the fluorescent screen, the photocathode, the electrostatic lenses and the output screen?

6. What is the formula used for determining brightness gain?

7. What is the purpose of the automatic brightness control?

8. What is the primary limitation of resolution of the fluoroscopic image?

9. What are the basic components of the tube used in a video camera?

10. What are the types of dynamic and static filming systems used to record the fluoroscopic image?

11. What radiation protection practices should be adhered to by the radiographer during fluoroscopy?

REFERENCES AND RECOMMENDED READING

Barnes, Gary T., and Jack M. Tishler. Fluoroscopic image quality and its implications regarding equipment selection and use. *The Physical Basis of Medical Imaging*. 93–106. Editors: Coulam, Craig M., John J. Erickson, F. David Rollo, and A. Everette James, Jr. New York: Appleton-Century-Crofts, 1981.

Beekmans, A. G. Image quality aspects of x-ray image intensifiers. *Medicamundi* 27, 25, 1982.

Birken, H., and C. I. Bejczy. A new generation of x-ray image intensifiers. *Medicamundi* 18:3, 120, 1978.

Bushong, Stewart. *Radiologic Science for Technologists: Physics, Biology, and Protection*. 4th ed. St. Louis, MO: C. V. Mosby Co., 1988.

Curry, Thomas S., James E. Dowdey, and Robert C. Murry, Jr. *Christensen's Physics of Diagnostic Radiology*. 4th ed. Philadelphia, PA: Lea & Febiger, 1990.

Fuchs, Arthur W. Edison and roentgenology. *The American Journal of Roentgenology* 57:2, 145–156, 1947.

Gould, R. G. Video communication systems in radiology. *Electronic Imaging in Medicine*. 326–347. Editors: Fullerton, Gary D., William R. Hendee, John C. Lasher, William S. Properzio, and Stephan J. Riederer. New York: American Institute of Physics for the American Association of Physicists in Medicine, 1984.

Gray, Joel E., John G. Stears, Francisco Lopez, and Merrill A. Wondraw. Fluoroscopic imaging: Quantitation of image lag or smearing. *Radiology* Feb., 563, 1984.

Gray, Joel E., Norlin T. Winkler, John Stears, and Eugene D. Frank. *Quality Control in Diagnostic Imaging*. Baltimore, MD: University Park Press, 1983.

Kuhl, W., and J. E. Schrijvers. 5 XG—A new 14 in. x-ray image intensifier tube. *Medicamundi* 22:3, 1977.

Seeram, Euclid, *X-Ray Imaging Equipment*. Springfield, IL: Charles C. Thomas Publisher, 1985.

Seeram, Euclid. Some characteristics of the cesium iodide x-ray image intensifiers. *The Canadian Journal of Radiology, Radiotherapy, and Nuclear Medicine* 9:1, 42–43, 1978.

Siedband, Melvin P. Fluoroscopic imaging. *The Physical Basis of Medical Imaging.* 75–92. Editors: Coulam, Craig M., John J. Erickson, F. David Rollo, and A. Everette James, Jr. New York: Appleton-Century-Crofts, 1981.

Stears, John G., Joel E. Gray, and Eugene D. Frank. Radiologic exchange (dose reduction with 105 mm spot films). *Radiologic Technology* 60:6, 515–516, 1989.

Sturn, R. E., and R. H. Morgan. Screen intensification systems and their limitations. *American Journal of Roentgenology* 62, 613, 1949.

THE CASE OF THE DRIPPING FILM

What caused the horizontal lines and drip marks on this radiograph?

(Images courtesy of E. D. Frank and J. G. Stears, Mayo Clinic/Foundation)

Answers to the case studies can be found in Appendix E.

38 TOMOGRAPHY

. . . there exists between (tube and plate), in space, a single fixed plane, in which each point always has a corresponding image point on the plate; hence, only the organs contained in this plane are in focus.

André-Edmund-Marie-Bocage, from *Method of, and apparatus for, radiography on a moving plate.*

OUTLINE

THE TOMOGRAPHIC PRINCIPLE
TOMOGRAPHIC QUALITY
TYPES OF MOTION
TOMOGRAPHIC PROCEDURES

OBJECTIVES

Upon completion of this chapter, the student should be able to:

1. Define tomography.
2. Explain the tomographic principle.
3. Explain the relationship of tomographic amplitude to exposure amplitude.
4. Describe the effects of tomographic amplitude, distance from the fulcrum, distance from the image receptor and the orientation of tube motion on image blur.
5. Explain the causes of tomographic phantom images.
6. Explain the function of the fulcrum.
7. Describe the dimensions of the focal plane.
8. Correlate changes in exposure amplitude with their effect on section thickness.
9. Describe a section interval.
10. Evaluate linear tomographic quality parameters.
11. Compare various types of linear, circular and complex tomographic motions.
12. Establish a tomographic procedure, including section thickness and interval, for a clinical problem.

13. Describe the specialized tomographic techniques.
14. Select appropriate exposure factors for a tomographic examination after a satisfactory preliminary scout radiograph has been produced.

Tomography is a radiographic technique that employs motion to show anatomical structures lying in a plane of tissue while blurring or eliminating the detail in images of structures above and below the plane of interest. It primarily demonstrates coronal sections, although sagittal sections of most body parts and transverse sections of the head may be accomplished through positioning.

First developed in 1921, and long the premier investigative procedure for removing superimposing structures, tomography is now used in only a few limited areas. Since the advent of modern computerized sectional imaging techniques (i.e., computed tomography and magnetic resonance imaging) its use has declined rapidly, although it is still considered of value for routine examination of the kidneys during intravenous pyelography. Tomography has also been found useful when computerized modalities are too costly or unavailable.

Although many have claimed credit for the development of tomography, only nine investigators actually had a part in its development, beginning with André Edmund Bocage (French dermatologist 1892–1953) and including the American radiographer Jean Kieffer. Tomography has been called planigraphy, stratigraphy and laminography over the years, and it is still sometimes called body section radiography.

THE TOMOGRAPHIC PRINCIPLE

The principle of tomography is based on synchronous movement of two of the three elements in a tomographic system: the x-ray tube, the object and the image receptor. Most tomographic units synchronize the movements of the x-ray tube and the image receptor in op-

posite directions around a stationary fulcrum (pivot point) during the exposure. Their alignment is maintained by a rigid attachment, such as a metal rod. The object to be examined is placed at the fulcrum (Figure 38–1). The result is a tomographic image in which the area located at the fulcrum is sharp because it has not moved in its relationship to the tube and the image receptor during the exposure (Figure 38–2). However, structures above and below, which would have been superimposed, are now blurred due to the motion. The reduced

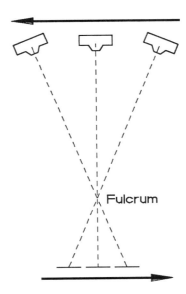

Figure 38–1. The tomographic principle—the interrelationships. The x-ray tube and image receptor are attached so they move in opposite directions while maintaining their alignment. The fulcrum, as the point around which the movement occurs, remains the single unmoving point. Objects placed at the fulcrum are imaged sharply while all other objects are blurred.

A

B

C

Figure 38–2. A tomogram of the maxillary sinuses in an AP projection with the fulcrum (A) 19 cm from the table, (B) 20 cm and (C) 21 cm. The structures that are sharp are located within the fulcrum focal plane. Structures above and below the focal plane are blurred. Note the opacification of the right maxillary sinus and the thickening of the mucosal wall in the inferior left sinus.

density permits visualization of the sharp details of the area of interest through their blurred images.

Although tomography is a dynamic process, it can be understood by careful consideration of the tomographic concept. Oblique projections or tube angle projections are used to project objects away from one another. Tomography builds on this geometry in a dynamic manner (Figure 38–3). As the tube proceeds through the tomographic motion, the projected images are first at a severe tube angle, which gradually decreases to a perpendicular beam, which then increases to a severe tube angle in the opposite direction. The resulting projection of superimposed objects first to one side, then to the other, causes their projected image to be streaked, or blurred, across the length of the image receptor. The longer the blurring, the less opportunity to create a sharp image. The shorter the blurring, the sharper the image. Therefore, there is a direct relationship between distance from the fulcrum and blurring. The greater the distance from the fulcrum, the greater the blurring and vice versa.

Those images that lie in the plane of the fulcrum will be projected onto exactly the same location on the image receptor because

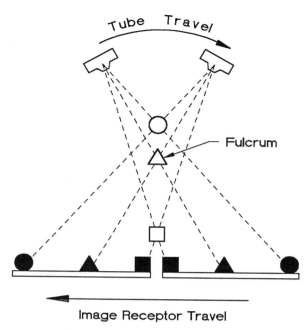

Figure 38–3. The tomographic concept. The ball is projected to the right of the triangle as the exposure begins but is blurred completely across the triangle to appear at the left by the end of the exposure. Also note that the box goes through the same blurring, but in the opposite direction.

the image receptor is moving at exactly the proper rate to maintain their location. Objects located above and below the fulcrum will be projected onto varying locations on the image receptor as it moves, thus blurring their images. The further the object is from the fulcrum, the greater the difference between its projected motion and the motion of the image receptor. This causes its image to be projected at various locations. The more its image is blurred, the easier it is to visualize sharp, unblurred structures through the blurring.

Because the creation of a section of sharply defined tissue is similar to cutting slices out of the body for examination, terms such as "cuts" and "slices" have evolved. Because these phrases can easily cause immense

distress when overheard by patients, the radiographer should strive to adhere to the term "section," avoiding "cut" and "slice."

TOMOGRAPHIC QUALITY

Tomographic Amplitude

The tomographic amplitude, arc or angle is the total distance the tube travels (Figure 38–4). The x-ray tube does not have to be engaged in an exposure for the entire tomographic angle. However, the tomographic amplitude is always greater than or equal to the exposure amplitude. There is an inverse relationship between the tomographic amplitude and the section thickness, as discussed below.

Exposure Amplitude

The exposure amplitude, arc or angle is the total distance the tube travels during the

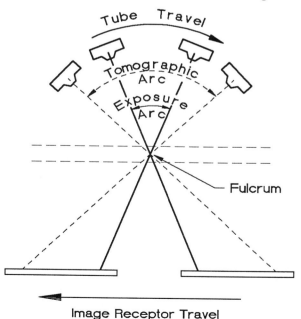

Figure 38–4. Tomographic and exposure amplitude, arc or angle.

exposure (Figure 38–4). The x-ray tube is engaged in an exposure for the entire exposure angle. The exposure amplitude is always equal to or less than the tomographic amplitude.

Blur

Blur is the streaking or smearing that results in the loss of nearly all recorded detail of objects outside the focal plane. There is an inverse relationship between blurring and the image density of objects. Increased blurring causes decreased density, thus making an object more transparent. This permits objects within the focal plane to be seen through the blurring. Blur is affected by the tomographic amplitude, distance from the fulcrum, distance from the image receptor and orientation of tube motion.

Tomographic Amplitude The tomographic amplitude has a direct linear relationship to blur width. As the tomographic amplitude increases, blur increases in direct proportion. For example, doubling the tomographic amplitude will double image blur.

Distance from the Fulcrum The distance from the fulcrum has a direct relationship to blur width. As the distance of an object from the fulcrum increases, blur increases.

Distance from the Image Receptor The distance from the image receptor has a direct relationship to blur width. As the distance of an object from the image receptor increases, blur increases. For example, blurring of superimposed structures around a pulmonary lesion is greater when the affected side is positioned down for lateral decubitus tomograms because this positions the unaffected lung farther from the image receptor.

Orientation of Tube Motion The orientation of tube travel has a direct relationship to

blur width. As the orientation of tube travel approaches perpendicularity, blur increases. Figure 38–5 shows the difference between an image of a structure that is perpendicular to a linear tomographic motion and one that is parallel.

Figure 38–5. The effect of the orientation of tube motion on the long axis of the object. The tomographic phantom has a star pattern of wires. When the fulcrum is 1 cm below the wires, blurring occurs. This image was produced with a linear motion from the top to the bottom of the radiograph. Arrows illustrate where the wire perpendicular to the direction of motion is projected with maximum blurring. The wire parallel to the direction of motion is projected with no lateral blurring. (The linear motion causes blurring only as elongation at the ends of the wire.) The wires at 45° are projected with intermediate amounts of blurring. (Courtesy of Suellen Chandler, Philips Medical Systems.)

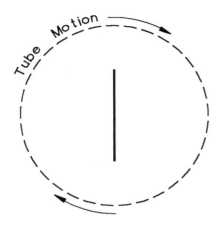

Figure 38–6. Phantoms caused by circular tomographic motion. Although the top and bottom of the circle produce motion that is perpendicular to the long axis of the object, the sides produce parallel motion. During the time the parallel motion occurs, the image blurring is decreased, thus producing a sharper and more dense image. This sharper and more dense image is the phantom, blur edge or blur margin.

Phantoms

Phantoms are sometimes called blur edges or blur margins. They are images that do not correspond to existing structures. They are false images and, as such, are dangerous to the diagnostic process. Phantoms are produced during complex tomographic motions, especially circular, when the tube motion is parallel to the long axis of the structure (Figure 38–6). They are also caused by blur overlap (Figure 38–7) and displacement of blur margins due to the tomographic motion. For example, a dense bony structure may have its blur margin projected into a soft tissue area. Especially in cranial and chest tomography, the decreased blur density may simulate a pathological soft tissue condition. Reduced section thickness and increased exposure amplitude decrease phantom images.

Fulcrum

The fulcrum is the pivot point around which the motions of the tube and the image receptor are centered. It determines the focal plane and thereby controls the section level. The fulcrum may be fixed so that the patient is moved up and down to change the section level (the Grossman principle). More commonly, the fulcrum is adjustable so that it

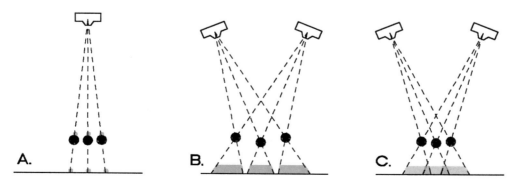

Figure 38–7. Tomographic blur overlap phantoms. (A) The sharp image of three wires produced by a static radiograph. (B) The blurred image of three wires produced by a small exposure amplitude. (C) The blur overlap that produces two phantom images from three wires imaged with a large exposure amplitude.

moves up and down while the patient remains stationary.

Focal Plane

The focal plane is often referred to as the section, although the terms section level, layer height, object plane and depth of focus have also been used. It is the region within which the image exhibits satisfactory recorded detail and is controlled by the level of the fulcrum. The focal plane is not an exactly defined region. Objects located near the fulcrum are less blurred while objects located further from the fulcrum are more blurred. Consequently, gradually increasing recorded detail eventually reaches a point where it is considered of diagnostic sharpness. This point defines the margins of the focal plane.

Section Thickness

Section thickness is the width of the focal plane and is controlled by the exposure angle (Figure 38–8). Exposure angle is inversely proportional to section thickness. As the exposure angle increases, section thickness decreases. Conversely, as the exposure angle decreases, section thickness increases.

Section thickness occurs in a plane parallel to the image receptor (Figure 38–9). Although there is an increase in magnification due to the increased OID of object C as the x-ray tube moves to the left, there is also a corresponding increase in the SOD and SID. The ratio of SID to SOD, the magnification ratio, remains the same, as do the ratios for objects A and B. Therefore, although magnification has an effect on the detail and sharpness of to-

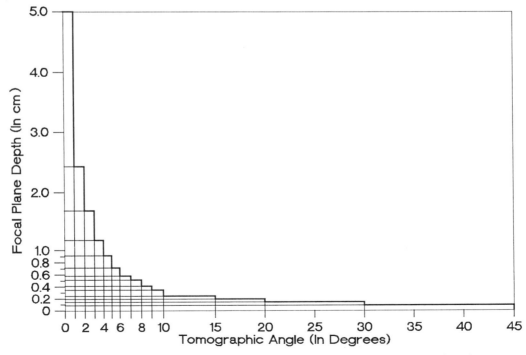

Figure 38–8. The effect of exposure angle on section thickness. (Reprinted with permission from Dowdell, Lois C., *The Joy of Sectioning*, Railfare Enterprises Limited, West Hill, Ontario, 1984.)

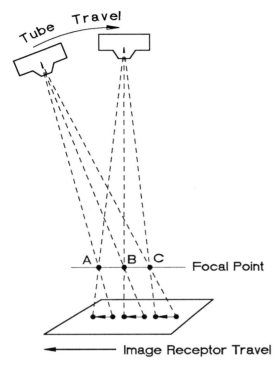

Figure 38–9. The effect of tomographic movement on magnification of objects in the focal plane.

mographed objects, tomographic motion does not change the total effect from that seen in a static radiograph of the same area.

Most tomographic images exhibit less contrast than static images of the same regions because of the decreased tissue density that is being imaged with a single section. The decreased difference in subject density also constitutes decreased subject contrast. Additionally, the blurring of structures above and below the fulcrum increases the base density of the image. Increased base density decreases contrast because fewer densities remain within the diagnostically visible range of densities.

Section Interval

The distance between fulcrum levels is the section interval. During tomographic pro-

cedures, the section interval should not exceed the section thickness. Tomographing an object with section intervals greater than the section thickness creates gaps of unexamined tissue that may permit misdiagnosis.

A procedure must be planned to establish appropriate section intervals. At least one full section above and below the area of interest is required to prove completion of the sectioning. Careful consideration of section thickness permits the use of section intervals that create a slight overlapping of sections. For example, an exposure amplitude that produces a 0.5 mm section thickness should be used with fulcrum changes of 0.4 mm to permit a 0.1 mm overlap (0.05 mm at the top and bottom of each section).

TYPES OF MOTION

Tomography was first achieved with a linear motion. However, numerous types of complex or pluridirectional tube motions have been developed which provide a total distance of tube travel up to nearly five times that of a linear motion although, to avoid excessive shape distortion, their amplitude does not exceed 48°. In addition, they provide motion significantly different from the shape of the subject, thus increasing perpendicular movement and reducing phantom images. Essentially, these motions add a second dimension to linear tomography (Figure 38–10B–G). Tomographic motion can be visualized by quality assurance pinhole tracings.

Complex motions require equipment that counter-rotates the grid as the tube moves. The image receptor is moved but is not counter-rotated since it must remain aligned to the anatomical structures of the patient. Counter-rotation of the grid eliminates the need for a reciprocating mechanism to blur the grid lines.

Linear

Linear tomography occurs when the movement of the tube and image receptor are

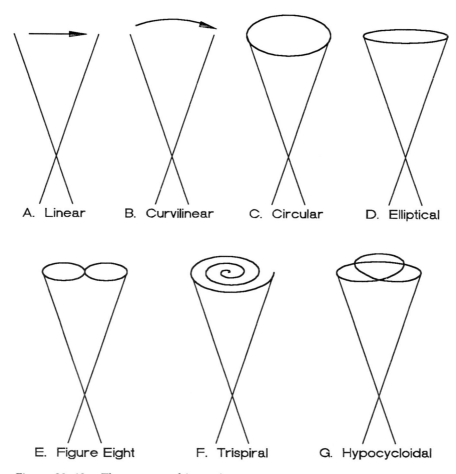

Figure 38–10.   The tomographic motions.

along a straight line (see Figure 38–10A). Linear motion has a major quality problem because the SID and OID change as the tube moves. Both SID and OID are greater at the extreme left and right positions than at the center position. During the tomographic motion the distances are in constant fluctuation.

Linear tomography also has a significant decrease in image quality because blurring is dependent on the orientation of the structure to the linear motion. Structures that are parallel to the motion are not so much blurred as they are streaked. Figure 38–5 illustrates the blurring of lines perpendicular to linear motion and the streaking (elongating) of parallel lines. Linear streaking causes sharp images from structures as much as several centimeters away from the fulcrum. Elongated linear streaking is not a phantom image; it is the image of structural margins that were not blurred.

Linear motion places severe limitations on the total tomographic amplitude. Because the angle of the tube to the object and the image receptor has limits beyond which shape

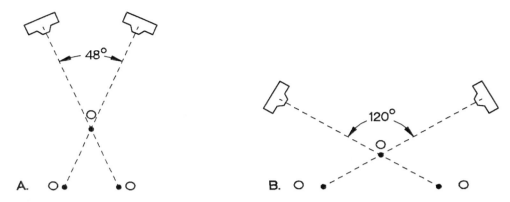

Figure 38–11.   Limitations to total linear tube amplitude.

distortion is objectionable, the thinness of the tomographic section is also limited (Figure 38–11). Total tomographic arc is limited to 48°. The only method of decreasing section thickness is to develop complex tomographic motions that permit greater amplitude.

Linear tomography remains popular because it is an inexpensive addition to a diagnostic x-ray unit. It requires a rod to attach the x-ray tube and the Bucky tray, an adjustable fulcrum through which the rod may pivot, and a motor to drive the x-ray tube stand. All other tomographic motions require specialized units designed to provide the desired motion through complicated tracks, gears, pivots, etc.

Because the motion of the tomographic unit creates the tomographic sectional image, it is critical to maximize the motion. This is accomplished by aligning the long axis of the part of interest to the direction of the tube motion. For example, tomograms of the sternum should be done with the long axis of the patient's body perpendicular to the length of the x-ray table. Inability to accomplish this type of positioning for numerous areas of the body is a disadvantage of linear tomography.

Curvilinear

Curvilinear tomography improves on the linear motion by maintaining SID and OID and

reducing magnification differences (see Figure 38–10B). It is still of limited value due to the single, linear direction of the motion.

Circular

Circular tomographic motions (see Figure 38–10C), although a vast improvement over linear motions, do not eliminate edge phantoms (see Figure 38–6). They require specialized equipment and exposure times of 3–6 seconds. Consequently, they are seldom used because most units capable of circular motions are also capable of more complex motions, as discussed below.

Elliptical

Elliptical tomographic motions (see Figure 38–10D) eliminate some of the edge phantoms of circular motions, especially when the long axis of the ellipse is perpendicular to the long axis of the object of interest. As with circular motions, they are seldom used because most units capable of elliptical motions are also capable of more complex motions.

Figure Eight

Some tomographic units provide a motion that forms a figure eight (see Figure 38–10E) while others are more random in nature. These motions eliminate most phantom images, although their total tomographic amplitude is not as great as that of trispiral or hypocycloidal motions.

Trispiral

The trispiral motion (see Figure 38–10F) provides maximum tomographic amplitude, thus producing the thinnest possible section.

Hypocycloidal

The hypocycloidal motion (see Figure 38–10G) also provides maximum tomographic amplitude, thus producing the thinnest possible section.

TOMOGRAPHIC PROCEDURES

Tomography is most often used to localize objects that are difficult to see due to superimposed structures. Because the section thickness determines how much tissue is visualized for each section, each examination must be evaluated to determine an appropriate series of tomographic sections. Routine procedures often begin with a preliminary scout exposure for diagnostic comparisons. This image is also useful in establishing exact structural locations and verifying exposure factors.

Exposure Factors

Choosing proper technique exposure factors for tomography requires special attention to compensate for the time needed for the tomographic amplitude.

Time It is critical that the time be set first. The exposure time must match the length of time required for the x-ray tube to complete the tomographic amplitude. An exposure time that is less than the amplitude will not permit full blurring and will project erratic phantoms. An exposure time that is greater than the amplitude will increase the density of the image at the final tube position, thus increasing the

recorded detail while decreasing the blurring of structures outside the focal plane. Complex tomographic motions often require 3 or 6 second exposures.

Milliamperage Dedicated tomography unit generators provide special stations below 100 mA to permit appropriate mAs to be set with the long times required for complex tomographic motions. Stations of 10, 15, 20, 25, 30, 40 and 50 mA are extremely helpful in these situations. Approximately 30 percent more mAs is required for a wide angle tomogram due to the loss of scatter density caused by the air gap at the extremes of the tomographic motion. Zonographic tomograms usually require the same mAs as static radiographs.

Kilovoltage All fine density adjustments must be accomplished by variations of kVp because of the limitations imposed by the fixed time settings. The 15 percent rule is a critical tool in determining these adjustments. It is also useful to recall that a 5 percent change in kVp is required to produce a visible density difference in most images. Because these adjustments tend to increase kVp to the point where contrast may become a problem, every possible device that will eliminate scatter radiation should be employed. These include maximum collimation (to the exact area of interest), lead masks at the tabletop, high ratio grids and compression bands.

Specialized Techniques

Narrow Angle Tomography or Zonography

Zonography or narrow angle tomography (exposure amplitudes of less than 10°) is used when localization is necessary because the exact location of a structure is unknown or when a survey is being performed, for example, on a lesion of the lung or on the kidneys. A small exposure amplitude is

Figure 38–12.   The effect of exposure amplitude on section thickness. (A) A small exposure amplitude to produce a thick section for localization or as a survey examination. (B) A larger exposure amplitude to produce thin sections for detailed examination. (Reprinted with permission from Littleton, J.T., *Tomography: Physical Principles and Clinical Applications*, Section 17: Golden's Diagnostic Radiology Series, © 1976 the Williams & Williams Co., Baltimore, MD.)

used to produce a thick section (Figure 38–12A). Zonography has reasonable contrast but poor recorded detail because of the thick section.

Wide Angle Tomography Wide angle tomography is used when a lesion has been localized or a specific structure has been determined to require a more detailed examination. A series of thinner sections may then be used (see Figure 38–12B). Wide angle tomography has inherently low contrast but a reasonable amount of recorded detail because of the thin section. It is useful in the examination of small bone structures, such as the inner ear, although computed tomography now has much to offer in this area of diagnosis.

Multifilm Tomography Multifilm tomography uses a series of films placed at regular intervals by spacers or intensifying screens within a book cassette and uses OID in place of fulcrum changes to achieve the tomographic effect. Although a significantly greater exposure is required to provide sufficient photons for the last film, the single exposure is usually less than the total of the exposures necessary to produce the same information in a series of separate images. Its primary advantage is that the entire series for lung tomography is achieved at the same breathing phase.

Panoramic Tomography Specialized equipment has been developed to permit slit scan radiography of the curved surfaces of the face and head, especially of the mandible (Figure 38–13). The terms pantomography, orthopantomography and panoramic tomography have been used to describe this type of x-ray unit. Slit scan radiography uses only the perpendicular photons of the primary beam by using a lead mask to collimate the beam to a narrow slit. Both the x-ray tube and the film rotate past the slit during the exposure to lay out the structure of interest, much like rolling paint from a roller onto a wall (Figure 38–14).

SUMMARY

Tomography is a radiographic technique employing motion to show structures lying in a plane of tissue while blurring or eliminating the detail in images of structures in other planes. It primarily demonstrates coronal sections, although sagittal sections of most body parts and transverse sections of the head may be accomplished through positioning.

Figure 38–13.   A panoramic projection of the mandible.

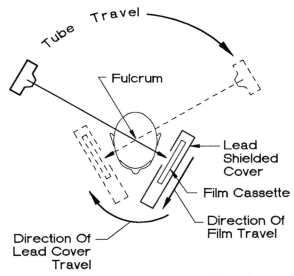

Figure 38–14.   Panoramic tomographic equipment.

The principle of tomography is based on synchronous movement of two of the three elements in a tomographic system: the x-ray tube, the object and the image receptor. Most tomographic units synchronize the movements of the x-ray tube and the image receptor in op-

posite directions around a stationary fulcrum during the exposure. Those images that lie in the plane of the fulcrum will be projected onto exactly the same location on the image receptor because the image receptor is moving at exactly the proper rate to maintain their location. Objects located above and below the fulcrum will be projected onto varying locations on the image receptor as it moves, thus blurring their images.

The tomographic amplitude, arc or angle is the total distance the tube travels. The exposure amplitude, arc or angle is the total distance the tube travels during the exposure. The exposure amplitude is always equal to or less than the tomographic amplitude. Blur is the streaking or smearing that results in the loss of nearly all recorded detail of objects outside the focal plane and is affected by the tomographic amplitude, distance from the fulcrum, distance from the image receptor and orientation of tube motion. Blur edges and blur margins are called phantoms.

The focal plane is often referred to as the section, although the terms section level, layer height, object plane and depth of focus have also been used. It is the region within which the image exhibits satisfactory recorded detail and is controlled by the level of the fulcrum. Section thickness is the width of the focal plane and is controlled by the exposure angle. The distance between fulcrum levels is the section interval. During tomographic procedures, the section interval should not exceed the section thickness.

Tomography was first achieved with a linear motion. Complex or pluridirectional tube motions have been developed, which include circular, elliptical, figure eight, trispiral and hypocycloidal.

Choosing proper exposure factors for tomography requires consideration of exposure time, milliamperage and kilovoltage. Specialized tomographic techniques include narrow angle, wide angle, multifilm and panoramic tomography.

REVIEW QUESTIONS

1. Define tomography.

2. How does a basic tomographic system operate?

3. What is the difference between tomographic amplitude and exposure amplitude?

4. What factors affect tomographic blur?

5. What is the function of the fulcrum?

6. How is section thickness controlled?

7. Which of the tomographic motions alters distance during the exposure arc?

8. What are the advantages of complex tomographic motions?

9. Why is it important to establish the exposure time prior to setting the other exposure factors for a tomogram?

10. Differentiate between the uses of narrow-angle and wide-angle tomography.

REFERENCES AND RECOMMENDED READING

Barnes, Gray T., and Richard F. Moreland. A linear tomographic alignment test object. *Radiology* Oct., 247, 1981.

Bushong, Stewart C. *Radiologic Science for Technologists: Physics, Biology, and Protection.* 4th ed. St. Louis, MO: C. V. Mosby Co., 1988.

Coulam, Craig M., John J. Erickson, and S. Julian Gibbs. Image and equipment considerations in conventional tomography. *The Physical Basis of Medical Imaging.* 123–140. Editors: Coulam, Craig M., John J. Erickson, F. David Rollo, and A. Everette James, Jr. New York: Appleton-Century-Crofts, 1981.

Curry, Thomas S., James E. Dowdey and Robert C. Murry. *Christensen's Physics of Diagnostic Radiology.* 4th ed. Philadelphia, PA: Lea & Febiger, 1990.

Dowdell, Lois C. *The Joy of Sectioning.* Toronto: Railfare, 1984.

Dowell, Lois C. Today's typical tomography: A guide for everyone. *The Canadian Journal of Medical Radiation Technology* 11:4, 188, 1980.

Durzich, M. L. *Technical Aspects of Tomography.* Baltimore, MD: Williams & Wilkins, 1978.

Forster, E. *Equipment for Diagnostic Radiography.* Lancaster, England: MTP Press Ltd., 1985.

Littleton, Jesse T., and Mary Lou Durzich. *Sectional Imaging Methods: A Comparison.* Baltimore, MD: University Park Press, 1983.

Littleton, J. T. *Tomography: Physical Principles and Clinical Applications.* Section 17: Golden's Diagnostic Radiology Series. Baltimore, MD: Williams & Wilkins, 1976.

Lockery, Robert M. Principles of body-section radiography. *Radiologic Technology* 42:5, 335, 1971.

National Bureau of Standards. *Methods of Evaluating Radiological Equipment and Materials: Handbook 89.* Washington, D.C.: National Bureau of Standards, 1963.

Smith, Wendy V. J. A review of tomography and zonography. *Radiography* 37:433, 5, 1971.

Soni, Vinod Paul. A review of tomography. *Canadian Journal of Radiography, Radiotherapy, and Nuclear Medicine* 8:4, 172–189, 1977.

Tomographic exposure angle. *Radiography* 50:594, 291, 1984.

Tyndol, Donald A., and Susan M. Bedsale. Exposure reduction and image quality for pantomographic radiography. *Radiologic Technology* 59:1, 51, 1988.

THE CASE OF DO YOU KNOW YOUR WHOLE GRAINS?

What common grain is this?

(Reprinted by permission of the International Society of Radiographers and Radiological Technicians from the K. C. Clark Archives, Middlesex Hospital, London, England)

Answers to the case studies can be found in Appendix E.

39 SPECIALIZED TECHNIQUES
Roger Smith

"Put your arms about it," he said, "Embrace the board—pretend it's something else, if you like. Press your breast against it, as though it filled you with rapture. Like that. Draw a deep breath. Hold it!" he commanded. "Now, please!" Hans Castorp waited, blinking, his lungs distended. Behind him the storm broke loose: it crackled, lightened, detonated—and grew still. The lens had looked into his inside.

Thomas Mann, *Der Zauberberg* (*The Magic Mountain*).

OUTLINE

STEREORADIOGRAPHY
MAGNIFICATION OR MACRORADIOGRAPHY
DUPLICATION
SUBTRACTION
XERORADIOGRAPHY

OBJECTIVES

Upon completion of this chapter, the student should be able to:

1. Describe the principles of stereoradiography.
2. Describe the basic methods of producing stereoradiographs.
3. Draw diagrams showing the basic principles of magnification.
4. Calculate the enlargement factor for a given technique.
5. Discuss the significance of focal spot size in magnification techniques.
6. Describe the characteristics of duplicating film.
7. Draw a diagram of a typical duplication unit.
8. Explain the process of duplicating an image.
9. Describe the principles of photographic subtraction.
10. Explain a typical subtraction procedure in step form.
11. Describe the principles of the xeroradiographic image processing system.
12. Describe, in step form, the xeroradiographic process.

STEREORADIOGRAPHY

When Röntgen discovered x-rays in 1895 the science of photography was already well advanced. In fact, the first public projection of moving images took place about the time he was giving his paper, "On a New Kind of Rays" (Appendix A). Three-dimensional imaging was shown by Wheatstone's stereo viewer in 1838. Stereoradiography involves the three-dimensional viewing of radiographs. It was developed almost immediately following the discovery of x-rays and was so popular that most radiography between 1900 and 1930 was stereo. Eventually the radiation dangers inevi-

tably associated with double exposing changed stereoradiography to a special technique and it is used today only on rare occasions.

The Principles of Stereo Imaging

The principle of human visual three-dimensional viewing involves each eye seeing a slightly different view. The optic nerve fibers divide in the chiasma so that some retinal signals from each eye are shared with those of the other eye, as well as crossing over, before being interpreted in the visual cortex (Figure 39–1A). The brain processes these signals together

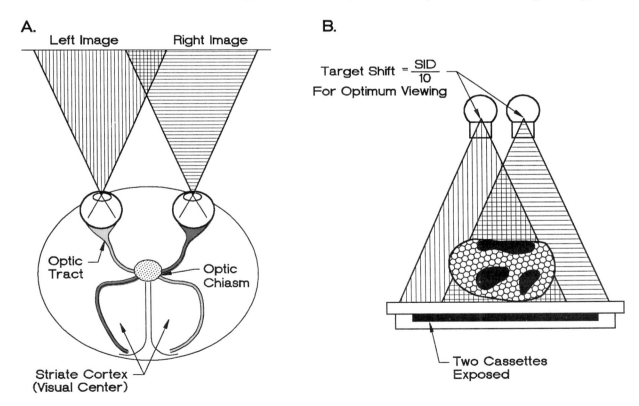

Figure 39–1. Principles of stereoradiography. (A) How the brain perceives three-dimensional images. (B) How the x-ray system reproduces three-dimensional images.

and produces depth perception, which is a learned process. Radiographers and radiologists live in a two-dimensional imaging world, but we are reminded that the patient is three-dimensional, and we use that knowledge to help position the patient into lateral and oblique views for optimum information.

To achieve true three-dimensional radiography, two separate images must be presented to the brain. This requires two exposures of the object. For comfortable viewing perception, the target must be separated by at least the average human interpupillary distance (2.5" or 6 cm). In fact, a relationship exists between the SID and this shift (see Figure 39–1B). The rule that has developed is 10 percent of the SID for the total shift of the x-ray target between exposures. Separate cassettes are exposed to each target position and the films viewed by the appropriate eye (right eye sees right image, left eye sees left image). Care must be taken when doing Bucky stereoradiography because of the possibility of grid cut-off. It is best to shift parallel to the grid lines when possible.

Since the brain should be presented with nearly equal images to blend, the same speed screens, exposure technique, film speed and processing must be used for both radiographs. Care must be taken to instruct the patient not to move between exposures. Lead marking is important and must identify both the patient side and the direction of the tube shift. This can be done by using double markers (RR, right side right shift, and RL, right side left shift) or normal side markers and lead arrows to show direction (R ↑ and R ↓). Stereo can be simulated by taking the second projection after rotating the object by about 6°–8°. Geometrically, this produces the same effect as moving the target between exposures. It is important to note that the central ray can be left at right angles to the film for achieving stereo, but this means the collimator must be opened slightly to avoid cutting off the image, thus possibly irradiating the patient unnecessarily. A safer technique is to angle the tube back to film center and collimate to film size.

Methods of Viewing

Images viewed as if seen from the target are called orthoscopic (normal view), and images viewed as if seen from behind the cassette are called pseudoscopic (false view). Figure 39–2A shows a simple arrangement where each eye can be trained to see its own image by blocking overlap with a screen or by using stereo binoculars. With the latter, the films must be reversed on the view boxes since the images are reflected once via a prism. Other stereo viewing units may still be found, such as the Wheatstone (see Figure 39–2B) and Stanford stereoscopes, both of which use mirrors to present each eye with a separate image. In all these methods the reward, after a moment of adjustment to the system, is a truly three-dimensional perspective of the body.

Other Stereo Applications

Stereoradiography has been preempted, over the years, by tomography and, now, by computed tomography and magnetic resonance imaging, and is no longer a popular technique in routine radiography. Other stereo applications do exist, however, and include the following:

1. Some centers have investigated the heart and brain with stereocinefluorography, using either two parallel x-ray tubes mounted close together or a special stereo x-ray tube with targets which are activated separately on opposite sides of the same anode. Images are displayed to special monitors via image intensifiers. The stereo presentation for the eyes can be achieved using polarizing filters or color filters. It is also possible via film imaging, using polarizing glasses or alternate pulsed liquid crystal lenses, to

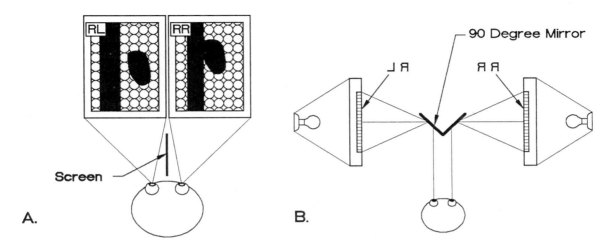

Figure 39–2. Three-dimensional viewing systems. (A) An alternative three-dimensional viewing method using stereo binoculars. (B) A Wheatstone stereoscopic viewer.

view the images. Such systems are extremely complex and costly to operate.

2. A 3-D fluoroscopy unit has been manufactured, for GI work, that images onto a TV monitor with a plastic gridded screen for direct 3-D effect.

3. Stereo lateral skull images are still produced in some radiology departments, but with one of the images a true lateral, as part of the skull routine, and the other taken after the full shift of 10 percent of the SID.

MAGNIFICATION OR MACRORADIOGRAPHY

All radiographic images are magnified, if by only a small amount. Accepting that the focal spot is nearly a point, then even contact radiography, such as that of extremities, will be slightly enlarged.

Magnification Factor (MF)

In the majority of radiography the goal is to minimize the OID. However, there are times when deliberately placing the object closer to the target will increase the details for improved diagnosis, not just by enlarging the part, but by moving detailed structures away from other objects and opening up the view of such things as the vasculature of the brain.

The concept is simple, as shown in Figures 26–2 and 26–3. Magnification factor (MF) is calculated as:

$$MF = \frac{SID}{SOD}$$

Example: If the SID = 40″ (100 cm) and the SOD = 15″ (38 cm), what is the magnification factor?

Answer:

$$MF = \frac{SID}{SOD}$$

$$MF = \frac{40″}{15″}$$

$$MF = 2.7$$

It is clear that an object can be projected twice its natural size by placing it at half the normal

SID, (i.e., 20" [50 cm]). This is the most common type of macroradiography currently in use, although techniques that permit up to 4× magnification are also used.

Focal Spot Size

Figure 39–3 shows the reality of a finite focal spot. It produces inherent unsharpness in the form of edge gradient or penumbra. From the object and film point of view, the focal spot has two dimensions, and its sides produce a double shadow.

Magnification increases penumbra and reduces image quality to an unacceptable level. Therefore, it is essential to use fractional focal spots for magnification radiography. Many tubes, especially fluoroscopic tubes with image intensifiers, will have fractional focal spots to permit macroradiography. Focal spots from 0.3 mm^2 to 0.5 mm^2 are in common use. Macroradiography is used in skeletal radiography for detecting arthritic or osteoporotic changes, in mammography for detecting microcalcifications and in enlargement angiography for small vessel detail.

The radiographer's responsibilities during macroradiography include:

1. Immobilizing the patient, since the slightest motion will be greatly exaggerated.
2. Precise centering (it is better to center the beam to the cassette first, then center the object to the beam).
3. Tight collimation to protect the patient from excessive exposure.
4. Since there is a considerable air gap with macroradiography, scattered radiation contributes much less to film density. This permits elimination of a grid, while requiring significantly more total exposure.

The exposure adjustment varies from about two to four times the mAs. Placement of the part closer to the focal spot increases the entrance skin dose during macroradiography. From the clinical standpoint, the user of this technique must carefully consider the benefit versus the costs of radiation exposure. Experimental entrance skin dose measurements from the techniques mentioned above are shown in Table 39–1.

Attempting to decrease exposure by the use of very high speed film/screen combinations would defeat the purpose of macroradiography because sufficient detail would not be

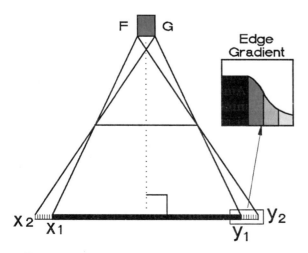

Figure 39–3.   The reality of a finite focal spot.

TABLE 39–1			
RELATIVE ENTRANCE SKIN DOSES FOR MACRORADIOGRAPHY			
		Entrance Skin Dose	
Examination	Routine	Macro-radiography	Increase
Navicular	8.4 mR	48.0 mR	5.7×
C-spine	378.0 mR	1,520.0 mR	4.0×

All doses are calculated to maintain radiographic density with a lucite and human bone phantom.

recorded. It is possible to achieve macroradiography at lower exposures by reducing the SID overall to 24″ (60 cm).

It is important to remember that the size of the effective focal spot varies with the technical factors used. Higher kVp tends to maintain a smaller focal spot because the electron beam is more parallel in passing from cathode to anode. Conversely, higher mA tends to produce a larger focal spot.

Microfocus Tubes

There is a need for much better control over the effective focus in macroradiography, so special tubes have been designed. These tubes may be radically different from traditional designs. One tube brings the electron beam under the guidance of an electron lens, which can focus the beam to about 0.1 mm², which is close to the theoretical point.

Some tubes attempt to improve energy distribution in the beam by having an angle of 45° to the target surface (thus eliminating the anode heel effect). The tubes often employ stationary anodes for stability. In these situations there must be additional measures to remove heat from the post-target area, such as forced oil or water cooling. It is important to remember that all small focal spots have severe heat unit limits, and it should be understood that anatomical details in the object that are smaller than the effective focus will not form sharp images on the macroradiograph.

DUPLICATION

Duplication is the process by which a nearly exact copy, the same size, or miniaturized, is made of a radiographic image. Duplicates arose from the need to share visual information with other institutions, with other hospital departments for educational purposes, and for volume storage and medical legal purposes. Film manufacturers have made duplication relatively easy by producing ready-to-use duplicating film that is processed in automatic processors, and devices for exposing it (Figure 39–4).

Solarization Effect

The solarization effect is a technique from the early days of photography that produces prints by exposure to sunlight. If an ordinary silver halide emulsion is exposed long enough, it will reach the reversal phase and actually lose density (Figure 39–5).

Duplicating Film

Modern duplicating film has a single emulsion and is presolarized; it is chemically fogged to D-Max by the manufacturer. Therefore, further exposure decreases optical density.

Duplicating film has an average gradient of OD 1.0 to 1.5 and is sensitized to about 350 nm, which is in the ultraviolet range. It is possible to post a simple technique chart by a duplicating unit after a brief trial with duplicating film and a control radiograph.

Various authors have written of techniques used to save overexposed radiographs in order to avoid having to repeat the examination. Diagnostic information from images that are overexposed as much as 75 percent can often be saved via duplication with long exposure times. This technique is limited to original radiographs with a density of about OD 3.1 or less.

With some of the faster emulsions now available, the exposure requirements may be so low that the copying unit cannot accurately time them. In these instances, the duplicating system can be slowed down to match the emulsion by blocking part of the unit's ultraviolet tube with blackened film, black electrical tape or by an orange/yellow filter.

Very large institutions and other mass users of radiographic images, such as the military and survey units, often need to reduce the size

Figure 39–4.   A radiographic duplication/subtraction unit. A radiograph is duplicated by the following steps:

1. A clean radiograph requiring duplication is placed on the glass plate and centered using the view light control.
2. The view light is switched off and, under safelight, a duplicating film of appropriate size is placed emulsion down on the original radiograph to be duplicated. (Placing the notches on the film in the lower left (LL) corner places the emulsion down.)
3. The lid is latched tightly to achieve good film-to-film contact.
4. The timer is set and an exposure is made in the duplication mode.
5. Both films are removed from the glass plate; the duplicating film is processed and the original is returned to storage.

Exposure adjustments are made by comparing the duplicate to the original. Because duplicating film is a positive emulsion, exposure adjustments are the opposite of those used for radiographic film. For example, a darker duplicate is produced by decreasing exposure time.

The duplicate image will be slightly less sharp than the original because of the divergence of light as it travels through the two emulsions of the original onto the single emulsion of the duplicate. In addition, the duplicate image will have significantly higher contrast because the slope of the solarized D log E curve is always steeper than with radiographic films.

of images because of limited storage facilities. In these situations a copy-stand device with a roll-film camera can be used. These units use 16 mm to 100 mm photographic roll-film.

SUBTRACTION

Subtraction began as a photographic technique that was used to overcome the superimposition of opacified arteries and various bone structures in lateral cerebral angiograms. Subtraction attempts to remove all densities on the finished image except the opacified vessels. This is accomplished by subduing or subtracting bone densities to a neutral gray, leaving the contrast-medium-filled vasculature in high contrast to the subtracted background.

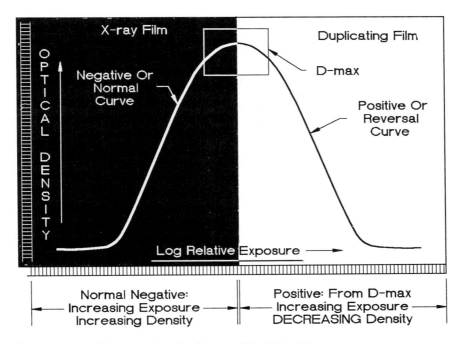

Figure 39–5.   The complete duplication film D log E curve.

Procedure

The subtraction procedure is shown in Figure 39–6. It requires:

1. A preliminary scout image without contrast medium.
2. A contrast medium image in exactly the same position and with the same technical factors.
3. A special mask and subtraction film.
4. A special subtraction exposure unit installed in a darkroom. (It is possible to perform subtraction on a darkroom bench or with a glass-fronted cassette, using a carefully controlled light source.)

As in all photography, testing is necessary to derive the best results. The density of the mask is the key, since the contrast-medium-injected images should not be repeated. Once a routine is established with fixed techniques, the subtraction procedure exposures should vary little.

Second-Order Subtraction

Second-order subtraction may be used if the first mask is insufficiently dense. The preliminary film is superimposed over the light mask and another mask is produced from the two.

Unsharp Mask Technique

The unsharp mask technique interposes a thick sheet of optical quality glass between the original image and the subtraction film to produce a very blurred mask. The blurred mask can enhance images, particularly for reproduction photography for publication.

Figure 39–6. The subtraction process. A subtracted radiograph is produced by using a duplication/subtraction unit in the following steps.

A mask image is produced to subdue or cancel the bone image:

1. Place the preliminary scout radiograph on the glass plate of the duplication/subtraction unit.
2. Under safelight conditions, place an unexposed subtraction mask film emulsion down (notch in LL or UR corner) over the scout radiograph. Close and latch the lid to achieve good film-to-film contact and expose the film in the subtraction mode.

3. Both films are removed from the glass plate; the subtraction mask film is processed and the scout radiograph is returned to storage.
4. The mask film is evaluated for sufficient density. Since this is a positive print of the scout radiograph the bones will appear black. Insufficient bone density will not subtract enough density during the subtraction process. Exposure adjustments are made as for diagnostic film (i.e., a darker image is achieved by increasing exposure time).

A subtraction image is produced by selecting the contrast medium radiograph from which a subtraction print is desired and using the following procedure:

1. Place the mask film emulsion up on the glass plate of the duplication/subtraction unit and turn on the view light.
2. Place the contrast medium radiograph over the mask film and align the two images until the maximum subtraction of densities is achieved. Most densities should appear as a uniform density from the combination of the two opposite emulsions with only the contrast medium remaining in high contrast. Secure the alignment of the two images with masking tape.
3. Under safelight conditions, place an unexposed subtraction print film emulsion down (notch in LL or UR corner) over the two aligned films. Close and latch the lid to achieve good film-to-film contact and expose the film in the subtraction mode.
4. All three films are removed from the glass plate; the subtraction print film is processed while the mask film and contrast medium radiograph are returned to storage.
5. The subtraction print film is evaluated for sufficient density and exposure adjustments are made if necessary (i.e., if a darker image is desired the exposure time should be increased). Subtraction print film produces black vasculature. White vasculature can be produced by substituting duplication film for subtraction print film during the final exposure (step 3).

XERORADIOGRAPHY

Xeroradiography was developed from the original dry paper technology copiers of the Xerox Corporation in the early 1950s to provide a waterless processing system for radiography in cold-war bomb shelters. The basic unit in xeroradiography is a reusable cassette consisting of a simple plastic light-tight case enclosing a smooth, thin plate coated with selenium on an aluminum base. Selenium is a semiconducting material that becomes conductive when it is irradiated. This makes the selenium plate a sensitized surface that will respond to light or x-ray exposure; it can be used in place of a film and screen cassette (Figure 39–7).

The xeroradiography system consists of a conditioning unit that prepares the cassette for exposure and a processing unit that derives a permanent image from the charged selenium plate. There are no film, screen or wet processing involved in xeroradiography. The finished image is a blue print on thick, plastic-coated paper.

Conditioning

The xeroradiographic plate must be conditioned by removing all traces of previous exposures. This is done by heating the plate to remove residual charges and brushing off residual image powder (see Figure 39–7A). The plate is then cooled and stored in a magazine until needed. When a plate is required, it is passed very close to a high-voltage wire carrying a positive current. The corona discharge from this wire creates a uniform positive charge on the plate surface, thus sensitizing it for exposure. The cassette is then closed and ejected for use.

Exposure

The cassette is exposed to ionizing radiation exactly like a film/screen cassette (see Figure 39–7B). The radiation pattern from the

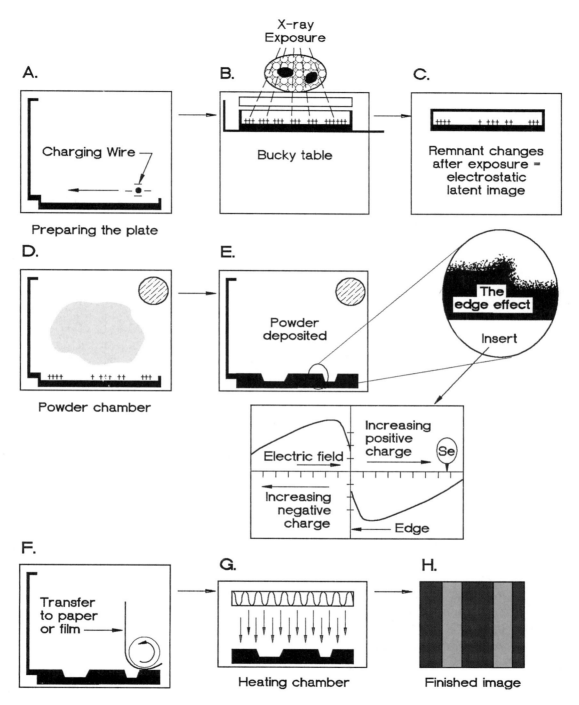

Figure 39–7.   The xeroradiographic process.

patient, impinging on the charged selenium surface, causes ionization, which in turn causes the differential discharge from the plate. This creates the latent image (see Figure 39–7C).

Processing

To produce a visible image after exposure, the cassette is placed in the processing unit. The unit opens the cassette in a light-tight chamber, removes the selenium plate, and transports it to a powder chamber (see Figure 39–7D). A very fine blue powder is blown into the chamber through a charging grill. Depending on the charge selected by the operator for the powder, a positive or negative image is produced. The powder adheres to the remnant charges on the selenium plate, thus creating an image in blue (see Figure 39–7E). A density control on the unit permits regulation of the amount of powder blown onto the plate. The plate is then transported to the next stage, where a plastic emulsion paper is rolled across the plate, transferring the blue powder onto the emulsion (see Figure 39–7F). The paper then passes into a warming chamber, where the plastic emulsion is heated to blend the powder into the plastic to create a permanent image (see Figure 39–7G). The paper is ejected to be viewed by reflected light (see Figure 39–7H). The cassette is returned to a storage box, which is placed in the conditioning unit to prepare the selenium plate for reuse.

Edge Enhancement

One of the effects of the xeroradiographic imaging method is the phenomenon of edge enhancement. The xeroradiographic system is inherently very low in contrast (and therefore extremely wide in latitude). Where there is an abrupt change in the charge pattern on the plate (i.e., an anatomical subject contrast edge) the powder tends to be deposited on the other side of the edge (somewhat like drifting snow or sand forming down-wind of a fence) (see Figure 39–7E insert).

This advantage made xeroradiography the method of choice for low subject contrast investigations, such as mammography, during the 1970s and 1980s. The charge phenomenon also produces a forbidden zone in wide areas next to an edge, where powder cannot deposit. This edge is sometimes referred to as the halo effect. The wide latitude and range of densities available in xeroradiography demonstrate details from ribs or humerus, to the borders of the breast (Figure 39–8).

The radiation dose levels required for xeroradiography are higher than single-screen and film mammography. This slow speed has

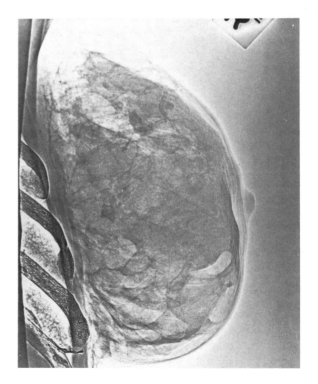

Figure 39–8.   A xeroradiographic mammogram (xeromammogram).

reduced the use of the xeroradiographic system for mammography in recent years, despite the inherent contrast enhancement.

Associated Systems

Other alternatives to silver-based imaging have been developed using charged plate and image transfer principles, based on the magazine-loaded table. A base of thermoplastic film supplied in rolls is used with the density on the image produced by black carbon powder. In some units, the exposing chamber is pressurized with a gas to increase attenuation and improve charge transfer. Such systems are called ionography or electron radiography.

SUMMARY

Stereoradiography involves the three-dimensional viewing of radiographs. The principle of human visual three-dimensional viewing involves each eye seeing a slightly different view. The optic nerve fibers divide in the chiasma so that some retinal signals from each eye are shared with those of the other eye, as well as crossing over, before being interpreted in the visual cortex. To achieve true three-dimensional radiography, two separate images must be presented to the brain.

In the majority of radiographs the goal is to minimize the OID. Macroradiography deliberately places an object closer to the target. This process increases the details for improved diagnosis by moving detailed structures away from other objects and opening up the view of such things as the vasculature of the brain. The magnification factor (MF) is calculated as SID/SOD. It is essential to use fractional focal spots for this work.

Duplication is the process by which a nearly exact copy, the same size, or miniaturized, is made of a radiographic image. Duplicates arose from the need to share visual information with other institutions, with other hospital departments for educational purposes, and for volume storage and medical legal purposes. Film manufacturers have made duplication relatively easy by producing ready-to-use duplicating film that is processed in automatic processors, and devices for exposing it. Modern duplicating film has a single emulsion and is presolarized; it is chemically fogged to D-Max by the manufacturer.

Subtraction began as a photographic technique that was used to overcome the superimposition of opacified arteries and various bone structures in lateral cerebral angiograms. Subtraction attempts to remove all densities on the finished image except the opacified vessels. This is accomplished by subduing or subtracting bone densities to a neutral gray, leaving the contrast-medium-filled vasculature in high contrast to the subtracted background.

Xeroradiography was developed to provide a waterless processing system for radiography. The basic unit involves a reusable cassette consisting of a simple plastic light-tight case enclosing a smooth, thin plate coated with selenium on an aluminum base. Selenium is a semiconducting material that becomes conductive when it is irradiated. This makes the selenium plate a sensitized surface that will respond to light or x-ray exposure. A conditioning unit prepares the cassette for exposure and a processing unit derives a permanent image from the charged selenium plate. The finished image is a blue print on thick, plastic coated paper.

REVIEW QUESTIONS

1. How is tube shift determined for stereoradiography?

2. What factors contributed to the decline in the use of stereoradiography?

3. Describe the phenomenon of edge gradient.

4. What are the common sizes of focal spots used for macroradiography?

5. What is solarization?

6. What type of light source is used to expose the duplication emulsion?

7. What is the purpose of the use of subtraction?

8. What are the components of the reusable cassette in xeroradiography?

9. How is the edge enhancement effect advantageous in xeroradiography?

REFERENCES AND RECOMMENDED READING

Bushong, Stewart C. *Radiologic Science for Technologists: Physics, Biology, and Protection.* 4th ed. St. Louis, MO: C. V. Mosby Co., 1988.

Chesney, D. N., and M. O. Chesney. *X-Ray Equipment for Student Radiographers.* London: Blackwell Scientific Publications, 1984.

Cullinan, Angeline M. *Producing Quality Radiographs.* Philadelphia, PA: J. B. Lippincott Company, 1987.

Curry, Thomas S., James E. Dowdey, and Robert C. Murry. *The Physics of Diagnostic Radiology.* 4th ed. Philadelphia, PA: Lea & Febiger, 1990.

Fodor, Joseph III, and Jack C. Malott. Magnification radiography. *Radiologic Technology* 58:4, 313–318, 1987.

Jenkins, David. *Radiographic Photography and Imaging Processes.* Lancaster, England: MTP Press, 1980.

Jenkins, David, and S. M. Latham. The duplication of chest radiographs. *Radiography* 45:539, 244–248, 1979.

Martin, Allan J., and Andrew K. Poznanski. A simple approach to lightening an overexposed film with a Blue Ray copier. *Radiologic Technology* 49:1, 39, 1977.

Mathias, Jerome L., and James R. Marquis. Radiographic duplication: A simple method of minimizing radiation dosage to the patient. *Radiologic Technology* 48:3, 293, 1976.

Pruneau, Donna, Susan Faszold, David Sostarich, Kris Weinshillbaum. A practical approach to direct magnification radiography. *Radiologic Technology* 59:2, 121, 1988.

Ridgway, Arthur, and Walter Thumm. *The Physics of Medical Radiography.* Reading, MA: Addison-Wesley Publishing Co., 1973.

Roberts, Derrick P., and Nigel L. Smith. *Radiographic Imaging—A Practical Approach.* Lancaster, England: Churchill Livingstone, 1988.

Seeram, Euclid. *X-Ray Imaging Equipment.* Springfield, IL: Charles C. Thomas Publisher, 1985.

Snopek, Albert M. *Fundamentals of Special Radiographic Procedures.* 2nd ed. Philadelphia, PA: W. B. Saunders Co., 1984.

Wilson, Peter. Some application problems and solutions in xeromammography. *Radiologic Technology* 48:4, 389–403, 1977.

40 DIGITAL IMAGE PROCESSING

. . . the digital computer has revolutionized virtually every element of diagnostic imaging . . . diagnostic imaging is one of the most exciting and rapidly evolving fields of medicine, and without question is leading all of medicine into the computer-electronic era.

William R. Hendee, Preface to Christopher C. Kuni's *Introduction to Computers and Digital Processing in Medical Imaging.*

OUTLINE

THE COMPUTER
IMAGE PROCESSING
DIGITAL IMAGE QUALITY
DIGITAL RADIOGRAPHY AND FLUOROSCOPY
DIGITAL PICTURE ARCHIVING AND COMMUNICATION
   SYSTEMS (PACS)

OBJECTIVES

Upon completion of this chapter, the student should be able to:

1. Describe the differences between analog and digital computers.
2. Describe the differences between programs and data.
3. State reasons why binary machine code is used in place of other languages.
4. Describe the basic function of a central processing unit, read only memory and random access memory.
5. Describe the basic function of various memory storage, input and output devices.
6. Explain the basic function of an array processor.
7. Describe the process of digital image data acquisition.
8. State reasons why Fourier transformation and inverse Fourier transformation are used in digitization of imaging data.
9. State the function of convolution and deconvolution.
10. Describe the effects of frequency, contrast and noise on digital image quality.

11. Explain the function of digital image window level and width controls.
12. Describe various factors that directly affect digital image resolution.
13. Explain the digital subtraction process and various filtering techniques.
14. Describe the photostimulable imaging process.
15. Describe a digital picture archiving and communication system (PACS).

The future of medical imaging lies unquestionably in computerized applications of the numerous modalities that currently exist, as well as in the integration of those now on the horizon. The explosion of the imaging sciences that has taken place since the early 1970s was caused by the first wave of digital computerization in computed tomography (CT) and ultrasound. Computed tomography has captured the imagination of the public; digital processing has now been successfully applied to nuclear medicine, subtraction angiography and magnetic resonance imaging (MRI), and is currently being explored for its application to electroencephalography.

The method by which these imaging modalities have been computerized is digital processing of imaging information. The resulting sectional images have enabled radiographers to understand anatomy from transverse, sagittal and coronal perspectives. Those who work in the digital computerized modalities must often visualize anatomy as a dynamic three-dimensional tilting, rotating and tumbling process due to computer manipulation of imaging data.

THE COMPUTER

Computers are devices that process information. The earliest computer device, the abacus, dates to around 3,000 B.C., and calculating machines were developed in the 1600s. The modern electronic computer, ENIAC, was developed in 1945 at the University of Pennsylvania. The addition of the mathematical theories of Baron Jean Fourier (1768–1830) and George Boole (1815–1864), solid state electronics in the 1940s, and microchip technology in the 1960s were all required prior to the first digital computer applications in medical imaging.

Analog and Digital Computers

Analog computers handle data composed of continuously varying electrical currents. Digital computers handle data composed of definite quantities of current (i.e., current on versus current off). For example, an analog watch displays time with hands while a digital watch uses a numerical readout. All medical imaging is achieved with digital computers, often from information that has been processed by an analog-to-digital converter (ADC). Digitization of analog information, such as the vast number of incident photons that comprise a radiographic image, always reduces the quantity and quality of the remaining information. Figure 40–1 illustrates the digitization process. Digital-to-analog converters (DAC) are sometimes used to permit faster transmission of data. After transmission, an ADC is used to convert the data for digital display or processing.

Programs and Data

Computers use two types of information: operating instructions, called the **program** and collected facts, called **data**. Programs provide specific instructions for calculations and sequential steps to be followed. Special computer languages, such as FORTRAN (FORmula TRANslation) and BASIC (Beginner's All-purpose Symbolic Instruction Code) are used

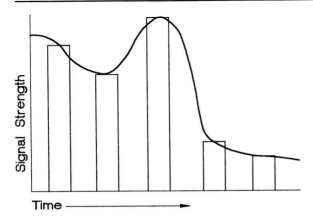

Figure 40–1.   Analog-to-digital conversion of imaging information. The line represents the input data; the blocks represent the digitization of the data.

for programming. Programs are called **software** while computer equipment is called **hardware**. One of the most useful programming techniques is the ability to program a computer to do problem solving, such as an if-then statement in which a computer can determine if a condition has been met, and then perform various operations depending on the exact conditions.

1	read memory 1
2	if memory 1 is less than 5 then go to line 5
3	if memory 1 equals 5 then go to line 6
4	if memory 1 is greater than 5 then go to line 7

For example, this program provides three alternative actions depending on the value of the information stored in memory 1. Complex programs have many alternative functions that

can be performed as variables are processed by the computer.

Binary Machine Language

Computers operate from a **binary machine language**. Just as English has a 26 letter symbol alphabet, the binary system operates with a two symbol alphabet. Because electrical currents are most easily understood as being either on or off, the binary system consists of information recorded as either a zero for off or a one for on. Each binary number is called a **bit**, for **binary digits**. Nominal numbers function on a base 10 system instead of base 2. Table 40–1 illustrates how the numbers 1 through 10

TABLE 40–1	
BINARY CODE NUMBERS	
Arabic	Binary
1	1
2	10
3	11
4	100
5	101
6	110
7	111
8	1000
9	1001
10	1010
.	.
.	.
.	.
16	10000
.	.
.	.
32	100000
.	.
.	.
etc.	

are written in binary code. An eight bit word is required to form the 26 letters of the English alphabet. As a convenience, an eight bit word is called a **byte**. Computer memory is often rated in terms of the total byte memory (rounded off). For example, a 10 megabyte magnetic hard disk will store over 10,000,000 bytes (80,000,000 bits) of information.

Central Processing Unit (CPU)

The CPU is the heart of every computer. It directs information to and from the various components that make up the computer system. For example, when a computer is turned on, the CPU may extract information from a permanent memory that loads an operating system program into the working memory. This operating system may then display instructions on a cathode ray tube (CRT) monitor. When a keyboard is used to input information, the CPU may then extract a program from memory and begin to carry out its instructions to operate imaging equipment.

The electrical connections between the CPU and the components run along a system of parallel conductors called a **bus**. Parallel connections permit simultaneous transmission of information but they are expensive because a separate conductor must exist for each channel of information. Serial connectors are less expensive but require significantly more transmission time because information must be transmitted sequentially instead of simultaneously. Peripheral devices, such as memory storage units, printers, modems and imaging systems, also use parallel and serial connectors.

Memory

Information can be stored in a computer's memory as magnetic variations and can be transferred as voltage. Magnetic field direction or greater and lesser voltage represent "on," or 1, and "off," or 0 indications. Memory is also classified as **read** memory or **write** memory. Read memory simply extracts information without alteration. Write memory replaces (deletes) old memory with new information.

ROM and RAM Memory is classified as read only memory (ROM) or random access memory (RAM). Both standard ROM and programmable ROM (PROM) usually contain basic operating instructions that are rarely, if ever, changed. The RAM usually functions as temporary storage for programming and operating instructions during their use and is constantly changed. When the main power to the computer is turned off, RAM is erased while ROM is maintained.

Peripherals

Peripheral devices permit input and/or output of information to and/or from the CPU. Some peripherals may appear to be a physical part of the computer, such as an input memory disk drive, while others may appear to be separate devices, such as a paper printer.

Memory Storage Devices A number of memory storage devices for data have become popular. These include **magnetic** and **optical** recording on both **tape** and **disk**. Information can be stored by optical (laser) recording and reading as well as by electronic and magnetic fields. Magnetic tape is often called mag tape and, although inexpensive, is difficult to access because data is stored serially. Magnetic disks have evolved from large (8") to small (5¼") **floppy disks** and then to even smaller (3½") **diskettes**. For large amounts of data a **hard disk** (Winchester drive) is required. Although they are more expensive, disks have become extremely popular because random access storage permits extremely short access times. Optical tape and disks permit the storage of significantly more data, but the recording equipment is much more expensive and the tape or disk cannot be rerecorded. Medical imaging modalities have used all of these devices for storing images and their associated data.

Input Devices The most familiar computer input device is a keyboard with a CRT for visualization of information before it is sent into the CPU. For example, a CT unit may wait for an entire examination protocol to be entered before it is sent to the CPU. In addition to keyboards, some units provide a visual marker known as a **cursor** on the CRT screen. The cursor can be moved by keyboard arrows, a joystick, track ball, pad and pen, light or ultrasonic pen or a specialized sliding control unit called a **mouse**. Some radiographic equipment uses a CRT touch screen for input, and voice-activated units will be feasible some day. Input via these devices can be remarkably simple. For example, ultrasound units will place a centimeter ruler through the anatomical image from a cursor location and CT units will provide radiation attenuation coefficient numbers (CT numbers) for the tissue at the cursor location. Image receptors, such as television cameras, ultrasonic transducers, CT ion detectors and MRI radiofrequency detectors also input information signals to CPUs for processing into visual images.

Output Devices The most familiar output devices are CRT screens and paper printers. Computerized imaging systems often send output information directly to CRT or laser film recording systems for the production of visual images. Most computerized imaging systems incorporate both input and output CRTs into their control consoles. Some computers use a single CRT for both input and output information.

Array Processors An array processor is a specialized computer that functions as a peripheral. It uses its CPU memory to perform simultaneous mathematical operations in a parallel fashion at extremely high speed instead of performing them sequentially. Array processors are useful when vast numbers of repetitive calculations are required, as in the processing of image detector data from CT or MRI equipment.

IMAGE PROCESSING

Digital Image Acquisition

A digital image is one that has been converted into numerical values for transmission or processing. A detector of some type must be used to acquire the image information. There are many types of detectors for various types of input information—ionizing radiation, ultrasonic waves, radiofrequencies, etc. Detectors acquire information either by **scanning** an area for information or by area or **array** detection, in which information is received from an entire area at once. For example, a fluoroscopic image is digitized by the plumbicon™ camera for transmission to the display monitor CRT. Although the CRT image is of significantly less resolution than the original image, it is simply a matter of numbers. The CRT is limited to 525 or 1,050 lines of resolution while the primary photon beam has millions of incident photons. If the CRT could display millions of lines of data, the image would exhibit comparable resolution. Most CRTs are capable of only 1–2 lp/mm.

Although digital images currently have diagnostic limits due to resolution, as display capabilities increase diagnostic confidence will also increase. Computerized digital images are described in terms of the number of values displayed per image side. A **matrix** is a square series of boxes that gives form to the image (Figure 40–2A). Each box of an image matrix will display a numerical value which can be transformed into a visual brightness or density level (Figure 40–2B & C). The individual matrix boxes are known as picture elements or **pixels**. The greater the matrix size the better the resolution because a larger matrix provides

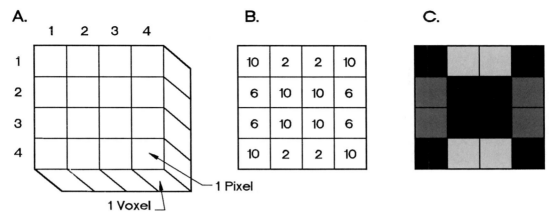

Figure 40–2. Digital image matrix expressions. (A) A matrix. (B) A matrix with numerical values. (C) A matrix with visual density values corresponding to the numerical values in B.

smaller pixels. Pixel size determines resolution (Figure 40–3A–E). CT and MRI images are usually displayed on a 512 × 512 matrix (262,144 pixels). Each pixel location is determined by its address (for example, in Figure 40–2A the address of the labeled pixel is 4-4). In medical imaging each pixel value corresponds to a three-dimensional volume of tissue known as a **voxel** (see Figure 40–2A).

Fourier Transformation

The primary mathematical method used in the creation of computerized medical images is the Fourier transformation. Transformations are simply conversions of data to more useful forms, as when radiation doses are changed from rems to mSv. Visual transformations can also be useful, as when a decubitus abdomen radiograph is viewed horizontally to facilitate detection of air-fluid levels.

Fourier's mathematics accomplishes transformations of extremely complex functions into separate but simpler functions. Kuni uses an example of a Fourier transform applied to separate music into functions of varying amplitudes, frequencies and timing phases. This data can then be recorded on magnetic tape for use in a tape player. The Fourier transform per-

mits the reconstruction of portions of the data when the other portions and their relationships are known. It is also possible to use the inverse Fourier transform to change back to the original data.

In computerized imaging, the Fourier transform is used on data representing image intensities at specific locations. For example, Figure 40–4 demonstrates different attenuation coefficients at specific image receptor locations. The inverse Fourier transformation can then be used to mathematically back-project an image of the structures that produced the attenuation coefficients (Figure 40–5).

Convolution and Deconvolution

It is sometimes useful to modify the value of each pixel to enhance or suppress a visual characteristic of the image. This process is actually mathematical filtering. **Convolution is the process of modifying pixel values by a mathematical formula**. It is sometimes called a **mask** because a set of mathematical operations is placed over each pixel, the pixel value is changed, the mask is then applied to the next pixel and so on. The total process is one of sliding the mask over all the pixel data and then displaying the modified image. **Deconvo-**

INFINITE

512 × 512

128 × 128

Figure 40–3. The effect of matrix size on resolution. (Photographs courtesy of Doug Raver, Lima Technical College.)

64 × 64

32 × 32

lution is the process of returning the pixel values to their original level by a reverse process.

DIGITAL IMAGE QUALITY

Data Characteristics

The quality of the data acquired from the image receptor is measured by its frequency, contrast and noise.

Frequency The frequency data is the raw data to which a Fourier transformation is applied to create the digital image. The acquired frequency is a measure of the total amount of contrast within the image. A high contrast image has high frequency, while a low contrast image has low frequency.

Contrast As with any image contrast, the acquired contrast is a measure of the differences between the data values. A **direct** relationship exists between subject contrast and acquired data contrast. When the subject contrast is high, the acquired data contrast will be high.

Noise Image noise is random background information that is detected but does not contrib-

Figure 40–4.   Image receptor data correlated to specific spatial locations. (Reprinted with permission from Greenfield, George B. and Lincoln Hubbard, *Computers in Radiology,* Churchill Livingstone, New York, 1984.)

ute to image quality. It is congruent with audio noise, such as the static "white noise" heard on frequencies between radio stations. White noise is visualized as "snow" on frequencies between television stations. It is measured as the **signal-to-noise ratio** (S/N). A high S/N indicates little noise in the image. Most fluoroscopic image noise is from electronic sources (i.e., the television chain). Background noise can be seen when the unit is used without a subject, although static digital images also contain visual noise. The noisiest component of most digital systems is the television camera. Commercial systems often have an S/N of 200 but the high resolution systems used in digital fluoroscopy have an S/N between 500 and 1,000.

Although noise looks like quantum mottle, the effect of the noise level on the digital image is more like the effect of base plus fog on radiographic film. Image noise has a **direct** relationship to contrast. Increased noise decreases image contrast. Conversely, increased image contrast tends to obscure or decrease noise. The effect of image noise on density is irrelevant in digital imaging because the computer can easily compensate for lack of density

Figure 40–5.   The concept of back-projection. (Reprinted with permission from Coulam, Craig M., and John J. Erickson, "Equipment considerations in computed tomography," *The Physical Basis of Medical Imaging,* 213–229. New York: Appleton-Century-Crofts, 1981.)

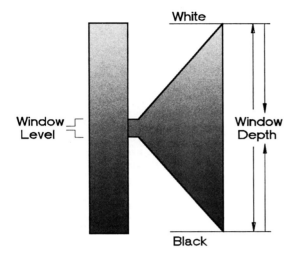

Figure 40–6.   Digital image windows. The window level can be moved up and down the density scale. The window width can be expanded and contracted.

as long as sufficient contrast exists to differentiate diagnostic data from noise.

Display Qualities

The density and contrast of the digital image are controlled by varying the numerical values of each pixel. The human visual range encompasses 32 or fewer shades of gray, while the photon beam that exits the patient encompasses over 1,000 shades. Most digital image detectors are sensitive to the majority of these 1,000 differences. Because the range of stored densities is so much wider than the visual range, any digital image is only a small part of the total data obtained by the computer. Each image is only a "window" on the total range of data (Figure 40–6). The computer can easily change the level and width of the display window by mathematical recalculations.

The quantity of information stored for each pixel varies depending on the gray scale imaging abilities of the system. For example, if a black and white image is desired with no

intermediate shades of gray, each pixel will require a single bit. Each pixel will either be turned on for white or off for black. When shades of gray are required, as for all diagnostic images, as many as 12 bits may be required per pixel. A 512 × 512 CT image could require 3,145,728 bits (393,216 bytes or 394 Kb). A single CT image requires more memory than the 256 Kb available in a common personal microcomputer.

The radiographer usually controls which portion of this vast amount of information will be seen by controlling the display image density and contrast recorded on the hard copy from which many radiologists diagnose. Although argument has been made for encouraging diagnosis from CRT displays, the majority of radiologists continue to read transilluminated film hard copy images for most examinations. This practice makes the radiographer responsible for choosing the appropriate density and contrast ranges to be displayed. It is critical that radiographers who are required to produce digital images be familiar with the manner in which the computer determines what portion of the image information will be displayed. Careful image processing is critical to avoid obscuring diagnostically critical information from the radiologist.

Window Level   When the values of each pixel are changed by addition or subtraction, the total value of the entire image changes. Because a computer can express a vast range of values, it can "see" image densities far below and beyond the range of human vision. One of the most important values of digital imaging is the ability of the computer to mathematically bring density differences into the visual range from extremely low input doses that would produce densities far below the normal range of vision.

The window level controls image density. There is a **direct** relationship between window level and image density (see Figure

40–6). When the window level is increased, image density increases. The window level must be adjusted to the proper level to display diagnostically relevant information. Information outside the chosen window level is lost from diagnosis. In some instances two images may have to be produced to visualize an appropriate range of densities. For example, in routine chest CT an image with appropriate densities for the mediastinum and chest wall must be recorded in addition to a second image with appropriate densities for the lung fields (Figure 40–7).

Window Width When the values of each pixel are changed by multiplication or division, the value range of the entire image changes. A computer can expand or compress image densities to fill the range of human vision. Window width changes are sometimes called gray scale expansion or compression. Another important value of digital imaging is the ability of the computer to mathematically expand the visual density differences from similar input

doses that would produce contrast far below the normal range of vision.

The window width controls image contrast. There is a **direct** relationship between window width and image contrast (see Figure 40–6). When the window width is increased, image contrast increases. Figure 40–8 illustrates different window levels and widths. An extremely wide window width requires the com puter to ignore fine contrast differences in order to display the entire range of data. An extremely narrow window width requires the computer to ignore a large amount of data outside the chosen range. For this reason, **window width can be said to control visibility of detail**. Extremely narrow window widths may cause an objectionable increase in the image noise level. Information outside the chosen window width is lost from diagnosis. The window width must be adjusted to display a maximum amount of diagnostically relevant contrast.

Resolution Resolution is controlled by the matrix size, as discussed above. There is a

Figure 40–7A & B. A clinical example of window level and width changes. Computed tomography of the chest requires two images to demonstrate the entire range of diagnostic densities. (A) High window level and narrow window width to demonstrate the mediastinum and chest wall. (B) Low window level and wide window width to demonstrate the lung fields. (Courtesy of Van Wert County Hospital, Van Wert, Ohio.)

Figure 40–8A–F. Window levels and widths. The same chest CT as in Fig. 40–7, with window width changes. (A) Extremely narrow. (B) Moderate. (C) Extremely wide. The same chest with window level changes. (D) Extremelylow. (E) Low. (F) Normal. The gray scale at the right of each image has a line to demonstrate where the high and low densities are extracted from the available data, illustrating both the window width and level. It is advisable to set the window level (density) first and then determine an appropriate window width (contrast). (Courtesy of Van Wert County Hospital, Van Wert, Ohio.)

direct relationship between matrix size and image resolution (see Figure 40–2). When matrix size is increased, image resolution increases. Matrix size is not variable within a system. It is controlled by the quantity of image detectors and the accompanying electronics built into the system.

As discussed previously, the primary limitation on digital images is the raster scan pattern of the display CRT. Commercial units achieve only 525 lines of interlaced scanning in which only 262.5 lines are scanned in one pass. This produces only 1–2 lp/mm for diagnostic imaging. The frequency response of the

incoming signal is termed the **bandwidth.** The bandwidth also affects the resolution. In the United States, commercial television is broadcast at 4 MHz, which produces about 320 lines of resolution.

Progressive scanning increases resolution slightly by scanning all 525 lines in order. **Slow scanning** also increases resolution but cannot be used in real-time dynamic studies with digital fluoroscopy. High resolution video is now available commercially and has been used in radiological applications for some time. The raster pattern is increased to 1,050 lines (often called a 1,000-line system) and the bandwidth is increased to 20 MHz, which produces about 800 lines of resolution. The result is a resolving ability of about 3–4 lp/mm.

Filtering Digital filtering of images utilizes the computer to extract more diagnostic information. It is usually accomplished by transforming the image into frequencies, mathematically altering the frequency by convolution and then using deconvolution and an inverse Fourier transformation to reproduce the image. The computer either accentuates or suppresses selected frequencies during the filtering process. Digitized image filters are classified as low-pass, band-pass or high-pass. The term **masking** is sometimes applied to the filtering process to indicate which frequencies have been suppressed. Masking of high frequencies produces low-pass filtering and vice versa.

Low-pass filtering either amplifies or deletes all but the low frequencies. It frequently appears to reduce image contrast and is often used to remove high frequency noise, especially when very little data is available (Figure 40–9). Low-pass filtering can also be accomplished by averaging each pixel's value with that of adjacent pixels. This type of low-pass filtering is sometimes called **smoothing.** Nine point smoothing averages each pixel with the eight adjacent pixels to accomplish a nine pixel average. Low radiation count nuclear medicine studies often use smoothing techniques.

Band-pass filtering either amplifies or deletes all but a selected range or band of frequencies. It is useful in the elimination of characteristic emission peaks, or in nuclear medicine, when a particular characteristic emission permits the localization of an injected radioisotope.

High-pass filtering either amplifies or deletes all **but** the high frequencies. It often appears to increase image contrast and is sometimes called **edge enhancement** filtering or **sharpening** (Figure 40–10). When the frequencies that represent structures of interest can be identified, as in contrast medium filled vessels, amplification of their frequencies can

A   B

Figure 40–9.   Low-pass filtering or smoothing. Transverse brain sections from a nuclear medicine study. (A) Smoothed. (B) Noisier filter. (Courtesy of Mike Ballistrea, Department of Nuclear Medicine, Meridia Hillcrest Hospital, Mayfield Heights, Ohio.)

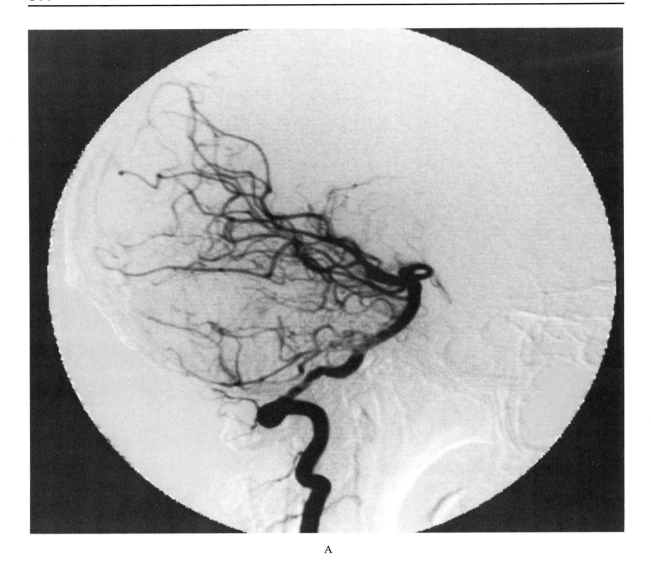

A

Figure 40–10.   High-pass filtering or sharpening. Edge enhancement is demonstrated on these digital sub-traction angiograms. (A) Normal image. (B) With high-pass filtering. (Courtesy of Rick Halker, Lima Memorial Hospital, Lima, Ohio.)

produce an edge enhancement effect while other frequencies are actually suppressed. The result is an image with edge enhancement and greatly increased contrast. This type of high-pass filtering is useful in digital vascular imag-ing and in digital mammography. However, extremely small structures can sometimes be buried in an edge, and undesirable edges are usually enhanced as well as those that are of diagnostic value.

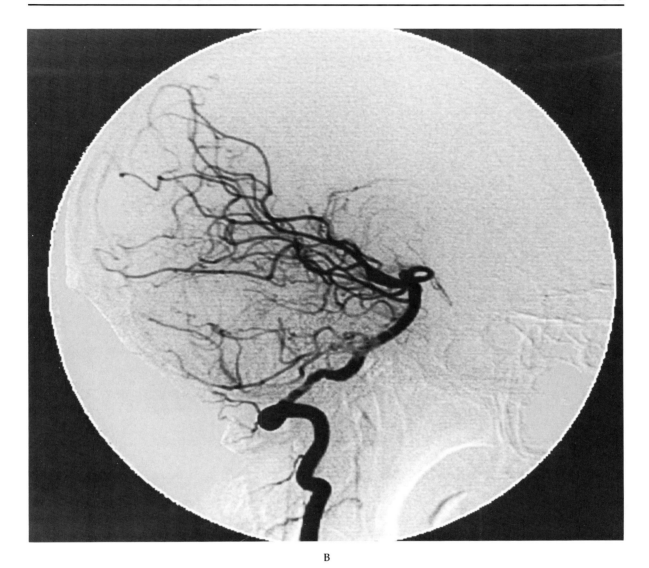

B

DIGITAL RADIOGRAPHY AND FLUOROSCOPY

Digital fluoroscopic systems began clinical trials in the early 1970s and gained acceptance for angiographic subtraction studies during the 1980s. Although several digital radiographic systems have been developed, image quality, cost and memory storage limits continue to confine their clinical applications. An exception is the use of a scanned projection image for orientation with CT studies.

Digital Subtraction Radiography

Digital subtraction radiography (DSR) combines the digitization of an image with subtraction techniques. The most common use of DSR is with fluoroscopic angiography as a substitute for static serial angiographic films produced by a rapid film changer. As a result of this primary use, DSR is also known as digital subtraction angiography (DSA), digital subtraction imaging (DSI), digital vascular imaging (DVI) and digital fluoroscopy (DF), although the last two do not necessarily use subtraction.

Imaging Procedure

The x-ray tube used for digital fluoroscopy operates in pulses at diagnostic range mA (100–300 mA) to avoid quantum mottle. A high-resolution image intensifier with a low lag plumbicon™ tube or CCD camera is used as the image receptor in a DSR system. Its function is to digitize the incoming photon beam. Formation of the DSR image requires that a scout image be obtained. The scout image is then reversed to form a **mask.** The mask is then superimposed on subsequent images containing an injected contrast medium. The result is subtraction of all the densities that were present in the scout image, leaving only the densities that were added by the injected contrast medium. For example, a cerebral angiogram can be modified by DSR to produce dynamic images of the cerebral vasculature with the cranial structures removed. The technique is particularly useful in demonstrating small vessels that would otherwise be obscured by superimposed bony structures.

A DSR system does not use mathematical reconstruction such as the Fourier transformation. Instead it simply manipulates the digitized information mathematically. Because manipulation must be accomplished very quickly (about 30 images per second), an array processor is required.

Temporal Subtraction Temporal subtraction is the basic subtraction procedure discussed above but within a limited time. It is used to reduce subject noise, thus increasing contrast between opacified vessels and other structures. The term **mask subtraction** is applied to the simplest form of temporal subtraction, which consists of real-time display and storage of subtracted images.

Time interval difference (TID) subtraction is designed to permit visualization of the difference between two different phases of vascular injection. It is accomplished by setting a time interval that is maintained between the mask and the injection image. Consequently, the mask continues to change. For example, if the time interval corresponds to the difference between 5 images, exposure 1 would become the mask for exposure 6, exposure 2 would mask exposure 7, etc. The resulting image can demonstrate early vascular filling in one color (usually black) and late filling in another color (usually white). TID subtraction presents an abbreviated dynamic study. The primary advantage of the technique is that motion is often eliminated because the time interval between the mask and the injection image is very short.

Matched filtering uses the sum of several images obtained when the contrast medium is at its maximum (during the arterial phase of an injection). The mask is then subtracted from the combined image of maximum contrast material.

Recursive filtering combines several injected images to form a subtraction, as with matched filtering. Recursive filtering is much more sophisticated in that the images are density weighted, or given greater emphasis according to a time scheme. The time scheme or **time filter** can be set by the operator to enhance structures of interest.

Dual Energy Subtraction Dual energy subtraction techniques can be used to separate the K-shell characteristic edge of iodine (at 33 keV) from surrounding bone and soft tissue. Essentially the technique subtracts a high kVp image and a low kVp image. Dual energy subtraction is useful because all images can be acquired during the injection phase, thus sufficiently reducing the time between exposures to eliminate most motion. It is of little value by itself, but it is useful in hybrid subtraction.

Hybrid Subtraction Hybrid subtraction is a combination of energy subtraction with one of the temporal subtraction techniques. It has the advantage of reducing patient motion while providing a more normal image than with time interval difference subtraction.

Pixel Shifting Pixel shifting is used to help overcome patient motion, which is especially a problem with temporal subtraction. Motion disrupts the alignment, or registration, of the mask and renders the image useless.

When high pressure injection techniques are used, as in most angiographic studies, it is extremely difficult for patients to avoid movement. **Pixel shifting** or **linear translation** is possible when attempting to resolve motion problems. The computer can compare pixel values while shifting either the mask or the injected image until overall pixel values are as close to one another as possible to create the closest possible visual alignment. Pixel shifting is effective only for linear motion; it is not effective with rotary motion, such as swallowing.

Photostimulable Radiography

Photostimulable radiography, also known as computed radiography or diagnostic digital radiography, uses image receptors with barium fluorohalide screens that function quite differently from intensifying screens in that a latent image is stored upon exposure to ionizing radiation (in a manner similar to the xeroradiographic process). The latent image can be released upon stimulation by light, permitting the photostimulable screens to be exposed in cassettes with diagnostic radiographic equipment (see Figure 24–1).

The incident photon beam produces a latent image within the fluorohalides. The fluorohalides are stimulated by a laser, which causes them to emit light. The light is then detected by a photomultiplier tube which digitizes the image. Display and storage then proceed as with any other digital image. Although resolution continues to be a problem, patient dose is dramatically reduced, and digital contrast and latitude control are superior. It appears that photostimulable detectors may offer a feasible method of producing digitized images with existing diagnostic radiographic equipment.

DIGITAL PICTURE ARCHIVING AND COMMUNICATION SYSTEMS (PACS)

Picture archiving and communication systems (PACS) are computerized storage and transmission systems for digitized images of all types, including static diagnostic, ultrasound, CT, MRI, DSR, etc. The first advances in PACS technology were made with long distance transmission systems for clinics in remote areas (such as northern Canada) and for specialist consultations in rural areas. Some hospitals use PACS so radiologists can receive images and provide immediate consultation at satellite centers and when on call at home.

Although concerns continue to be expressed over the resolution of PACS images, in most instances a preliminary reading can be provided. In addition, PACS images can be manipulated by window level and width adjustments, enlargements, tissue density readings and subtractions, permitting the radiologist to obtain more information than any film image can provide and without additional exposure dose to the patient.

Archiving

A major problem for all radiology departments is the storage of film as required by local legal precedents. Many institutions store all films for five to seven years, with pediatric and litigation films retained indefinitely. Many hours of staff time and immense amounts of space are required to maintain these files. A PACS system eliminates the need for most of the space for storage and reduces the time requirements. Misfiling becomes much less likely and acquisition time can be reduced tremendously. In addition, PACS terminals permit access to images from remote locations (for example, surgery, emergency units, etc.).

Image storage requires immense amounts of memory. Digitization of static radiographic images requires at least a 1,050 × 1,050 matrix with 12 bits of gray scale density per pixel (high resolution chest digitization has been done with a 4,096 × 4,096 matrix). Most other modalities (CT, ultrasound, MRI, etc.) require a 512 × 512 matrix with 6–8 bits per pixel. This means that an average examination requires 1–6 Mb of memory for storage. Complete digitization cannot occur until sufficient inexpensive memory becomes available to make PACS possible. For example, a 500-bed hospital that performs 75,000 examinations per year would require over 400,000 Mb (400 gigabytes) of image storage per year. Although this memory would normally be available by hard disk storage, the routine retrieval of images three to five years old in most departments would require immediate access memory of over 1,500,000 Mb (1,500 gigabytes) in our example hospital.

Communication

Communication of PACS images involves transmitting images with voice and/or word processing to distant locations. Whether the location is removed from the radiology department by a floor, a building, a block or hundreds of miles, radiologist consultation becomes available more efficiently than before.

Thinking has also begun on linking PACS images to programming that would permit radiological diagnosis. In the early 1960s a radiological diagnostic program was proven to be accurate, but no method has yet been accom-plished to acquire the complex pattern recognition that is necessary. This development is in the distant future, after artificial intelligence programming has been developed.

SUMMARY

The future of medical imaging lies in computerized applications of the numerous modalities. The method by which these imaging modalities have been computerized is digital processing of imaging information.

Computers are devices that process information. Analog computers handle data composed of continuously varying electrical currents. Digital computers handle data composed of definite quantities of current (for example, current on versus current off). All medical imaging is achieved with digital computers, often from information that has been processed by an analog-to-digital converter (ADC). Computers use two types of information: operating instructions, called the program and collected facts, called data. Programs are called software while computer equipment is called hardware.

Computers operate from a binary machine language with a two symbol alphabet. Because electrical currents are most easily understood as being either on or off, the binary system consists of information recorded as either a 0 for off or a 1 for on. Each binary number is called a bit, for binary digits. An eight-bit word is called a byte. Computer memory is often rated in terms of the total byte memory.

The CPU directs information to and from the various components that make up the computer system. Information is stored in a computer's memory and is classified as read only memory (ROM) or random access memory (RAM). Peripheral devices permit input and/or output of information to and/or from the CPU and include memory storage devices, along with a variety of input and output devices.

A digital image is one that has been converted into numerical values for transmission or processing. A detector of some type must be used to acquire the image information. A matrix is a square series of boxes that gives form to the image. The individual matrix boxes are known as picture elements or pixels. Pixel size determines resolution. In medical imaging each pixel value corresponds to a three-dimensional volume of tissue, known as a voxel.

The primary mathematical method used in the creation of computerized medical images is the Fourier transformation. Convolution is the process of modifying pixel values by a mathematical formula. Deconvolution is the process of returning the pixel values to their original level by a reverse process.

The quality of the data acquired from the image receptor is measured by its frequency, contrast and noise. The density and contrast of the digital image are controlled by varying the numerical values of each pixel. The window level controls image density. Window width changes the gray scale expansion or compression and therefore controls contrast. Resolution is controlled by the matrix size.

Digital filtering of images is usually accomplished by transforming the image into frequencies, mathematically altering the frequency by convolution and then using deconvolution and an inverse Fourier transformation to reproduce the image. The computer either accentuates or suppresses selected frequencies during the filtering process. Digitized image filters are classified as low-pass, bandpass or high-pass.

Digital subtraction radiography (DSR) combines the digitization of an image with subtraction techniques. The most common use of DSR is with fluoroscopic angiography as a substitute for static serial angiographic films produced by a rapid film changer.

Photostimulable radiography uses photostimulable image receptors made of barium fluorohalide screens that can store a latent image which can be released upon stimulation by light. They can be exposed in cassettes with diagnostic radiographic equipment.

Picture archiving and communication systems (PACS) are computerized storage and transmission systems for digitized images of all types.

REVIEW QUESTIONS

1. What is the difference between analog and digital computers?

2. Why do computers operate from a binary machine language?

3. What is the function of the central processing unit?

4. What is the most common input device?

5. How is a digital image acquired?

6. What is image noise?

7. How do the window level and the window width affect the digital image display?

8. What are the three types of digital image filtering methods?

9. What is the principle application of digital subtraction radiography?

10. What is the purpose of pixel shifting during digital subtraction?

11. What are the advantages of PACS?

REFERENCES AND RECOMMENDED READING

Berland, Lincoln L. *Practical CT Technology and Techniques*. New York: Raven Press, 1987.

Brody, William R. *Digital Radiography*. New York: Raven Press, 1984.

Brody, William R., and Albert Macovski. Dual-energy digital radiography. *Diagnostic Imaging* 3, 18–25, 1981.

Bushong, Stewart C. *Radiologic Science for Technologists: Physics, Biology, and Protection.* 4th ed. St. Louis: C.V. Mosby Co., 1988.

Coulam, Craig M., and John J. Erickson. Equipment considerations in computed tomography. *The Physical Basis of Medical Imaging,* 213–229. New York: Appleton-Century-Crofts, 1981.

Curry, Thomas S., James E. Dowdey, and Robert C. Murry. *Christensen's Physics of Diagnostic Radiology.* 4th ed. Philadelphia, PA: Lea & Febinger, 1990.

De Brusk, Peter D. Digital x-ray imaging: The basics. *Radiologic Technology* 54, 280, 1983.

Dobbins, James T., and Allen O. Powell. Variable compensation technique for digital radiography of the chest. *Radiology* 157, 451, 1989.

Gould, R. G. Digital hardware in radiography and fluoroscopy. *Applied Radiology* 13, 137–140, 1984.

Greenfield, George B., and Lincoln Hubbard. *Computers in Radiology.* New York: Churchill Livingstone, 1984.

Hindel, R. Digital imaging—the technology of the future. *The Canadian Journal of Medical Radiation Technology* 14:4, 128, 1983.

Hunter, Tim B. *The Computer in Radiology.* Rockville, MD: Aspen, 1986.

Kuni, Christopher C. *Introduction to Computers and Digital Processing in Medical Imaging.* Chicago, IL: Yearbook Medical Publishers, Inc., 1988.

Kushner, David C. Radiation dose reduction in the evaluation of scoliosis: An application of digital radiography. *Radiology* 154, 175, 1986.

Long, Bruce W. Computed radiography: Photo-stimulable phosphor image plate technology. *Radiologic Technology* 61:2, 107–112, 1989.

Mistretta, Charles A., and Andrew B. Crummy. Digital fluoroscopy. *The Physical Basis of Medical Imaging.* 107–122. Editors: Coulam, Craig M., John J. Erickson, F. David Rollo, and A. Everette James, Jr. New York: Appleton-Century-Crofts, 1981.

Noz, M. E., W. A. Erdman, G. Q. McGuire, et al. Modus operandi for a picture archiving and communication system. *Radiology* 152, 221–223, 1984.

Pratt, W. K. *Digital Image Processing.* New York: John Wiley and Sons, 1978.

Price, Ronald R., F. David Rollo, W. Gordon Monahan, and A. Everette James, Jr. *Digital Radiography: A Focus on Clinical Utility.* New York: Grune & Stratton, 1982.

Riederer, S. J., and R. A. Kruger. Intravenous digital subtraction: A summary of recent developments. *Radiology* 147, 633–638, 1983.

Smith, C. B. Physical principles of digital radiography. *Radiography* 50:590, 41–44, 1984.

41 COMPUTED TOMOGRAPHY

The physicians seem to be quite keen on it.

Allan Cormack upon being informed that he and Godfrey Hounsfield were to share the 1979
Nobel Prize for Medicine for the invention of computed tomography.

OUTLINE

THE INVENTION OF COMPUTED TOMOGRAPHY
GANTRY
TABLE
X-RAY TUBES
DETECTORS
COMPUTER
DISPLAY CONSOLE
IMAGE STORAGE UNITS
COMPUTED TOMOGRAPHY NUMBERS (HOUNSFIELD UNITS—HU)
IMAGE RECONSTRUCTION
IMAGE QUALITY
SCANNING PROCEDURES
RADIATION PROTECTION

OBJECTIVES

Upon completion of this chapter, the student should be able to:

1. Relate the invention of computed tomography.
2. Describe typical gantry components.

3. Explain the basic features of each generation of CT scanners, especially third and fourth generation units.
4. Explain why CT tabletops have patient weight limits.
5. Compare the requirements for a CT x-ray tube with those of a routine diagnostic tube.
6. Explain the operation of a scintillation crystal and photomultiplier tube CT detector.
7. Explain the operation of a xenon gas-filled ionization chamber CT detector.
8. Discuss the importance of detector alignment and calibration.
9. Discuss the use of a CT computer menu or index.
10. Describe the major display features possible with advanced software.
11. Describe the calculation and use of Hounsfield units.
12. Explain reformatting image reconstruction.
13. Explain how CT display image density and contrast are controlled.
14. Describe the factors affecting resolution, including voxel, pixel and matrix size.
15. Discuss methods of reducing CT image noise and motion.
16. Illustrate section shape, partial volume effect and scan arc to scanning procedures.
17. Discuss radiation protection of the patient and others during CT examinations.

Computed tomography (CT) produces a digital tomographic image from diagnostic x-rays. The basic principle of CT involves digitizing an image received from a slit scan projection of the patient's body and then back-projecting the image through mathematical algorithms.

Although CT scanning is usually performed transversely, digital processing of information can produce sagittal and coronal sections (Figure 41–1). Because the CT x-ray beam is confined to a slit, much scatter radiation is eliminated from the image. The combination of the transverse sectioning procedure with slit scanning produces an image of significantly better quality than that available with other imaging methods. Primarily the image differentiates various types of soft tissues (e.g., gray matter, white matter, blood, tumor, cerebrospinal fluid, etc.). When digital image data manipulation is added, CT provides more diagnostic information than any other ionizing radiation imaging modality.

As with other tomographic modalities, the terms "cut" and "slice" are used in clinical practice. Because these phrases can easily cause distress when overheard by a patient, the radiographer should strive to adhere to the term "section," avoiding "cut" and "slice."

THE INVENTION OF COMPUTED TOMOGRAPHY

The invention of computed tomography has been credited to Godfrey N. Hounsfield for his work in 1970–71, although preliminary work was done by Oldendorf in 1961 and Cormack in 1963, and all three based their work on the investigations of the Austrian mathematician J. Radon, who proved in 1917 that an image of a three-dimensional object could be produced from its mathematical projections. Hounsfield was a research engineer with Electro-Musical Instruments Ltd. (EMI), the English firm that gained international renown as the Beatles' music publishers during the 1960s. His original scanner was built on a lathe bed and required nine days to produce a single section image. Although the company sold its CT business, it continues to operate American and British EMI record labels. Hounsfield and Cormack were awarded the 1979 Nobel Prize for Medicine. Hounsfield's invention parallels

Figure 41–1. Computed tomography sections: A. sagittal, B. transverse, C. coronal.

Röntgen's discovery of x-rays as the two most outstanding contributions to medical imaging.

Early CT units were capable of only axial tomography, and the term computerized axial tomography (CAT) scanning became a popular acronym. Modern CT units are capable of diverse modes much more complex than simple axial scanning. However, the term CAT scanning may endure, as have other antiquated radiologic terms (e.g., flat plate and wet reading). A modern CT unit includes a gantry, table, x-ray tube, detectors, computer, display console and image storage units (Figure 41–2).

GANTRY

The gantry is the movable frame of the CT unit. It contains the x-ray tube and detectors and is the most visible part of the unit. The gantry frame maintains the alignment of the tube and detectors and contains the equipment necessary to perform the scanning movements. The gantry includes a 50–85 cm (20"– 34") aperture for the patient. Obese patients who exceed the tabletop weight limits must never be forced into the aperture. They may become stuck.

Most gantrys can be angled up to 30° to permit positioning for partial coronal images. This is especially desirable in obtaining transverse scans perpendicular to the vertebral column. Table angulation can sometimes be used in place of gantry angulation. Scanners with the x-ray beam placed near the table side of the aperture permit more comfortable positioning of the patient and may permit coronal or sagittal scanning of some body parts, especially of the head. Both magnetic resonance imaging and CT reconfiguration software may be used in place of positions designed to achieve coronal or sagittal sections.

Positioning lights are usually mounted on the gantry as well. Intense white halogen lights and low-power red laser lights are used

Figure 41–2.   A computed tomography unit. (Courtesy of GE Medical Systems).

for positioning. The body part of interest must be properly centered to the aperture because the extreme edge of the scanning field produces a severely degraded image. There are often three positioning lights for accurate sagittal, coronal and transverse centering.

Scanner Generations

Computed tomography technology advanced very rapidly after Hounsfield's discovery. Scanners are often described by their generation, with the original EMI head scanner considered to be the first. Although there are no distinct lines between the generations, Table 41–1 illustrates the major characteristics of each.

First Generation First generation CT scanners were designed for examination of the head only and are no longer available (Figure 41–3). The head was surrounded by a water bag to eliminate air interfaces. A single x-ray tube and a pair of detectors were aligned on a fixed C-arm. The detectors were sodium iodide scintillation crystals with photomultiplier tubes. A pencil-thin slit field, 3 mm × 26 mm, scanned a 180° arc around the patient's head. Each detector was exposed to a 3 mm × 13 mm field. First generation units used a rotating scan and index system that scanned the head linearly (from one side to the other), indexed 1°, repeated the scanning process, indexed another 1°, etc., for the entire 180° (Figure 41–4).

TABLE 41–1

MAJOR CHARACTERISTICS OF CT UNIT GENERATIONS

First generation
head only
linear scan and rotate (180 scans, 1° rotations)
paired detectors (160 measurements per scan)
4.5–5 minute scan time
pencil beam
single detector

Second generation
fan-shaped beam (permitting whole body scanning)
up to 30 detectors
10–90 second scan time
linear scan and rotate (6 scans, 30° rotations)

Third generation
fan-shaped beam
up to 300 detectors
2–10 second scan time
360° rotation of x-ray tube and detectors
crude dynamic capabilities

Fourth generation
fan-shaped beam
360° ring of stationary detectors
2–10 second scan time
360° rotation of x-ray tube
dynamic capabilities

Others
nutating detector ring
multiple anode ring (cardiac system)
    50 msec scan time
multiple x-ray tube to video (DSR system)
    16 msec scan time

This is also called a translate (scan) and rotate (index) system. The x-ray tube was on during scanning and off during indexing. Although the pair of detectors did not decrease the 180° scanning time, they permitted two anatomical sections to be scanned simultaneously, thus reducing the total examination time by half.

The detectors measured the attenuation coefficient of the exit radiation beam at overlapping 1.7 mm intervals 240 times during each scan. The unit required 4.5 minutes to complete a pair of full 180° scans and 5 minutes to reconstruct the images. Each section was derived from 43,200 measurements (180° × 240) and was displayed on an 80 × 80 matrix. Each display pixel represented a voxel of tissue 3 mm × 3 mm × 13 mm although a 1.5 mm pixel display became available. A common examination routine for the head consisted of 10–12 sections, which required 25–35 minutes to obtain.

Second Generation Second generation CT units used a fan-shaped beam instead of a pencil slit and a linear array of as many as 30 detectors (Figure 41–5). They too are no longer available. The fan-shaped beam and increased number of detectors permitted scanning and

Figure 41–3. A first generation CT head scanner.

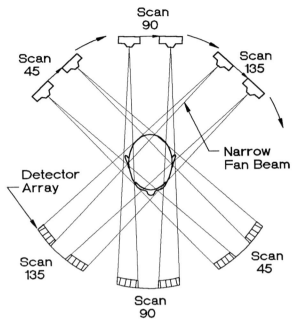

Figure 41–4. First generation CT scan and rotate system. Only three scans (the 45th, 90th, and 135th) are shown to simplify the illustration. A single scan and rotate required 180 scans, each 1° apart.

rotation with fewer linear movements. For example, a 30 detector unit could complete the 180° linear movement in only six rotations of 30° each. However, the loss of collimation increased the amount of scatter radiation detected. This is a major disadvantage of all fan beam scanners. A lead mask was added to the detectors to assist in reducing the scatter reaching the detectors. Scan time was reduced to between 10 and 90 seconds, a reasonable respiratory suspension time, thus permitting examination of the whole body.

Third Generation Third generation CT units used a wider fan-shaped beam and a curved array of 250–500 detectors (Figure 41–6). The fan-shaped beam was wide enough to include the entire body in a single exposure

and rotated 360° within the gantry, thus eliminating the linear scan and rotate system. A typical third generation scanner might produce 700,000 measurements per section. Various scanning arcs were usually possible, for example 220° or 360°. Scan time was reduced to between 1 and 12 seconds, permitting sequential images to crudely approximate dynamic functions. Third generation units that featured dynamic scanning usually performed at about four scans per minute, which equals the routine scanning time of a fourth generation unit.

Fourth Generation Fourth generation CT units were developed as a result of a competitive contract awarded to the American Science and Engineering Company (AS&E) by the United States National Institutes of Health

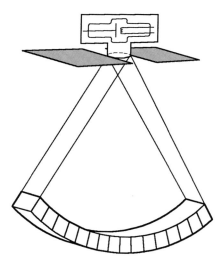

Figure 41–5.   A fan-shaped beam.

Figure 41–6.   A third generation CT scanner.

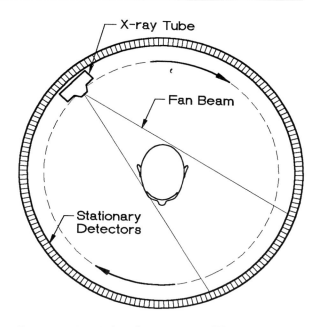

Figure 41–7.   A fourth generation CT scanner.

ing calibration requirements. As many as 1,200,000 measurements may be processed per section. A wider range of scan arcs, including arcs over 360°, are usually possible with scan times ranging from 0.5 to 10 seconds.

Some fourth generation scanners are capable of dynamic scanning rates in the range of 15 scans per minute. The limiting factor is the interscan time and the computer processing time, not the actual scanning time. Dynamic scanning is usually achieved by reducing the interscan time to 1–2 seconds and not indexing the gantry. Scanning occurs first in a clockwise direction, then counterclockwise, etc. Another technique, called overscan, may also be available. Overscanning uses a scan of more than 360°. The overscan may be displayed as segmented data from 2, 3 or 4 scans as a single image.

Fifth Generation Designs
Other CT designs have been produced. A **nutating** unit is one in which a 360° ring of detectors wobbles

(NIH). They use a fan-shaped beam with 600–2,000 stationary detectors arrayed in a 360° ring (Figure 41–7). The ring of detectors eliminates movement of detectors, thereby decreasto continually intercept a perpendicular beam from a tube which is also rotating 360°. The term nutating is derived from a similar motion observed in astronomy. This unit is capable of dynamic scanning. Two other designs also exist: the cardiac and the dynamic spatial reconstructor (DSR).

The **cardiac scanner** replaces the x-ray tube with a huge electron gun that directs an electron beam in a circular pattern at a 360° anode ring. The fan beam that is produced is intercepted by a 360° detector array. The patient is placed within the anode ring, somewhat akin to being inside the x-ray tube itself. This unit is a dynamic scanner as it can produce four sections simultaneously within 50 msec. The **dynamic spatial reconstructor** (DSR) was developed at the Mayo Clinic in Rochester, Minnesota. It uses 14 x-ray tubes with fluorescent screens and video cameras and is capable of producing an image in 16 msec.

TABLE

The CT table may be either flat or curved. It is usually made of carbon graphite fiber to decrease beam attenuation. Because the top must extend beyond the table to move the patient into the gantry aperture, it must be capable of supporting the entire weight of the patient without sagging when fully extended. Tabletops are rated for maximum weight and it is critical that the radiographer make sure that this weight is not exceeded. Extensive damage to the table may result when attempts are made to examine very large patients who exceed the tabletop weight limit. Physicians must be informed if the CT unit cannot move obese patients into the aperture for examination. Examinations of patients over the weight limit may remove the CT unit from clinical use for all patients for a considerable time while the top is replaced. The top is motor-driven to permit the patient to be moved the exact desired

distance between sections. Section intervals may be controlled automatically by a program initiated at the control console. The table must also be capable of vertical movement, both for positioning within the aperture and for ease of patient transfer.

X-RAY TUBES

The rapid sequential exposures required to produce CT images produce massive amounts of heat in the x-ray tube. Most CT x-ray tube difficulties have revolved around attempts to solve this problem. The early scanners used a stationary anode with a 2 mm × 16 mm focal spot operating at 120 kVp and 30 mA. This reduced image resolution significantly. However, since first generation images were usually displayed on an 80 × 80 matrix, the x-ray tube was not the problem in this system.

As matrix size increased to 512 × 512, rotating anode tubes with focal spots as small as 0.6 mm × 1.2 mm came into use. Small focal-spot scanners use a pulsed beam to reduce the heat load. Modern pulsed scanner tubes operate at 120 kVp, 1–5 msec pulses, and up to 1,000 mA. Some units permit 80 and 140 kVp to be selected, sometimes in alternate pulses, for dual-energy scanning in which comparisons can be made between images at different kVp values. In addition, 0.5–5.0 million heat unit anodes of layered alloys, cylindrical anodes and liquid-cooled and air-cooled tube housing designs have been developed. A CT tube may produce 30 exposures per examination. Because most CT units are scheduled for 10–20 examinations per day, a tube may accumulate 10,000 exposures in a single month. It is not unusual for a CT tube to fail after several months. Only a few last a full year.

The radiation beam is double collimated, once at the tube exit and again at the detector entrance. This assists in eliminating scatter information. Collimation controls the voxel length. Collimation is variable from 1 mm to 13 mm and is usually controlled by the software program. The dimension of the collimation width determines the voxel length, or section thickness.

DETECTORS

Detectors must be capable of responding with extreme speed to a signal, without lag, must quickly discard the signal, and prepare for the next. They must also respond consistently and be small in size. They are usually placed with a source-to-image receptor distance of 44″ (110 cm). Development of solid-state detectors may be the next major refinement in CT imaging.

Scintillation Crystals and Photomultiplier Tubes

Early detectors consisted of a scintillation crystal in contact with a photomultiplier tube (Figure 41–8). This system was used in nuclear medicine for many years prior to the advent of CT. A sodium iodide (NaI) crystal absorbs an x-ray photon and produces light flashes (scintillations) in proportion to the energy of the

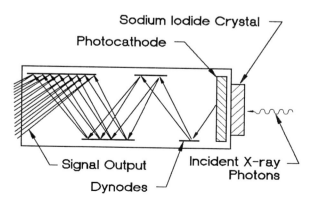

Figure 41–8. A scintillation crystal and photomultiplier tube detector.

photon and at the exact location where the photon struck within the crystal. This light (photo) is then amplified (multiplied) by the photomultiplier (PM) tube. The light photon strikes the cathode of the PM tube, where it is converted into electrons. The electrons are then amplified by a series of dynodes as they move through the tube. Each dynode has a higher voltage, thereby increasing the number and voltage of the electrons as they move toward the anode. Upon striking the anode, the electrons are converted into a digital signal which can be processed by the computer.

Although sodium iodide scintillation crystals are nearly 100 percent efficient within the diagnostic x-ray range, they exhibit phosphorescent afterglow, or lag. This makes them useless with the rapid sequential exposures in the later generation scanners. Some units have been produced using bismuth germinate, cesium iodine, and cadmium tungstate scintillation crystals, which, although less efficient ($\approx$ 90 percent), have minimal afterglow. A major disadvantage of scintillation-PM detectors is their size and interspace material, which prohibit packing them closer in the detector array. This reduces their total detection efficiency to less than 50 percent.

Xenon Gas-Filled Ionization Chambers

The most common CT detector is a xenon gas-filled ionization chamber (Figure 41–9). It operates on the same principle as an ionization chamber. Essentially, it measures ionization in air by attracting to an electrode the ions created by x-ray photons in the air. The electrodes are usually thin tungsten plates spaced 1.5 mm apart. This spacing determines the maximum detector (and therefore display pixel size) resolution. The electrodes are alternately charged with positive and negative voltages. The quantity of ionic charge at the electrode is

Figure 41–9. A xenon gas-filled ionization chamber CT detector. The tungsten plate electrodes are alternately charged with positive and negative voltages.

proportional to the energy of the photons detected between the electrodes. The detected energy comprises a digital signal that is sent to the computer.

Gas detectors range in efficiency from 60 to 90 percent but exhibit no lag. Ion chamber detectors were not used in the original EMI scanner because they were not sensitive enough. This disadvantage was overcome by using a long ion chamber and filling it with krypton or xenon, the heaviest inert gas, at high compression (20 atmospheres or more).

Although gas-ion detector efficiency may be only 60 percent, these detectors can be packed extremely close in the detector array, permitting a detection efficiency of slightly less than 50 percent, which is similar to that of scintillation-PM detectors.

Alignment

Tube and detector alignment is critical in CT because of the tight collimation of the tube and the collimator mask at the detector. The slightest misalignment may produce a concentric ring artifact image that completely overrides clinical information.

Rotating anode tubes are aligned with their long axis perpendicular to the scanning plane. This prevents the anode heel effect within the useful beam while eliminating the gyroscopic effect on the rotating anode.

Calibration

Detectors must remain in close calibration at all times. Some scanners calibrate detectors one per day while others calibrate them during scanning. One fourth generation scanner calibrates each detector immediately before and after it detects the fan beam. Detectors that are out of calibration may cause artifacts that destroy image quality.

COMPUTER

The CT computer is designed to control data acquisition, process and display, and storage. The computer itself is usually enclosed in a room that has controlled temperature and humidity. The CT console provides the radiographer with access to the software program that controls data acquisition, processing and display. Remote consoles may also be linked to the system to permit display and storage functions. Control of data storage may be available at the control console, remote consoles or at the storage units themselves.

A systems program is used to start up the CT unit. This program turns on and performs quality assurance checks on numerous components in both the x-ray equipment and computer hardware systems, warms up the x-ray tube, etc. It also permits the radiographer to record various problems that need the attention of the service engineer. One of its main functions is to perform calibration checks on the detectors, although this may be an ongoing process during scanning. A diagnostics program with specific quality assurance tests is used by service engineers to troubleshoot the systems.

The CT console operates from a "menu" or index directory of operations. The radiographer simply uses a keyboard, light pen or other input device to indicate the desired operation. At the beginning of each examination, patient information, such as identification, history, etc., is entered. This information permits retrieval of the images at a later date and will also be displayed adjacent to each image.

Data Acquisition

The data acquisition program controls a variety of operations, including tube and detector collimation (pixel size), matrix size, gantry angle, tabletop entrance into the gantry aperture, section increment movements of the tabletop, x-ray tube voltage and amperage, scan speed (the scanning operation itself) and the direction of detector signals to the digital image processing section of the computer.

DISPLAY CONSOLE

The processing and display program controls the digital image production process, including the series of mathematical formulas (algorithms) that compile the image and the display parameters, such as window level and width.

The display console is often part of the main console and appears as a separate CRT with controls (Figure 41–10). Also available are separate reporting consoles that permit radiologists to display images and electronically report the results, and independent consoles that contain their own CPU to retrieve and display images from the memory storage units and to receive images from examinations in progress.

Features

Most CT display units permit a wide range of display features to enhance diagnosis.

Figure 41–10.   CT main console with display CRT. (Courtesy of Siemens Medical Systems, Inc.)

These vary by manufacturer but often include the following.

Scanogram A localization image or **scanogram** is often displayed as the first image of an examination. It is achieved prior to the examination by slit scanning as the tabletop moves the patient through the tightly collimated primary beam. The resolution of the image is affected by the speed of the scan and the exposure output of the tube. The poorer the scan, the less the patient dose. Because these images are used primarily for localization, image quality is seldom important. The radiographer should advocate the highest-speed scan and the lowest exposure output possible. The addition to the slit scan of dotted lines corresponding to the section intervals provides a convenient reference guide when viewing the sectional images. The scanogram can serve as a diagnostic tool in radiation therapy treatment planning by using a cursor to delineate the margins of a tumor on a series of transverse sections. The scanogram can then compile the cursor delineations to provide a coronal and sagittal outline of the tumor. The scanogram is sometimes called by one of a number of trademark names.

Grid Application A grid pattern may be added to any image. Radiographers use the grid to confirm exact centering of the patient; radiologists use the grid pattern to describe precise structural locations.

Cursor A cursor can be used to outline an area of interest. The area can be recorded on film and the Hounsfield unit mean or standard deviation can be displayed for the tissue within the marked area. Hounsfield units (HU) are discussed below. A line can be drawn between any two cursor locations, displaying the area's measurement within the patient. A cursor can also be used by itself to mark an area of interest.

Density Contouring Software is available that permits selection of a single point by a cursor, with the program highlighting all pixels of matching HU. This feature can be used to outline a tumor or other object.

Radiation Therapy Planning Special software is available to facilitate radiation therapy treatment planning through the use of cursors and integration with dosimetric data from a dosimetry computer.

Reverse Display Reverse display is available to reverse the image from left to right and/or reverse the density display so that blacks appear white and whites appear black.

Magnification Although nearly unlimited magnification may be accomplished, distortion usually becomes objectionable beyond 3×.

Suppression Originally designed to suppress the information from surgical clips, this feature permits a problem area, such as a surgical clip, to be outlined and then deleted from the reconstruction data.

Annotation Text may be added to images for descriptions or anatomical labeling.

Histograms A histogram is a bar graph which may provide useful diagnostic data in some instances. Software is available to produce these graphs by Hounsfield units and by time versus motion. Volumetric analysis is possible with some histographic data.

Hounsfield Units (HU) (CT Number) A histogram of the Hounsfield units along a line drawn between two cursor points may be useful in some diagnoses.

Time-Motion Histograms of various motions versus time may also be displayed for diagnosis of vascular flow or heart motion. These histograms are of limited value in CT because other modalities, especially ultrasonography and nuclear medicine, produce more accurate information.

Three-Dimensional Imaging Software and separate image processing units are available that will reconstruct CT data into a three-dimensional image (Figure 41–11) that can be manipulated in a manner similar to a draftsman's CAD/CAM computer graphics system. The image can be rotated, tumbled or tilted to demonstrate structures that would otherwise be hidden. Images can be adjusted to various degrees of translucency and can be divided. For example, an image of the head may have soft tissue density reduced to 25 percent, bone density reduced to 50 percent, and the right half of the image removed to permit viewing of the left side of the sella turcica.

IMAGE STORAGE UNITS

A number of memory storage devices are in use with CT units. The most popular are magnetic hard disks and tape, although magnetic floppy disks, optical disks and optical tape are also available. The magnetic hard disks will store 5–500 Mb. The most popular storage is magnetic tape, which, although difficult to access, is capable of storing over 100 examinations per tape.

Figure 41–11.   Three-dimensional CT reconstructions. (A) Pelvis. (B) Spine. (Courtesy of GE Medical Systems.)

COMPUTED TOMOGRAPHY NUMBERS (HOUNSFIELD UNITS—HU)

The true linear attenuation coefficients of the tissue voxels are not exactly represented by the data received by the CT computer. Therefore a series of tissue density values has evolved for CT measurements. Originally named computed tomography numbers, they were renamed Hounsfield units (HU) after the Nobel Prize was awarded to Godfrey Hounsfield in 1979. These numbers are calculated by comparing the linear attenuation coefficient of each pixel to the linear attenuation coefficient of water, according to the following formula:

$$\text{CT Number} = \frac{1,000 \ \mu_p - \mu_w}{\mu_w}$$

where: μ_p = linear attenuation coefficient of measured pixel, and

μ_w = linear attenuation coefficient of water.

Therefore the HU of water is always 0, average bone +1,000, and air −1,000. Table 41–2 illustrates the HU of other tissues. The CT unit can display the HU of any given volume of tissue. Most units use a cursor to delineate the pixels to be measured and then display the HU on the CRT next to the image. Radiologists may use HUs occasionally to assist in diagnosis even though the original hope of defining HUs for specific pathologies has not been realized. The attenuation data received by CT detectors is accurate ± 0.2 percent; therefore HUs are accurate ±2.

IMAGE RECONSTRUCTION

The detectors send information proportional to the attenuation coefficient of the voxel

TABLE 41–2	
HOUNSFIELD UNITS (HU) (CT NUMBERS) OF VARIOUS TISSUES	
Bone, petrous	+ 3,000
Bone, average	+ 1,000
Bone, cortical	+ 800
Blood, clotted	+ 55–75
Spleen	+ 50–70
Liver	+ 40–70
Pancreas	+ 40–60
Kidney	+ 40–60
Aorta	+ 35–50
Muscle	+ 35–50
Brain, white matter	+ 36–46
Cerebellum	+ 30
Brain, gray matter	+ 20–40
Blood	+ 13–18
Cerebrospinal fluid	+ 15
Tumors	+ 5–35
Gallbladder	+ 5–30
Water	0
Orbits	− 25
Fat	− 100
Lungs	− 150–400
Air	− 1,000

of tissue lying between the detector and the x-ray tube. The CT image is then reconstructed using a mathematical algorithm (Fourier transformation or back-projection) of the digitized information received by the computer.

The programs used by CT scanners compensate for numerous intrinsic and extrinsic factors, including the emission spectrum of the beam, and weighting factors for the geometrical aberrations caused by beam divergence and semicircular detector arrangement. Reconstruction often requires up to 30 seconds. However, when an array processor is used, reconstruction time can be decreased to less than one second, which is desirable for dynamic studies.

Reformatting

Reconstruction software is available that permits reformatting the information from a series of sectional images to produce an image of a section not actually scanned. For example, the extracted coronal image could be formed by reconstruction of only the appropriate voxels from each of the transverse sections. A typical reformatted CT image is shown in Figure 41–12.

Reformatting may also be used for a magnification technique called **targeting**, which permits an area of interest to be selected for reformatting. The reformatting process reconstructs the image data in a smaller pixel size to permit magnification with less distortion. This technique is used for regions in which extremely fine detail is necessary, such as the inner ear.

IMAGE QUALITY

Computed tomography image quality is primarily controlled by resolution and noise considerations. Density and contrast, as with any digitized image, can be manipulated by the computer. The prime consideration of the radiographer when making decisions regarding how to perform a particular CT examination must involve obtaining the necessary resolution while limiting noise.

Density and Contrast

Display density and contrast differences are varied with window level and width controls. Most CT images can demonstrate contrast differences of as little as 4 percent (4 HU), as compared to a minimum of 10 percent for a diagnostic radiograph. Appropriate CT window widths are shown in Table 41–3.

Figure 41–12. A reformatted CT image. The upper image is a coronal reconstruction from data acquired during axial transverse scanning of the cervical spine. Note the square bone fragment from the fracture. It is against the left side of the circular dens of C–2 at the center of the image. (Courtesy of Barbara Imber and St. Rita's Medical Center, Lima, OH.)

Resolution

The resolution of the CT image depends on pixel, voxel and matrix size. High contrast objects 1.5 times the pixel size or larger can be imaged reliably. For example, a pixel size of 0.5 mm can resolve an object 0.75 mm in size. Low contrast objects may require a larger pixel size to permit the detectors to provide sufficient data to reach a visible difference between the attenuation coefficients. Therefore low contrast objects may actually be seen better with a larger pixel size, although the total resolution is reduced. The current spatial resolution possible is about 0.35 mm, as compared to

TABLE 41–3	
APPROPRIATE COMPUTED TOMOGRAPHY WINDOW WIDTHS	
Area of Interest	**Window Width**
Head	70–200
Spine	350–750
Orbits	350–700
Heart	250–350
Abdomen	250–450
Thorax for lungs	1,200–1,400
Inner ear	2,000–4,000

0.25 mm and better with diagnostic radiography. However, this resolution is not possible under routine scanning conditions.

Voxel, Pixel and Matrix Size Discussion of CT imaging detail must consider voxel, pixel and matrix size. It is possible to have pixels and matrix size equal yet the voxel width may have a considerable effect on image quality. Matrix sizes offered on CT units have included 256 × 256, 320 × 320, 360 × 360, and 512 × 512. Because most CT images are processed and displayed with a circular field, the actual number of image pixels is less than if the matrix were square. For example, a 512 × 512 circular field matrix has slightly over 200,000 pixels. Most radiologists consider the diagnostic information available from matrix sizes of 256 × 256 and less to be inferior.

Voxel width may be varied between 8 mm and 13 mm. A common voxel size might be 1 mm × 1 mm × 10 mm with 10 mm representing the voxel width. The 20 percent additional tissue volume of a 13 mm voxel requires 60 percent more radiation exposure to produce an image of comparable quality. Therefore patient dose considerations in CT are similar to those in diagnostic radiography. Improved image quality can only be achieved through increased exposure to the patient.

Interface Artifacts Depending on the mathematical algorithm used, imaging aberrations displayed as density differences may occur when two objects have more than a 60 percent difference in attenuation coefficients. These artifacts are called undershoot and overshoot. Any object of greatly different contrast, such as metallic surgical clips, bullets, an old contrast medium and air, is likely to cause a star pattern artifact. The effect can be somewhat modified by using a larger matrix. However, different reconstruction algorithms that mathematically filter or compensate for the effect have been designed for various body

parts. For example, a soft tissue algorithm is useless during examination of the inner ear. A special bone algorithm is required to produce useful information when a number of small bony structures are in close proximity to one another.

Magnification The **display or reconstruction field of view** (FOV) is different from the scan field of view. True CT magnification is achieved by choosing a smaller display field of view. This produces an image with less tissue per voxel, which in turn provides higher resolution and a larger image of a smaller area of interest. Magnification of the matrix field size has no effect on image resolution. When a CT image matrix is magnified it may be possible to perceive individual pixels. This causes the image to appear less sharp. Therefore most radiologists prefer to diagnose from images of a smaller size that are sharp.

Noise

All digital images have noise problems. Noise on a CT image is directly related to the amount of data collected by the detector. It appears as quantum mottle (best seen in an image of a water phantom) and normally comprises 3–5 percent of the image. Most CT image noise is a result of statistical fluctuation in the information recorded by the detector, not a result of computer reconstruction mathematics. **The amount of noise controls the low contrast resolving ability of the CT unit.** A standard CT quality assurance measurement is a daily noise evaluation that is done by imaging a phantom and using a cursor to read the HUs for control areas. Each reading should average at least 100 pixels (10 × 10 matrix).

Motion Motion on a CT image is a function of exposure time, just as in diagnostic radiography. The exposure time in CT is controlled by the quantity of data detected. Because insufficient data results in a poor quality image, motion during a CT scan is displayed as a series of very poor quality images. For example, a rib that moves is recorded in a series of locations due to the movement instead of in a stationary location if respiration had been suspended. Each of the movement images is of poor quality because the detector received too little data to permit reconstruction of a normal quality image. Some CT units are capable of analyzing a motion image, deleting the portion of the data that made up the motion, and then reconstructing a stationary image from the remaining data. Although these images do not contain as much information as originally planned, they do eliminate the motion (Figure 41–13).

SCANNING PROCEDURES

Section Interval and Thickness

The section interval is the distance between scan sections. The section thickness is the width of the volume of tissue being examined (the voxel). Section thickness is usually slightly less than voxel width because of the divergence of the beam. Both the section interval and the thickness are determined by the section shape and the partial volume effect.

Section Shape Although section thickness is equivalent to voxel width, or slightly less, a section does not have parallel sides due to the divergence of the x-ray beam. Figure 41–14 illustrates the section shape problem that either overlaps or excludes tissue between sections. The scanning procedure must take this geometry into account. Overlapping, which occurs with section intervals equal to voxel width, is desirable. For example, a voxel width of 13 mm should use section intervals of 13 mm. In most procedures it is important that no sections of tissue miss examination. Overlap and exclusions must be considered when designing the section interval sequence for the scanning procedure. Most CT unit programs have standardized scanning procedures for the various examinations, although they can be modified to fit specific circumstances and institutional requirements.

Figure 41–13.   Computer correction of motion. (A) Motion artifacts obscuring information. (B) Separate images for each third of the scan time reveal all the motion that occurred during the final third of the scan. (C) Reconstruction using only the first two-thirds of the scan time produces a diagnostic quality image.

Figure 41–15.   The partial volume effect.

Figure 41–14. Section shape due to divergent beam geometry. (A) The first scan produces a wedge-shaped volume of scanned tissue. (B) The final scan produces a concave volume of double scanned tissue with a convex volume of single scanned tissue at the edges.

Partial Volume Effect Because the data from an entire section thickness is averaged together to form the image, the exact location of a section may cause small structures or portions of large structures to be hidden when they comprise only a small percentage of the total section. This is a common concern during CT of the vertebral column when a section interval happens to produce a section where an intervertebral disc comprises a small percentage of the total section volume (Figure 41–15). This is called the partial volume effect. It may obscure any object that is smaller than the voxel width (section thickness) when that object is scanned by two sections. Compensation for the partial volume effect may be overcome in some instances by slightly overlapping sections.

Scan Arc

Third and fourth generation scanners permit selection of the scanning arc. Common scan arcs are 220°, 360°, and 400° or 440° overscan on fourth generation units. The scan arc is sometimes called **half scan**, **full scan or overscan**. Wider scan arcs require more time to reconstruct the image and provide higher resolution.

Exposure Factors

Most CT scanning is performed at 120 kVp. Time is not a factor, as it must be controlled by the scanning program to provide sufficient exposure dose to the detectors (much as in fluoroscopy and conventional tomography). The CT radiographer usually varies the mA to control the primary beam. However, dual energy scanning units require scanning with different kVp values, usually 80 kVp or 140 kVp.

Algorithm

As discussed earlier under image reconstruction techniques, the proper reconstruction algorithm must be used to mathematically filter unwanted artifacts. The CT console often combines the proper algorithm with the scanning procedure. As with digital subtraction radiography, high-pass and low-pass filters and other mathematical manipulations can also be performed to improve image quality.

Scan Field Size

The scan field size, or field of view, is set to accommodate the size of the part under examination. The smaller the scan field size, the better the image resolution and the faster the scan time. Common field sizes are 25 cm for the head and magnification of the spine, 35 cm for small bodies and 48 cm for large bodies.

RADIATION PROTECTION

Patient Exposure Dose

Because of the strictly collimated primary beam, most CT examinations have a patient exposure dose similar to that of the same part in diagnostic radiography examinations. The original EMI head scanner averaged 1.0 rad per examination, which was less than in a radiographic examination of the skull. Subsequent generations of scanners deliver two to six times this dose because they use and detect more radiation to produce higher quality images. The exposure dose is quite low because the exposure for each section is not compounded. Each sectional exposure represents one portion of the total exposure. In diagnostic radiography each projection exposes the entire part. Therefore, although a single CT section exposure is similar to the exposure dose for an entire radiographic projection, the fact that they are not compounded results in a total exposure less than would be expected (although not compounded, scatter is received by adjacent sections). Scanogram doses have been reported between 5 and 100 mrads.

Filtration Filtration is used in CT in a manner similar to that in diagnostic radiography. A special "bow tie" filter has been developed for CT that matches the beam divergence and shape of the patient's body in transverse section (Figure 41–16).

Exposure to Others

Exposure dose to other persons in the scanning room results primarily from scatter from the patient, as during fluoroscopy. Lead aprons and other appropriate protective equipment should be used by anyone in the scanning room during examinations. A routine scan might produce a scatter dose of 2 to 5 mrads per section at one meter from the patient. Unless absolutely necessary, no one should be present in the scanning room while the unit is in operation. When someone must be present, he or she should remain as far

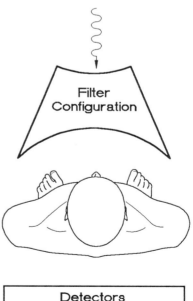

Figure 41–16. A CT bow tie filter.

from the patient as possible to take best advantage of the inverse square law. Standard radiation protection procedures should be followed: the most desirable person to stay with a patient is a relative, then a nonradiology staff member. A radiology department member is the last to be considered. Although use of a remotely controlled power injector is preferred, persons who must manually inject a contrast medium during scanning procedures should stand behind a lead shield, as far from the gantry as possible.

SUMMARY

Computed tomography (CT) produces a digital tomographic image from diagnostic x-rays. The basic principle of CT involves digitizing an image received from a slit scan projection of the patient's body and then back-projecting it through mathematical algorithms.

A modern CT unit includes a gantry, table, x-ray tube, detectors, computer, display console and image storage units. The gantry is the movable frame of the CT unit. It contains the x-ray tube and detectors and is the most visible part of the unit. The gantry frame maintains the alignment of the tube and detectors and contains the equipment necessary to perform the scanning movements. CT tables are usually made of carbon graphite fiber to decrease beam attenuation and must support the entire weight of the patient without sagging when fully extended. They are rated for maximum weight. Modern pulsed scanner x-ray tubes operate at 120 kVp, 1–5 msec pulses, and up to 1,000 mA. The most common CT detector is a xenon gas-filled ionization chamber which measures ionization in air by attracting to an electrode the ions created by x-ray photons in the air.

The CT computer is designed to control data acquisition, process and display, and storage. The CT console operates from a "menu" or index directory of operations. The radiographer uses a keyboard, light pen or other input device to indicate the desired operation. The data acquisition program controls a variety of operations, including tube and detector collimation (pixel size), matrix size, gantry angle, tabletop entrance into the gantry aperture, section increment movements of the tabletop, x-ray tube voltage and amperage, scan speed and direction of detector signals to the digital image processing section of the computer. The processing and display program controls the digital image production process. The display console permits a wide range of display features, including the scanogram, grid pattern, cursor, density contouring, radiation therapy planning, reverse display, magnification, suppression, annotation, histograms and three-dimensional imaging. Hounsfield units (HU), or CT numbers, represent the tissue density values for each pixel.

Computed tomography image quality is primarily controlled by resolution and noise considerations. Density and contrast, as with any digitized image, can be manipulated by the computer and are varied with window level and width controls. The resolution of the CT image depends on pixel, voxel and matrix size. Imaging aberrations (artifacts) displayed as density differences may occur when two objects have more than a 60 percent difference in attenuation coefficients. Noise on a CT image is directly related to the amount of data collected by the detector. Motion on a CT image is a function of exposure time, just as in diagnostic radiography.

The section interval is the distance between scan sections. Its determination is effected by the section shape and the partial volume effect. Section thickness is equivalent to voxel width, or slightly less. Because the data from an entire section thickness is averaged together to form the image, the exact location of a section may cause small structures or portions of large structures to be hidden when they comprise only a small percentage of the total section. This is called the partial volume effect.

Because of the strictly collimated primary beam, most CT examinations have a patient exposure dose similar to that of the same part in diagnostic radiography examinations. Filtration is used in CT in a manner similar to that in diagnostic radiography. Exposure dose to other persons in the scanning room results primarily from scatter from the patient, as during fluoroscopy. Lead aprons and other appropriate protective equipment should be used by anyone in the scanning room during examinations.

REVIEW QUESTIONS

1. What are the major components of a modern CT unit?

2. What is the gantry?

3. Why are tabletops rated for maximum weight?

4. What is the purpose of the detectors in a CT unit?

5. What operations are controlled by the data acquistion program?

6. What is a scanogram?

7. How are Hounsfield units (HU) (CT numbers) calculated?

8. What controls the density, contrast and resolution of the CT image?

9. Explain the partial volume effect.

10. How does exposure dose in CT compare to the exposure doses for routine radiography?

REFERENCES AND RECOMMENDED READING

Ambrose, J., and G. Hounsfield. Computerized transverse axial tomography. *British Journal of Radiology* 46:148, 1023–1047, 1973.

Berland, Lincoln L. *Practical CT Technology and Techniques*. New York: Raven Press, 1987.

Brooker, M. J. *Computed Tomography for Radiographers*. Lancaster, England: MTP Press Limited, 1986.

Brooks, R. A., and G. DiChiro. Slice geometry in computer assisted tomography. *Journal of Computer Assisted Tomography* 1:2, 191–199, 1977.

Bushong, Stewart C. *Radiologic Science for Technologists: Physics, Biology, and Protection*. 4th ed. St. Louis, MO: C. V. Mosby Co., 1988.

Curry, Thomas S., James E. Dowdey, and Robert C. Murry. *Christensen's Physics of Diagnostic Radiology*. 4th ed. Philadelphia, PA: Lea & Febiger, 1990.

Davison, Malcolm. X-ray computed tomography. *Scientific Basis of Medical Imaging*. 54–92. Editor: Wells, P. N. T. Edinburgh: Churchill Livingstone, 1982.

General Electric. *Introduction to Computed Tomography*. Milwaukee, WI: General Electric Company, Medical Systems Division, Publication 4691, 1976.

Greenfield, George B., and Lincoln B. Hubbard. *Computers in Radiology*. New York: Churchill Livingstone, 1984.

Haaga, J. R., F. Miraldi, W. MacIntyre, J. P. LiPuma, P. J. Bryan, and E. Wiesen. The effect of mAs variation upon computed tomography image quality as evaluated by in vivo and in vitro studies. *Radiology* 138, 449–454, 1981.

Haughton, Victor M., and Alan L. Williams. *Computed Tomography of the Spine*. St. Louis, MO: C. V. Mosby Co., 1982.

Hendee, William R. *The Physical Principles of Computed Tomography*. Boston, MA: Little, Brown and Company, 1983.

Hounsfield, G. N. Computed tomography—past, present and future. *Medical Imaging*. 1–9. Editors: Kreel, Louis, and Robert E. Steiner. Chicago, IL: Yearbook Medical Publishers, Inc., 1979.

Hounsfield, G. N. Computerized transverse axial scanning (tomography): Part I. Description of system. *British Journal of Radiology* 46, 1016–1022, 1973.

Hunter, Tim B. *The Computer in Radiology*. Rockville, MD: Aspen, 1986.

Knapp, Robert H., Michael W. Vannier, and Jeffrey L. Marsh. Generation of 3-D images from CT scans: Technological perspective. *Radiologic Technology* 56:6, 391–398, 1985.

Kuni, Christopher C. *Introduction to Computers and Digital Processing in Medical Imaging*. Chicago, IL: Yearbook Medical Publishers, Inc., 1988.

McCullough, E. C., and J. T. Payne. X-ray transmission computed tomography. *Medical Physics* 4, 85–, 1977.

Morgan, Carlisle Lee. *Basic Principles of Computed Tomography*. Baltimore, MD: University Park Press, 1983.

Seeram, Euclid. *Computed Tomography Technology*. Philadelphia, PA: W. B. Saunders Company, 1982.

Seijo, Charles A. A CT scanning protocol for a Q.A. program. *Radiologic Technology* 52:5, 497, 1981.

Short, Alec J. Reconstructions in computerized transverse axial radiography. *Radiography* 47: 557, 119, 1981.

Ter-Pogossian, Michel M. Physical principles and instrumentation. *Computed Body Tomography*. 1–7. Editors: Lee, Joseph K. T., Stuart S. Sagel, and Robert J. Stanley. New York: Raven Press, 1983.

Ter-Pogossian, Michel M., Michael E. Phelps, Gordon L. Brownell, Jerome R. Cox, Jr., David O. Davis, and Ronald G. Evens, Editors. *Reconstruction Tomography in Diagnostic Radiology and Nuclear Medicine*. Baltimore, MD: University Park Press, 1977.

Wallace, Ronald P. The application of computerized tomography in radiation treatment planning. *The Canadian Journal of Medical Radiation Technology* 11:3, 146, 1980.

Yaffe, M., A. Fenster, and H. E. Johns. Xenon ionization detectors for fan beam computed tomography scanners. *Journal of Computer Assisted Tomography* 1:2, 419–428, 1977.

Yoshizumi, Terry T., Sudhir K. Suneja, and James S. Teal. Practical CT dosimetry. *Radiologic Technology* 60:6, 505, 1989.

42 MAGNETIC RESONANCE IMAGING

We are dealing not merely with a new tool but with a new subject, a subject I have called simply nuclear magnetism . . . the history of ordinary magnetism . . . has been rich in difficult and provocative problems, and full of surprises. Nuclear Magnetism . . . is like that too.

Edward M. Purcell from his Nobel Lecture,
December 11, 1952.

OUTLINE

THE PHYSICS OF MAGNETIC RESONANCE
PRODUCTION OF THE MAGNETIC RESONANCE IMAGE
MAGNETIC RESONANCE IMAGING EQUIPMENT
IMAGE QUALITY
SAFETY AND BIOLOGICAL HAZARDS

OBJECTIVES

Upon completion of this chapter, the student should be able to:

1. Describe the source of the magnetic fields within the body that are used during MRI.
2. Describe the properties of proton precession as used in MRI.
3. Define TI, TR, TE, T1 and T2.
4. Explain the functions of x, y, and z gradient coils in selecting an image section by the use of the Larmor equation and a gradient magnetic field.
5. Describe the use of RF pulses in the various MRI pulse sequences.
6. Analyze the various events during a spin-echo pulse sequence.
7. Describe the components of an MRI unit, including the stationary magnet, gradient and RF coils, table, and computer consoles.
8. Explain how MRI image contrast is controlled.
9. Describe the use of paramagnetic contrast agents.
10. Discuss methods of reducing MRI image noise.
11. Discuss safety measures for protection of all persons who approach the MRI unit magnetic field.

Magnetic resonance imaging (MRI) uses magnetism and radio frequencies (RF) to create diagnostic sectional images of the body (Figure 42–1). Because magnetism and radio frequencies are applied according to principles of nuclear physics and quantum mechanics, the process was originally called nuclear magnetic resonance (NMR); this term is still used in some instances.

THE PHYSICS OF MAGNETIC RESONANCE

In 1924 Wolfgang Pauli suggested that some nuclei spin. It was not until 1946 that nuclear magnetic resonance was first reported by Swiss physicist Felix Bloch (1905–1983) at Stanford and American physicist Edward Purcell (1912–) at Harvard. These men shared the 1952 Nobel Prize in physics for their work. In the late 1960s and early 1970s the basis for diagnostic MRI was developed by several researchers. In 1967 Jasper Jackson produced the first MR signals from a live animal, in 1971 Raymond Damadian reported NMR differences between normal tissue and tumors, in 1972 Paul Lauterbur produced the first magnetic

Figure 42–1. A sagittal MR image of the head. (Courtesy of GE Medical Systems.)

resonance image, in 1975 Damadian produced the first live animal MR images, and by 1977 the first diagnostic human images had been obtained.

Nuclear Magnetism

The nucleus of an atom is a tiny but highly charged piece of matter. Most atoms measure in the range of one angstrom in diameter. If the nucleus is spinning, it has angular momentum, or **nuclear magnetic moment**. This rotating charge acts as a current loop and produces a magnetic field, thus causing the nucleus to behave as a microscopic spinning bar magnet; it rotates and flips within the atom like a tiny gyroscope on perfect bearings. When nuclei having magnetic moments are placed in a magnetic field, they tend to align with the field, as does any magnet.

In addition to having a charge, a nucleus also has mass. The spinning mass has a moment of inertia as well as a magnetic moment. The moment of inertia resists changes to angular momentum, thus inhibiting the nucleus from aligning in a magnetic field. This inhibiting factor is measured as the ratio of the magnetic moment to the moment of inertia and is called the gyromagnetic (or magnetogyric) **ratio**. It is represented by the Greek letter gamma (γ) and is measured in units of **megahertz per tesla (MHz/T)**. Each isotope has a specific gyromagnetic ratio, which allows it to be differentiated during MR imaging (Table 42–1).

It was originally hoped that variations in gyromagnetic ratios and in the length of relaxation time after the application of an RF pulse would permit the differentiation of healthy tissue from diseased; however, the molecular basis that determines relaxation times has proven extremely complex and until sufficient knowledge is acquired in this area of biochemistry, MRI data cannot accurately diagnose tissue pathology. Consequently, the considerable value

TABLE 42–1	
MAGNETIC RESONANCE PROPERTIES OF DIAGNOSTICALLY IMPORTANT NUCLEI	
Nucleus	Gyromagnetic Ratio (MHz/T)
^{1}H	42.6
^{2}H	6.5
^{13}C	10.7
^{19}F	40.0
^{23}Na	11.3
^{31}P	17.2
^{39}K	2.0

$$\Omega = \gamma B_O$$

where: Ω = rate of precession
γ = gyromagnetic ratio
B_O = static magnetic field strength

The rate of precession (Ω) is also known as the angular velocity of the nuclear magnetic field.

Larmor Frequencies The gyromagnetic ratio (γ) is fixed for each element. Therefore the precessional frequency is fixed for a given magnetic field strength. This means that in a static homogeneous magnetic field, all protons in a nucleus of a given type element will rotate with exactly the same frequency. This frequency is called the **Larmor frequency** and is critical to MR imaging. Only those elements with nuclear angular momentum have nuclear magnetic moments and are capable of producing nuclear magnetic resonance signals. The most important of those that do is the proton, which is also the major isotope of hydrogen (^{1}H), because it is abundant in the human body and has a high gyromagnetic ratio (γ). **The precessional frequency is the Larmor frequency. It is the RF that induces magnetic**

of MRI continues to depend on the visual diagnostic abilities of the radiologist.

Precession of Nuclei Although the dynamics of rapidly rotating objects are quite complex, several of their properties are easily understood. The most important property is that of a rapidly spinning nucleus when it is subjected to a magnetic field; not only will the nucleus's magnetic field align with the external magnetic field, but it will also begin to wobble. This wobbling, like that of a spinning top when it begins to lose momentum, is actually a rotation of the axis of rotation, or precession (Figure 42–2). The rotational precession of the nucleus causes the magnetic field itself to precess. Therefore the direction of precession indicated in Figure 42–2 also represents the precession of the rotational magnetic field. MR imaging is accomplished through various measurements of this movement of the nuclear magnetic field.

The nuclear magnetic field is continually changing direction as it rotates around the axis of the external magnetic field's lines of flux. The **rate of precession** is indicated by the Greek letter omega (Ω) and is calculated as:

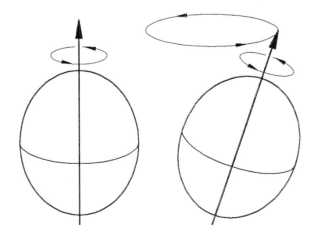

Figure 42–2. Precession.

resonance as well as the RF of the emitted nuclear magnetic resonance signal.

Production of the Nuclear Magnetic Resonance Signal

The laws of quantum mechanics permit protons to align either with the external magnetic field or against it. This creates two populations of proton orientations, those with spin up (parallel) and those with spin down (antiparallel). When an electromagnetic RF field that is alternating, or resonating, at the Larmor frequency is applied in addition to the static field, protons will alternate from spin up to spin down. This phenomenon is called **magnetic resonance**. Protons that are in the spin down state have excessive energy, which they emit as electromagnetic radiation in the **radio frequency (RF)** range. The Larmor equation predicts the exact RF that will be emitted by a specific element. When the RF is detected with an antenna and a radio receiver that is tuned to the proper frequency, magnetic resonance imaging is possible.

Production of the nuclear magnetic resonance signal requires applying a Larmor frequency alternating RF and then listening to the RF emissions from the protons. Digital imaging reconstruction techniques are then used to create sectional and three-dimensional images.

Magnetic resonance imaging data is accumulated by measuring detection differences of only one millionth of a percent (0.000001 percent). When a large number of protons are subjected to a magnetic field, the nuclear magnetic moments immediately begin lining up with the field; some line up in the same direction as the magnetic field while others line up in the opposite direction. For every 200,000,000 hydrogen atoms, about two more will align themselves *with* the predominate external magnetic field. In other words, 100,000,001 atoms will align with the field while 99,999,999 will align against it. This means that the body tissue has become almost imperceptibly magnetized.

MRI Parameters The primary parameters used to modify and control the MRI process include **proton spin density (PD, SD, or ρ), repetition time (TR), echo time (TE), inversion time (TI), spin-lattice or longitudinal relaxation time (T1), and spin-spin or transverse relaxation time (T2)**. The parameters that are used vary depending on the pulse sequence used.

Proton spin density (PD, SD, or ρ) is the quantity of resonating spins in a tissue. It is expressed as a percentage of the proton density of water and determines the MR signal strength (sometimes called image brightness) (Table 42–2). Various authors refer to it as pro-

TABLE 42–2

EFFECT OF PARAMETER VARIATION ON MR IMAGE DENSITY (BRIGHTNESS)

Image Weighting	TR	TE	Effect on MR Image Density Density (Brightness) With:		
			ρ Increased	Longer T1	Longer T2
Proton Spin Density (ρ)	long	short	+	−*	+*
T1	short	short	+	−	+*
T2	long	long	+	−*	+

* = some tissues only

ton density (PD), spin density (SD), or by the Greek letter rho (ρ). Proton density weighted images are achieved by using a long repetition time (TR) between pulses. This permits the RF signal from a larger number of protons to be detected, thus creating the image from a greater number, or density, of spinning protons. Proton density images have relatively low contrast due to the slight differences between the percentages of hydrogen present in various tissues (Table 42–2).

Repetition time (TR) is the time interval between pulse sequences. It is usually between 300 and 3,000 ms.

Echo time (TE) is the time between a 90° pulse and the echo during a spin-echo pulse sequence. It is usually between 10 and 100 ms. When more than one echo is recorded, the TE is designated as TE1, TE2, etc.

Inversion time (TI) is the time between a 180° pulse and a 90° inversion pulse in an inversion recovery pulse sequence. It is usually between 200 and 2,000 ms.

Spin-lattice relaxation time (T1) is the time required for precessing spins to align with the constant external magnetic field to 63 percent of the maximum possible strength. It is also known as longitudinal relaxation time and is sometimes called thermal relaxation time.

T1 is the time required for the sum of the magnetic moments, or M_O, to regain its original orientation following a 90° RF pulse. It varies depending on thermal interactions between resonating protons and other nuclear magnetic fields in the atomic lattice. The value of T1 increases with the strength of the magnetic field. The term longitudinal was originally applied in reference to the time required for precessing to cease and the proton spin to reorient with the original "longitudinal" magnetic field.

The T1 of hydrogen is approximately three seconds in water but this time varies considerably for hydrogen in different types of tissues. This phenomenon provides the contrast necessary for the MR image. T1 relaxation characteristics for various body tissues are shown in Table 42–3. Relaxation times vary with the amount of water available. In fact, dehydrated tissues will demonstrate significantly different relaxation times.

| TABLE 42–3 | | | | |

EXAMPLE T1 AND T2 RELAXATION TIMES IN A 0.15 TESLA FIELD

Relaxation times vary considerably depending on numerous factors, including the specific conditions surrounding the tissue and external magnetic field strength.

Tissue	T1	T2	T1/T2	Proton Density (Percent ρ Water)
Fat	170 ms	80 ms	2.1	9.6
Muscle	580 ms	40 ms	14.5	9.3
Brain, white matter	350 ms	80 ms	4.4	10.6
Brain, gray matter	500 ms	100 ms	5.0	10.6
Blood	720 ms	175 ms	4.1	
Cerebrospinal fluid	1,500 ms	260 ms	5.8	10.8
Water	2,500 ms	2,500 ms	0.0	11.0

T1/T2 is an indication of contrast differences between T1 and T2 weighted images.
(Adapted with permission from Elster, Allen D., *Magnetic Resonance Imaging: A Reference Guide and Atlas*. Philadelphia: J. B. Lippincott Company, 1986.)

When a magnetic field is applied, almost all the proton spins will have aligned after several T1 times have passed. Magnetic resonance imaging uses only those spins that have not been cancelled out by a corresponding spin in the opposite direction. Although these protons occur in only one out of 100,000,000 atoms, the vast quantity of atoms in even a small voxel of tissue produce a large number of eligible protons. Only these protons are capable of producing an RF when subjected to a magnetic field at the appropriate Larmor frequency.

The mechanism by which protons emit RF is especially complex because it occurs in three dimensions. However, careful consideration of a few simple illustrations will reveal that once the three-dimensional aspect is understood, the basic principle is not so difficult. The sum of the magnetic moments, or M_O, is always in the same direction as B_O (the static magnetic field strength) when the body is within the static external magnetic field. When M_O precesses, it produces a rotating magnetic field which is perpendicular to the original direction of M_O (Figures 42–3A and B). To cause protons to emit an RF, another magnetic field (B_1) must be applied for a brief moment. In Figure 42–3B the magnetic field in the x^1–y^1

Figure 42–3. Proton emission of radio frequencies (RF). (A) B_O is the direction of the static external magnetic field. M_O is the direction of the sum of the predominant proton magnetic moments. (B) When M_O is tipped slightly off the z axis, it immediately begins precessing around the z axis at its Larmor frequency. This causes a perpendicular magnetic field to rotate in the x–y plane, also at the Larmor frequency. (C) If an alternating magnetic field (B_1) is applied in the direction of x, it causes M_O to rotate further away from z toward y. B_1 is pulsed so that it is applied only during the moment that x is aligned with x^1 during every rotation. Because x is precessing at the Larmor frequency, the applied magnetic field must also be pulsed at the Larmor frequency.

plane is precessing synchronously with M_O (at the same angular speed). This precessing magnetic field is stationary in its relationship with M_O. This relationship is more easily understood by comparing it to riding on a carousel. Although the carousel is spinning (like M_O), when one rides on one of the horses the other horses appear to be stationary (x^1–y^1) while objects outside the carousel appear to be spinning around (x–y). If an alternating magnetic field (B_1) is applied in the direction of x, it will simply cause M_O to rotate further away from z toward y (Figure 42–3C). In order to apply B_1 in the direction of the moving x axis, it is simply pulsed so that it is applied only during the moment that x is aligned with x^1 during every rotation (Figure 42–3C). The concept of T1 as M_0 returns to equilibrium after an RF pulse is shown graphically in Figure 42–8. Because x is rotating at the Larmor frequency with M_0, **the applied magnetic field must be pulsed at the Larmor frequency**.

The Larmor frequency is very high, usually in the MHz range, for the 0.5–3.5 Tesla fields used in MR imaging. For example, the Larmor frequency for hydrogen in a 1.5 T field is 64 MHz, which is within RF bands of the electromagnetic spectrum (see Figure 2–10 and the end pages at the back of the book). The MHz frequency magnetic field for MRI is produced by a properly tuned radio transmitter coil, very similar to the coil used to receive UHF frequency television signals.

Spin-spin relaxation time (T2) is the time required, after precessing spins have aligned at an angle to the external magnetic field due to an RF pulse, for them to lose 63 percent of their coherence (alignment with each other) due to interactions between the spins. It varies depending on the tissue. It is also known as transverse relaxation time. T2 is always shorter than T1. The symbol **T2*** is used to indicate T2 due to inhomogeneities in the magnetic field and due to spin-spin relaxation. T2* is always shorter than T2.

Nuclear Magnetic Resonance Pulses

The distance that M_O precesses from the z axis is determined by the strength of B_1 and by the duration of the pulse. It is measured by the angle of the precession. For example, a 45° pulse tips the rotational axis of M_O 45° away from the z axis. The most common MRI pulses are 90° and 180°. A 180° pulse aligns M_O with the $-z$ axis or, in other words, aligns it perfectly in the opposite direction. A 360° pulse would return the rotational axis to its original position and therefore have no effect. During all pulsing only the protons spinning at the Larmor frequency that matches the pulse frequency will respond. The actual response of proton spin to an RF pulse is to change M_O in a precessing corkscrew motion (Figure 42–4).

A 90° pulse is used to tip the rotational axis of the protons so that they are spinning around the z axis in the x–y plane. Because the protons are functioning as spinning magnets, an electromagnetic force is produced when a coil of wire is positioned within the lines of flux. **The voltage that is detected from this**

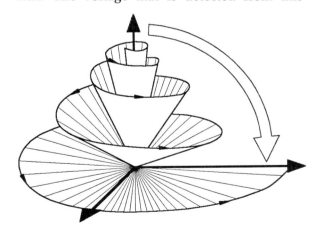

Figure 42–4. The precessing corkscrew motion of proton spin to an RF pulse. (Used by permission from Edelman, Robert R., and Hesselink, John R., *Clinical Magnetic Resonance Imaging*. Philadelphia: W. B. Saunders, 1990.)

arrangement is the magnetic resonance imaging signal. The coil is aligned to detect only precession in the x^1–y^1 plane. The frequency of the voltage matches the Larmor frequency of the precessing protons, thus making it possible to detect which element emitted the signal.

Nuclear Magnetic Resonance Decay

The signal that is emitted by the precessing protons decays exponentially. This occurs because the protons' magnetic fields are not exactly the same, even though they are all within the Larmor frequency range. Just as individual atoms of the same element have slight differences, precessional rates also differ slightly. For example, if a hydrogen proton is spinning at its Larmor frequency of 64,000,000 rotations per second and a second proton is spinning at 64,000,001 rotations per second, in 0.5 second the two protons will be exactly opposite one another. When this occurs, their magnetic fields cancel one another. The millions of protons that comprise M_O quickly become out of phase with each other by this process, which is called dephasing. **When a tissue sample has dephased, M_O ceases to exist and the magnetic resonance signal disappears.**

Free induction decay (FID) is the simplest example of this process. It produces the most basic type of MRI signal, as shown in Figure 42–5. Because an FID signal will vary depending on how many protons are spinning in the tissue volume, it is known as a **proton spin density (ρ) image**. Because proton density does not vary much in soft tissue, FID produces an extremely low contrast image.

PRODUCTION OF THE MAGNETIC RESONANCE IMAGE

The localization of information for the MR image occurs very differently from computed tomography or any other digital imaging modality, although the final computerized digital image reconstruction algorithms are very similar. Three electromagnetic coils are required to produce magnetic field gradients corresponding to the x, y, or z axis to be imaged. The RF that are detected from these gradient coils, as they are called, can then be analyzed to determine not only the type of atom they came from but also the atom's precise location within the imaging matrix.

Gradient Coils

Data localization in MRI is accomplished through the use of a gradient magnetic field that is superimposed on the static external magnetic field. The gradient coil field system was developed by the American physicist Paul Lauterbur in 1972 at the State University of New York (SUNY) at Stony Brook. Gradient coils can be resistive or superconducting and are located within the bore of the stationary magnet. They superimpose their magnetic fields on the uniform magnetic field produced by the stationary magnet. A gradient field coil produces a magnetic field somewhat like a magnetic penetrometer in that it grows in strength from one end to the other. The field strength varies in proportion to distance, usually between 1 and 10 mT/m (0.1–1.0 G/cm).

Since the strength of the magnetic field affects the precessional frequency of the proton spins, the result is different precessional frequencies according to location along the gradient field. This technique permits the MRI computer to determine the location of an RF signal with digital imaging calculations. It also permits the calculation of T1 and T2 as a function of distance along the axis of the magnetic field. Changing the x axis permits detection from an opposite direction and the use of many of the digital reconstruction algorithms employed in computed tomography (see Chapters 40 and 41). Other variations between the three gradient coils also permit various oblique

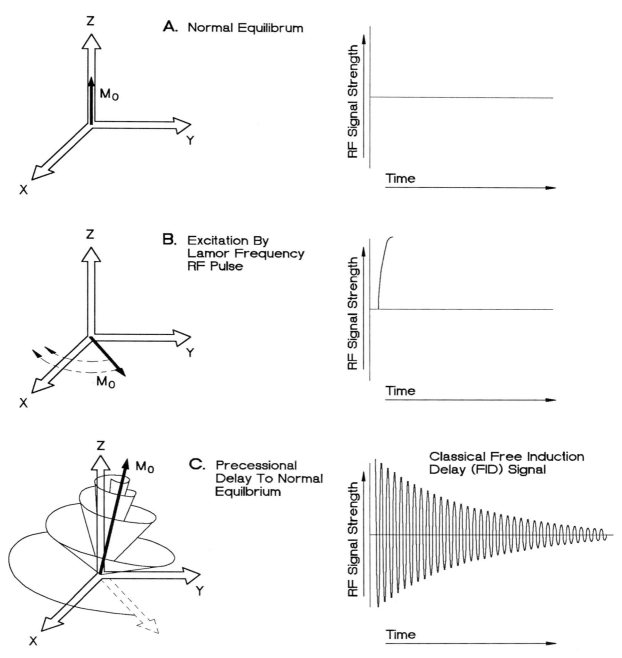

Figure 42–5.   Classical free induction decay (FID) signal. (A) Normal spin equilibrium. (B) When a Larmor frequency RF pulse is applied, M_O precesses 90° into the x–y plane, thus producing a maximum strength MR signal. (C) As M_O emits RF, it loses energy and precesses in a corkscrew back to normal equilibrium, emitting a gradually decaying RF signal.

sections to be constructed. The basic algorithm in MRI is a two-dimensional Fourier transform (2DFT) method. It is often expanded to a 3DFT to permit faster data acquisition.

Magnetic resonance imaging requires the use of three gradient coils, one each for the x, y, and z axes (Figure 42–11B). Each coil must be linear and uniform to within a few percentage points. **The gradient coils determine the section thickness as well as the resolution and contrast of the image**.

The z axis coil is called the section selection gradient because it determines the exact location of the section and its thickness. A thicker section is produced by increasing the RF band width or by increasing the magnitude (or slope) of the gradient. The z axis coil can be set to produce transverse, coronal, or sagittal sections.

The y axis coil is called the phase encoding gradient because it selectively precesses the protons to define the x–y coordinates within the section. This phase gradient must be repeated for each x coordinate in the matrix array. For example, a 256×256 matrix requires the phase gradient to be repeated 256 times to collect data for the entire matrix. This is the basic process of a two-dimensional Fourier transform (2DFT) data projection method.

The x axis coil is called the frequency encoding gradient or the readout gradient because it is applied for each value of the y axis coil. Three-dimensional MR imaging uses the z axis coil to cause a large volume of tissue to begin precessing. X and y encoding gradients are then compared and the collected data is reconstructed in three dimensions.

Although these phasing methods are not always applied to the x and y axes in the order described, spatial location is achieved by phase encoding for one axis while frequency encoding for the other. Variations in the use of all three gradient coils permit the acquisition of various oblique sections through the subject.

Magnetic Resonance Imaging Operations Sequence

The production of MR imaging data varies depending on the pulsing sequence used and on the manufacturer. As an example, a spin-echo pulse sequence of operations might include the following steps to produce an MR image:

1. A gradient is applied along the z axis. A 90° pulse is applied at a desired Larmor frequency. The z gradient selects an x–y plane (section selection). The z gradient is turned off. This produces a precessing M_O in the selected plane. The M_O in the other planes are still aligned along the z axis (Figure 42–6A).

2. A gradient is applied along the y axis for a short time. This produces precessing M_O at various rates depending on their location along the y axis gradient. The phasing of the precessing spins now indicates their location in the y–z plane (phase encoding) (Figure 42–6B).

3. A gradient is applied along the z axis again and a 180° pulse is applied with a frequency that will affect only the x–y plane that is being imaged. The z gradient is then turned off.

4. A gradient is applied along the x axis. This causes the precessing M_O to return a T2 spin-echo at differing frequencies that will indicate their positions along the x axis (readout frequency encoding) (Figure 42–6C). The RF receiver is then turned on and the signals received are sent to the MRI computer for digital image reconstruction.

Most MRI images are produced from 128 phase-encoded lines in the y axis. Each of these lines is frequency encoded for 256 points in the x axis. This produces a total of 32,768 spatial points in the x–y axis per image.

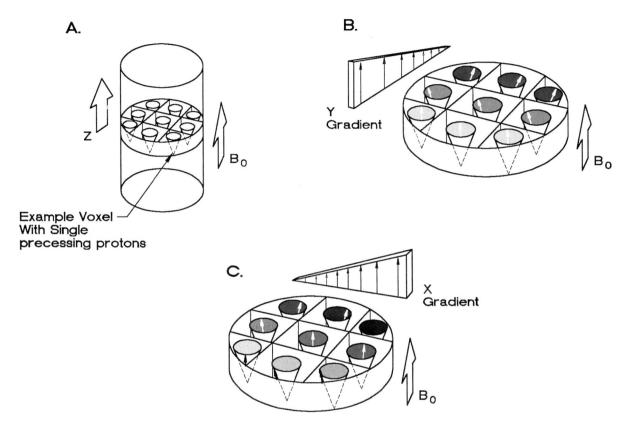

Figure 42–6.   Spatial location by gradient fields. (A) Application of the z gradient field produces precession within the selected section (the z axis). (B) Application of the y gradient field produces phase encoding along the y axis. Note that there is still no differentiation of spatial location along the x axis. (C) Application of the x gradient field produces frequency encoding along the x axis. Note that each voxel now has a different precession rate, thus permitting spatial location in the x, y, and z axes.

Radio Frequency Pulse Sequences

The primary variable in the data collection procedure during MRI is the sequence of RF pulses that are used to cause the protons to precess. There is a dramatic difference in the information that becomes visible with the various sequences. The operator must select the appropriate pulsing sequence as well as the proper intervals for the specific examination. As with most computed tomography units, the MRI control console includes programmed selections of sequences for various examinations. However, the knowledgeable MRI technologist can increase the quantity and quality of diagnostic information by understanding which sequences and intervals are best for specific tissues. The sequences are a series of various magnetic fields from the x, y, and z gradients, RF pulses at various angles, repetition times (TR), inversion times (TI), and echo times (TE). Most MRI units collect 256 pulse sequences per sectional image. All of the sequences are identical except for a change in the y magnetic field gradient, which controls the spatial localization of the RF signal received.

Partial Saturation Partial saturation is also referred to as saturation recovery (SR) or repeated free induction decay (repeated FID). The pulse sequence is a series of 90° RF pulses with the signal measured after each (Figure 42–7A). Note that the y gradient is changed for each pulse sequence to record data from a different anatomical section. The TR is set according to the tissue of interest.

If a 90° pulse is repeated before M_O is fully re-established along the z axis, the angle of M_O precession will depend on the first time interval (T1). Images produced with data collected at this point are known as partial saturation images because they vary with both proton density and the length of T1. Because different tissues have different T1 values, contrast can be varied by changing the repetition time (TR). However, when very short recovery times are encountered, the M_O is weak and this produces a very weak RF signal. When long recovery times are encountered, the M_O has time to recover and the T1 contrast is lost. For this reason partial saturation is not used for most MR imaging. However, short TR T1 partial saturation sequencing is useful in demonstrating cysts and subdural fluids and has been used for blood flow studies as well.

Inversion Recovery Inversion recovery is a two pulse sequence. It consists of a 180° pulse followed by the partial saturation sequence (Figure 42–7B). Because of the time required to accumulate data, it is seldom used in current clinical imaging. Note that the y gradient is changed for each pulse sequence to record data from a different anatomical section. The TR and TI are set according to the tissue of interest.

The first pulse is an inverting pulse to invert M_O into the −z axis. TI is an interpulse time delay that permits M_O to begin to recover, becoming less and less negative, reaching 0, then rising along the +z axis. No signal is generated during this process because M_O is not in the x–y plane. However, at a set interval a 90° pulse rotates M_O into the x–y plane, producing precession and an RF signal. The strength of this signal at the time of the 90° pulse will depend on the TI recovery time that was allowed. Because this is different for each tissue, useful MRI data can be collected. Inversion recovery provides good anatomical contrast because TI values for normal tissues vary considerably.

Because of the reversal of M_O, the RF signal decreases with a short TI, then flips and increases as TI increases (Figure 42–8). The MR unit is usually programmed to display the reversed (negative) range of M_O so that it is shown to be returning to its original equilibrium. This permits the image to be displayed lighter as the negative signal decreases and then to continue lighter as the positive signal increases. Short TI inversion recovery techniques are sometimes called STIR imaging.

Spin-Echo Spin-echo is the most popular pulse sequence because it reduces scan time significantly. It was first described by Carr and Purcell and is therefore also known as the Carr-Purcell (CP) sequence. The basic spin-echo sequence consists of a 90° pulse which initiates a partial saturation sequence. However, it is followed by a 180° pulse (the refocusing pulse) at 50 percent of the TE. The refocusing pulse flips the proton precession and produces a spin-echo RF signal that grows, then fades in intensity. The y gradient is changed for each pulse sequence to record data from a different anatomical section. The TR and TE are set according to the tissue of interest.

Figure 42–7. Magnetic resonance pulse sequences. (A) Partial saturation is a simple series of 90° RF pulses sequenced with short y and z gradient pulses and a long x gradient pulse. The RF signal is classical free induction decay. (B) Inversion recovery uses a 180° RF pulse sequenced with a z gradient pulse prior to a partial saturation sequence. The RF signal is a classical free induction decay that occurs with the 90° pulse. TI is measured between the two RF pulses. (C) Spin-echo uses a partial saturation sequence followed by a 180° (refocusing) RF pulse sequenced with an x and z gradient pulse but without a second y gradient pulse. The refocusing pulse flips the proton precession and produces the spin-echo RF signal. The RF signals that are received are a free induction decay followed by the spin-echo that begins faintly, increases to maximum strength, then fades away. TE is measured between the first and the echo RF signals.

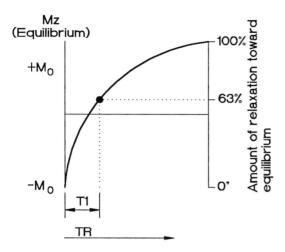

Figure 42–8. Relaxation after reversal of M_O during an inversion recovery pulse. Although the precession is decaying back toward equilibrium, it flips from the $-z$ axis to $+z$ at the solid horizontal line. By definition, T1 occurs when 63 percent of the return to the maximum field strength (equilibrium) has been attained.

The decay or dephasing process is used to advantage in spin-echo imaging by allowing dephasing to continue until it is nearly undetectable. This permits the faster spinning protons to precess further and further out of synch. When the 180° refocusing pulse is used to flip M_O in the opposite direction, the protons that have precessed faster and are the furthest out of synch now begin precessing back into synchrony with those that were slower. At an equal time after the 180° pulse, all the precessions will again be equal. This has the effect of an echo and produces the spin-echo signal. The process operates exactly as if the Indianapolis 500 auto race were begun and allowed to run for one hour. If each car were stopped at the end of the hour, turned around and run for a second hour at exactly the same speed, the race would end with all the cars crossing the finish line together. Although this would be a very boring race, in MRI it provides

enough time to measure the differences between the precessional rates.

The T2 term is used during spin-echo MRI to describe where the data collection occurs after the second time interval when 63 percent of the spins have lost their alignment with each other as they decay back toward equilibrium. The T2 relaxation characteristics for various body tissues are shown in Table 42–4.

Spin-echo pulses are weighted for T1 by using short TR and TE (Figure 42–13B). Although a T1 image is valuable when used in conjunction with a T2 image, it is not considered useful information by itself. Spin-echo pulses are weighted for T2 by using long TR and TE (Figure 42–13C).

Other Pulse Sequences Numerous other pulse sequences have been developed to increase the amount of data collected or to decrease the scanning time. Increased data collection sequences include a modification of Carr and Purcell's spin-echo sequence by Meiboom and Gill that is known as the CPMG sequence and stimulated echo acquisition method (STEAM). Fast MR imaging via decreased scanning time (20–50 ms) has been achieved by using gradient refocused echo (GRE) sequences (gradient-echo techniques) known as fast low-angle shot (FLASH), fast-imaging steady-state precession (FISP), gradient-recalled acquisition steady state (GRASS), and contrast-enhanced fast imaging (FAST). Because moving fluid produces no MR signal, the decreased scan time se-

TABLE 42–4		
EXAMPLE T1 AND T2 RELAXATION TIMES		
Tissue	**T1**	**T2**
Fat	170 ms	80 ms
Example tumor	580 ms	80 ms
Muscle	580 ms	40 ms

quences have received much attention as work proceeds on dynamic MR imaging for cardiac and blood flow studies. Reduction of motion artifacts in blood flow studies has been achieved with gradient motion rephasing (GMR), gradient motion nulling (GNR), motion artifact suppression technique (MAST), and presaturation (dark blood sequence).

Multisection and Multiecho Acquisition

Because many T1 relaxation times are relatively long, most MRI units begin to acquire data from additional sections while the first section is still proceeding through the pulse sequence. Most of the other pulse sequences, such as CPMG, follow this format. Both multisection and multiecho techniques are used. They are also called three-dimensional Fourier transform (3DFT) after the algorithm used during the compilation of the data. The TR interval between pulses is used to begin the pulse sequencing of other sections. Sections adjacent to those undergoing a pulse sequence are not imaged in order to avoid overlapping information. Instead, an alternating sequence is used to permit adjacent sections additional relaxation time.

MAGNETIC RESONANCE IMAGING EQUIPMENT

The typical MRI unit looks similar to a CT unit (Figure 42–9). However, its internal construction is unique, consisting of a stationary magnet within which are fitted gradient and radio frequency (RF) coils (Figure 42–10). The stationary magnet must be extremely strong; field strengths for clinical imaging range from 0.3–4.0 T. A table for the patient and a large computer for image processing, display, and storage complete the MRI system.

Figure 42–9. A typical MRI unit. A solenoid RF coil for the head is shown on the table. (Courtesy of GE Medical Systems.)

Stationary Magnet

Magnetic resonance imaging has been achieved with resistive, permanent, and superconducting magnets. Each has significant differences in potential field strength, stability, uniformity, and cost.

Resistive Resistive magnets produce a strong field in the range of 0.02–0.4 T from the flow of current in large numbers of turns of wire or conducting ribbons. These magnets are called resistive because of the large amount of resistance produced by this type of wiring configuration. The heat produced by the resistance is so great that resistive magnets are severely limited by their cooling requirements.

Resistive magnets provide good uniformity of magnetic field and are relatively inexpensive. However, their field strength is limited

RF Coil

Gradient Coils

Stationary Magnet

Figure 42–10. A typical MRI unit, with the relationship of the stationary magnet, gradient coil, and RF coil to the patient illustrated.

and somewhat unstable, they often exhibit longitudinal fringe field problems, and they consume a large amount of electrical power.

Permanent Permanent magnets of up to 0.3 T have been produced by inducing a strong magnetic field in ferromagnetic materials during manufacturing. These magnets are extremely heavy and may weigh up to 200,000 pounds (100 tons). Attempts have been made to use rare earth alloys to reduce the total magnet weight.

Permanent magnets are inexpensive to maintain and offer transverse field imaging. They also exhibit minimal fringe field problems. Because the strength of permanent magnets is limited by the number of magnetic domains available in the material, they have been used only for relatively low field strength MRI units, of up to approximately 0.15 T. Their

weight and temperature sensitivity can be a problem.

Superconductive Superconductive magnets may produce field strengths of up to 4 T. They use liquid cryogens to produce extremely low temperatures that permit some conductors to become superconductive. Much effort is currently being devoted to the development of room temperature superconductors. If these efforts are successful, MRI will become much less expensive and much more important as a diagnostic imaging tool.

Strong magnetic fields require enormous quantities of wire loops. For example, a 1.5 T magnet might require 1,000 loops, each carrying 1,000 A. This amperage in so many loops in the same circuit would produce a large quantity of heat and consume a great deal of power. In fact, a magnet of this strength cannot be produced because of these physical limits. The heat would melt the conducting wire and destroy the circuit.

At temperatures near absolute zero (0° Kelvin) some conductors lose nearly all resistance, thus becoming superconductors. This permits the construction of magnets with the strength necessary to permit MRI at 1 T and higher field strengths. Superconduction has been observed as a basic property of atoms, where electrons have been spinning in tiny electromagnetic fields, apparently since the creation of the universe, without losing rotational energy as heat and slowing down.

Special cooling agents, called **cryogens**, must be used to achieve the extremely low temperatures necessary for superconductive magnets. The electromagnetic coils are placed in an insulated chamber called a **dewar**, or **cryostat**, which contains **liquid helium**. A dewar is constructed much like an insulated Thermos bottle, with the electromagnet inside. Liquid helium has a boiling point of 4° K (−269° C or −452° F) and is used to maintain the coil temperature below 9.5° K (−264° C or −443° F). The liquid helium is then surrounded by another dewar, this one containing **liquid nitrogen**, which has a boiling point of 77° K (−196° C or −320° F). The nitrogen serves as another insulator to help maintain the temperature necessary for the helium to remain liquid. The process of bringing the superconducting magnet to the necessary temperature by using cryogens is called **ramping**.

Superconductive magnets are capable of very high field strengths. They typically produce very stable and uniform fields. However, they are expensive and require expensive site preparation and maintenance. In addition, the high field strengths may cause fringe field problems.

If the temperature of the cryogens rises to the boiling point of helium, both liquids will vaporize into gases. Neither gas can maintain the necessary environment for superconduc-

tion and the electromagnetic coil will rapidly overheat. This process is known as **quenching** and is a serious hazard to the electromagnet, the patient, and personnel during superconductive MRI. The rapid vaporization of the gases can replace the oxygen in areas around the MRI unit. Although safety release valves are designed to vent these gases outside the unit, audible oxygen monitors are required to warn personnel in the event of quenching. Although helium and nitrogen are not poisonous, if the gases displace the air in the examination areas asphyxiation becomes a danger and an explosion is also possible. A patient or technologist would lose consciousness quickly and could die within minutes. A mask and nonmagnetic O_2 tank are required to permit the technologist to remove a patient from the unit as rapidly as possible if the alarms sound. The technologist must put on an oxygen mask before attempting to help a patient or anyone else. If the technologist were to lose consciousness there might be no one else to help others.

In addition to these hazards, the heat buildup that occurs in the electromagnet during a quench usually does severe damage to the coil windings and requires extensive repairs or replacement of the entire coil. Quenching is therefore not only dangerous but also prohibitively expensive. Failure to maintain sufficient cryogenic pressures through regular replacement of natural evaporation is the most likely cause of a quench. Therefore, the dependability of the cryogenic supply company to the MRI unit is of critical importance.

Shim Coils All stationary magnets have irregularities in their fields due to the shape and construction of the magnets themselves, the location of ferromagnetic materials near the MRI unit, and the materials used in the construction of the MRI room. These irregularities are compensated for by adding a series of corrective magnetic coils, called **shim coils**, inside

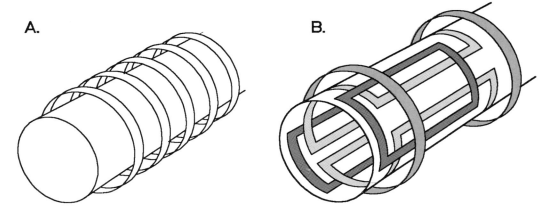

Figure 42–11.   (A) Shim coils and (B) gradient coils, both surrounding the bore of the stationary magnet.

the bore of the main stationary magnet. Shim coils can be resistive or superconducting and are custom fitted for each unit by adjusting the current to each (Figure 42–11A).

Magnetic Field Strength Magnetic field strength decreases inversely with the cube of the distance. This is much faster than the effect of distance (the inverse square law) that is so important in diagnostic radiography. The inverse cube law is complex but is based on the fact that both magnetic north and south poles are always present. The two poles affect each other with increasing significance as distance increases, the result being that the poles begin to cancel each other. This has the effect of reducing the magnetic field strength exponentially, as compared to the inverse square law.

This rapid fall-off of magnetic field strength makes it difficult to establish and maintain a homogeneous field for imaging. Because distance has such a dramatic effect on field strength, it becomes extremely difficult to perform MRI over a large area, even one the size and thickness of the human body.

The basic principles of magnetism are directly involved in determining magnetic field strength (see Chapter 4). The degree of alignment of induced magnetic domains in a material depends on the strength of the magnetic field that is inducing them and the inverse cube of the distance between them. This is expressed as:

$$M_I = \frac{M_O}{D^3}$$

where: M_I = induced magnetic field
M_O = original magnetic field
D = distance

This is of critical importance in understanding how magnetic attraction occurs. Not only does the attraction increase by the inverse cube with distance, but the number of magnetic domains also increases by the inverse cube. These two factors function mathematically so that their product represents the total attraction. In other words, the actual increase is not the inverse cube of the distance but rather the inverse cube of the distance times the inverse cube of the number of magnetic domains. Therefore, attraction occurs by the inverse sixth power. Moving ten times closer to the magnet actually causes the magnetic field strength attraction to increase by 1,000,000 times.

A free magnet will move to align itself in a magnetic field. For example, the needle of a compass aligns itself on a north-south axis because it experiences the torque of the earth's magnetic field. Torque can be a powerful force in a strong magnetic field. For example, this principle of inducing torque is used to activate the motors that move trains and lift elevators. However, torque also acts on the nucleus of an atom and can cause a nucleus to align with a magnetic field. This is a basic principle in MRI.

Gradient Coils

There are three sets of gradient coils, one each for the x, y, and z axes (Figure 42–11B). They can be operated as required to achieve the appropriate pulse sequence and spatial localization within the anatomical section.

Radiofrequency Coils

Radiofrequency (RF) coils may serve as both the transmitter and the receiver of the MRI signal (although some units use separate RF coils for each function). Because it is desirable to position RF coils as close as possible to the body part to be imaged, they are often sized and shaped to fit specific body parts. This type of coil is known as a **surface coil**. **Head, neck, and body** surface coils are commonly used in either **saddle** or **solenoid** shapes (a solenoid head coil is shown on the table in front of the magnet bore in Figure 42–9). **Solenoid (or birdcage) coils are used in a transverse magnetic field. Saddle coils are used in a longitudinal magnetic field. However, the best images are produced with ring-shaped surface (or local) coils that are placed directly on the patient, as close to the region**

of interest as possible. Body coils permit resolution to the depth of the entire body section but higher noise signals can be a problem. Surface coils permit thinner sections and lower noise signals, but they are limited to a depth of resolution of 5–6 cm.

It is important to select the RF coil appropriate to the structure being examined. For example, a small birdcage coil would image the entire knee quite well but a small surface coil would produce the best image of a single meniscus.

Table

The MRI table is usually slightly curved for patient comfort and to conform to the circular shape of the bore of the magnet. As with CT units, tabletops are rated for maximum weight and it is critical that this weight not be exceeded. Extensive damage to the table may result when attempts are made to examine very large patients who exceed the limit. The top is motor-driven to move the patient smoothly into the bore of the magnet.

Computer

Data acquisition sequences are complex in most MRI units. The computer must precisely control the gradient and RF coils and their pulsing sequences, as well as collect and process the received RF data. Most data is collected by sampling the received signal during a series of RF windows. All data and images can be stored electronically on magnetic or optical tape or disk. The operator can access the computer through two consoles, one for operating the MRI unit to acquire data, the other for manipulation of images for which data has been collected.

Operating Console The MRI unit operator controls the scanning procedure by specifying the radio frequency, RF pulse sequence, pulsing time intervals, matrix size, proton spin density, number of excitations (NEX) or acquisitions, field of view, and section parameters.

The radio frequency is adjusted by tuning the system to the proper Larmor frequency for the tissue to be examined and by tuning the RF coils to receive the desired RF signal that will be emitted from the tissues.

The RF pulse sequences are classified as partial saturation, inversion recovery, spin-echo, or one of the other fast data sequences discussed above. The MRI computer is programmed to initiate the RF and magnetic field pulses to accomplish the selected sequence. These sequences are usually extremely complex as they commonly use multisection and multiecho techniques to reduce scan time by acquiring data for numerous sections simultaneously. Although the operator does not have to initiate the various pulses, an appropriate sequencing method for the particular examination must be selected.

The most common variable in operating an MRI unit is the time interval (TI, TE, and TR) used to enhance image quality. Appropriate intervals determine T1 and T2 and vary depending on the tissue of interest, suspected pathology, and clinical experience (Table 42–3). The time intervals directly affect the total scan time.

As in all digital imaging, the matrix size controls the resolution of the image. The matrix size that is selected also has a direct effect on the total scan time, with a larger matrix producing higher resolution but requiring longer scan times. This is often set as the number of views, with 128 or 256 being common selections.

The quantity of protons precessing and emitting RF determines the proton spin density (ρ). This is determined by the number of excitations or acquisitions per scan. The longer the TR, the more time is available for RF emission. The larger the tissue sample or the greater the number of precessing protons in the tissue, the greater is the proton spin density. These factors determine the strength of the RF signal and therefore the density (brightness) of the image.

The number of signals used to create the image also has a direct effect on the total scan time. This is measured by the number of excitations (NEX) or acquisitions. It also determines the strength of the RF signal and the image brightness.

The field of view (FOV) also affects scan time and resolution. A larger FOV requires longer scan time and decreases resolution.

The section, the interval between sections, and the section thickness can all be controlled by the operator.

Display Console The image reconstruction algorithms used for MRI are similar to those used in CT (see Chapters 40 and 41). However, there are differences because of the increased data that is collected during the MRI pulse sequences. Depending on the pulse sequence and quantity of data collected, this permits oblique sections as well as routine sagittal, coronal, and even 3D reconstructions.

Most display consoles also permit the addition of software **filters**. Smoothing filters average pixel values but decrease resolution. Noise reduction filters eliminate image densities below a selected level. Edge (contour) enhancement filters accentuate the differences between pixels when those differences exceed a selected value. Other filters for special uses may be created with custom algorithms.

MRI display consoles permit density windows and contrast widths to be set as with any digital image processing technology. However, MRI units collect significantly more data than CT units and they have the ability to perform more complex data analysis as well. When sufficient TR is used, both T1 and T2 images can be produced. Reformatting of data to display transverse, sagittal, and coronal images, as well as oblique and three-dimensional images, is also possible without additional data collection (Figure 42–12). Region of interest (ROI) controls permit calculations of pixel values, histograms, and highlighting of specific regions. Scanograms for anatomical reference, grid application, reverse display, annotation, and simultaneous image display (collaging) are all possible. Electronic magnification of the field of view (FOV) is often used when filming MRI studies.

IMAGE QUALITY

Numerous factors directly affect image quality. The primary visual factor is often called brightness, which is actually the density of the MR image. The RF signal strength determines brightness, although other factors affect it.

Field Strength

Higher strength magnetic fields produce a stronger RF signal. There is a dramatic difference between the imaging parameters and the resultant image for the same tissues when examined under different strength magnets. Although the most efficient field strength has not yet been determined, it most likely is between 1 and 3 T.

Section Thickness

Section thickness is determined by the size (or depth) of the tissue voxel. It is the primary factor of image quality because all signals from a single voxel are mathematically combined to give a single image value for the voxel. Therefore the voxel size determines the smallest tissue differences that can be imaged.

The dimension of a voxel is determined by dividing the size of the field of view by the matrix size:

$$d = \frac{F}{M}$$

where: d = voxel dimension
F = field of view
M = matrix size

Example: What is the voxel dimension for a 256 × 256 matrix showing a field of view of 22 cm?

Answer: $d = \dfrac{F}{M}$

$$d = \frac{22 \text{ cm}}{256}$$

$$d = 0.0859 \text{ cm} = 8.59 \text{ mm}$$

Effect of MRI Parameters

The effects of the major MRI parameters, proton spin density (ρ), repetition time (TR), echo time (TE), inversion time (TI), spin-lattice relaxation time (T1), and spin-spin relaxation time (T2) are summed in Table 42–2.

The present state of MRI diagnosis demands that each examination include at least

Figure 42–12. A coronal MR image of the abdomen and pelvis. (Courtesy of GE Medical Systems.)

one T1 weighted image and at least one T2 weighted image. This is because proton precession (and therefore the frequency of the RF signal emitted) varies depending on adjacent tissues. As an example, a tumor might have a T1 and T2 as shown in Table 42–4. If the tumor were imbedded in fat, a T1 weighted image would provide the contrast to permit its detection; the tumor would be hidden in a T2 image because the T2 relaxation times of the tumor and of fat are identical, making them appear at the same image density. However, if the same tumor were imbedded in muscle, a T2 weighted image would be required to provide contrast; the tumor would be hidden in a T1 image because the T1 of the tumor and of muscle are identical.

A calculated pure T1 image can be reconstructed by software using an algorithm to compare two spin-echo scans of the same section. The second scan is performed with the same TE used in the first but TR is varied. There is some question about the diagnostic accuracy of scans produced by this method.

A calculated pure T2 image can also be reconstructed by software using an algorithm to compare two spin-echo scans of the same section. In this case, the second scan is performed with the same TR used in the first but TE is varied. There is some question about the diagnostic accuracy of scans produced by this method, as well.

Motion

Motion (temporal resolution) is a special problem in MRI because of the extremely long scan times that must be used. Good communication with the patient is the best method of assuring cooperation in reducing motion artifacts. Much has been written about patient claustrophobia due to the small diameter and long length of the bore of most MRI units. However, only about 5 percent of all patients cannot be examined due to claustrophobia.

Cardiac gating procedures that use an electrocardiographic wave to trigger scanning pulses have proven effective in reducing motion in thoracic, cardiac, and cervical spine imaging. Some patients can be led through a breath holding technique in which the technologist activates the pulse sequence at expiration to eliminate diaphragmatic motion. This technique is valid only with pulse sequences of ten seconds or less.

Spatial Resolution

Spatial resolution is determined by the homogeneity of the static external magnetic field, the steepness of the gradient fields, and the scan time. Its quality is limited by noise, or the signal-to-noise ratio; when this ratio becomes high, image quality begins to decrease. Current MRI units are capable of resolving objects as small as 1 lp/mm.

Signal-to-Noise Ratio

Noise, or extraneous visual information, is known as the signal-to-noise ratio (S/N). It is determined by the voxel size and detection volume, the quantity of precessing protons, the pulse sequence, and the field strength. It is undesirable because it reduces the visibility of low contrast structures. **The S/N is enhanced by reducing TE and using optimal TR.** It can also be enhanced by **averaging** a series of RF signals and by the use of a **stronger magnetic field**.

RF coils are sensitive enough that they can detect the tiny electrical currents produced by normal Brownian motion of body electrolytes. Because the quantity of Brownian motion increases with body temperature, it is referred to as **thermal noise**.

Scan Time

As with all digital imaging methods, scan time depends on the quantity of data that must be processed by the computer. In MRI it depends primarily on the pulse sequences TE and TR and the number of projections. For example, a 256 × 256 matrix with a TR of 2 seconds for 2 excitations might require a 17-minute scan time. For three-dimensional MRI, the scan time is usually much greater. For example, a 0.5 cm section thickness in a 15 cm volume might require a two-hour scan time. Multisection and multiecho pulse sequences are the prime methods of reducing scan time.

Image Contrast

Although different tissues have inherent contrast, it may not be demonstrated on the MR image unless proper imaging techniques are used. As MRI continues to develop, the techniques are constantly being researched and improved. In the future it may become the responsibility of the MRI technologist to apply the proper signal sequencing technique and reconstruction algorithm.

Image contrast can be controlled to a great extent by the manipulation of the sequence of radio frequency pulses, ρ, TI, TR, and TE. Maximum contrast is obtained when the RF signal strength is at its greatest difference between two tissues. For example, in Figure 42–13A, the T1 relaxation curves become further apart as time increases. Therefore, the contrast increases with increasing time.

A **T1 weighted image** is usually produced with a **short TR** (300–800 ms) to maximize T1 and a short TE to minimize T2 (Figure 42–13B). A **T2 weighted image** is usually produced with a **long TR** (2–3 sec) to minimize T1 and a **long TE** to maximize T2 (Figure 42–13C). However, there are some situations in which image density actually reverses (Figure 42–13A). In these instances a short TE produces greater T1 contrast while a long TE produces greater T2 contrast. When TE is set at the crossover point, no contrast is produced.

Subject contrast is primarily due to differences in proton densities. A **proton spin density image (ρ)** is produced with a **long TR** and a **short TE** to minimize both T1 and T2. It is primarily an FID signal and exhibits relatively low contrast due to the slight differences in proton density between tissues (Table 42–3). The subject contrast of a T1 image varies with the magnetic field strength, while T2 values remain essentially constant.

Whereas CT uses Hounsfield units, there are no standardized units for tissue measurements in MRI because subject contrast depends on the differences between the signals received from the tissues. There are so many different pulse and frequency sequences and algorithms in use that no unit system is yet feasible.

Most pathologies increase both T1 and T2. This produces a black, negative contrast image on a T1 weighted image and a white, positive contrast image on a T2 weighted image. This contrast disappears when images are not weighted toward either T1 or T2. Consequently, efforts should be made to produce weighted images when pathological conditions are to be demonstrated.

The effects of the most common parameter weighting, proton spin density (ρ), T1, and T2, on image density (brightness) are shown in Table 42–2.

Chemical Shift Artifact

The chemical shift is the slight difference between the resonating frequencies of similar protons. The differences are so slight that they are expressed in parts per million (ppm). For example, hydrogen in fat resonates at a slightly higher frequency than hydrogen in water (about 3 ppm). This produces a bright band next to a dark band on the MR image at water-fat interfaces and is considered an imaging artifact, although some studies have indicated that proper manipulation of the RF spectrum data

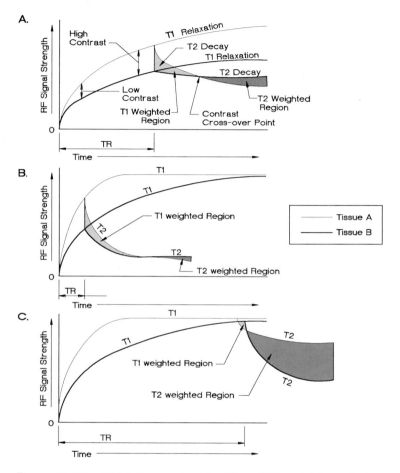

Figure 42–13. Obtaining contrast by T1 and T2 weighting during spin-echo imaging. The T1 curves demonstrate recovery back toward equilibrium after the first pulse. The T2 curves demonstrate decay from the refocusing pulse back toward equilibrium. (A) Relatively equal T1 and T2 weighting with a medium TR. Note the contrast crossover point. A short TE after the TR would produce a T1 weighted image. A long TE after the TR would produce a T2 weighted image. (B) T1 weighting occurs with a short TR. The shorter the TE after the TR, the greater the signal difference (contrast) between the tissues. (C) T2 weighting occurs with a long TR. The longer the TE before the TR, the greater the signal difference (contrast) between the tissues. (Adapted by permission from Friedman, Barry, R., et al., *Principles of MRI*. New York: McGraw-Hill, Inc. 1989.)

can produce useful information from chemical shift. Chemical shift artifacts can be reduced or eliminated by increasing the strength of the gradient fields, although this will also increase the visible noise in the image.

Paramagnetic Contrast Agents

Magnetic resonance imaging contrast agents are primarily **paramagnetic agents designed to enhance the T1 and T2 relaxation times of adjacent hydrogen nuclei.** Some agents are classified as T1 active or T2 active. They produce complex effects that vary depending on the RF pulsing sequence. For example, T1 shortening increases the RF signal intensity but T2 shortening decreases it. In many instances paramagnetic contrast agents permit the visualization of lesions with shorter TR, thus decreasing scan time.

Paramagnetic contrast agents have been developed for oral, intravenous, and inhalation administration, and although this is an active research area in MRI, at the present time the IV agents have predominated. Gadolinium^{+3} (Gd^{+3}), which has seven unpaired electrons, has the strongest relaxation rate properties and has proven effective in demonstrating various types of lesions. However, it is extremely toxic and is administered in a complex with DTPA (diethylenetriaminepentaacetic acid) (Gd-DTPA) to ensure detoxification.

SAFETY AND BIOLOGICAL HAZARDS

As yet, there is no known biological risk from the magnetic field of an MRI unit. However, magnetic resonance imaging units require special consideration of the environment in which they are installed because of possible interactions between their extremely strong magnetic fields with ferromagnetic materials and electromagnetic devices. Included among devices that are affected by MRI units are cath-

ode ray tubes, gamma cameras, cardiac pacemakers, and radio broadcasting and receiving equipment. This includes computers (including the MRI computer itself), x-ray tubes, image intensification systems, computed tomography units, ultrasound units, electron microscopes, credit cards, analog watches, and any other devices that operate on electromagnetic principles. Safe operating distances for these devices depend on the strength of the MRI magnet and may range up to 500 feet for a 1.5 T magnet.

The MRI unit itself can be seriously affected by moving ferromagnetic devices, such as elevators and automobiles, and by strong electromagnetic devices, such as power transformers and radio broadcasting antennas. Although ferromagnetic sheets can be used to shield the MRI unit and the main resonance frequency can be adjusted slightly to avoid ranges conflicting with other equipment, these measures can compromise the imaging ability of the unit.

Safety Factors

Because magnetic fields change so dramatically with distance, it is easy for someone who is not knowledgeable about them to be misled on safety considerations. Accidents around MRI units occur when ferromagnetic materials such as oxygen tanks, IV poles, mop buckets, scissors, and personal items such as earrings and belt buckles enter the field. These items can become lethal projectiles. Magnetic media, such as computer and audio disks, and magnetized information strips on credit cards may be erased.

Other electronic devices, such as cardiac pacemakers and pocket pagers, and physiologic monitors, such as electrocardiographic monitors, may be damaged or turned off and will not work properly in a strong magnetic field. It is also possible that metal objects that have been surgically implanted, such as replacement hips, aneurysm clips and surgical staples, or foreign objects, such as buckshot or metallic debri in the eye, may be torqued during MRI examinations with catastrophic consequences. For example, torquing an aneurysm clip could open an artery and cause a fatal hemorrhage. Careful histories and, in some cases, fluoroscopic screening, are safety precautions that must be taken before MRI. Patients with histories of surgical implants or with employment histories in metal working must be interviewed with special care. The objects considered to contraindicate MRI examination are listed in Table 42–5.

A few steps closer to an MRI unit will increase the magnetic field attraction by the inverse cube law. A distance of as little as one inch can make the difference between being able to hold onto an object and having it fly at incredible speed directly to the bore of the MRI unit. Remembering that an industrial electromagnet is capable of lifting an automobile or railroad car may help in understanding the power of an extremely strong magnetic field.

Within 10–20 feet of the magnet, wheelchairs and carts may begin to roll toward the MRI unit and within 5–10 feet, hairpins and pens may become projectiles. A cart may begin to roll from 20 feet away, but as it approaches the bore of the magnet the field may become strong enough to cause an oxygen tank or other object on the cart to become a projectile.

TABLE 42–5
OBJECTS THAT CONTRAINDICATE MRI EXAMINATION
Pacemakers
Ferromagnetic cranial aneurysm clips
Shrapnel or other metallic objects in vital locations
Cochlear implants

It is important to emphasize to others that the magnetic field is operating at all times. Many persons assume that, as with most electromagnetic devices, the magnetic field is on only when the unit is in operation. The doors to the MRI scanning room should not only be locked, but padlocked during hours the unit is closed. This procedure prevents entry by persons with master passkeys during these hours.

Because of the cryogenically established superconductive conditions, superconductor magnets maintain their fields at all times and are therefore hazardous at all times. The extremely strong field must be treated with respect. The attractive force on an object as large as an oxygen tank makes it possible to fatally injure a patient or technologist if he or she is caught between the object and the MRI unit.

Biological Factors

The United States Food and Drug Administration (FDA) issued MRI operating guidelines in 1982 that suggested limiting whole body exposure to 2.0 T for static magnetic fields, 6.0 T/sec for gradient fields, and a specific absorption rate (SAR) of 0.4 W/kg for RF fields. The SAR is the standard measurement of RF dose. Although there have not been any published reports of harmful effects due to the use of MRI, the issue is under intense study and much additional information is expected in the years to come. In the United States, the FDA requires prominent posting of triangular warning signs at the 5 G (0.0005 T) line. There are two signs, one indicating a strong magnetic field, the other with markings and wording prohibiting pacemakers or loose metal objects.

Static magnetic fields appear to augment the T wave amplitude of the heart. This may occur when conductive fluids, such as blood, pass through the static magnetic field, thus generating low potentials that may affect the biopotentials of the heart. No arrhythmias or other heart rate alterations have yet been produced in laboratory animals or observed in patients undergoing MRI.

Intense gradient magnetic fields have been shown to induce electrical currents in body tissues such as nerve, muscle, skeletal, and heart. Light flashes due to physiological stimulation of the retina have also been observed. However, these field strengths are far above that used in MRI.

Radio frequency magnetic fields are known to produce thermal effects. Potential biological damage would depend on the ability of the specific biological system to metabolically absorb and distribute heat. Some effects, including ocular cataractogenesis due to thermal heating of the eye and testes, have been recorded, although again at field levels well above those used in MRI.

Because of the lack of definitive data on the biological effects of MRI, pregnant women are seldom examined. However, when necessary, MRI studies are considered less hazardous to the fetus than computed tomography studies.

SUMMARY

Magnetic resonance imaging (MRI) uses magnetism and radio frequencies (RF) to create diagnostic sectional images of the body. If the nucleus is spinning, it has angular momentum, or nuclear magnetic moment. This rotating charge acts as a current loop and produces a magnetic field. When a rotating nucleus is subjected to a magnetic field, it will begin to precess. MR imaging is accomplished through various measurements of this movement of the nuclear magnetic field.

The frequency of precession is called the Larmor frequency and is critical to MR imaging. Production of the nuclear magnetic resonance signal requires applying a Larmor frequency alternating RF and then listening to the RF emissions from the protons. Digital imaging reconstruction techniques are then used to create sectional and three-dimensional images.

The primary parameters used to modify and control the MRI process include proton spin density (PD, SD, or ρ), repetition time (TR), echo time (TE), inversion time (TI), spin-lattice or longitudinal relaxation time (T1), and spin-spin or transverse relaxation time (T2). The parameters that are used vary depending on the pulse sequence used.

The localization of information for the MR image requires three electromagnetic coils to produce magnetic field gradients corresponding to the x, y, and z axes to be imaged. The RF that are detected from these gradient coils can then be analyzed to determine not only the type of atom they came from but also the atom's precise location within the imaging matrix.

The primary variable in the data collection procedure during MRI is the sequence of RF pulses that are used to cause the protons to precess. Partial saturation, inversion recovery, and spin-echo are the major sequences, although most MRI is done with spin-echo pulse sequences. There are many modifications of spin-echo sequences, including multisection and multiecho sequences.

A typical MRI unit consists of a stationary magnet within which are fitted gradient and radio frequency (RF) coils. The stationary magnet must be extremely strong; current field strengths range from 0.5–3.0 T. A table for the patient and a large computer for image processing, display, and storage complete the system.

The primary image quality factor is often called brightness, which is actually the density of the MR image. The RF signal strength determines brightness, although it is also affected by field strength, section thickness, the MRI parameters (ρ, TI, TE, TR, T1, T2), motion, spatial resolution, S/N, and scan time. Image contrast is controlled by manipulating the MRI parameters to produce T1 and T2 weighted images. Chemical shift artifacts may occur at fat-water interfaces although chemical shifting may provide useful diagnostic information in the future. Paramagnetic contrast agents are used to enhance image contrast. As yet, there is no known biological risk from the magnetic field of an MRI unit. However, magnetic resonance imaging units require special restrictions to their access because of possible interactions between their extremely strong magnetic fields and ferromagnetic materials and electromagnetic devices. Accidents around MRI units occur when ferromagnetic materials such as oxygen tanks, IV poles, mop buckets, scissors, and personal items such as earrings and belt buckles enter the field. These items can become lethal projectiles.

The Food and Drug Administration suggests limiting whole or partial body exposure to 2.0 T for static magnetic fields, 3.0 T/sec for gradient fields, and a specific absorption rate (SAR) of 0.4 W/kg for RF fields.

REVIEW QUESTIONS

1. What is the source of the magnetic fields within the body that are used during MRI?

2. What is precession?

3. What is TI? TR? TE? T1? T2?

4. How do the gradient coils select an image section?

5. What is accomplished by an RF pulse during a pulse sequence?

6. What occurs at each step during a spin-echo pulse sequence?

7. How is MR image contrast increased? decreased?

8. How can MR image noise be reduced by improving the S/N?

9. Describe appropriate safety measures for protection of all persons who approach the MRI unit magnetic field.

REFERENCES AND RECOMMENDED READING

Andrew, E.R. Nuclear magnetic resonance imaging. *Scientific Basis of Medical Imaging*, 212–36. Editor: Wells, P.N.T. Edinburgh: Churchill Livingstone, 1982.

Atkinson, Dennis J. Pulse sequence design. *Clinical Magnetic Resonance Imaging*, 313–40. Editors: Edelman, Robert R., and John R. Hesselink. Philadelphia, PA: W. B. Saunders Company, 1990.

Axel, Leon. Chemical shift imaging. *Magnetic Resonance Imaging*, 229–43. Editors: Stark, David D., and William G. Bradley, Jr. St. Louis, MO: C. V. Mosby Co., 1988.

Barrafate, Diane, and Mark Henkelman. MRI and surgical clips. *The Canadian Journal of Medical Radiation Technology* 16:3, 101, 1985.

Bloch, Felix, W. W. Hansen, and M. E. Packard. Nuclear induction. *Physics Review* 69, 127, 1946.

Bloch, Felix. Nuclear induction. *Physics Review* 70, 460–74, 1946.

Bloch, Felix. The principle of nuclear induction. *Nobel Lectures in Physics: 1942–1962.* New York: Elsevier Publishing Company, 1964.

Bushong, Stewart C. *Magnetic Resonance Imaging: Physical and Biological Principles.* St. Louis, MO: C. V. Mosby Co., 1988.

Curry, Thomas S., James E. Dowdey, and Robert C. Murry. *Christensen's Physics of Diagnostic Radiology.* 4th ed. Philadelphia, PA: Lea & Febiger, 1990.

Damadian, Raymond. Tumor detection by nuclear magnetic resonance. *Science* 171, 1151–53, 1971.

Damadian, Raymond, Keen Zaner, Doris Hor, Theresa DiMaio, Lawrence Minkoff, and Michael Goldsmith. Nuclear magnetic resonance as a new tool in cancer research: Human tumors by NMR. *Annals of the New York Academy of Science* 222, 1048–76, 1973.

Damadian, Raymond, M. Goldsmith, and L. Minkoff. NMR in cancer XVI: FONAR image of the live human body. *Physiological Chemistry and Physics* 9, 97–100, 1977.

Damadian, Raymond. *NMR in Medicine*. Berlin: Springer-Verlag, 1981.

Davis, P. Potential hazards in NMR imaging: Heating effects of changing magnetic fields and RF fields on small metallic implants. *American Journal of Roentgenology* 137, 857–60, 1981.

Edelman, Robert R., and John R. Hesselink. *Clinical Magnetic Resonance Imaging*. Philadelphia, PA: W. B. Saunders Company, 1990.

Edelman, Robert R., Klaus U. Wentz Kleefield, and Dennis J. Atkinson. Basic principles of magnetic resonance imaging. *Clinical Magnetic Resonance Imaging*, 3–38. Editors: Edelman, Robert R., and John R. Hesselink. Philadelphia, PA: W. B. Saunders Company, 1990.

Edelman, Robert R., Frank G. Shellock, and Joseph Ahladis. Practical MRI for the technologist and imaging specialist. *Clinical Magnetic Resonance Imaging*, 39–73. Editors: Edelman, Robert R., and John R. Hesselink. Philadelphia, PA: W. B. Saunders Company, 1990.

Engelstad, Barry L., and Gerald L. Wolf. Contrast agents. *Magnetic Resonance Imaging*, 761–81. Editors: Stark, David D., and William G. Bradley, Jr. St. Louis, MO: C. V. Mosby Co., 1988.

Elster, Allen D. *Magnetic Resonance Imaging: A Reference Guide and Atlas*. Philadelphia, PA: J. B. Lippincott Co., 1986.

Friedman, Barry R., Jerome P. Jones, German Chaves-Muñoz, Ann P. Salmon, and Christopher R. B. Merritt. *Principles of MRI*. New York: McGraw-Hill, 1989.

Fullerton, Gary D. Physiologic basis of magnetic relaxation. *Magnetic Resonance Imaging*, 36–54. Editors: Stark, David D., and William G. Bradley, Jr. St. Louis, MO: C. V. Mosby Co., 1988.

Grey, Michael L., and Charles W. Coffey, II. Methods for evaluating image quality in magnetic resonance imaging. *Radiologic Technology* 58:4, 339, 1987.

Hendrick, R. Edward. Image contrast and noise. *Magnetic Resonance Imaging*, 66–83. Editors: Stark, David D., and William G. Bradley, Jr. St. Louis, MO: C. V. Mosby Co., 1988.

Hinshaw, W. S., P. A. Bottomley, and G. N. Holland. Radiographic thin-section image of the human wrist by nuclear magnetic resonance. *Nature* 270: 22/29 December, 722–23, 1977.

Kereiakes, James G. Magnetic resonance imaging physics. *Magnetic Resonance Intense Weekend Ortho Review*, November 3–5, 1989. Cincinnati, OH: MR Education Foundation, Inc., and The Christ Hospital.

Kneeland, J. Bruce. Instrumentation. *Magnetic Resonance Imaging*, 56–65. Editors: Stark, David D., and William G. Bradley, Jr. St. Louis, MO: C. V. Mosby Co., 1988.

Lauterbur, Paul C. Image formation by induced local interactions: Examples employing nuclear magnetic resonance. *Nature* 242: March 16, 190–91, 1973.

Lipcamon, James D., Lee C. Chiu, Jeffrey J. Phillips, and Pradip M. Pottany. MRI of the upper abdomen using motion artifact suppression technique. *Radiologic Technology* 59:5, 415, 1988.

Martin, Joel F., and Robert R. Edelman. Fast MR imaging. *Clinical Magnetic Resonance Imaging*, 183–220. Editors: Edelman, Robert R., and John R. Hesselink. Philadelphia, PA: W. B. Saunders Company, 1990.

Morgan, Christopher J., and William R. Hendee. *Introduction to Magnetic Resonance Imaging*. Denver, CO: Multi-Media Publishing, 1984.

Pavlicek, William. Safety considerations. *Magnetic Resonance Imaging*, 244–57. Editors: Stark, David D., and William G. Bradley, Jr. St. Louis, MO: C. V. Mosby Co., 1988.

Philips Medical Systems. *Principles of MR Imaging*. The Netherlands: Philips Medical Systems Publication 1984-11, 1984.

Purcell, Edward M., H. C. Torrey, and R. V. Pound. Resonance absorption by nuclear magnetic moments in a solid. *Physics Review* 69, 37–83, 1946.

Purcell, Edward. Research in nuclear magnetism. *Nobel Lectures in Physics: 1942–1962*. New York: Elsevier Publishing Company, 1964.

Rollo, F. David, and James A. Patton. Nuclear magnetic resonance imaging. *The Physical Basis of Medical Imaging*, 243–52. Editors: Coulam, Craig M., John J. Erickson, F. David Rollo, and A. Everette James, Jr. New York: Appleton-Century-Crofts, 1981.

Roth, Klaus. *NMR–Tomography and Spectroscopy in Medicine: An Introduction*. Berlin: Springer-Verlag, 1984.

Saunders. Biologic effects of NMR clinical imaging. *Applied Radiology*, September/October, 43–46, 1982.

Sigal, Robert. *Magnetic Resonance Imaging: Basis for Interpretation*. Berlin: Springer-Verlag, 1988.

Smith, Hans-Jørgen, and Frank N. Ranallo. *A Non-Mathematical Approach to Basic MRI*. Madison, WI: Medical Physics Publishing Corporation, 1989.

Sprawls, Perry. Spatial characteristics of the MR image. *Magnetic Resonance Imaging*, 24–35. Editors: Stark, David D., and William G. Bradley, Jr. St. Louis, MO: C. V. Mosby Co., 1988.

Stark, David D., and William G. Bradley, Jr., editors. *Magnetic Resonance Imaging*. St. Louis, MO: C. V. Mosby Co., 1988.

Stetter, Eckart. Instrumentation. *Clinical Magnetic Resonance Imaging*, 355–76. Editors: Edelman, Robert R., and John R. Hesselink. Philadelphia, PA: W. B. Saunders Company, 1990.

Wehrli, Felix W. Principles of magnetic resonance. *Magnetic Resonance Imaging*, 3–23. Editors: Stark, David D., and William G. Bradley, Jr. St. Louis, MO: C. V. Mosby Co., 1988.

Wolfe, Gerald L., and Carol Popp. *NMR: A Primer for Medical Imaging*. Thorofare, NJ: Slack Book Division, 1984.

Young, Stuart W. *Nuclear Magnetic Resonance Imaging: Basic Principles*. New York: Raven Press, 1984.

APPENDIX A: "ON A NEW KIND OF RAYS" by W. C. RÖNTGEN

(1) A discharge from a large induction coil is passed through a Hittorf's vacuum tube, or through a well-exhausted Crookes' or Lenard's tube. The tube is surrounded by a fairly close-fitting shield of black paper; it is then possible to see, in a completely darkened room, that paper covered on one side with barium platinocyanide lights up with brilliant fluorescence when brought into the neighbourhood of the tube, whether the painted side or the other be turned towards the tube. The fluorescence is still visible at two metres distance. It is easy to show that the origin of the fluorescence lies within the vacuum tube.

(2) It is seen, therefore, that some agent is capable of penetrating black cardboard which is quite opaque to ultra-violet light, sunlight, or arc-light. It is therefore of interest to investigate how far other bodies can be penetrated by the same agent. It is readily shown that all bodies possess this same transparency, but in very varying degrees. For example, paper is very transparent; the fluorescent screen will light up when placed behind a book of a thousand pages; printer's ink offers no marked resistance. Similarly the fluorescence shows behind two packs of cards; a single card does not visibly diminish the brilliancy of the light. So, again, a single thickness of tinfoil hardly casts a shadow on the screen; several have to be superposed to produce a marked effect. Thick blocks of wood are still transparent. Boards of pine two or three centimetres thick absorb only very little. A piece of sheet aluminium, 15 mm. thick, still allowed the x-rays

By W. C. Röntgen. Translated by Arthur Stanton from the *Sitsungsberichte der Würsburger Physik-medic. Gesellschaft*, 1895.

(as I will call the rays, for the sake of brevity) to pass, but greatly reduced the fluorescence. Glass plates of similar thickness behave similarly; lead glass is, however, much more opaque than glass free from lead. Ebonite several centimetres thick is transparent. If the hand be held before the fluorescent screen, the shadow shows the bones darkly, with only faint outlines of the surrounding tissues.

Water and several other fluids are very transparent. Hydrogen is not markedly more permeable than air. Plates of copper, silver, lead, gold, and platinum also allow the rays to pass, but only when the metal is thin. Platinum .2 mm. thick allows some rays to pass; silver and copper are more transparent. Lead 1.5 mm. thick is practically opaque. If a square rod of wood 20 mm. in the side be painted on one face with white lead, it casts little shadow when it is so turned that the painted face is parallel to the x-rays, but a strong shadow if the rays have to pass through the painted side. The salts of the metals, either solid ir in solution, behave generally as the metals themselves.

(3) The preceding experiments lead to the conclusion that the density of the bodies is the property whose variation mainly affects their permeability. At least no other property seems so marked in this connection. But that the density alone does not determine the transparency is shown by an experiment wherein plates of similar thickness of Iceland spar, glass, aluminium, and quartz were employed as screens. Then the Iceland spar showed itself much less transparent than the other bodies, though of approximately the same density. I have not remarked any strong

fluorescence of Iceland spar compared with glass (see below, No. 4).

(4) Increasing thickness increases the hindrance offered to the rays by all bodies. A picture has been impressed on a photographic plate of a number of superposed layers of tinfoil, like steps, presenting thus a regularly increasing thickness. This is to be submitted to photometric processes when a suitable instrument is available.

(5) Pieces of platinum, lead, zinc, and aluminium foil were so arranged as to produce the same weakening of the effect. The annexed table shows the relative thickness and density of the equivalent sheets of metal.

	Thickness	Relative thickness	Density
Platinum	.018 mm.	1	21.5
Lead	.050 "	3	11.3
Zinc	.100 "	6	7.1
Aluminium	3.500 "	200	2.6

From these values it is clear that in no case can we obtain the transparency of a body from the product of its density and thickness. The transparency increases much more rapidly than the product decreases.

(6) The fluorescence of barium platinocyanide is not the only noticeable action of the x-rays. It is to be observed that other bodies exhibit fluorescence, *e.g.* calcium sulphide, uranium glass, Iceland spar, rock-salt, &c.

Of special interest in this connection is the fact that photographic dry plates are sensitive to the x-rays. It is thus possible to exhibit the phenomena so as to exclude the danger of error. I have thus confirmed many observations originally made by eye observation with the fluorescent screen. Here the power of the x-rays to pass through wood or cardboard becomes useful. The photographic plate can be exposed to the action without removal of the shutter of the dark slide or other protecting case, so that the experiment need not be conducted in darkness. Manifestly, unexposed plates must not be left in their box near the vacuum tube.

It seems now questionable whether the impression on the plate is a direct effect of the x-rays, or a secondary result induced by the fluorescence of the material of the plate. Films can receive the impression as well as ordinary dry plates.

I have not been able to show experimentally that the x-rays give rise to any calorific effects. These, however, may be assumed, for the phenomena of fluorescence show that the x-rays are capable of transformation. It is also certain that all the x-rays falling on a body do not leave it as such.

The retina of the eye is quite insensitive to these rays: the eye placed close to the apparatus sees nothing. It is clear from the experiments that this is not due to want of permeability on the part of the structures of the eye.

(7) After my experiments on the transparency of increasing thicknesses of different media, I proceeded to investigate whether the x-rays could be deflected by a prism. Investigations with water and carbon bisulphide on mica prisms of 30° showed no deviation either on the photographic or the fluorescent plate. For comparison, light rays were allowed to fall on the prism as the apparatus was set up for the experiment. They were deviated 10 mm. and 20 mm. respectively in the case of the two prisms.

With prisms of ebonite and aluminium, I have obtained images on the photographic plate, which point to a possible deviation. It is, however, uncertain, and at most would point to a refractive index 1.05. No deviation can be observed by means of the fluorescent screen. Investigations with the heavier metals have not as yet led to any result, because of their small transparency and the consequent enfeebling of the transmitted rays.

On account of the importance of the question it is desirable to try in other ways whether the x-rays are susceptible of refraction. Finely powdered bodies allow in thick layers but little of the incident light to pass through, in consequence of refraction and reflection. In the case of the x-rays, however, such layers of powder are for equal masses of substance equally transparent with the coherent solid itself. Hence we cannot conclude any regular reflection or refraction of the x-rays. The research was conducted by the aid of finely-powdered rock-salt, fine electrolytic silver powder, and zinc dust already many times employed in chemical work. In all these cases the result, whether by the fluorescent screen or the photographic method, indicated no difference in transparency between the powder and the coherent solid.

It is, hence, obvious that lenses cannot be looked upon as capable of concentrating the x-rays; in effect, both an ebonite and a glass lens of large size prove to be without action. The shadow photograph of a round rod is darker in the middle than at the edge; the image of a cylinder filled with a body more transparent than its walls exhibits the middle brighter than the edge.

(8) The preceding experiments, and others which I pass over, point to the rays being incapable of regular reflection. It is, however, well to detail an observation which at first sight seemed to lead to an opposite conclusion.

I exposed a plate, protected by a black paper sheath, to the x-rays, so that the glass side lay next to the vacuum tube. The sensitive film was partly covered with star-shaped pieces of platinum, lead, zinc, and aluminium. On the developed negative the star-shaped impression showed dark under platinum, lead, and more markedly, under zinc; the aluminium gave no image. It seems, therefore, that these three metals can reflect the x-rays; as, however, another explanation is possible, I repeated the experiment with this only difference, that a film of thin aluminium foil was interposed between the sensitive film and the metal stars. Such an aluminium plate is opaque to ultra-violet rays,

but transparent to x-rays. In the result the images appeared as before, this pointing still to the existence of reflection at metal surfaces.

If one considers this observation in connection with others, namely, on the transparency of powders, and on the state of the surface not being effective in altering the passage of the x-rays through a body, it leads to the probable conclusion that regular reflection does not exist, but that bodies behave to the x-rays as turbid media to light.

Since I have obtained no evidence of refraction at the surface of different media, it seems probable that the x-rays move with the same velocity in all bodies, and in a medium which penetrates everything, and in which the molecules of bodies are embedded. The molecules obstruct the x-rays, the more effectively as the density of the body concerned is greater.

(9) It seemed possible that the geometrical arrangement of the molecules might affect the action of a body upon the x-rays, so that, for example, Iceland spar might exhibit different phenomena according to the relation of the surface of the plate to the axis of the crystal. Experiments with quartz and Iceland spar on this point lead to a negative result.

(10) It is known that Lenard, in his investigations on kathode rays, has shown that they belong to the ether, and can pass through all bodies. Concerning the x-rays the same may be said.

In his latest work, Lenard has investigated the absorption coefficients of various bodies for the kathode rays, including air at atmospheric pressure, which gives 4.10, 3.40, 3.10 for 1 cm., according to the degree of exhaustion of the gas in discharge tube. To judge from the nature of the discharge, I have worked at about the same pressure, but occasionally at greater or smaller pressures. I find, using a Weber's photometer, that the intensity of the fluorescent light varies nearly as the inverse square of the distance between screen and discharge tube. This result is obtained from three very consistent sets of observations at distances of 100 and 200 mm. Hence air absorbs the x-rays much less than the kathode rays. This result is in complete agreement with the previously described result, that the fluorescence of the screen can be still observed at 2 metres from the vacuum tube. In general, other bodies behave like air; they are more transparent for the x-rays than for the kathode rays.

(11) A further distinction, and a noteworthy one, results from the action of a magnet. I have not succeeded in observing any deviation of the x-rays even in very strong magnetic fields.

The deviation of kathode rays by the magnet is one of their peculiar characteristics; it has been observed by Hertz and Lenard, that several kinds of kathode rays exist, which differ by their power of exciting phosphorescence, their susceptibility of absorption, and their deviation by the magnet; but a notable deviation has been observed in all cases which have yet been investigated, and I think that such deviation affords a characteristic not to be set aside lightly.

(12) As the result of many researches, it appears that the place of most brilliant phosphorescence of the walls of the discharge-tube is the chief seat whence the x-rays originate and spread in all directions; that is, the x-rays proceed from the front where the kathode rays strike the glass. If one deviates the kathode rays within the tube by means of a magnet, it is seen that the x-rays proceed from a new point, *i.e.* again from the end of the kathode rays.

Also for this reason the x-rays, which are not deflected by a magnet, cannot be regarded as kathode rays which have passed through the glass, for that passage cannot, according to Lenard, be the cause of the different deflection of the rays. Hence I conclude that the x-rays are not identical with the kathode rays, but are produced from the kathode rays at the glass surface of the tube.

(13) The rays are generated not only in glass. I have obtained them in an apparatus closed by an aluminium plate 2 mm. thick. I purpose later to investigate the behaviour of other substances.

(14) The justification of the term "rays," applied to the phenomena, lies partly in the regular shadow pictures produced by the interposition of a more or less permeable body between the source and a photographic plate or fluorescent screen.

I have observed and photographed many such shadow pictures. Thus, I have an outline

Fig. 1.   Photograph of the bones in the fingers of a living human hand. The third finger has a ring upon it.

Fig. 2. Photograph of a compass card and needle completely enclosed in a metal case.

of part of a door covered with lead paint; the image was produced by placing the discharge-tube on one side of the door, and the sensitive plate on the other. I have also a shadow of the bones of the hand (Fig. 1), of a wire wound upon a bobbin, of a set of weights in a box, of a compass card and needle completely enclosed in a metal case (Fig. 2), of a piece of metal where the x-rays show the want of homogeneity, and of other things.

For the rectilinear propagation of the rays, I have a pin-hole photograph of the discharge apparatus covered with black paper. It is faint but unmistakable.

(15) I have sought for interference effects of the x-rays, but possibly, in consequence of their small intensity, without result.

(16) Researches to investigate whether electrostatic forces act on the x-rays are begun but not yet concluded.

(17) If one asks, what then are these x-rays; since they are not kathode rays, one

might suppose, from their power of exciting fluorescence and chemical action, them to be due to ultra-violet light. In opposition to this view a weighty set of considerations presents itself. If x-rays be indeed ultra-violet light, then that light must possess the following properties.

(a) It is not refracted in passing from air into water, carbon bisulphide, aluminium, rock-salt, glass or zinc.

(b) It is incapable of regular reflection at the surfaces of the above bodies.

(c) It cannot be polarised by any ordinary polarising media.

(d) The absorption by various bodies must depend chiefly on their density.

That is to say, these ultra-violet rays must behave quite differently from the visible, infra-red, and hitherto known ultra-violet rays.

These things appear so unlikely that I have sought for another hypothesis.

A kind of relationship between the new rays and light rays appears to exist; at least the formation of shadows, fluorescence, and the production of chemical action point in this direction. Now it has been known for a long time, that besides the transverse vibrations which account for the phenomena of light, it is possible that longitudinal vibrations should exist in the ether, and, according to the view of some physicists, must exist. It is granted that their existence has not yet been made clear, and their properties are not experimentally demonstrated. Should not the new rays be ascribed to longitudinal waves in the ether?

I must confess that I have in the course of this research made myself more and more familiar with this thought, and venture to put the opinion forward, while I am quite conscious that the hypothesis advanced still requires a more solid foundation.

This article was reprinted from Nature, No. 1369, Vol. 53, January 23, 1896.

APPENDIX B: AGFA's TROUBLESHOOTING THE RADIOGRAPHIC SYSTEM Symptoms and Possible Causes

LOW DENSITY

A. Underexposure
1. Wrong Exposure Factors
   a. Too low kilovoltage
   b. Too low milliamperage
   c. Too short exposure
   d. Too great focal-film distance
2. Meters out of calibration
3. Timer out of calibration
4. Inaccurate setting of meters or timer
5. Drop in incoming line voltage
   a. Elevators, welders, furnaces, blowers, etc. on same curcuit
   b. Insufficient size of power line or transformers
6. Photocell timer out of adjustment
7. Incorrect centering of patient to photocell
8. Central ray of X-ray tube not directed on film
   a. X-ray tube rotated in casing
9. Distance out of grid radius
10. Bucky timer inaccurate
11. One or more valve tubes burned out (Full wave rectifying machines)

B. Underdevelopment
1. Improper development
   a. Time too short
   b. Temperature too low (Hydroquinone inactive below 55° F, or 13° C)
   c. Combination of both
   d. Inaccurate thermometer

2. Exhausted developer
   a. Chemical activity used up
   b. Activity destroyed by contamination
3. Diluted developer
   a. Water overflowed from wash tank
   b. Insufficient chemical mixed originally due to tank actually larger than rating
   c. Improper additions
4. Incorrectly mixed developer
   a. Exact capacity of tank unknown
   b. Mixing ingredients in wrong sequence
   c. Omission of ingredients
   d. Unbalanced formula composition

HIGH DENSITY

A. Overexposure
1. Wrong exposure factors
   a. Too high kilovoltage
   b. Too high milliamperage
   c. Too long exposure
   d. Too short focal-film distance
2. Meters out of calibration
3. Timer out of calibration
4. Inaccurate setting of meters or timer
5. Surge in incoming line voltage
6. Photocell timer out of adjustment
7. Incorrect centering of patient to photocell

B. Improper development
1. Time too long

2. Temperature too high
3. Combination of both
4. Inaccurate thermometer
5. Insufficient dilution of concentrated developer
6. Omission of bromide when mixing

C. Fog—see section on "FOG"
1. Light struck
2. Radiation
3. Chemical
4. Film deterioration

LOW CONTRAST

A. Overpenetration from too high kilovoltage
1. Overmeasurement of part to be examined
2. Incorrect estimate of material or tissue density
3. Meters out of calibration
4. Meters inaccurately set
5. Surge in incoming line voltage
6. Undermeasurement of focal-film distance

B. Scattered radiation
1. Failure to use Bucky diaphragm
2. Failure to use stationary grid
3. Failure to use cutout diaphragm
4. Failure to use suitable cones
5. Failure to use lead backing cassette

C. Too short exposure
1. Timer out of calibration
2. Timer inaccurately set
3. Overload relay kicked out

D. Improper development

HIGH CONTRAST

A. Underpenetration from too low kilovoltage
1. Undermeasurement of part to be examined
2. In parts of varying thickness, setting of kilovoltage for thinner sections
3. Meters out of calibration
4. Meters inaccurately set
5. Drop in incoming line voltage
   a. Elevators, welders, furnaces, etc. on same line
   b. Insufficient size of power line or transformer
6. Overmeasurement of focal-film distance

B. Too long exposure
1. Timer out of calibration
2. Timer inaccurately set

C. Improper development

FOG

A. Unsafe light
1. Light leaks into processing room
   a. Leaks through doors, windows, etc.
   b. Poorly designed labyrinth entrance
      1) Bright light at outer entrance
      2) Reflection from white uniforms of persons passing through
   c. Sparking of motors
      1) Ventilating fans
      2) Dryer fans
      3) Mixers-barium
      4) Light leaks in film carrying box
2. Safelights
   a. Bulb too bright
   b. Improper filter
      1) Not dense enough

      2) Cracked
      3) Bleached
      4) Shrunken
  3. Luminous clock and watch faces
  4. Lighting matches in darkroom
  5. Where film is carried from machine to darkroom in containers, container may leak light

B. Radiation

  1. Insufficient protection
    a. During delivery or transportation in laboratory or shop
    b. Film storage bin
    c. Loaded cassette racks—steel back should face toward source of radiation
    d. Not enough protection for loading darkroom
  2. Improper storage
    a. Radium
    b. Isotopes
    c. X-ray machines

C. Chemical

  1. Prolonged development (See item B under "HIGH DENSITY")
  2. Developer contaminated
    a. Foreign matter of any kind (Metals, etc.)
  3. Contaminated chemicals

D. Deterioration of film

  1. Age (Use oldest film first)
  2. Storage conditions
    a. Too high temperatures
      1) Hot room
      2) Cool room but near radiator or hot pipe
    b. Too high humidity
      1) Damp room
      2) Moist air
      3) Ammonia or other fumes present in darkroom or other work area

  3. Delivery conditions
    a. Moisture precipitation when cold box of film is opened in hot, humid room
    b. Fresh boxes should be stored overnight at room temperature before opening

E. Excessive pressure on emulsions of unprocessed film

  1. During storage
  2. During manipulation in darkroom

F. Loaded cassettes stored near heat, sunlight or radiation

STAINS ON RADIOGRAPHS

A. Yellow

  1. Exhausted, oxidized developer
    a. Old
    b. Covers left off
    c. Scum on developer surface
      1) Oil from pipelines
      2) Impure water used when mixing
      3) Dust
  2. Prolonged development
  3. Insufficient rinsing
  4. Exhausted fixing bath

B. Dichroic

  1. Old, exhausted developer
    a. Colloidal metallic silver
  2. Nearly exhausted fixer
  3. Developer containing small amounts of fixer or scum
  4. Films partially fixed in weak fixer, exposed to light and refixed
  5. Prolonged intermediate rinse in contaminated rinse water

C. Green tinted
1. Insufficient fixing or washing

DEPOSITS ON RADIOGRAPHS

A. Metallic
1. Oxidized products from developer
2. Silver salts reacting with hydrogen sulfide in air to form silver sulfide
3. Silver loaded fixer

B. White or crystalline
1. Milky fixer
   a. Hardener portion added too fast while mixing
   b. Hardener portion added when too hot
   c. Excessive acidity
   d. Developer splashed into fixer
   e. Insufficient rinsing
2. Prolonged washing

C. Grit
1. Dirty water
2. Dirt in dryer

MARKS ON EMULSION SURFACES

A. Runs
1. Insufficient fixing
   a. Weakened fixer
   b. Unbalanced formula
   c. Exhausted ingredients
   d. Low acid content
      1) Deficient when fresh
      2) Diluted from rinse water
      3) Neutralized by developer because of insufficient or no rinsing
2. Drying temperature too high
3. Contact with hot viewing box

B. Blisters
1. Formation of gas bubbles in gelatin
   a. Carbonate of developer reacting with acid of fixer
   b. Unbalanced processing temperatures
      a. Combination of hot fixer and cool developer
      b. Combination of cool fixer and hot developer
   c. Excessive acidity of fixer
   d. No agitation of film when first placed in fixer

C. Reticulation
1. Non-uniform processing temperatures
   a. Developer (Hot)
   b. Fixer (Cool)
   c. Wash
2. Weakened fixer with little hardening action

D. Frilling
1. Weakened fixer with little hardening action
2. Hot processing solutions
   a. Developer
   b. Fixer
   c. Wash

E. Drying marks from uneven drying of gelatin
1. Excessive drying temperatures
2. Extremely low humidity
3. Puddies (Buckshot marks)
   a. Drops of water striking semi-dried emulsion surface
4. Streaks
   a. Drops of water running down semi-dried emulsion surface
      1) Water splashes
      2) Drying air flow too rapid
      3) Insufficient or uneven squeeze last roller pair waterrack

F. White spots
1. Screens pitted
2. Grit or dust present on film or screens
3. Chemical dust settling on film or screens (Particles of certain chemical dusts will also cause black spots)

G. Artifacts
1. Crescents—rough handling
2. Smudge marks—fingerprints or finger abrasions
3. Bands in marginal areas usually due to screen mounting medium

SLOW DRYING

A. Waterlogged films
1. Insufficient hardening in fixer
   a. Too short fixing period
   b. Weakened fixer from splashing
   c. Exhausted fixer
   d. Insufficient acidity (carry over dev. fixer)
2. Wash water too warm

B. Incoming air too humid

C. Incoming air too cold

D. Air velocity too low

STREAKS ON RADIOGRAPHS

A. Insufficient agitation while processing

B. Fog

C. Chemically active deposits (Dried chemicals)

D. Pressure fog

E. Scratches
1. Careless handling
2. Grit present in air, cassettes, or on illuminator

F. Exposure to white light before complete fixing

G. Uneven drying due to high temperature and low humidity

LACK OF DETAIL OR FUZZINESS

A. Motion (Tube, film, subject)
1. Inadequate immobilization
2. Too long exposure
3. Vibration of floor
4. Slipping of subject on mount
5. Stepping on and off operator's platform during exposure where control and tube are mounted on common mobile base
6. Failure to arrest tube vibration after positioning before making exposure

B. Poor contact of intensifying screens

C. Improper distance relationship
1. Object film distance too great
2. Target film distance too short

D. Improper focal spot
1. Too large
2. Damaged (Cracked or pitted)

STATIC

A. Low humidity

B. Insulation

1. Use of rubber gloves, shoes, finger cots, etc.
2. Insulated flooring

C. Improper handling in:

1. Removal from box
2. Removal from interleaving paper
3. Loading cassette
4. Unloading cassette
5. Loading hanger
6. Films stacked before processing

Reprinted with permission from Agfa Matrix Division of Agfa Corporation, 100 Challenger Road, Ridgefield Park, NJ 07660.

APPENDIX C: DU PONT BIT SYSTEM

WHAT THE BIT SYSTEM DOES

The Bit System helps to change techniques, create new exposure and processing conditions, estimate patient skin exposure, and understand the factors affecting radiographic quality. It supplements practical experience by helping you make changes quickly and accurately.

HOW IT WORKS

Bit values are relative exposure units common to all radiographic variables and assigned according to the effect of the variable on film density. They serve the same trading purpose as money. Values are arranged in tables so that reading up the column increases film exposure and density and vice versa. A + 1.0 Bit increase doubles exposure and a − 1.0 Bit decrease halves exposure (see Table "T").

The Bit System has these versatile features. You can:
- make changes with the speed and mathematical accuracy of simple addition and subtraction.
- use either centimeter or inch distances; Fahrenheit or Centigrade temperatures.
- be compatible with existing technique change methods. Table T lists equivalent % and mAs factor changes.
- incorporate new radiographic variables as their control becomes desirable.
- put the Bit System into a computer as we have done in the Micro Quality Manager® computerized quality control system.

Bit tables are accurate under average conditions of use. However, normal generator variations in beam quality, milliampere seconds and other variables introduce errors into the Bit System as well as all other technique conversion systems. Usually an exposure or processing variation of .2 Bits (15%) is not recognized in a radiograph because of the latitude of the system. A .4 Bit (32%) variation is obvious and may require a repeat exposure.

OPTIMIZING TECHNIQUES

Technique charts frequently need to be changed due to individual preference, new equipment, film, screens, processing conditions, etc. Some of the typical changes that can be made with the Bit System and their benefits follow:
- Convert to Rare Earth film-screen systems to optimize image quality/skin exposure.

- Raise kVp and shorten time to stop motion.
- Change from no grid to grid and raise kVp to increase exposure latitude.
- Use faster screens and shorter time to reduce skin exposure.
- Increase illuminator brightness and mAs to increase radiographic contrast.
- Increase distance and kVp to reduce penumbra unsharpness.
- Increase screen speed and reduce focal spot size to reduce penumbra unsharpness.
- Lower developer temperature and increase mAs to reduce quantum mottle.

WAYS TO USE THE BIT SYSTEM

1. CHANGE TECHNIQUES BY MEASURING ON THE TABLES

All radiographic variables are spaced on this card so that a distance change on one table will have the same effect on exposure as the same distance on another table.

Example: Increase kVp from 64 to 85 and Decrease Time from 2/5 sec. to Reduce Contrast

(1) PLace edge of a piece of paper beside kVp Table H.
(2) Mark the paper edge at 64 and 85 kVp in this case.
(3) To indicate a kVp increase, piace an up arrow between the marks on the paper.
(4) Move paper edge to "time" Table K and place the mark beside the original 2/5 sec. and extending in the down direction.
(5) Read new exposure time (1/10 sec.) at the other mark.

2. CHANGE THE TECHNIQUES WITH SLIDE RULE SUPPLEMENT

The Slide Rule Supplement contains time, mAs and kVp tables in inverted form. When one of these scales is placed beside one on the fold out card with known original factors side-by-side, other combinations providing the same radiographic density can be read direct. Use as in the following example:

Example: Change from Original Technique of 64 kVp and 2/5 sec. to 85 kVp and New Time to Reduce Contrast

(1) Place kVp scale of supplement beside time scale (Table K) of this folder.
(2) Move scales vertically until original technique, 64 kVp and 2/5 sec., are beside each other.
(3) Read new time, 1/10 sec., beside new kVp — 85 kVp.
(4) Read any other combinations desired.

3. CHANGE TECHNIQUES BY TOTALING BITS

As with phototiming, it should not make any difference to the film what combination of technical factors within reason are selected to make an exposure as long as a certain total number of exposure units (Bits) are provided.

Assuming you want the same film density as the original, total the Bits of the **original** factors to be changed and subtract the Bit Value of the **new** factor to be used. The remainder will be the Bit Value of the other new factor.

Example: kVp Increase and Time Decrease to Reduce Contrast

Original kVp	: 64 =	6.4 Bits
Original sec.	: 2/5 =	+ 11.0
Original Total		17.4
New kVp	: 85 =	± 8.4
Unknown sec.		9.0 Bits or 1/10 sec.

4. CREATE NEW TECHNIQUES USING BIT TOTALS PROVIDED

This extension of the totaling method discussed on the opposite page is used when techniques are non-existent. A technique is selected to exactly meet the Guide Bit Total provided. Two applications of this principle follow:

- **Correct exposure** exists when kVp Bits + mAs Bits + Film-Screen Bits + Grid Bits + F-F Distance Bits + Anatomical Thickness Bits = Guide Bit Total.

    Guide Total may be obtained by totaling Bits on all important variables used to expose excellent radiographs. These Totals are then used when new techniques are needed.

BIT SYSTEM SLIDE RULE TABLES

% Increase (+)
% Decrease (−)

+3100%	
+2720%	
+2360%	
+2040%	**TO USE**
+1760%	
+1500%	1. Select one factor above
+1310%	and another factor to be
+1130%	changed from the
+ 970%	folding bit card.
+ 812%	
+ 700%	2. Lay **original** techniques
+ 592%	side by side.
+ 503%	
+ 425%	3. Read any new technique.
+ 357%	
+ 300%	
+ 247%	
+ 200%	
+ 163%	
+ 130%	
+ 100%	
+ 74%	
+ 51%	
+ 32%	
+ 15%	
0	
− 13%	
− 24%	
− 34%	
− 42%	
− 50%	
− 56%	
− 62%	
− 67%	
− 71%	
− 75%	
− 78%	
− 81%	
− 83%	
− 86%	
− 87%	
− 89%	
− 91%	
− 92%	
− 93%	
− 94%	
− 95%	
− 95.5%	
− 96%	
− 96.5%	
− 97%	

kVp	mAs	Seconds	
25 —	.63 —	− 1/1000 =	.0010
26 —	.72 —	− 1/860 =	.0012
27 —	.83 —	− 1/780 =	.0013
28 —	.94 —	− 1/666 =	.0015
29 —	1.08 —	− 1/560 =	.0017
30 —	1.25 —	− 1/500 =	.0020
31 —	1.45 —	− 1/430 =	.0023
33 —	1.66 —	− 1/360 =	.0026
34 —	1.80 —	− 1/333 =	.0030
35 —	2.16 —	− 1/280 =	.0035
37 —	2.50 —	− 1/250 =	.0040
38 —	2.90 —	− 1/215 =	.0046
39 —	3.33 —	− 1/180 =	.0053
41 —	3.75 —	− 1/160 =	.0063
42 —	4.4 —	− 1/140 =	.0072
43 —	5.0 —	− 1/120 =	.0083
44 —	5.7 —	− 1/105 =	.0095
45 —	6.6 —	− 1/90 =	.0110
46 —	7.5 —	− 1/80 =	.0125
47 —	8.7 —	− 1/72 =	.0143
49 —	10 —	− 1/60 =	.0166
50 —	11.2 —	− 1/50 =	.019
51 —	13 —		.022
53 —	15 —	− 1/40 =	.025
54 —	17.5 —		.029
55 —	20 —	− 1/30 =	.033
56 —	23 —	− 1/24 =	.038
58 —	26 —		.044
60 —	30 —	− 1/20 =	.050
62 —	35 —		.057
64 —	40 —	− 1/15 =	.066
66 —	45 —		.075
68 —	52 —	− 1/12 =	.087
70 —	60 —	− 1/10 =	.100
72 —	70 —		.115
74 —	80 —	− 2/15 =	.132
76 —	92 —	− 3/20 =	.151
78 —	105 —		.175
80 —	120 —	− 1/5 =	.200
82 —	140 —		.230
85 —	160 —	− 1/4 =	.265
88 —	182 —	− 3/10 =	.300
91 —	210 —		.350
94 —	240 —	− 2/5 =	.400
98 —	280 —	− 1/2 =	.455
102 —	320 —		.525
106 —	365 —	− 3/5 =	.600
110 —	420 —		.700
115 —	485 —	− 3/4 =	.800
120 —	550 —		.920
125 —	640 —	− 1 =	1.05
130 —		− 1-1/5 =	1.20
135 —			1.40
141 —		− 1-1/2 =	1.60
147 —			1.83
153 —		− 2 =	2.10
		− 2-1/2 =	2.50
			2.80
		− 3 =	3.20
			3.70
		− 4 =	4.20
		− 5 =	5.00
			5.50
		− 6 =	6.32

TABLE E
Generator Output*
80 Kvp & 20 inches Distance

	mr/mAs	=	Bits
	60	=	4.4
	52	=	4.2
	45	=	4.0
	40	=	3.8
	35	=	3.6
Av. 3 phase	30	=	3.4
	26	=	3.2
	23	=	3.0
	20	=	2.8
	17.5	=	2.6
Av. 1 phase	15	=	2.4
	13	=	2.2
	11.2	=	2.0
	10	=	1.8

*mr measured in air at 80 Kvp
20″ distance and normal filtration

TABLE F
FOCAL-FILM DISTANCE

Inches	=	Bits	=	Centimeters
6.7	=	12.0	=	17
7.3	=	11.8	=	18.5
7.7	=	11.6	=	19.5
8.3	=	11.4	=	21
9.0	=	11.2	=	22.5
9.5	=	11.0	=	24
10.0	=	10.8	=	25.5
10.6	=	10.6	=	27
11.4	=	10.4	=	29
12.2	=	10.2	=	31
13	=	10.0	=	33
14	=	9.8	=	35
15	=	9.6	=	38
16	=	9.4	=	40
17	=	9.2	=	43
18	=	9.0	=	46
19	=	8.8	=	48
21	=	8.6	=	53
22	=	8.4	=	56
24	=	8.2	=	61
25	=	8.0	=	64
27	=	7.8	=	69
29	=	7.6	=	74
31	=	7.4	=	79
33	=	7.2	=	84
36	=	7.0	=	91
39	=	6.8	=	99
41	=	6.6	=	104
44	=	6.4	=	112
48	=	6.2	=	122
51	=	6.0	=	130
55	=	5.8	=	140
58	=	5.6	=	147
63	=	5.4	=	160
67	=	5.2	=	170
72	=	5.0	=	183
77	=	4.8	=	196
83	=	4.6	=	211
88	=	4.4	=	224
95	=	4.2	=	241
102	=	4.0	=	259
109	=	3.8	=	277
116	=	3.6	=	295
125	=	3.4	=	318
136	=	3.2	=	345
144	=	3.0	=	366
154	=	2.8	=	391
165	=	2.6	=	419
176	=	2.4	=	447
180	=	2.2	=	457
203	=	2.0	=	516
218	=	1.8	=	554

TABLE G
ANATOMICAL THICKNESS

Centimeters	=	Bits
1	=	10.8
2	=	10.6
3	=	10.4
4	=	10.2
5	=	10.0
6	=	9.8
7	=	9.6
8	=	9.4
9	=	9.2
10	=	9.0
11	=	8.8
12	=	8.6
13	=	8.4
14	=	8.2
15	=	8.0
16	=	7.8
17	=	7.6
18	=	7.4
19	=	7.2
20	=	7.0
21	=	6.8
22	=	6.6
23	=	6.4
24	=	6.2
25	=	6.0
26	=	5.8
27	=	5.6
28	=	5.4
29	=	5.2
30	=	5.0
31	=	4.8
32	=	4.6
33	=	4.4
34	=	4.2
35	=	4.0
36	=	3.8
37	=	3.6
38	=	3.4
39	=	3.2
40	=	3.0
41	=	2.8
42	=	2.6
43	=	2.4
44	=	2.2

TABLE H

kVp	=	Bits
153	=	11.4
147	=	11.2
141	=	11.0
135	=	10.8
130	=	10.6
125	=	10.4
120	=	10.2
115	=	10.0
110	=	9.8
106	=	9.6
102	=	9.4
98	=	9.2
94	=	9.0
91	=	8.8
88	=	8.6
85	=	8.4
82	=	8.2
80	=	8.0
78	=	7.8
76	=	7.6
74	=	7.4
72	=	7.2
70	=	7.0
68	=	6.8
66	=	6.6
64	=	6.4
62	=	6.2
60	=	6.0
58	=	5.8
56	=	5.6
55	=	5.4
54	=	5.2
53	=	5.0
51	=	4.8
50	=	4.6
49	=	4.4
47	=	4.2
46	=	4.0
45	=	3.8
44	=	3.6
43	=	3.4
42	=	3.2
41	=	3.0
39	=	2.8
38	=	2.6
37	=	2.4
35	=	2.2
34	=	2.0
33	=	1.8
31	=	1.6
30	=	1.4
29	=	1.2
28	=	1.0
27	=	.8
26	=	.6
25	=	.4

TABLE I

mAs	=	Bits
640	=	22.0
550	=	21.8
485	=	21.6
420	=	21.4
365	=	21.2
320	=	21.0
280	=	20.8
240	=	20.6
210	=	20.4
182	=	20.2
160	=	20.0
140	=	19.8
120	=	19.6
105	=	19.4
92	=	19.2
80	=	19.0
70	=	18.8
60	=	18.6
52	=	18.4
45	=	18.2
40	=	18.0
35	=	17.8
30	=	17.6
26	=	17.4
23	=	17.2
20	=	17.0
17.5	=	16.8
15	=	16.6
13	=	16.4
11.2	=	16.2
10	=	16.0
8.7	=	15.8
7.5	=	15.6
5.7	=	15.2
5.0	=	15.0
4.4	=	14.8
3.75	=	14.6
3.33	=	14.4
2.90	=	14.2
2.50	=	14.0
2.16	=	13.8
1.80	=	13.6
1.66	=	13.4
1.45	=	13.2
1.25	=	13.0
1.08	=	12.8
.94	=	12.6
.83	=	12.4
.72	=	12.2
.63	=	12.0

TABLE J

mA	=	Bits
2100	=	11.4
1840	=	11.2
1600	=	11.0
1400	=	10.8
1200	=	10.6
1060	=	10.4
900	=	10.2
800	=	10.0
700	=	9.8
600	=	9.6
530	=	9.4
450	=	9.2
400	=	9.0
350	=	8.8
300	=	8.6
260	=	8.4
225	=	8.2
200	=	8.0
175	=	7.8
150	=	7.6
130	=	7.4
112	=	7.2
100	=	7.0
87	=	6.8
75	=	6.6
65	=	6.4
56	=	6.2
50	=	6.0
43	=	5.8
38	=	5.6
33	=	5.4
28	=	5.2
25	=	5.0
22	=	4.8
19	=	4.6
16	=	4.4
14	=	4.2
12	=	4.0
11	=	3.8
9.5	=	3.6
8.3	=	3.4
7.2	=	3.2
6.3	=	3.0
5.4	=	2.8
4.7	=	2.6
4.1	=	2.4
3.6	=	2.2
3.2	=	2.0
2.7	=	1.8
2.35	=	1.6
2.05	=	1.4
1.80	=	1.2
1.55	=	1.0
1.35	=	.8
1.17	=	.6
1.02	=	.4

TABLE K

Fraction Seconds =	Bits =	Decimal Seconds
6 =	15.0 =	6.32
	14.8 =	5.50
5 =	14.6 =	5.00
	14.4 =	4.20
4 =	14.2 =	3.70
	14.0 =	3.20
3 =	13.8 =	2.80
2-1/2 =	13.6 =	2.50
	13.4 =	2.10
2 =	13.2 =	1.83
	13.0 =	1.60
1-1/2 =	12.8 =	1.40
1-1/5 =	12.6 =	1.20
	12.4 =	1.05
1 =	12.2 =	.920
	12.0 =	.800
3/4 =	11.8 =	.700
3/5 =	11.6 =	.600
	11.4 =	.525
1/2 =	11.2 =	.455
2/5 =	11.0 =	.400
	10.8 =	.350
3/10 =	10.6 =	.300
	10.4 =	.265
1/4 =	10.2 =	.230
1/5 =	10.0 =	.200
	9.8 =	.175
3/20 =	9.6 =	.151
2/15 =	9.4 =	.132
	9.2 =	.115
1/10 =	9.0 =	.100
	8.8 =	.087
1/12 =	8.6 =	.075
1/15 =	8.4 =	.066
	8.2 =	.057
1/20 =	8.0 =	.050
	7.8 =	.044
1/24 =	7.6 =	.038
1/30 =	7.4 =	.033
	7.2 =	.029
1/40 =	7.0 =	.025
1/50 =	6.8 =	.022
	6.6 =	.019
1/60 =	6.4 =	.0166
1/72 =	6.2 =	.0143
1/80 =	6.0 =	.0125
1/90 =	5.8 =	.0110
1/105 =	5.6 =	.0095
1/120 =	5.4 =	.0083
1/140 =	5.2 =	.0072
1/160 =	5.0 =	.0063
1/180 =	4.8 =	.0053
1/215 =	4.6 =	.0046
1/250 =	4.4 =	.0040
1/280 =	4.2 =	.0035
1/333 =	4.0 =	.0030
1/360 =	3.8 =	.0026
1/430 =	3.6 =	.0023
1/500 =	3.4 =	.0020
1/560 =	3.2 =	.0017
1/666 =	3.0 =	.0015
1/780 =	2.8 =	.0013
1/860 =	2.6 =	.0012
1/1000 =	2.4 =	.0010

TABLE L
TECHNIQUE CHANGES REQUIRED FOR PATHOLOGY

RESPIRATORY SYSTEM

Increase kVp	Bits
Atelectasis	+.4
Bronchiectasis	+.4
Carcinoma (advanced)	+.4
Edema	+.4
Empyema	+.6
Hydropneumothorax	+.6
Pleural Effusion	+.6
Pneumoconiosis	+.5
Pneumonia	+.5
Thoracoplasty	+.6
Tuberculosis (calcific-miliary)	+.4

Decrease kVp	Bits
Emaciation	—.5
Emphysema	—.6

OTHER SYSTEMS

Increase kVp	Bits
Acromegaly	+.4
Ascites	+.6
Arthritis (Rheumatoid)	+.4
Cirrhosis of Liver	+.4
Charcot Joint	+.4
Edema	+.4
Hydrocephalus (without air)	+.4
Metastasis (Secondary to prostatic carcinoma)	+.4
Osteochondroma	+.4
Osteoma	+.4
Osteomyelitis (healed)	+.4
Osteopetrosis	+.4
Paget's Disease	+.4

Decrease kVp	Bits
Arthritis (degenerative)	—.5
Atrophy	—.5
Bowel Obstruction	—.5
Cystic Diseases	—.5
Emaciation	—.5
Gout	—.5
Hydrocephalus (with air study)	—.5
Hyperparathyroidism	—.5
Leprosy	—.5
Multiple Myeloma	—.5
Necrosis	—.5
Osteomyelitis (active)	—.5
Pneumoperitoneum	—.5
Sarcoma	—.5
Syphilis (advanced)	—.5

(mAs may be changed instead of kVp.)

TABLE N

Collimation	mAs Bits
8" X 10" or larger	0
5" X 7"	+.3
Cylinder Collapsed	+.5
Cylinder Extended	+.7

TABLE S
GRID TRANSMISSION (80 kVp)

Ratio	% Trans =	Bits
None	100 =	10.0
	87 =	9.8
6 in. Air Gap	76 =	9.6
	66 =	9.4
	58 =	9.2
4:1 60L	50 =	9.0
	44 =	8.8
	38 =	8.6
5:1 80L, 6:1 103L	33 =	8.4
8:1 103L	29 =	8.2
8:1 80L, 10:1 103L	25 =	8.0
10:1 80L	22 =	7.8
12:1 103L	20 =	7.6
5:1 Cross Hatched	17 =	7.4
16:1 80L	14 =	7.2
8:1 Cross Hatched	13 =	7.0

PERCENTAGES

TABLE T

Bit Change	% Increase (+) % Decrease (—)	Dosage or mAs Factor*	Relative mAs or Arithmetic Speed
+ 5.0	+ 3100%	32.00X	3200
+ 4.8	+ 2720%	28.20X	2820
+ 4.6	+ 2360%	24.60X	2460
+ 4.4	+ 2040%	21.40X	2140
+ 4.2	+ 1760%	18.60X	1860
+ 4.0	+ 1500%	16.00X	1600
+ 3.8	+ 1310%	14.10X	1410
+ 3.6	+ 1130%	12.30X	1230
+ 3.4	+ 970%	10.70X	1070
+ 3.2	+ 812%	9.12X	912
+ 3.0	+ 700%	8.00X	800
+ 2.8	+ 592%	6.92X	692
+ 2.6	+ 503%	6.03X	603
+ 2.4	+ 425%	5.25X	525
+ 2.2	+ 357%	4.57X	457
+ 2.0	+ 300%	4.00X	400
+ 1.8	+ 247%	3.47X	347
+ 1.6	+ 200%	3.00X	300
+ 1.4	+ 163%	2.63X	263
+ 1.2	+ 130%	2.30X	230
+ 1.0	+ 100%	2.00X	200
+ .8	+ 74%	1.74X	174
+ .6	+ 51%	1.51X	151
+ .4	+ 32%	1.32X	132
+ .2	+ 15%	1.15X	115
0	0	1.00X	100
— .2	— 13%	.87X	87
— .4	— 24%	.76X	76
— .6	— 34%	.66X	66
— .8	— 42%	.58X	58
—1.0	— 50%	.50X	50
—1.2	— 56%	.44X	44
—1.4	— 62%	.38X	38
—1.6	— 67%	.33X	33
—1.8	— 71%	.29X	29
—2.0	— 75%	.25X	25
—2.2	— 78%	.22X	22
—2.4	— 81%	.19X	19
—2.6	— 83%	.17X	17
—2.8	— 86%	.14X	14
—3.0	— 87%	.13X	13
—3.2	— 89%	.11X	11
—3.4	— 91%	.09X	9
—3.6	— 92%	.08X	8
—3.8	— 93%	.07X	7
—4.0	— 94%	.06X	6
—4.2	— 95%	.05X	5
—4.4	— 95.5	.045	4.5
—4.6	— 96%	.04X	4
—4.8	— 96.5	.035	3.5
—5.0	— 97%	.03X	3

*New mAs = Old mAs X mAs Factor

Reprinted with permission from:

**E. I. DU PONT DE NEMOURS & CO. (INC.)
MEDICAL PRODUCTS DEPARTMENT
CUSTOMER TECHNOLOGY CENTER
WILMINGTON, DELAWARE 19898
PHONE 1-800-527-2601**

APPENDIX D: BASIC EXPOSURE TABLE SIEMENS POINT SYSTEM

Guideline values for free setting

The exposure guideline values given apply for optimum development conditions and when a 12 pulse generator or a DC voltage generator is used. If there is a deviation from the given exposure parameters, the required change of the exposure parameters must be made according to the correction and conversion table.

* *For units with undertable tube: 70 cm*
For units with overtable tube: 115 cm
** *Cassette on tabletop*

Object		Thickness (cm)	SID (cm)	Screen (Typ)	Grid (Pb 12/40)	Points	kV	mAs
Skull								
Skull survey	p.a./a.p.	19				30	70	50
Face bones	lat.	16	115	Special/TU	with	26	66	25
Skull	lat.	16				27	66	32
Skull	axial	22				35	85	63
Petrous bone	sag.	17	115	Special/TU	with	33	73	80
Petrous bone, Stenvers	view	17				32	70	80
Nasal								
Sinuses	p.a.	22	115	Special/TU	with	32	70	80
Orifice of optic nerve after Rhese		17	115	Special/TU	with	29	66	50
Mandible	lat.	11	105**	Titan D	without	20	57	12,5
Chest								
Ribs 1–7	p.a./a.p.	20				28	66	40
Ribs 8–12	p.a./a.p.	22	115	Titan D	with	34	70	125
Sternum	p.a.	21				31	63	100
Sternum	lat.	30				32	66	100
Clavicle	p.a./a.p.	14	115	Titan D	with	25	60	32
Scapula	a.p.	17				28	63	50
Scapula	a.p.	14	115	Titan D		31	63	100
Lung	p.a./a.p.	21	185	Ruby	with	33	125	8
Lung	p.a./a.p.	21	185	Ruby		33	150	4
Lung (in bed)	p.a./a.p.	21	115		without	18	60	6,3
Lung, heart	lat.	30	150	Titan D	with	29	125	4
Lung, heart	lat.	30	185		with	32	150	3,5
Lung, heart	lat.	30	115	Titan D	without	21	77	4
Oesophagus	obl.	28	70/115*	Titan HS	with	24/28	90	4/10
Abdomen								
Kidney, gallbladder	lat.	27				35	81	80
Kidney, gallbladder	a.p.	19	115	Special/TU	with	29	66	50
Urinary bladder	a.p.	19				29	66	50

Object		Thickness	SID	Screen	Grid	Points	kV	mAs
Urinary bladder	axial	21	115	Special/TU		33	70	100
Gravid uterus	lat.	28	115	Titan HS	with	36	125	20
Content study of stomach p.a.		22	70/115*	Special/TU		28/32	102	6,3/16
Bulbus	p.a.							
Gastrointestinal tract, survey sup.		22	70/115*	Special/TU	with	28/32	102	6,3/16
Stomach, relief	p.a.							
Spinal column								
Cervical vertebrae, 1–3	oral	13						
Cervical vertebrae, 4–7	a.p.	13	150	Titan D	with	33	70	100
Cervical vertebrae, 1–7	lat.	12						
Cervical vertebrae, 1–7	obl.	13	150	Titan D		33	70	100
Thoracic vertebrae	a.p.	21	115	∓Graduated	with	35	73	125
Thoracic vertebrae	lat.	30	115	±Graduated		35	81	80
Lumbar vertebrae, 1–4	a.p.	19		Special/TU		31	77	40
Lumbar vertebrae, 1–4	lat.	27	115	∓Graduated	with	39	90	125
Lumbar vertebrae, 1–4	obl.	22		Special/TU		33	81	50
Lumbar vertebrae, 5	a.p.	22	115	Titan/TU	with	38	77	63
Lumbar vertebrae, 5	lat.	33	115			38	90	100
Pelvis								
Pelvis, hip	a.p.	20				30	73	40
Sacrum, coccyx	a.p.	19	115	Special/TU	with	31	73	50
Sacrum, coccyx	lat.	33				37	90	80
Upper extremities								
Shoulder joint	a.p.	11	115		with	26	63	32
Shoulder joint	axial	11	105**	Titan D	without	20	60	10
Upper arm	a.p./lat.	8	105**		without	16	55	6,3
Elbow	a.p.	6				14		4
Elbow	lat.	8	105**	Titan D	without	15	55	5
Forearm	a.p.	6				14		4
Forearm	lat.	7				15	55	5
Wrist	p.a.	4	105**	Titan D	without	9	46	3,2
Wrist	lat.	6				12	52	3,2
Hand	p.a.	3				7	42	3,2
Hand	lat./obl.	6	105**	Titan D	without	10	48	3,2
Finger		2				4	40	2,5
Lower extremities								
Neck of femur	axial	22	105*		without	29	70	40
Femur	sup.	13	115	Titan D	with	30	70	50
Femur	inf.	12	115		with	27	60	50
Knee joint	a.p.	12	115		with	24	60	25
Knee joint	lat.	10	115	Titan D	with	23	60	20
Knee joint fissure		12	105**		without	17	57	6,3

Object		Thickness	SID	Screen	Grid	Points	kV	mAs
Patella	axial	7				16		6,3
Tibia	a.p.	11	105**	Titan D	without	16	55	6,3
Tibia	lat.	9				15		5
Ankle	a.p.	9				17	55	8
Ankle	lat.	7	105**	Titan D	without	15	50	8
Oscaleis	lat.	7				14	50	6,3
Oscaleis	axial	10				18	55	10
Metatarsus	d.pl./p.a.	5	105**	Titan D	without	13	50	5
Metatarsus	obl.	6				12	50	4
Foot	lat.	7	105**	Titan D	without	13	50	5
Toes		3				8	44	3,2

Correction Values

In exposure points[†] for deviations from the starting conditions

SID	cm	65	75	85	95	105	115	130	145	160	185	210	235	260	290	325	360	400
	Points	−5	−4	−3	−2	−1	0	+1	+2	+3	+4	+5	+6	+7	+8	+9	+10	+11

Screen[‡]	Type	Titan HS/2 HS	Titan U/2 U/Tit.-Grad./Special	Titan D/2 D	Sapphire/Sapph.-Grad.	Ruby	Ruby Super
	Points (50–90 kV)	−7	−3	0	0	+3	+6
	(90–150 kV)	−8	−4	−1	0	+3	+6

Generator	Type	DC voltage	12-pulse	Multipulse	Six-pulse	Two-pulse
	Points in kV	0	0	0...+1	+1	+3

Grid	Type	withoout	Pb 8/40	Pb 10/40	Pb 12/40
	Points	−6	−2	−1	0

Object	State	Thin	Thick	Close collimation	Plaster half-shell	Plaster, dry	Plaster, wet
	Points	−3...−1	+1...+3...	+2	...+3	...+5	...+7

Tomography	Pattern	—	◯	◯	16°	
	Points	+2	+3	+3	+3	+4

[†] An exposure point difference of three causes doubling or halving of the dose. An exposure point difference of one causes a blackening change of $\triangle_s \approx 0.25$ on the X-ray film.

[‡] Guideline Values for the dose requirement of Siemens intensifier screens for the same blackening

Correction Values *(continued)*

Zonography	Pattern	—	○
	Points	+1	+1

Screen	Titan HS/2 HS violet	Special Titan U/2 U Graduated green	Sapphire Titan D/2 D Graduated blue	Ruby orange	Ruby Super yellow
dose require- ment	$\frac{1}{5}$	$\frac{1}{2}$	1	2	4

Conversion Table

From Exposure points * into mAs or kV values

kV	Points	mAs		kV	Points	mAs		kV	Points	mAs
—	−10	0,1		46	4	2,5		90	18	63
—	− 9	0,125		48	5	3,5		96	19	80
—	− 8	0,16		50	6	4		102	20	100
—	− 7	0,2		52	7	5		109	21	125
—	− 6	0,25		55	8	6,3		117	22	160
—	− 5	0,32		57	9	8		125	23	200
—	− 4	0,4		60	10	10		133	24	250
—	− 3	0,5		63	11	12,5		141	25	320
—	− 2	0,63		66	12	16		150	26	400
—	− 1	0,8		70	13	20		—	27	500
40	0	1		73	14	25		—	28	630
41	1	1,25		77	15	32		—	29	800
42	2	1,6		81	16	40		—	30	1000
44	3	2		85	17	50				

APPENDIX E: ANSWERS TO CASE STUDIES

The Case of the Unidentified Flying Object in the Skull

Chapter 2, p. 42

This patient was shot in the left temporal region by an arrow. The shaft was broken off prior to the time the radiograph was taken.

The Case of the Wierd X-Ray Machine

Chapter 3, p. 62

This is an old full-wave tube rectification unit with each rectifier placed as shown in the circuit drawings in Chapter 6.

The Case of the Black Mediastinum

Chapter 5, p. 118

The cassette was not lightproof because of a warped back and damage to the felt light seal in the bottom center of the film. The light that entered the cassette through the damaged felt seal flashed directly upward where the warped cassette back had destroyed the film/screen contact. Because the other regions of the cassette maintained good film/screen contact, no light affected them.

The Case of the Metal Fence

Chapter 7, p. 163

The radiographer who produced this mobile image was using a grocery cart to transport cassettes from the patient room to the x-ray department. This particular cassette was against the side of the cart when an excessive amount of scatter from another exposure reached it.

The Case of the Double Row of Capsules

Chapter 8, p. 173

This is a pack of fire crackers from Taiwan.

The Case of the Deep Sea Rodeo

Chapter 11, p. 207

A seahorse

The Case of the Ghostly Plants

Chapter 13, p. 235

A peony.

The Case of the Dark Line in the Abdomen

Chapter 15, p. 258

The radiographer failed to verify that the patient had followed instructions to remove everything between the waist and feet. The patient's underwear had a thick elastic band that redistributed the fatty tissue above and below the band. The band pushed tissue above and below the band, making those parts of the image light, while less tissue directly under the band made that part of the image dark.

The Case of the Injured Animal

Chapter 16, p. 275

This is a rodent, a muskrat. The cause of death was a severed thoracic vertebral column, the result of being caught in a trap in the Ohio woods.

The Case of the White Snakes

Chapter 20, p. 340

The radiographer failed to observe that the high-voltage cables were within the primary beam field. Observe the sheath of grounding net inside the upper cable.

The Case of Lumpy

Chapter 21, p. 350

Theodore Bear

The Case of the Colon in the Spider's Web

Chapter 25, p. 411

This patient was unable to hold the barium within the colon and the sheet has become barium soaked. The wrinkled sheet is dense enough to make a distinct image under the patient.

The Case of the Line in the Stomach

Chapter 27, p. 437

The stomach is half filled with liquid barium. The line is an air-fluid level between the air and barium.

The Case of the Missing Lower Pelvis

Chapter 29, p. 467

This patient is quite obese and the large volume of soft tissue that has fallen down over the pelvis is demonstrated with an appropriate density. However, these technical factors produce much too much density for the pelvis. A second radiograph to demonstrate the pelvis, shown here, fails to demonstrate the abdomen. A case of "You can't have your cake and eat it too."

The Case of the Animal with the Large Calcified Tumor-like Mass

Chapter 31, p. 493

A chicken's egg about to be laid

The Case of the Last Dinner

Chapter 32, p. 500

There are no skeletal remains of the snake's last dinner on this image, but it's good practice to always examine your radiographs with careful attention to detail; the last dinner could have been demonstrated if it had been eaten more recently.

The Case of the Very Dense Object

Chapter 33, p. 509

The object is a bullet that was absorbed by the patient, a Chicago policeman, many years previous. Because it did not cause any discomfort, it was never removed. Notice the fragments lodged in the soft tissue down the right side of the thoracic vertebral column.

The Case of the Dripping Film

Chapter 37, p. 572

The horizontal lines are pi lines, so called because they are spaced apart by pi times the diameter of the first film processing roller. They are caused when developer precipitates onto the top rollers at the level of the chemistry when left in the tank overnight. When the first film is processed, the precipitate is deposited on the film emulsion each time the roller turns. The drip marks are most likely from developer solution that was splattered onto the film while it was being held vertically before processing.

The Case of Do You Know Your Whole Grains?

Chapter 38, p. 587.

Wheat

INDEX

A

Abdomen
    attenuation, decreased, 253
    pathological problems of,
        247, 250
    increased attenuation, 250
Abdominal radiography, film/
        screen selection and,
        348
Abscess, defined, 247
Absolute value, algebra and,
        9–10
AC *See* Alternating current (AC).
Acetic acid, film development
        and, 296
Acromegaly, defined, 250
Active osteomyelitis, defined,
        253
Added filtration, 176
Addition
    approximate values, 7
    decimals, 5
    fractions, 4
    like terms, algebraic expres-
        sions and, 12–13
Adhesive, radiographic film
        and, 278–79
Aerophagia, defined, 253
Air
    attenuation and, 237–38
    core transformers, 106
Algebra
    absolute value and, 9–10
    division and, 10
    equations, 14–15
        addition, 15
        division, 15–16
        multiplication, 15–16
        subtraction, 15
    expressions in, 11–14
    multiplication and, 10

number, negative of, 10
order of operation, 10–11
signed numbers and, 9–10
subtraction and, 10
variation and, 16–17
Algebraic expressions, 11–16
    addition, like terms, 12–13
    distributive law, 11–12
    evaluating, 14
    exponents and, 13
    subtractions, like terms, 12–13
Alternating current (AC), 73
    dynamometers and, 104
    generators, 98–99
        illustrated, *98*
    impedance, 100
    inductive reactance of, 96
    motors, 103–4
        induction, 103–4
        synchronous, 103
    production of, illustrated, *99*
Aluminum, as filtering material,
        175
Ammonium thiosulfate, 296
Amplitude, tomography and,
        576
AMU. *See* Atomic mass units.
Anatomical part, contrast and,
        393
Anatomically programmed
    exposure systems, 463–64
    radiography, 507
Aneurysm, aortic, 250
Angiography
    film/screen selection and, 347
    film/speed selection and, 347
Angulations, 423–24
    source-to-image receptor
        distance (SID),
        comparisons, *423*
Annihilation reaction, 202
Anode
    described, 112
    video camera tubes and,
        563–64

Anode assembly
    x-ray tube, 145–53
        anode, 146–51
Anode heel effect
    contrast and, 392
    density and, 369
    projections and, *369*
    x-ray tube and, 150–51
Anode screens, fluoroscopy
        and, 557
Anorexia nervosa, defined, 252
Aortic aneurysm, 250
Aperture diaphragm
    beam restriction and, 228–30
        field size determination,
        230
Archaeological radiography,
        212, 214
Archiving
    digital, 617–18
    radiographic films, 296–97
Arithmetic
    decimal numbers and, 5–6
    decimals, 4–5
    dimensional analysis, 8–9
    exponents and, 7
    fractions, 4
    graphing, semilogarithmic,
        17
    measurement, units of, 17–21
    powers of ten, 7
    rounding off and, 6–7
    significant digits and, 6
    values, computation with,
        6–7
Armature, defined, 97
Array processors, 606
Art restoration, radiography
        and, 212
Arthritis, degenerative, defined,
        253
Artificial permanent magnets,
        89
Ascites, aortic, 250
Aseptic necrosis, defined, 253

Italic page numbers indicate illustrations.